Nurses Making Policy

D1572895

Rebecca M. Patton, MSN, RN, CNOR, FAAN, is the past, two-term president of the American Nurses Association (ANA; 2006–2010), and currently holds the inaugural Endowed Perioperative Nursing Chair, Atkinson Scholar in Perioperative Nursing at Frances Payne Bolton School of Nursing, Case Western Reserve University, where she is obtaining her doctor of nursing practice (DNP) degree. As a nurse, author, and lecturer, Ms. Patton has presented extensively throughout the world. Between 2006 and 2010, she logged over 330,000 miles as president of the ANA. Ms. Patton has testified before Congress and met with major policy makers—including Presidents Obama, Bush, and Clinton—when she lobbied on health care issues affecting nurses and the general public. She was invited by President Bush to tour and meet with the soldiers and nurses at the Guantanamo Detainee Camp in Cuba. Ms. Patton was selected twice by the U.S. State Department to serve on the U.S. delegation at the World Health Assembly in Geneva, Switzerland. Ms. Patton serves on the *American Nurse Today* (*ANT*) editorial board and has written chapters for books on medical–surgical nursing and for nursing journals. She has received numerous recognitions, including the ANA Distinguished Membership Award; Sigma Theta Tau International Founder Dorothy Garrigus Adams Award for Excellence in Fostering Professional Standards, 2013; *Modern Health Care* "Top 100 Most Influential Persons in Healthcare" in 2009 and 2010; and Community Involved Political Action Award from the Sigma Theta Tau, Delta Xi Chapter at Kent State University. She is a fellow of the American Academy of Nursing.

Margarete L. Zalon, PhD, RN, ACNS-BC, FAAN, is a professor in the Department of Nursing at the University of Scranton, Scranton, Pennsylvania, and an adult health clinical nurse specialist. She is a past chair of the American Nurses Foundation (2006–2011) and a former board member of the American Nurses Association. She also served as vice president, American Nurses Credentialing Center (2005–2006), and is a past president of the Pennsylvania State Nurses Association. Dr. Zalon is a fellow of the American Academy of Nursing, and a member of its Acute and Critical Care Expert Panel. Her research focuses on vulnerable elders, and she has had her research funded by the National Institute of Nursing Research. She has authored book chapters, as well as articles in *Nursing Research, Applied Nursing Research, Journal of Nursing Scholarship, Journal of Nursing Measurement, Journal of Nursing Education*, and *Nurse Educator*, and numerous articles in other professional publications. She has made research and health policy presentations at the local, state, national, and international levels.

Ruth Ludwick, PhD, RN-BC, CNS, FAAN, is director of Nursing Research, Robinson Memorial Hospital, Ravenna, Ohio; professor emeritus, Kent State University, College of Nursing; and an independent consultant. As leader, researcher, and educator, Dr. Ludwick has transformed standards of nursing care of older people and the gerontological preparation of nurses. She has a sustained record of research and publications focused on challenging and significant gerontological nursing issues such as restraint reduction, health literacy, and advance care planning. Her funding includes grants from the Agency for Healthcare Quality and Research, National Institute of Aging, Institute of Museum & Library Science, and the National Palliative Care Research Center. She has served on the editorial boards of the *Online Journal of Issues in Nursing* and the *International Journal of Older People Nursing*. She has authored over 100 articles, book chapters, editorials, and compilations appearing in a variety of renowned journals, such as *Nursing Research, Advances in Nursing Science, Journal of Gerontological Nursing, Journal of the American Geriatric Society, Nursing Ethics*, and *Journal of Pain and Symptom Management*.

Nurses Making Policy
From Bedside to Boardroom

Rebecca M. Patton, MSN, RN, CNOR, FAAN
Margarete L. Zalon, PhD, RN, ACNS-BC, FAAN
Ruth Ludwick, PhD, RN-BC, CNS, FAAN

Editors

*Co-Published With the
American Nurses Association*

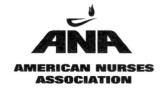

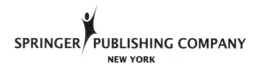

NEW YORK

Springer Publishing Company, LLC
11 West 42nd Street
New York, NY 10036
www.springerpub.com

Acquisitions Editor: Margaret Zuccarini
Composition: Integra Software Services Pvt. Ltd

ISBN: 978-0-8261-9891-4
E-book ISBN: 978-0-8261-9892-1
PowerPoint ISBN: 978-0-8261-2046-5

Instructors' Materials: Qualified instructors may request supplements by e-mailing textbook@springerpub.com

14 15 16 17/ 5 4 3 2 1

The author and the publisher of this Work have made every effort to use sources believed to be reliable to provide information that is accurate and compatible with the standards generally accepted at the time of publication. Because medical science is continually advancing, our knowledge base continues to expand. Therefore, as new information becomes available, changes in procedures become necessary. We recommend that the reader always consult current research and specific institutional policies before performing any clinical procedure. The author and publisher shall not be liable for any special, consequential, or exemplary damages resulting, in whole or in part, from the readers' use of, or reliance on, the information contained in this book. The publisher has no responsibility for the persistence or accuracy of URLs for external or third-party Internet websites referred to in this publication and does not guarantee that any content on such websites is, or will remain, accurate or appropriate.

Library of Congress Cataloging-in-Publication Data

Nurses making policy : from bedside to boardroom / Rebecca M. Patton, Margarete L. Zalon, Ruth Ludwick, editors.
    p. ; cm.
Includes bibliographical references and index.
ISBN 978-0-8261-9891-4—ISBN 978-0-8261-9892-1 (E-book)—ISBN 978-0-8261-2046-5 (Teacher PowerPoint)
I. Patton, Rebecca M., editor. II. Zalon, Margarete L., editor. III. Ludwick, Ruth, editor. IV. American Nurses Association, issuing body.
[DNLM: 1. Nursing—organization & administration—United States. 2. Policy Making—United States. 3. Health Policy—United States. 4. Leadership—United States. 5. Nurse's Role—United States. 6. Organizational Policy—United States. WY 16 AA1]
RT41
610.73--dc23

2014032181

Printed in the United States of America by Bradford & Bigelow.

To all nurses who have made policy an integral part of their lives

To future nurses who read this book and take action

To families, friends, and colleagues

To all who believe in nursing and the power of nurse advocacy

To the individuals who appreciate and value the need for a
Washington Fellows Program for Nurses

Contents

Contributors

Sheila A. Abood, PhD, RN   Adjunct Faculty, Grand Valley State University, Kirkhof College of Nursing, Grand Rapids, Michigan

Virginia Trotter Betts, MSN, JD, RN, FAAN   President, Health Futures, Inc., Nashville, Tennessee

Josepha E. Burnley, DNP, RN, FNP-C   Nurse Consultant/Project Officer, Nursing Practice and Workforce Development, Division of Nursing, Health Resources and Services Administration, U.S. Department of Health and Human Services, Rockville, Maryland

Pamela F. Cipriano, PhD, RN, NEA-BC, FAAN   President, American Nurses Association, Silver Spring, Maryland; Research Associate Professor, University of Virginia School of Nursing, Charlottesville, Virginia

Sean P. Clarke, PhD, RN, FAAN   Associate Dean for Undergraduate Programs; Professor, William F. Connell School of Nursing, Boston College, Boston, Massachusetts

Deborah Colton, MSW   Senior Vice President for Strategic Communication, Massachusetts General Physicians Organization, Boston, Massachusetts

Joanne Disch, PhD, RN, FAAN   Professor ad Honorem, University of Minnesota School of Nursing, Minneapolis, Minnesota

Marianne Ditomassi, MSN, MBA, RN   Executive Director for Patient Care Services Operations and Magnet Recognition, Massachusetts General Hospital, Boston, Massachusetts

Rose Iris Gonzalez, PhD, MPS, RN   Independent Consultant; Past Director, Government Affairs, American Nurses Association, Silver Spring, Maryland

Linda K. Groah, MSN, RN, CNOR, NEA-BC, FAAN   CEO/Executive Director, Association of periOperative Registered Nurses, Denver, Colorado

Amy L. Hader, JD   Director, Legal and Government Affairs, Association of periOperative Registered Nurses, Denver, Colorado

Debbie Dawson Hatmaker, PhD, RN, FAAN Executive Director, American Nurses Association, Silver Spring, Maryland

Jeanette Ives Erickson, DNP, RN, FAAN Senior Vice President for Patient Care and Chief Nurse, Massachusetts General Hospital, Boston, Massachusetts

Mathew Keller, BSN, JD, RN Regulatory and Policy Nursing Specialist, Minnesota Nurses Association, St. Paul, Minnesota

Ruth Ludwick, PhD, RN-BC, CNS, FAAN Independent Consultant; Director of Nursing Research, Robinson Memorial Hospital, Ravenna, Ohio; Professor Emeritus, Kent State University, College of Nursing, Kent, Ohio

Kathy Malloch, PhD, MBA, RN, FAAN President, KMLS, LLC; Associate Professor of Practice, Arizona State University College of Nursing and Health Innovation, Phoenix, Arizona; Clinical Professor, The Ohio State University College of Nursing, Columbus, Ohio; Clinical Consultant, API Healthcare, Hartford, Wisconsin

Suzanne Miyamoto, PhD, RN Director of Government Affairs and Health Policy, American Association of Colleges of Nursing, Washington, DC

Rebecca M. Patton, MSN, RN, CNOR, FAAN Past President, American Nurses Association; Lucy Jo Atkinson Scholar in Perioperative Nursing, Frances Payne Bolton School of Nursing, Case Western Reserve University, Cleveland, Ohio

Janice M. Phillips, PhD, RN, FAAN Director of Government and Regulatory Affairs, CGFNS International, Inc., Philadelphia, Pennsylvania

Tim Porter-O'Grady, DM, EdD, ScD(h), APRN, FAAN, FACCWS Senior Partner, Tim Porter-O'Grady Associates, Inc.; Associate Professor, Leadership Scholar, College of Nursing and Health Innovation, Arizona State University, Phoenix, Arizona; Clinical Professor, Leadership Scholar, The Ohio State University College of Nursing, Columbus, Ohio; Adjunct Professor, Dean's Advisor, Emory University, Atlanta, Georgia

Eileen M. Sullivan-Marx, PhD, RN, FAAN Dean and Erline Perkins McGriff Professor, New York University College of Nursing, New York, New York

Karen Tomajan, MS, RN, NEA-BC Director, Professional Practice, John Muir Medical Center, Concord, California

Susan Tullai-McGuinness, PhD, MPA, RN Adjunct Associate Professor, Case Western Reserve University, Frances Payne Bolton School of Nursing, Cleveland, Ohio

Eileen Weber, DNP, RN, PHN, JD Clinical Assistant Professor, University of Minnesota School of Nursing, Minneapolis, Minnesota

Loretta Alexia Williams, BSN, RN   Graduate Research Assistant and Instructor, Jonas Nursing Leadership Scholar (2012–2014), University of Tennessee Health Science Center College of Nursing, Memphis, Tennessee

Shanita D. Williams, PhD, MPH, APRN   Branch Chief, Nursing Practice and Workforce Development, Division of Nursing, Health Resources and Services Administration, U.S. Department of Health and Human Services, Rockville, Maryland

Kathleen M. White, PhD, RN, NEA-BC, FAAN   Director, Master's Entry Into Practice Program; Associate Professor, Johns Hopkins University School of Nursing, Baltimore, Maryland

Margarete L. Zalon, PhD, RN, ACNS-BC, FAAN   Professor, Department of Nursing, University of Scranton, Scranton, Pennsylvania

Foreword

The American Nurses Foundation (ANF) was founded in 1955 as the philanthropic arm of the American Nurses Association (ANA) for the purpose of improving health care and supporting registered nurses throughout the United States. As of 2012, the strategic direction of the ANF has been to invest in key initiatives to advance its mission: "Transforming the nation's health through the power of nursing."

This book, *Nurses Making Policy: From Bedside to Boardroom*, edited by Rebecca M. Patton, Margarete L. Zalon, and Ruth Ludwick, will be a key marker in the transformation of nursing. Patton, Zalon, and Ludwick designed this book with a clear goal in sight: the creation of a **Washington Fellows Program for Nurses**, administered through the ANA and supported through the book royalties. The legacy of this commitment is far-reaching, as each new fellow will build on the successes of his or her predecessors. This nursing influence, at the executive and legislative branches of our government, is viewed as a complement to existing policy programs. At the same time, it also takes the nursing agenda to a new level of influence.

Patton, Zalon, and Ludwick have gathered the experts in nursing policy development and implementation as chapter contributors—the best of the best in nursing. These contributors have provided key insights to move the nursing profession forward and position nurses in leadership roles in the health policy arena, locally, nationally, and globally.

The editors' generosity in supporting the ANF reflects their professional and personal commitments to the power of nurses' philanthropy. Each has played a key role in ensuring the Foundation's growth and success to ensure that nurses maximize their power.

Current Foundation initiatives designed to empower nurses include:

1. Leadership programs: Supporting ANA's Leadership Institute and increasing the number of nurses on key influential boards of directors in the following health care sectors: for profit, philanthropic, and health systems
2. Educational scholarships: Provided to undergraduate and graduate students focused on leadership and underrepresented groups
3. Promotion and advocacy: Promoting the contributions to health care by nurses through multiple media outlets

ANF initiatives that are focused on transforming health include:

1. Nursing research grants: Annual awards to nurses to provide seed money to beginning and experienced researchers to conduct studies that advance health science and the enhancement of patient care
2. Specific health programs: Development of a tool kit to assist nurses in recognizing posttraumatic stress disorders in the nation's veterans and military service members, and a sleep disorders program focused on helping nurses understand the deleterious effects of shiftwork
3. Health Nurse Project: Development of a mindfulness tool kit for nurses and sponsorship of other initiatives to highlight the need for improving nurses' health

The ANA's board is committed to transforming the nation's health by helping nurses solve key health issues. We will accomplish this mission by generating and providing the funds for nurses to influence and lead in these key areas central to health care. We applaud the work of our colleagues, the editors and contributors to this book, for taking the lead in telling nursing's story in health policy and advancing the skills of future generations of nurses who aspire to lead.

Joyce J. Fitzpatrick, PhD, MBA, RN, FAAN, FNAP
Elizabeth Brooks Ford Professor in Nursing
Frances Payne Bolton School of Nursing
Case Western Reserve University
Cleveland, Ohio
Chair, American Nurses Foundation Board of Trustees

Kate Judge, BA
Executive Director
American Nurses Foundation
Silver Spring, Maryland

Preface

This book uses a hands-on approach designed to help graduate students and nurses across a variety of settings develop health policy skills in order to advocate for patients and work empowerment at the bedside, boardroom, or in state and national politics. The textbook is divided into four units: Making the Case, Analyzing Policy, Strategizing and Creating Change, and Judging Worth and Advancing the Cause. The chapters of the book take the reader on a journey though the policy-making process, from identifying a policy issue, to initiating a plan, to, finally, evaluating it.

Unique features of this 15-chapter book are the steps to changing policy, which are presented in detail, and actual exemplars (Policy Challenge and Policy on the Scene) that are offered in every chapter as told by nurses working locally and nationally. These stories are written by direct-care nurses as well as high-profile nationally known leaders. Throughout each chapter, policy development is exemplified at both the big "P" and little "p" levels, from the grand scale of state or national work, to the local work environment. We believe both are essential and often the interplay between the two levels is not always recognized or acknowledged. Thus, health policy is every nurse's responsibility. Although the creation of the American Nurses Foundation **Washington Fellows Program for Nurses** endowed fund is designed to ensure nurses' placement at the highest policy tables, our commitment is to engage and foster nurses' policy activism at all levels. This will enable nurses taking one step at a time to realize the full power generated by more than 3 million nurses taking steps together to advance health.

The book's intended audience includes:

- Graduate nursing students; in particular students in doctoral programs
- Registered nurses enrolled in baccalaureate degree completion programs
- Registered nurses working to improve their practice environments
- Leaders of state nurses and specialty nurses associations

To enhance understanding of the policy process, each chapter introduces a real-life situation in a Policy Challenge, which is directly related to a specific aspect of the policy process, as well a number of Policies on the Scene that illustrate key points. Concluding each chapter is the Option for Policy Challenge that describes outcomes of the Policy Challenge. Each chapter includes Key Concepts to aid in learning. Learning Activities take readers through the steps of the policy process in order to enhance their policy expertise. Also included in each chapter are E-Resources. These consist of websites, social media links, important policy documents, policy tool kits from various organizations, and additional resources to expand understanding of the policy process. **A Power-Point presentation of the material, provided in a lecture/discussion format for each chapter, is available for instructors through Springer Publishing Company, by e-mailing *textbook@springerpub.com*.**

Rebecca M. Patton
Margarete L. Zalon
Ruth Ludwick

Acknowledgments

This book is a testament to collaboration among friends and colleagues and reflects the support of numerous family members. Support from family and collaboration and encouragement from friends and colleagues are essential ingredients to a commitment to policy, whether working late to write overdue policies, running for elected office, or writing a book on policy. As you read our acknowledgments we encourage you to thank those who are supportive to you.

We thank, in the Patton family, mother Mary Ellen, sister Betty Jane—both registered nurses—and brothers Bob and John. In the Zalon family, we thank husband John; and in the Ludwick family, we thank husband John, son Tom, and mother Bernice Potisuk.

We are grateful for the assistance of Lynn Barabach, MSN, RN, who initially assisted as part of her DNP coursework and continued because of her commitment to advocacy.

Without a doubt we owe endless thanks to the contributors—the esteemed authors of each chapter—and those who shared their real-life stories in the Policy Challenges and the Policies on the Scene.

Special Acknowledgments

We thank the colleagues who embraced the need for this book, the creation of the American Nurses Foundation (ANF) **Washington Fellows Program for Nurses**, and the establishment of the ANF endowed fund (www. anfonline.org). This book, *Nurses Making Policy: From Bedside to Boardroom,* launches the creation of this fund to ensure nurses' voices are heard at the highest level.

We are pleased to be part of a ground breaking publishing arrangement between Springer Publishing Company and the American Nurses Association. In particular, we thank Margaret Zuccarini, Publisher, Nursing, for her support and encouragement in the development of this project.

Abbreviations

AACN	American Association of Critical-Care Nurses
AAFP	American Academy of Family Physicians
AAMI	Association for the Advancement of Medical Instrumentation
AAN	American Academy of Nursing
AANA	American Association of Nurse Anesthetists
AANP	American Academy of Nurse Practitioners
AARP	American Association of Retired Persons
ACA	Affordable Care Act
ACNM	American College of Nurse-Midwives
ACNP	American College of Nurse Practitioners
ACO	Accountable Care Organization
ACOG	American College of Obstetricians and Gynecologists
ADHD	attention deficit hyperactivity disorder
ADM	automatic dispensing machine
AHA	American Hospital Association
AHCPR	Agency for Health Care Policy and Research
AHRQ	Agency for Healthcare Research and Quality
AIM	Adams Influence Model
AIR	assessment, intervention, reassessment
AMA	American Medical Association
AMIA	American Medical Informatics Association
ANA	American Nurses Association
ANAI	American Nurses Advocacy Institute
ANC	Army Nurse Corps
ANCC	American Nurses Credentialing Center
AORN	Association of periOperative Registered Nurses
APN	advanced practice nurse
APRN	advanced practice registered nurse
ASA	American Society of Anesthesiologists
ASC	ambulatory surgery center
ASPAN	American Society of PeriAnesthesia Nurses
ASPEN	American Society for Parenteral and Enteral Nutrition

ATSDR	Agency for Toxic Substances and Disease Registry
AzNA	Arizona Nurses Association
BCIS	Bureau of Citizenship and Immigration Services
BHB	B'more for Healthy Babies
BLS	Bureau of Labor Statistics
BON	board of nursing
BORN	Board of Registration in Nursing
CABSI	catheter-associated bloodstream infection
CAS	Complex Adaptive Systems
CAUTI	catheter-associated urinary tract infections
CCNA	Center to Champion Nursing in America
CCTP	Community-Based Care Transitions Program
CDC	Centers for Disease Control and Prevention
CEO	chief executive officer
CEPR	Center for Economic and Policy Research
CFAR	Center for Applied Research
CGFNS	Commission on Graduates of Foreign Nursing Schools
CHAPS	Coalition for Healthcare Worker and Patient Safety
CLABSI	central line-associated bloodstream infection
CMMI	Center for Medicare and Medicaid Innovation
CMS	Centers for Medicare and Medicaid Services
CNM	certified nurse midwife
CNN	Cable News Network
CNO	chief nurse officer
CNS	clinical nurse specialist
CPG	clinical practice guideline
CPR	Coalition for Patients' Rights
CRBSI	catheter-related bloodstream infection
CRNA	certified registered nurse anesthetist
CSDH	Commission on the Social Determinants of Health
CSH	Center for Spirituality and Healing
CTSA	Clinical and Translational Science Award
CVD	cardiovascular disease
DHHS	Department of Health and Human Services
DME	durable medical equipment
DNP	doctor of nursing practice
DOJ	Department of Justice
DOL	Department of Labor
DRA	Deficit Reduction Act

EBP	evidence-based practice
ED	emergency department
EHR	electronic health record
ENA	Emergency Nurses Association
EPC	evidence-based practice center
EVIPNet	Evidence-Informed Policy Network
FDA	Food and Drug Administration
FHBC	family health and birth center
FHSSA	Foundation for Hospices in Sub-Saharan Africa
FQHC	federally qualified health center
GNA	Georgia Nurses Association
GSA	Gerontological Society of America
HAI	hospital-acquired infection
HANYS	Healthcare Association of New York State
HCH	health care homes
HCUP	Healthcare Cost and Utilization Project
HHS	Health and Human Services
HIA	health impact assessment
HIE	health information exchanges
HIMSS	Health Information and Management Systems Society
HIPAA	Health Insurance Portability and Accountability Act
HIT	health information technology
HP	Healthy People
HRSA	Health Resources and Services Administration
HSA	Health Security Act
IBCLC	international board-certified lactation consultant
ICN	International Council of Nurses
IHIA	Indian Health Improvement Act
IHI	Institute for Healthcare Improvement
IMR	infant mortality rate
IOM	Institute of Medicine
IRB	institutional review board
ISMP	Institute for Safe Medication Practices
IV	intravenous
IWPR	Institute for Women's Policy Research
LACE	licensure, accreditation, credentialing, and education
LANO	Louisiana Alliance of Nursing Organizations
LBW	low birth weight

LDA	Lobbying Disclosure Act
LHHS	Labor, Health and Human Services
LOS	length of stay
LPN	licensed practical nurse
LPN/LVN	licensed practical/vocational nurses
LSNA	Louisiana State Nurses Association
LWBS	leaving without being seen
MAP	Measure Applications Partnership
MARN	Massachusetts Association of Registered Nurses
MMA	Medicare Prescription Drug, Improvement, and Modernization Act
MNA	Minnesota Nurses Association
NACNS	National Association of Clinical Nurse Specialists
NAHN	National Association of Hispanic Nurses
NAPNAP	National Association of Pediatric Nurse Practitioners
NAS	National Academy of Sciences
NASN	National Association of School Nurses
NCATS	National Center for Advancing Translational Sciences
NCMHD	National Center on Minority Health and Health Disparities
NCNR	National Center for Nursing Research
NCSBN	National Council of State Boards of Nursing
NDNQI	National Database of Nursing Quality Indicators
ND	nursing doctorate
NFP	nurse family partnership
NGO	nongovernmental organization
NHL	non-Hodgkin's lymphoma
NHTSA	National Highway Traffic Safety Administration
NIH	National Institutes of Health
NINR	National Institute of Nursing Research
NIWI	Nurses in Washington Internship
NLC	nurse licensure compact
NMHCs	nurse-managed health centers
NNCC	National Nursing Center Consortium
NOLF	Nursing Organization Liaison Forum
NOVA	Nurses Organization for Veterans Affairs
N-PAL	nurse political action leaders
NP	nurse practitioner
NPN	nurse politicians network
NPS	National Prevention Strategy
NPSF	National Patient Safety Foundation
NPUAP	National Pressure Ulcer Advisory Panel
NQF	National Quality Forum

NSNA	National Student Nurses Association
NSSRN	National Sample Survey of Registered Nurses
N-STAT	Nurses Strategic Action Team
NYONE	New York Organization of Nurse Executives
NYSNA	New York State Nurses Association
OAC	Obesity Action Coalition
OADPG	Office of the Associate Director for Program
OASIS	Outcome and Assessment Information Set
OCHE	Oregon Coalition for HealthCare Ergonomics
OECD	Organization for Economic Cooperation and Development
OHRP	Office for Human Research Protections
ONA	Ohio Nurses Association
ONL	Organization of Nurse Leaders
ONS	Oncology Nurses Society
OPCSA	Office of Policy, Communications and Strategic Alliances
OR	operating room
OSHA	Occupational Safety and Health Administration
PA	physician assistant
PAC	political action committee
PACE	Program of All-Inclusive Care for the Elderly
PACU	postanesthesia care unit
PCMH	patient-centered medical home
PCORI	Patient-Centered Outcomes Research Institute
PES	Practice Environment Scale
PEST	political, economic, sociocultural, technological
PEST(LE)	political, economic, sociocultural, technological, legal, environmental
PHI	protected health information
PICC	peripherally inserted central catheter
PPACA	Patient Protection and Affordable Care Act
PR	public relations
PSNA	Pennsylvania State Nurses Association
QR	quick response
QSEN	Quality and Safety Education for Nurses
RAC	regional action coalition
RCT	randomized controlled trial
RN	registered nurse
RNFA	registered nurse first assistant
RWJ	Robert Wood Johnson
RWJF	Robert Wood Johnson Foundation

SANE	sexual assault nurse examiner
SBAR	situation, background, assessment, and recommendation
SBHC	school-based health center
SBHP	school-based health program
SDOH	social determinants of health
SES	socioeconomic status
SNA	state nurses association(s)
SOPP	scope of practice partnership
SPHM	safe patient handling mobility
SPS	student policy summit
SRPP	social research, policy, and practice
SWOT	strengths, weaknesses, opportunities, and threats
TBNE	Texas Board of Nurse Examiners
TCM	Transitional Care Model
TNA	Tennessee Nurses Association
TNA	Texas Nurses Association
UAP	unlicensed assistive personnel
UCLA	University of California, Los Angeles
UTI	urinary tract infection
VA	Department of Veterans Affairs
VAE	ventilator-associated events
VAP	ventilator-associated pneumonia
VBP	value-based purchasing
VHA	Veterans Health Administration
VLBW	very low birth weight
VRU	voice response unit
WHO	World Health Organization
WWW or W3	World Wide Web

Nurses Making Policy

I

Making the Case

ONE

Leading the Way in Policy

Rebecca M. Patton
Margarete L. Zalon
Ruth Ludwick

... nurses must see policy as something they can shape rather than something that happens to them.—Institute of Medicine (2011)

OBJECTIVES

1. Explain the role of nurses in policy in a variety of settings.
2. Analyze the historical underpinnings for the role of nurses in policy.
3. Examine nurse's responsibilities to society in formulating policy.
4. Appraise the potential of nursing's influence and impact on health, quality, and safety.

As a registered nurse (RN), you make a difference in the lives of your patients. You have ideas to create change that will positively impact patient care or the nursing work environment. You picture yourself as an advocate improving quality, access, or value. However, you do not know where to begin. You have advocated for a change in patient care and made a case by searching and evaluating the evidence, or completing research, or teaching information that was prerequisite to carrying out your vision of change. In spite of your diligence, have you found you did not see the results you expected? Maybe you became discouraged with policies within your organization or felt powerless to make a change? Or perhaps you did not see the results expected in the time frame you projected. Did you persist? Maybe you achieved the expected change but found you could not account for the success of the plan. Key to the success in making your vision become reality is understanding the policy-making process and using it to help translate your change into the reality of everyday practice; in this way, you can become a policy advocate. Nurses are vital to leading the way in policy from the bedside to the boardroom.

We make the case beginning with this chapter and throughout the book that once policy skills are understood and practiced, nurses can successfully engage in policy making. These skills are essential to nurses in the trenches, performing direct care across all settings, as well as for nurses in leadership, education, and research positions. Thus, policy making permeates every aspect of nursing practice, whether or not we realize it.

Given that nurses comprise the largest sector of health care providers, spend the most time with patients, and share a unique intimacy with patients related to functional care activities, nurses bring critical understanding and potential solutions to many high-profile complex health care issues such as access, quality, cost, and value. Nurses "… practice at the intersection of public policy and personal lives; they are, therefore, ideally situated and morally obligated to include sociopolitical advocacy in their practice" (Falk-Rafael, 2005, p. 222). Every day, nurses see how health policy decisions such as access to care based on preexisting conditions impact patients and their families, and how organizational staffing policies may harm patients and adversely affect them and their work environment.

Creating and maintaining a health policy is everyone's job. Some believe that one's position defines policy involvement. We argue that health policy is everyone's responsibility. Nurse managers, educators, and administrators are often viewed as having more obvious roles in the successful articulation of federal and state regulations and implementation of institutional policies. Direct-care nurses live at the edge of those policies and regulations every day. "Nursing skills are political skills" (Feldman & Lewenson, 2000, p. 58). Nurses are uniquely qualified to assume important roles in policy. See the Policy Challenge, which illustrates one nurse's policy journey as trustee of a community hospital board.

POLICY CHALLENGE: Becoming a Hospital Trustee
Mary Jane K. DiMattio, PhD, RN, Scranton, PA

I became a hospital trustee in my mid-thirties. My appointment to the Board resulted from a combination of connections, credentials, and personal characteristics. My brother-in-law works in the financial sector and is a visible member of the community, serving on many nonprofit boards. Through him, my husband and I were invited to a dinner party at the home of a local physician. The guest of honor was a Catholic bishop from another state, and I recall becoming engaged in a discussion about Catholic health care. I must have felt the need either to promote or to defend nursing's role. Apparently, our physician host was taking note of my participation in the lively exchange because he later nominated me to serve on the board of the local, Catholic hospital. At the time, the hospital, which was owned by a larger health system, was seeking diversity among its trustees, so my gender and age likely worked in my favor during the vetting process, in addition to my being Catholic, holding a doctoral degree from an Ivy League university, and having had prior community-board experience.

As a nurse, I brought a voice to the board. I am fortunate to have had a doctoral leadership course with the late Dr. Margaret Sovie, RN, FAAN, who emphasized the necessity to "marshal the evidence" when engaging in nursing advocacy. I gathered facts in advance of making a point or fact-checked afterward to correct anything I might have said in error. Depending on the agenda, I brought research articles to support points I wished to make. A strong research background served me particularly well when I chaired the Quality Committee of the board. My greatest accomplishments were to raise awareness about nursing among other trustees and to keep nursing on the administration's radar. When I first started, a fellow trustee—a business professional about my age—asked if we didn't have "bigger fish to fry" than nursing issues. By the time I finished my tenure, other trustees often asked how a particular initiative or decision might affect the nursing staff, and there was a chief nursing officer, who reported to the chief executive officer (CEO) instead of a director of nursing, who reported to the chief operating officer. Despite my efforts, certain staffing issues and an outmoded care delivery model persisted. One reason was the steep learning curve I faced in understanding hospital finance. Another is that the role of the trustee is to serve as an advisor and to ensure the overall mission and governance of the hospital. This means that trustees are not to involve themselves in daily operations, especially in the unionized environment where I served. I sometimes made the case that challenging the nursing organization was a part of upholding the mission and met with varying degrees of success, depending on who was the CEO.

See Option for Policy Challenge.

EVERY NURSE'S ROLE IN POLICY

Nurses' everyday practical lens, combined with nursing skills like problem solving and communication, makes health policy competence a smart and necessary fit for nursing now, as well as for its vitality in the future. Nurse leaders experienced in policy at the national, state, local, or organizational level know that nurses possess numerous essential skills that can be adapted to successful policy making. These skills include the ability to gather data rapidly and accurately, day-to-day experiences with people, skill at juggling opposing demands, and the capability to connect with and mobilize groups (Gebbie et al., 2000).

In a like manner, Warner (2003) interviewed nurse activists to explore the skill set necessary for political competence. These excerpts from the nurses, labeled Nurse C and Nurse D, echo and amplify Gebbie's findings:

"Nursing gives you observational skills, lots of information, and experience making quick decisions .... Nursing is balancing competing priorities and looking for ways for everyone to win" (Nurse D). Another discussed nursing as excellent preparation for the legislator role: "We are very versatile. We are able to grasp complex issues and keep many things on the plate at one time" (Nurse C). (Warner, 2003, p. 138)

Furthermore, accrediting organizations mandate that all nursing education programs have health policy education incorporated in the curriculum, and nursing organizations across the world advocate policy action. Shared governance and other forms of collective action (e.g., alliances and unions) at their core are about direct-care nurses and managers mutually making decisions and developing policies for practice. Yet, nurses frequently voice that they have no control over policy and that there is no time in the fast-paced world of health care, with the numerous rules and regulations, to become policy experts. If we don't speak up for the policies we need and want, we find there are many others willing to step in and speak for us, yet they may not represent our interests or needs with regard to patient care or our work environments. Being silent provides an unspoken endorsement of the status quo. It allows others to make their voices heard in the void of our silence.

While all nurses must be fully engaged in the policy process, the level of involvement (local, state, national, international, organizational) depends on education, skill, practice, and mentoring. A necessary skill in actualizing political power is to know and comprehend the basics of the policy process. Provisions of the American Nurses Association *Code of Ethics for Nurses* (ANA, 2001) call for practicing nurses in all roles and all settings to be involved in policy as part of their duty to their profession, patients, and society (see also Chapter 2, "Advocating for Nurses and for Health"). Involvement in policy may include the spectrum of work on government activities, institutional decisions, organizational positions, or professional standards.

The duty to be active in politics often seems foreign to nurses as they assume political activism means being involved in the official tasks of government like holding political office. This broad or top-down view of politics very often implies holding office in a major organization or government, working actively to pass state and federal laws related to safe patient care or some such similar activity. We refer to politics on this grand scale as Politics with a big "P." In 2014, six nurses held office in the U.S. House of Representatives, 113th Congress (American Nurses Association, n.d.) as compared with 20 members of the 113th Congress who were physicians. Eddie Bernice Johnson (D TX) is one of the nurses serving in the 113th Congress. When she took office for the first time over 20 years ago, she became the first RN elected to Congress. Obviously, more nurses are needed at this grander scale, given there are over 3 million licensed RNs in the United States.

Advocacy in nursing takes on different forms in different settings. Although we need more nurses to hold political office, this is only one of many arenas where nurses can work for the promotion of health and the elimination of health care disparities through the use of big "P" strategies for health care policy development and implementation. Nursing care is always provided within a social, economic, cultural, and political context, which includes the health care system and society (Ballou, 2000). To address social justice issues, nurses need to employ an "upstream" approach. This refers to approaches that address primary prevention and the root causes of disease and disability, whereas most nurses are in downstream positions in providing direct care instead of working to change harmful systems of care (Bekemeier, 2008). The familiar classic public health story is that of rescuers frantically working to pull people out of a river instead of going upstream to figure out why people are falling into the river and preventing that from happening in the first place (Zola, as told to McKinlay, 1986). Not only is an upstream approach necessary, but also the strategies to influence upstream decisions necessarily involve collaborative or team efforts and/or political action.

Although some nurses may assume significant advocacy roles by holding public office, or lobbying for political action, all nurses can advocate for and with patients. They can advocate for themselves and their work environment. Politics carried out at this micro level and those processes associated with nurses' work environments are also called politics, but the word is not capitalized; the term *politics* in these cases is referred to as politics with a little "p." Micropolitics does not mean less important; it is used to convey a difference in scope. Examples of little "p" politics might include implementing a "no lift" policy in a clinical agency, or ensuring that children within a certain school district are allowed to carry their asthma inhalers with them in accordance with the latest asthma self-management standards. Nurses may be more familiar with advocacy within the context of the nurse–patient relationship since we have traditionally focused our efforts and energies on encouraging nurses to be advocates at the individual level. However, we argue that the profession and the public need nurses to be advocates at all levels to achieve our health care goals, that they cannot be achieved without attention to disparities, and that the advocacy competencies learned at the micro or little "p" level can be readily transferred to other arenas.

POLICY ARENAS FOR NURSES

We believe that politics is a process that requires nurses who are savvy with both big "P" and little "p" politics. We, therefore, are using the following definition. Politics: "… is a process that includes not only that which is typically associated with political functions (e.g., government, police, and workers' unions) but also that which is involved in the regulation, structure, and action of all individuals' behavior" (O'Byrne & Holmes, 2009). All humans are political. We try every day to influence others based on our beliefs, values, and knowledge. Have you ever called fellow nurses before a meeting where you work to tell them about an idea you want them to support? Have you tried to influence other nurses to more actively support an initiative that you believe in, like breastfeeding, bedside shift reporting, or asking a manager to buy a product such as automated sphygmo-manometers? On a larger scale, look at the impact of two certified nurses, Jennifer Pallotta and Joan Banovic, who developed a major recycling program for the operating room (OR) where they work in New Jersey. After they read that many by-products in the OR could be recycled, they used an evidence-based approach, consulted with a medical waste company, and developed a plan that led to significant savings. In fact, they realized a 50% decrease in biohazardous waste, which on average is up to 10 times more expensive to dispose of than other hospital waste (Nurse-led, 2013).

While there are numerous examples of how nurses advocate daily, being political is still often misunderstood. Being political can be seen as less than desirable in a world where politics is associated with disingenuous elected officials and political campaigns are perceived as increasingly uncivil and negative. Recently, a staff nurse expressed hesitancy in writing a letter to the editor in response to a negative article on breastfeeding as she did not want to be viewed as "too political." Upon further exploration, she voiced she did not want to seem "too radical." Because of the perceptions of incivility in politics, nurses may see expressing political voice as upsetting the apple cart. In the software program Microsoft Word, the word *radical* is listed as a synonym for political. Nurses may also believe that they do not have the competencies necessary for taking political action. Sometimes it seems contradictory that nurses, who as a group are good at work-arounds and soothing hot-tempered families, patients, and coworkers, have trouble seeing that these skills are transferable to the policy-making process. With further discussion and exploration with a mentor about what it means to be political, editorial support, and general encouragement, the once hesitant nurse who was worried about being "too political" publicly demonstrated her advocacy by writing her first letter to the editor. In Policy on the Scene 1.1, see the example of another approach to advocating: that of a guest columnist, which was written by a doctorate of nursing practice (DNP) student. See also Chapter 10, "Working With the Media: Shaping the Health Policy Process."

POLICY ON THE SCENE 1.1: Guest Column, *The Plain Dealer,* Cleveland, Ohio
Lynn Barabach, MSN, RN

Now is the time to impact our children's mental health

March 24, 2013

One day your son comes home and says, "My brain is not working right." This scenario was posed by Governor John Kasich during his February 19, State of the State address. What would you do? Most families will start a journey into our nation's mental health care system. If your family receives Medicaid, there is a good chance you will have a 4- to 6-week wait for the first appointment. Or, you take your son to a local emergency department.

The Kaiser Family Foundation in 2007 reported that 66.2% of Ohio children between the ages of 2 and 17 received care for emotional, developmental, or behavioral problems in a 12-month period. This included a wide range of diagnoses, including autism, anxiety, depression, eating disorders, oppositional defiant disorder, attention deficit hyperactivity disorder (ADHD), and psychosis, to name a few. All of these diagnoses require professional assessment and treatment. Treatment includes inpatient and outpatient care, medication, and counseling for the child/adolescent and families. Treatment is specific to the child or adolescent and his or her diagnosis. Care is provided by large health care systems and community-based agencies.

Providing the appropriate care for these children and adolescents is very important. Everyone has heard of the school shootings at Chardon, Sandy Hook, and Virginia Tech and the impact the shooter's mental health had on each incident. While these are extreme examples, they do remind us of the importance of mental health care. Children and adolescents with emotional disturbances have the highest failure rates in school, with 50% of the students dropping out of high school. Children and adolescents who do not receive the appropriate treatment are at risk for homelessness, becoming involved with the criminal justice system, unemployment, and alcohol and drug abuse. Is this what we want for our children?

Access to mental health services for families on Medicaid is especially difficult and families continue to struggle. Currently, Ohio Medicaid allows recipients 25 visits per 12-month period, plus 8 hours of psychological testing per year for psychology services and/or counseling. There are many children who need more frequent care. Additionally, other services that are a benefit to children and adolescents with mental health needs are either paid at a very low rate or not covered at all. Such services include group therapy sessions and programs/classes that focus on issues like self-esteem, communication, and social interactions. Transitional services to assist young adults to become independently functioning adults are important and are usually provided by mental health agencies.

Governor Kasich, in his 2013 State of the State address, supported the expansion of mental health benefits for Medicaid recipients. Most Ohio citizens would agree with Governor Kasich. The Ohio Legislature must act to increase benefits for mental health care, especially for children and adolescents. Benefits need to include "wraparound" services. These would include group therapy, social services, transitional services, and family therapy.

(continued)

Ohio needs to provide educational funding for students interested in providing mental health services to children and adolescents. The demand for mental health professionals continues to grow. We must grow the number of professionals who can care for these children and adolescents.

With the expansion of Medicaid, Ohio is in a position to support our children and adolescents to overcome mental health concerns and grow into successful, productive adults. Ohioans are encouraged to write, call, or meet with their state legislators to support increasing mental health services and coverage to all of Ohio's children and adolescents.

Barabach is an RN with a master of science in nursing degree who lives in North Olmsted. Reprinted with permission from *The Plain Dealer*.

POLICY-MAKING PROCESS

Basic knowledge of the policy process is the first step in planning how to initiate your potential political power and influence real changes in your patients' lives, your work environment, or social policy change in your community and beyond. Policy making is a goal-oriented course of action that individuals or groups take on behalf of or as part of organizations, facilities, systems, and government in dealing with a problem or issue.

The basic phases of the policy-making process have much in common with the steps of the nursing process and the comparison is helpful in beginning to demystify the policy process. Like the steps of the nursing process, policy making is viewed as cyclical, involves continued feedback, and may take longer in certain phases depending on the project being undertaken. While this four-phase process is not fully comprehensive of all the steps in policy making, this comparison provides a solid starting point for nurses reviewing and developing policy. It starts much like the nurse work done every day with the identification of a problem after an assessment of a patient or a situation and then follows logically the problem-solving and decision-making steps used to solve everyday patient problems. A side-by-side comparison of the policy process with the nursing process is illustrated in Exhibit 1.1.

Using this type of comparison, the process becomes manageable and one can see how all nurses have the potential to identify, formulate, implement, and evaluate

EXHIBIT 1.1 NURSING PROCESS AND POLICY PROCESS COMPARISON

NURSING PROCESS	POLICY PROCESS
• Assess and diagnose • Plan interventions • Implement the care • Evaluate	• Recognize and identify a problem • Formulate policy • Implement the policy change • Monitor and evaluate the result

change based upon their work setting, their community, and their passion. However, the number of steps and the details involved in policy making vary. See Chapter 2 for an illustration of the problem-solving process. The most basic approach to policy identifies three policy development phases: recognition and identification, formulation, and implementation. Since policy making is an ongoing evolutionary process, we have added a critical but often overlooked step, monitoring and evaluating, which is consistent with the fourth phase of the nursing process. Policy making is easier to understand by breaking down the steps into pieces that are small enough to study and seeing the pieces helps us understand the whole.

Improving policy is a task that numerous individuals, groups, organizations, legislative bodies, and governments seek as a goal in order to improve health. As the world, health care, and nursing have become progressively multifaceted, uncertain, changeable, and interconnected, the policy-making process has become more complex. The potential complexity of the policy-making process is illustrated in Figure 1.1. Throughout the book, we will discuss more detailed steps, tools, and techniques that are necessary as the complexity of the policy process is more fully explored.

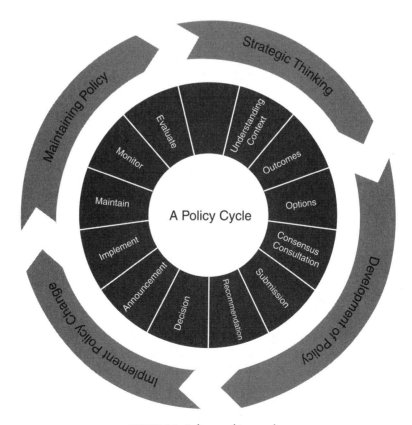

FIGURE 1.1 Policy-making cycle.

Reprinted with permission from Economic Policy Unit: Office of the First Minister and Deputy Minister (n.d.).

THE POLICY JOURNEY

Developing policy is a journey and that journey varies depending on the context of the situation. The processes associated with the journey can be both formal and informal. Whether working to pass legislation related to preventing workplace violence against nurses, developing a board policy that requires an RN to be a member, or reviewing a nursing policy within a hospital related to certification payment, the steps of policy making are the same but the journey for those involved in the process may vary depending on roles and the situation. Let's look at some of the different approaches used to stop workplace violence against nurses to show how the journey can vary. At the organizational level, both the Emergency Nurses Association (ENA) and the ANA have played instrumental roles in helping to raise awareness and support legislative initiatives aimed at preventing violence against nurses and prosecuting those who do act against nurses. At the individual level, nurses are vital to this process. When the State of New York was debating a law to protect nurses (Violence Against Nurses bill [A3103-A/S4018-A]), Fatima Saint-Vil, of Maimonides Medical Center in Brooklyn, used a letter to the governor, accompanied by supporting signatures from 150 nurses, to passionately describe her experience of being assaulted by a patient in the emergency room (Silk, 2010). This illustrates the important role that each of us may play in advancing a policy position.

Does your state have a law to protect nurses from violence? As of this writing, 21 states have passed legislation related to protecting nurses. The ANA tracks progress in state legislation for selected issues of importance to nurses (see Figure 1.2). If the final goal for an issue is federal legislation, then quite often legislation needs to be passed by a critical number of states before our federal legislators take it up for consideration. Tennessee, in June 2013, became the latest state to pass legislation against violence that specifically addresses assault against health care workers. This legislation illustrates the importance of being inclusive when possible and broadening the policy impact. However, nursing policy does not necessarily advocate exclusively for nurses. While a nursing lens is helpful in developing policy (see Chapter 11, "Applying a Nursing Lens to Shape Policy"), using a nursing lens to limit who we advocate for is shortsighted. Often, to move policy forward, nurses need to move their advocacy base beyond nursing and involve other colleagues as well as consumers who might benefit from the advocacy.

As part of their advocacy role, the ENA has developed a free tool kit for workplace violence that is available on the Internet (2010). In the tool kit, they identify five steps, similar to the steps discussed earlier, to tackle the problem of violence. These steps illustrate the tailoring of steps to a particular project.

As suggested in the recount earlier about the nurse who was assaulted, a key event that ignites a passion is often the reason that nurses become involved in advocacy and policy. Can you identify your passion? Are you motivated to prevent needlesticks, support health care reform, promote safe staffing, activate

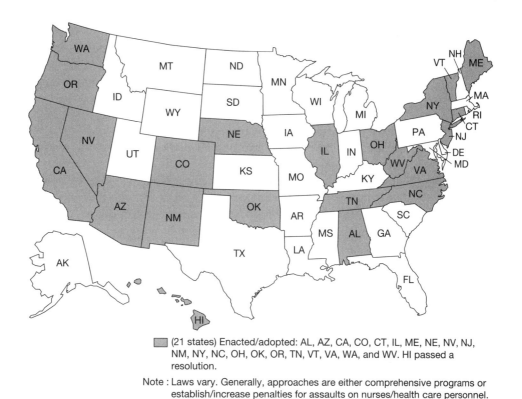

(21 states) Enacted/adopted: AL, AZ, CA, CO, CT, IL, ME, NE, NV, NJ, NM, NY, NC, OH, OK, OR, TN, VT, VA, WA, and WV. HI passed a resolution.

Note : Laws vary. Generally, approaches are either comprehensive programs or establish/increase penalties for assaults on nurses/health care personnel. Laws excluding nurses are not reflected.

FIGURE 1.2 The American Nurses Association statewide legislative agenda: workplace violence. Reprinted with permission from the American Nurses Association, 2014b.

safer patient handling policies, or advocate for laws to help prevent violence against nurses? Listen to ANA president Karen Daley, PhD, MPH, RN, FAAN, on YouTube (www.youtube.com/watch?v=UATLtR_27YE) tell how a needle-stick on the job as a staff nurse changed her life and intensified her commitment to nursing as an activist. Her story will be further referred to in other areas of the book as it is powerful. When federal needlestick legislation was finally voted on in 2000, Senator Ted Kennedy called Daley from the Senate floor to inform her of its passage with the commitment to ensure the president's immediate signature. Today, we need to be sure that nurses know how the law is applied in their practice settings and that nurses who use needles and sharps are involved in the decision making about such purchases for their institutions as mandated by the law.

These stories of passion also hold the key to nurse political activation, as they also provide rich stories that put faces to an issue and help outsiders, like legislators or board members, understand the richness and complexity of health care issues of frontline nurses as they provide care that impacts their constituents. The passion that often comes from personal experiences in professional caregiving or from within one's personal life may be a catalyst, but passion alone does not account for political activism. Many nurses indicate that their life experiences from education and family played a role in their political activism. A former staff member of the Ohio Nurses Association, who served as a legislative intern and also ran for state office, writes:

> The idea of running for elective office was far from my mind when I first became a nurse over 45 years ago. At that time, like so many young nurses, I was concerned about being able to skillfully care for my patients after graduating from a hospital-based diploma program. Of course, I also wondered if I would get that first job and be able to work through the sometimes complex relationships I encountered with my new work colleagues. As if that weren't enough, I was learning what it meant to be a mother of three children while orchestrating multiple moves necessitated by my husband's job. I barely had time to think beyond the moment, so the idea of taking on anything extra was far from my mind. (Lanier, 2012, p. 8)

Gebbie, Wakefield, and Kerfoot (2000) discussed the role of chance in political involvement and identified four common themes that emerged as the starting points for policy career trajectories: family, education, employment, and networking. Family is important in inculcating values and expectations and instilling confidence. Parents are important, especially parents who are involved in advocacy efforts much like Rebecca M. Patton, a past ANA president, who told people when she was in nursing school that one day she would be ANA president. She attributes much of her drive to her parents and specifically her mother, Mary Ellen Patton, RN, who was a strong staff nurse advocate, nurse union leader, and served on the ANA Board of Directors during Patton's adolescent years.

Education, both high school and nursing school, was also cited by many nurses in the development of their advocacy roles. For Kenya Haney, MSN, RN, past president of the National Student Nurses Association (2009–2010), her classes for her master's degree and the mandatory health policy courses were pivotal in her ongoing drive to be a political activist. As she stated, "I am at our state house [Missouri] all the time to advocate for health policies for our patients and our profession" (K. Haney, personal communication, June 20, 2013). Most of the nurses in Gebbie's study had a master's or doctoral degree.

Work environment features such as autonomy, reimbursement issues, and policy knowledge needs were identified in the study by Gebbie and colleagues (2000) as the impetus for policy involvement. Nurses in the Gebbie study wanted a role that would provide a conduit to a wider range of influences to improve patient care. The last influence for those with policy careers was networking with important people (nurses and non-nurses) in the community, organizations, and politics (Gebbie et al., 2000). This is corroborated by the CEO of the International Council of Nurses, David Benton, BS, MS, MPhil, RGN, RMN, "I was very lucky, I had very good role models" (D. Benton, personal communication, May 23, 2012).

Thus, nurses can be guided to influence policy in many ways. In the past 20 years, guidelines on education about policy, roles of nurses in shared governance, the calls for increased numbers of baccalaureate-prepared nurses, and an increased number of nurse role models are making a positive impact on nurse involvement in policy (see Chapter 11 for additional details). However, in spite of these strides, most would agree that extensive policy involvement by nurses is still lacking. Nursing education hasn't consistently provided nurses with tools to change the system, but rather to function within it (Koff, 2004, p. 132) and, often, nursing students view public policy as an inhibitor or barrier, as something that other people do (Rains & Barton-Kriese, 2001).

The lack of expertise in policy may contribute to the perception by some that nurses are not leaders. In over 1,500 interviews of American opinion leaders in the public and private sectors, academia, and trade organizations, government (75%) and health insurance executives (56%) were viewed as the groups most likely to exert a great deal of influence on health care reform in comparison with 14% for nurses (Khoury, Blizzard, Wright Moore, & Hassmiller, 2011). Although nurses are consistently rated as the most trusted professionals in Gallup polls (Newport, 2012), with 85% of respondents rating nurses as very high in honesty and ethical standards, they are not viewed as leaders in our health care system. Bekemeier (2008, p. 51) takes a more proactive stance in pointing out the consequences of this dichotomy, "While improving the health of the few we may serve as individuals, as nurses we are complicit in the illness and death of many." Our perspective on health from a nursing lens enables us to be leaders in the promotion of health and in addressing the factors that determine health in our communities by moving beyond our individual nurse–patient relationships and learn to advocate for change in our organizations, our communities, and our nation to promote health.

If you have been active in policy, what influenced you and where did you start? Often nurses report starting at a local level of involvement and then branching out as skills and resources are developed. See Figure 1.3 for strategies to enhance your readiness for influencing policy development.

Being apolitical is not acceptable, nor is it reality. As Florence Nightingale admonished, "… I think one's feelings waste themselves in words, they ought all to be distilled into actions, which bring results" (Cook, 1913, p. 94). Not being political limits what we do for patients. In 2011, the Institute of Medicine (IOM), as it noted in our introduction, made a clarion call for action for nurses to "have a voice in health policy decision making and be engaged in implementation efforts related to health care reform" (IOM, 2011, p. 8). This call to action is historic as it provides a plan for nursing advocacy in health care at the national level and is coupled with initiatives in each state that are designed to make it happen. We are at a unique juncture in the history of nursing with the alignment of forces that encourage and enhance nurses' opportunities to take on a more active role in advocacy across multiple settings. Expectations for workforce needs, quality and safety initiatives, interprofessional collaboration, health care reform, and

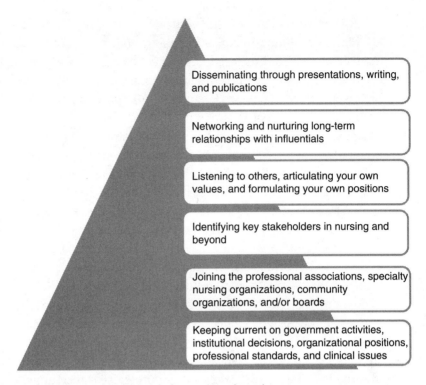

FIGURE 1.3 Getting ready for a role in the policy process.

environmental health are some of the confluence of forces that mandate nurses assume a leadership role in health at the little "p" and the big "P" levels. These expectations are briefly described in the following sections.

WORKFORCE NEEDS

Workforce needs are a critical arena for nursing policy development. In fact, workforce needs are linked to patient safety. According to the Lucian Leape Institute of the National Patient Safety Foundation (NPSF) (2013, p. 1), "If we expect the workforce to care for patients, we need to care for the workforce. Workplace safety is also inextricably linked to patient safety. Unless caregivers are given the protection, respect and support they need, they are more likely to make errors, fail to follow safe practice, and not work well in teams."

The years ahead indicate that the demand for nursing services is going to increase exponentially, and therefore work processes, workspace, work hours, staffing, and organizational cultures need to support the work of nurses to prevent errors, readily detect errors, and mitigate the effects of errors (Steinwachs & Hinshaw, 2004). The workforce needs of the profession can be broadly categorized into workforce development, safety, staffing, respect and civility, and conditions of employment. See Exhibit 1.2 for a listing of potential areas for nursing policy development. While not meant to be exhaustive, these areas provide opportunities for nurses to make improvements in their work environment

EXHIBIT 1.2 NURSING WORKFORCE NEEDS

Workforce development	Adequacy of the supply Distribution and utilization of nurses and advanced practice nurses Education International recruitment Role, practicing to scope of education and training Diversity
Workplace safety	Safe patient handling Safe needles, sharps, and devices Slips, trips, and falls Musculoskeletal injuries Occupational exposures to communicable diseases Occupational exposures to hazardous substances Work release during a disaster Reproductive rights and hazards Resources for impaired nurses
Adequacy of staffing and support services	Safe staffing levels Mandatory overtime Fatigue Healthy work hours and schedules Adequacy of support (pharmacy, housekeeping, etc.) Adequacy of access to medications, supplies, and equipment
Respect and civility	Bullying Blame-free environment, just culture Harassment, sexual harassment Physical and verbal abuse Respect for all team members
Conditions of employment	Wage compression Pay for performance Paid time off, overtime Family medical leave Sick time Preemployment screening (smoking, weight) Mandatory immunizations Discrimination Disabilities Union representation Continuing education Credentialing, privileging Reimbursement for advanced practice nurses Independent practice for advanced practice nurses

as well as to advance issues of relevance to the profession. In examining the range of these workforce needs, it is clear that there are opportunities for policy involvement at the little "p" level within organizations or at the big "P" level through local, state, federal, and even international initiatives.

Nurses have a long history of being at the forefront of policy initiatives to improve working conditions and to advance the profession. Nurse leaders established the ANA in 1896 to protect the public from untrained individuals claiming to be nurses. They also wanted to improve the poor working conditions of nurses. In 1934, the ANA House of Delegates approved a resolution calling for an 8-hour workday for nurses. Since then, the areas for nurse involvement in policy have grown exponentially.

The complexities of nurses' workforce needs are illustrated by the changing landscape of the workday that cuts across issues related to patient safety, staffing, fatigue, mandatory overtime, and overtime compensation. In the past 10 to 15 years, many hospitals transitioned to 12-hour shifts in order to provide an attractive incentive for recruiting and retaining nurses. This schedule flexibility was a boon for some facilities, allowed nurses to return to school, provided more days and weekends off, and so forth. Disadvantages include longer hours in addition to time for commuting, irregular pay weeks, adverse health effects, and challenges in providing coverage for absences and time for training. Now adding to these issues is research about fatigue and patient safety as well as legislative and regulatory initiatives related to overtime pay and mandatory overtime. In a landmark study, for example, it was found that nurses were three times as likely to make an error when working shifts lasting more than 12.5 hours (Rogers, Hwang, Scott, Aiken, & Dinges, 2004). These findings provided the foundation for the IOM recommendation that nurses do not work more than 12 hours per day and 60 hours per week (Page et al., 2004, pp. 12–13). We know that people will have considerable awake time before and after their shifts, which then results in a tendency to have chronic sleep restriction. Nurses who work more than 12.5 hours have twice the risk of a drowsy driving episode and have a 9% increased risk of such an episode for each hour of sleep lost (Scott et al., 2007).

For many years, nurses associations, including the ANA, and unions indicated that the nurse should be the one who determines whether she or he can safely work an additional shift, or accept an overtime assignment. This was predicated on nurses' knowledge of how long they were awake prior to the start of the shift, and their personal evaluation of their fatigue as well as control over working hours. The ANA's position statement indicates that nurses have an ethical obligation to consider their level of fatigue when accepting overtime assignments (ANA, 2006). While policy initiatives focused on mandatory overtime with 16 states restricting the use of mandatory overtime for nurses, more recently organizations have taken a more holistic approach in examining policy in relation to not only shift length, but also fatigue, sleep deprivation, human performance factors, and role expectations.

While nurses may bear partial responsibility for choices related to accepting longer shift assignments, employers also have an obligation to provide staffing levels that do not result in the use of overworked and fatigued nurses to provide care. This is significant in light of research that individuals are not able to accurately judge their own alertness when their sleep is restricted

(Zhou et al., 2012). Likewise, economic reasons may drive some nurses to accept overtime requests. And their proposed federal legislation to change practices with regard to overtime pay may influence nurses' decisions about the type of positions sought for employment. With some widely publicized errors and an acknowledgment that extended working hours can impact patient safety, the New York State Board of Nursing has taken the position that nurses working beyond their normally scheduled hours (except in declared emergencies) need to demonstrate their competence. Working more than 16 hours within 24 hours is considered by the board in deciding whether the nurse willfully disregarded patient safety (New York State Department of Education, 2013). While this is only one state's practice, it has implications for all nurses, particularly in cases of a serious lapse in safety or a sentinel event.

These issues about working hours illustrate the challenges in developing policies to address the workforce development needs of nurses. Staff nurses need and want fair scheduling of their work hours. In some settings, neonatal nurse practitioners, acute care nurse practitioners, OR nurses, and certified registered nurse anesthetists may be on call for 24 consecutive hours. Chief nurse executives need to provide optimal staffing for their facilities in a manner that does not compromise safe patient care. The public has a right to safe and high-quality care and expects that nurses will be able to provide it. Policies that are developed to address these issues and a host of other workforce development needs must be fair, be conducted using a deliberative process, and reflect the interests of diverse stakeholder groups. These efforts are ongoing and cut across the spectrum of policy development in health care from policy with the little "p" with regard to how a nurse handles the response to a supervisor's request to work overtime, to big "P" policy with the proposal of legislation to end mandatory overtime or change federal law for overtime to allow employees to choose between overtime and paid time off.

NURSES AT THE FOREFRONT OF QUALITY AND SAFETY

Nurses, by virtue of being with patients at the point of care, whether it is at the bedside in a hospital, at an elementary school, or at a primary care office, practice from the perspective of nursing in a holistic manner. We are the largest group of health care professionals, so our reach is pervasive and our potential for influence is wide. Nurses are at the sharp end of health care when they provide direct care. However, it is the blunt end where policy decisions are most often debated and made. However, any discussion of quality and safety and implementation of strategies to improve health must include nurses as the gatekeepers at the sharp end. The IOM now classic report, *To Err Is Human: Building a Safer Health Care System* (Kohn, Corrigan, & Donaldson, 1999), dramatically publicized the statistic that 98,000 deaths occur annually from medical errors. This number equates to a jumbo jet crash every day.

The IOM Committee on Quality Health Care in America felt that safety was an integral component of quality and that quality could not be improved without addressing safety (Kohn et al., 1999). While the IOM report did not begin the patient safety movement, its release put the spotlight on a number of safety organizations such as the Institute for Safe Medication Practices (ISMP), Institute for Healthcare Improvement (IHI), and the NPSF, and spawned the release of subsequent reports such as *Keeping Patients Safe: Transforming the Work Environment of Nurses* (Page, 2004). Patient safety advocate Lucian Leape (2010), David Marx, creator of the just culture movement (2003), and others have long advocated for a systems approach to patient safety, recognizing that major errors were most likely due to a series of faults within a system and that blaming individuals for major errors did not prevent them from happening again. These initiatives have certainly saved lives. However, we know that the adoption of safety initiatives and achieving successful outcomes is quite complex and frustratingly slow, as often there is a disconnect between point of care and policy decisions. We offer two examples of how nurses at the sharp end are important to policy.

One point-of-care challenge is illustrated by a process designed to improve medication safety. In 2008, the Centers for Medicare and Medicaid Services (CMS) adopted an interpretive guidance that time-critical scheduled medications needed to be administered within 30 minutes of their prescribed time (CMS, 2011). Technological advances made it possible to track the timing of medication administration and allowed linking hospital reimbursements to compliance with this 30-minute rule. It is most likely that every nurse learned in school that medications should be administered within 30 minutes of the scheduled time, one of the five rights of medication administration, and that it was considered an error when this rule was violated. Yet, clearly there is no supporting evidence for this long-standing dictum, which does not take into consideration individual patient needs and the nature of the medication. Many nurses did not complete error reports when this rule was violated. This rule was impractical, created undue hardships on nurses, and, in fact, created safety problems, which the interpretive guidance was intended to prevent.

The ISMP (2010) completed a survey of nearly 17,500 nurses affected by the 30-minute rule. The impressive response rate indicates that nurses were concerned about their abilities to deliver care safely. The ISMP found that 70% of the nurses worked in an organization that enforced such a policy and that only 5% were able to comply. Nurses felt that they were set up to fail by being forced to take unsafe shortcuts and found work-arounds. Nurses, for example, removed medications all at once for all assigned patients from an automatic dispensing machine (ADM), gave their identification badges to another nurse to scan for a double check of a medication such as insulin, delayed administering pain medications so that standing order medications were administered on time, and bypassed pharmacy review of orders (ISMP, 2010). Nurses, particularly direct-care nurses at the bedside in hospitals, were not represented in the initial development of the guidance. Sadly, this also indicates that, in a significant number of settings, nurses were powerless to stop such a change in policy that had a negative impact on their ability to deliver safe patient care.

Conversely, the overwhelming response of nurses to the ISMP survey illustrates the power in numbers and the power of evidence. The ISMP, the ANA, and other organizations marshaled their resources to reverse this guidance. We will never know how many patients were harmed and how many nurses were unfairly disciplined by their employers while the original CMS guidance was in place. In order to provide safe care, nurses, particularly those nurses at the sharp end of care, need to be recognized for their expertise in the formulation and execution of everyday policies and standards impacting patient care. See Figure 1.4 for examples of nurses' policy initiatives that have had an impact on patient safety and quality. In addition, nurses need advocacy skills in order to make these processes work so that their patients can benefit from safe and high-quality care.

Lack of input at various levels within and beyond the organization continues to be a challenge for nurses. While nurses have increased roles and responsibilities for decision making within health care organizations, recognizing nurses as autonomous professionals has been slow (Paynton, 2008). Understanding how nurses serve as the early warning system for infectious disease in their countries provides an example of how important it is for nurses to have input within their organization and beyond. While the impact of nursing on patient health outcomes is well documented through research, infectious disease and disasters are tragic reminders of what the world is like when nurses' voices go unheard. See Policy on the Scene 1.2 for the story of one nurse's efforts at the sharp end of the severe acute respiratory syndrome (SARS) epidemic.

The SARS epidemic and the response to it in Toronto provide lessons about the vital roles that nurses can and should play in planning and organizing resources to deal with this kind of an epidemic. Nurses are critical in raising the warning. However, the potential to avert disaster is diluted by poor working

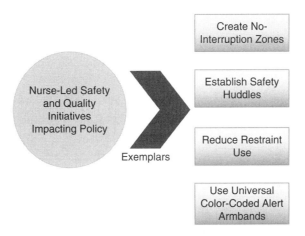

FIGURE 1.4 Exemplars of nurse-led safety and quality initiatives.

POLICY ON THE SCENE 1.2: Nurses' Early Warnings

In 2003, Anna Wong, an intensive care unit (ICU) nurse manager at a Toronto hospital, read in a Chinese-language daily newspaper about a family in Hong King who took a trip to mainland China, and then, the father and daughter became sick and two family members died (Gottlieb, Shamian, & Chan, 2004). When Ms. Wong had a patient in the ER whose mother had died recently, she asked the night nurse to check if the family had traveled to Hong King and, indeed, the mother had done so. It was her alert that set in motion an investigation of the epidemic that turned out to be caused by SARS. Although nurses warned that a second wave of SARS had arrived in Toronto, government officials announced that the transmission of SARS in Toronto had ceased. However, Canada, Ontario, and Toronto politicians and business leaders campaigned to overturn a World Health Organization (WHO) advisory against travel to Toronto (Parsons, 2003). Nurses did not know how deadly the SARS virus was and, in some instances, nurses were only provided surgical masks instead of N95 masks.

Here, the issue was one of a systematic failure to listen to nurses' concerns, problems ingrained in the blunt end of care, or latent or system factors that are not readily apparent to the casual observer. Various explanations were proffered regarding this failure, including the desire to indicate that Toronto was a safe destination for travelers. In this instance, it was a nurse who made the initial connection that something was seriously wrong at her hospital. Subsequently, it was thought that the danger from SARS had dissipated. Although the nurses raised their concerns again and again, they were told it was not SARS; not only did the nurses raise the alarm, but they also returned to work in the face of certain danger (The SARS Commission, 2006). Nurses engaged in public protests and, subsequently, leaders of the Registered Nurses Association of Ontario were instrumental in getting policies and procedures changed so that patients and those who cared for them would not be at risk. Unfortunately, this did not happen before two nurses and a physician lost their lives in the process.

conditions, a systemic lack of preparedness, and failure to include nurses in key policy decisions. When sorely tested systems running at capacity experience a surge in demand, the public's health is at risk. We cannot rely on what we have termed the little "p" alone. We must advocate for effective communication, planning, organizational support, and resources, knowing that minimal or half-hearted efforts are not going to achieve the health outcomes that we believe to be important to the nation and the health of the world.

INTERPROFESSIONAL COLLABORATION

Interprofessional collaboration will be an increasingly important arena in the health care systems of the future because of the evidence of its positive impact on patient outcomes through improved coordination and communication. The IOM calls for all health care professionals to be educated to deliver patient-centered care as members of interprofessional teams (Greiner & Knebel, 2003, p. 3) and is included in the Quality and Safety Education for Nurses (QSEN) project (Cronenwett et al., 2007). The call for increased interprofessional collaboration provides nurses opportunities for ongoing involvement in the development of little "p" policies within an organization such as the implementation of fall risk reduction protocols or rapid response teams, as well as opportunities for big "P" influence on health care through participation in major policy groups or organizations.

Opportunities for collaboration and influence at the big "P" level are sometimes the direct result of paid participation to obtain membership or seats at key policy tables. Some of these seats can range upward of $25,000 for one seat. For example, a number of nursing organizations hold seats at the National Quality Forum (NQF) (see Exhibit 1.3). NQF members also include representatives of other health professional groups (e.g., medicine and pharmacy), consumers, health plans, provider organizations, purchasers, public health/community groups, suppliers, and industry.

The NQF brings health care leaders together to build consensus on national priorities and goals for performance improvement, as well as provide the endorsement of standards for measuring performance. The NQF, through its Measure Applications Partnership (MAP), provides input to the Department of Health and Human Services on the selection of performance measures for public reporting and performance-based payment. Inclusion of a nurse-sensitive measure (e.g., pressure ulcers) as an NQF quality measure is important recognition for quantifying the daily work of nurses. Using recognized nurse-sensitive measures strengthens research, demonstrating the relationship between patient outcomes and nurse staffing. Norma Lang, PhD, RN, FAAN, a noted leader in quality who has served on the NQF and worked hard to make the work of nurses visible, noted that, "If you can't name it, you can't control it, finance it, teach it, or put it into public policy" (Clark & Lang, 1992). Sometimes, an organization can be a member of a policy group for years with seemingly little or no progress, but then an opportunity may arise to influence the agenda in a way that makes a dramatic difference for health care. Participation in the NQF provides the nurse leaders with not only opportunities for collaboration across professions, but also opportunities to collaborate with business leaders and consumer advocates.

Nurses are represented by the ANA at numerous other tables. These include the IOM, IHI, National Council of Patient Information and Education, National Coordinating Council for Medication Error Prevention and Reporting, and the e-Health Initiative, among others. Very often, the ANA provides the only nurse representation at a policy table. The ANA represents all nurses, focusing on issues across the broad spectrum of nursing care. It also has close relationships

EXHIBIT 1.3	NATIONAL QUALITY FORUM NURSE ORGANIZATION MEMBERS

Academy of Medical–Surgical Nurses

American Academy of Nursing

American Academy of Nurse Practitioners

American Association of Colleges of Nursing

American Association of Nurse Anesthetists

American College of Nurse-Midwives

American Nephrology Nurses Association

American Nurses Association

American Organization of Nurse Executives

Association of periOperative Registered Nurses

American Psychiatric Nurses Association

Association of Rehabilitation Nurses

Association of Women's Health, Obstetric and Neonatal Nurses

Emergency Nurses Association

Hospice and Palliative Nurses Association

Infusion Nurses Society

National Association of Pediatric Nurse Practitioners

National Council of State Boards of Nursing

NICHE-Nurses Improving Care for Healthsystem Elders

Nursing Alliance for Quality Care

Oncology Nursing Society

University of Kansas School of Nursing

Visiting Nurse Associations of America

Wound, Ostomy and Continence Nurses Society

with 21 nursing organizations that are its affiliates and over 60 nursing organizations through the Nursing Organizations Alliance. Specialty organizations may also represent nurses in interprofessional groups focused on their practice area. In addition, the ANA and other nursing organizations have the opportunity to make recommendations for appointments to key policy positions in governmental agencies (e.g., CMS) and nongovernmental organizations (e.g., The Joint Commission) (see Chapter 3, "Navigating the Political System").

It is important that we, as nurses, are proactive and that we are well positioned by being involved in interprofessional collaboration at numerous levels of important agenda-setting organizations. Interprofessional collaboration provides opportunities for building relationships when working together on areas of mutual interest and concern. Forging these relationships becomes important in crossing bridges and enabling organizations to address areas of policy disagreement in the future.

HEALTH CARE REFORM

Health care reform with the passage of the Patient Protection and Affordable Care Act (PPACA) provides nurses with numerous opportunities to intersect with health policy initiatives to transform our health care system. This legislation covers the broad spectrum of health care delivery, providing nurses with numerous opportunities to influence the development of health policy. See Exhibit 1.4 for areas covered by the PPACA that have particular relevance for nurses. Two examples of health care reform, in relation to the role of nurses in care coordination and

EXHIBIT 1.4   KEY PROVISIONS OF PPACA AND IMPLICATIONS FOR NURSES

AREA	KEY FEATURES
Primary care workforce	Scholarships and loan repayment; funding for National Health Service Corps and Public Health Service Corps
Workforce development programs	Title VII funding for advanced practice nurses, workforce diversity, education, quality and retention grants, loan repayment and scholarships for nursing students, nurse faculty, public health professionals, allied health professionals, health professionals in pediatric or geriatric settings, and graduate nurse education; redefining health professionals shortage areas; demonstration grants Indian Health; establishes National Healthcare Workforce Commission
National Practitioner Data Bank	Streamlining and standardizing processes for clinical privileging
Patient-centered medical homes	Grants program for community-based interdisciplinary, interperfessional teams to support primary care
Nurse-managed health centers	Grant support for nurse-managed health centers providing primary care to underserved and vulnerable populations
Certified nurse midwives (CNMs)	Increase in reimbursement rates for CNMs to provide parity with physicians

(continued)

EXHIBIT 1.4 KEY PROVISIONS OF PPACA AND IMPLICATIONS FOR NURSES (*CONTINUED*)

Payment for Medicare	Bonus payment for primary care providers in health professions' shortage areas (does not apply to CNMs)
Innovations Center at CMS	Development and testing of various innovative health care payment and service delivery models
Independence at Home	Demonstration program for chronically ill Medicare beneficiaries
School-based health centers (SBHCs)	Funding for new and existing SBHCs with preference to sites serving large number of children receiving medical assistance
Nursing home transparency	Public reporting of staffing and turnover data. Establishment of complaint resolution process. Mandated disclosure of ownership and wage and benefit wage data
Patient-centered outcomes research	Grants to support patient-centered comparative effectiveness research
State health insurance exchanges	All types of licensed health care professionals are included as providers
Essential health benefits package	Defines essential benefits covered under health insurance benefits packages
Accountable care organizations (ACOs)	Providers and suppliers working together to coordinate care for Medicare beneficiaries; reporting of quality improvement results; establishes nurses' roles in quality improvement and care coordination
Center for Quality Improvement and Patient Safety	Identification of best practices for quality improvement in the delivery of health care services

Source: American Nurses Association (2014a).

the removal of barriers to practice (advanced practice registered nurses [APRNs] and hospital staff nurses, respectively), are illustrated here for application to policy.

Nursing is taking a leadership role in care coordination—one of the profession's traditional roles and a vital element in health care reform. Care coordination helps ensure that patients' needs and preferences are met over time with regard to health services and information sharing, and involve the deliberate organization of patient care activities in order to facilitate the appropriate health care service delivery (ANA, 2012). However, the advancement of nurses' contributions to care coordination has met with resistance (American Academy of Family Physicians, 2012) as advanced practice nurses work for recognition as leaders in patient-centered medical homes (PCMH). PCMH is a care model that redesigns primary care so that it is patient centered and comprehensive, accessible, coordinated while maintaining quality and safety, and satisfying for the patient (Agency for Healthcare Research and Quality, n.d.). The PPACA, often shortened to ACA, makes funds available for PCMHs to transform primary care by paying care coordinators, who very often are nurses, for their work. A number of PCMH demonstration projects are using strategies such as team-based care, sustained partnerships, enhanced access, coordinated care, and system-based approaches to quality, all of which are promising for improving care processes. All nurses, including advanced practice nurses, can be involved in transforming primary care practices to PCMH models. An illustration of the big "P" in policy at work was when nurses, including the ANA president at the time, Rebecca M. Patton (2006–2010), were regularly involved in the discussions and development of PPACA with the president, White House staff, and members of Congress. Consequently, PPACA uses clinician-neutral language—specifically, primary care "practitioners" or "providers"—enabling advanced practice nurses to lead PCMH teams, depending on individual state laws and regulations. Although the winds of change are favorable to nursing and nurses have the opportunity to participate in the process at many levels, moving forward on these opportunities to capitalize on nursing's traditional roles requires continued organized and concerted collaborative efforts in order to achieve equitable access to high-quality care.

Barriers to practicing at the full scope of one's education and training still exist in many settings. While, typically, barriers to practice are discussed in the context of advanced practice nurses (clinical nurse specialists, certified nurse midwives, certified RN anesthetists, and nurse practitioners), RNs providing direct care are not immune from this phenomenon. For example, some hospitals may still have a unit charge nurse who will be responsible for all communications with physicians. The oft-cited reason is that nurses do not have the experience to make the decisions about calling physicians. This then creates a situation where nurses do not have the opportunity to learn and practice competencies related to interprofessional communication and collaboration. Using a third party for communication may result in unnecessary delays and possibly errors when important details are not communicated in either direction. Yet, when the charge nurse is not around, the nurse who was not allowed to communicate regularly with physicians is expected to handle the essential communications with skilled proficiency and aplomb. This type of ingrained hierarchical communication pattern limits professional autonomy and growth and can negatively impact patient safety. Gebbie (2011) describes the "socialized hesitation" of nurses to use critical thinking and decision making as a detriment to providing the highest level of care and calls upon organizations to upgrade their position descriptions to include expectations for professional decision making and the use of evidence-based practice.

Safe staffing, a major issue for nurses at the bedside, is also a barrier to practicing at the full scope of their education and training by creating conditions that make it difficult for nurses to deliver the care that they believe meets professional standards and is safe for their patients. When nurses are forced to work faster, when they don't have sufficient time to complete their work, when they have to work longer hours, and they don't have the resources to do their work, it creates stress for nurses. The evidence is substantial that these workload stressors have an impact on patient outcomes (Aiken et al., 2012; Trinkoff et al., 2011), and that inadequate nurse staffing has a more significant impact on older Black surgical patients (Carthon, Kutney-Lee, Jarrin, Sloane, & Aiken, 2012).

Barriers for advance practice nurses may also contribute to patient safety problems. For example, APRNs, including nurse practitioners, clinical nurse specialists, and certified nurse midwives, along with physician assistants, are not allowed to order home health services, yet APRNs coordinate the majority of skilled care to home health patients (ANA, 2011a). This leads to unnecessary delays for patients who need such services as well as delays in patient discharge from more expensive hospital settings (ANA, 2011a). In 2014, APRNs will not be able to order oxygen, home blood glucose monitors, and other durable medical equipment (DME) without a physician verification of a face-to-face encounter. Legislation was introduced in the House of Representatives of the 113th Congress to address this issue by amending Title XVIII of the Social Security Act (H. R. 3833) by allowing nurse practitioners, clinical nurse specialists, and physician assistants to document their own face-to-face encounters.

THE ENVIRONMENT AND HEALTH

Nurses have long recognized the role of the environment in maintaining health. Florence Nightingale emphasized that the environment should promote health and in no way be harmful. The provision of fresh air, light, a quiet environment, nutrition, warmth, clean water, sanitation, and cleanliness was essential to this vision. From a social justice perspective, these same environmental factors are central to the elimination of health care disparities around the world. Access to clean water is vital to preventing and treating life-threatening diarrhea, which kills yearly about 750,000 children younger than age 5 (WHO, 2013). Cleaner air in the community where we live and work means children are less likely to get asthma. The World Health Organization (WHO) estimates that as many as 24% of global diseases are caused by environmental exposures that can be averted, and more than 33% of the diseases in children younger than age 5 are caused by environmental exposures that can be modified (Prüss-Üstün & Corvalán, 2006). Every day we learn more about the relationship of certain diseases to the environment: asthma, allergies, emphysema, cancer, heart disease, stress. In fact, it is difficult in the course of a day to come across a patient whose health is not impacted by the environment. These numbers and everyday experiences with our patients are a call to action for policies that help make improvements to the environment and strengthen our public health so that everyone can live to their fullest potential.

Nurses are ideal natural advocates for environmental health. Nurses understand the issues and can articulate them to the public to garner support and build coalitions for action that can improve environmental health at work, in schools, in hospitals, and in communities. Recent natural disasters have shown the need for and provided the opportunity to address environmental health issues, and nurses have responded individually and collectively when disasters have hit. Hurricane Sandy, which struck in 2012, left thousands without clean water, electricity, or heat. All in a community suffer when this type of disaster hits, but the poor and often the elderly, who have fragile support systems, often bear the brunt of a disaster. Disasters, whether natural hurricanes and tornadoes or man-made terrorist attacks, often impact those with the least resource reserves the most. These socioeconomic and demographic inequities easily translate into increased health care disparities when disaster hits (see Chapter 14, "Eliminating Health Inequities Through Policy, Nationally and Globally").

The ANA (2010) has actively pursued examining and advocating for legal and ethical roles of nurses in natural disasters and, as a result, issued a brief, *A Nurse's Duty to Respond in a Disaster.* The ANA brief discusses some of the ethical and personal issues related to the duty of a nurse to respond to disasters and raises questions to consider before disaster strikes. Also contained in the Brief is information on how the ANA was involved with other interprofessional organizations (e.g., IOM's Forum on Medical and Public Health Preparedness for Catastrophic Events) in writing suggested principles for policy developers that need to be accounted for when planning standards of care for all health care providers involved in disasters.

OPTION FOR POLICY CHALLENGE: Advice for Assuming a New Role in Policy
Mary Jane K. DiMattio

A nurse vice president mentored me in the area of quality. I engaged in informal peer mentoring with some of the business professionals on the board. I shared my knowledge of clinical and quality issues, while they imparted their understanding of finance and business strategy. Also, my hospital had an excellent parent organization, which provided an orientation to the role of the trustee, a subscription to *Trustee Magazine*, and continuing education at yearly board retreats. I advise anyone considering the role of hospital trustee to inquire about similar educational opportunities (in addition to legal coverage under the Directors and Officers Policy). I encourage reading health care policy and trade journals, so as to articulate nursing's role within the larger health care enterprise, and strongly suggest either formal preparation or a mentor in the areas of health care economics and finance.

I started on the board with a "we versus them" attitude, but learned that most of the professionals who run health care organizations care deeply about delivering quality care and face enormous pressures to keep

(continued)

their organizations financially viable. Nurses must propose solutions that are cost conscious. I think that, today, the ideal nurse trustee can speak on the best ways to reconcile quality with cost. Most important, I suggest that patient advocacy is at the heart of serving as a hospital trustee.

Serving on a hospital board comes at the expense of one's time, particularly if the board's structure involves subcommittees. Also, a great deal of the real work is done outside of formal meetings. There can be a lot of stress and even heartache (I participated in selling our hospital to a for-profit company). But the positives of this type of professional service far outweighed any negatives for me. One of my proudest professional moments came on the airport shuttle to a board retreat. The woman seated across from me asked on which hospital board my husband served. I felt immensely fortunate to explain to her that I am a nurse, who serves as a hospital trustee.

While we have global and regional environmental health issues, we can also consider the familiar phrase that all politics is local. We need not look very far for an opportunity to improve environmental health. Nurses themselves, as briefly addressed in the chapter so far, may be at risk for harm from environmental hazards in their own work settings and may contribute to environmental harms by poor practices in their work settings. Not only do we have more research than ever that demonstrates the link between the work environment of nurses and patient outcomes but we have the link as well between the work environment and the health of nurses. Nurses can and should be at the forefront of efforts to ensure that their working conditions are safe.

Nurses may be informed about the hazards associated with chemotherapeutic agents, but they may not even know about the nature of hazards associated with chemicals such as cleaners, solvents, disinfectants, and pesticides despite ubiquitous safety data sheets. Hospitals and other health care organizations expose their employees to a wide range of hazards: biological, chemical, ergonomical, physical, and psychological. A 2007 survey of more than 1,500 nurses across the United States, sponsored by the ANA, the Environmental Working Group, Healthcare Without Harm, and the University of Maryland School of Nursing, indicates that one-third of nurses had high exposures, defined as being exposed at least twice a week to at least five chemicals and other hazardous substances for 10 or more years (Environmental Working Group, 2007). These data indicate the need for nurses to work to implement strategies at the little "p" level by marshaling forces to replace hazardous materials and institute engineering controls, as well as at the big "P" level to institute necessary legislative and regulatory action to ensure that nurses and their coworkers have a healthy and safe environment to deliver quality care.

It is not just hazardous chemicals that are a concern for nurses. A 2011 ANA survey of nurses about health and safety in their work environment indicates that on-the-job injuries increased slightly in comparison with 2001. In addition, nearly all nurses indicate they have worked despite experiencing musculoskeletal pain. The two top health and safety concerns are (1) the acute or chronic effects of stress and overwork and disabling musculoskeletal injury and (2) concerns about on-the-job assault, which have increased (ANA, 2011b). Also, approximately 10% of the nurses said they have had an automobile accident that was related to fatigue or shift work. The results of these surveys and the evidence drawn from the world around us indicate that we have much work to do and that each of us needs to be involved in making the environments in which we live, work, and play safer for all.

Nurses are also tackling broader issues of environmental concern. The Pennsylvania State Nurses Association (PSNA) submitted a proposal that was adopted by the ANA's House of Delegates in 2012 calling for a national moratorium on new permits of unconventional oil and natural gas extraction (fracking) until human ecological safety could be ensured (McDermott-Levy, Kaktins, & Sattler, 2013). This was a bold move by PSNA, which gave national voice to a problem experienced at the local level. It also illustrates the potential within the nursing community to address environmental health problems. In developing its proposal, PSNA drew upon the expertise of the members of its environmental health council, one of whom is Nina Kaktins, MSN, RN, a nurse and a geologist who has willingly shared her knowledge with health care professionals across Pennsylvania. Access to clean water for communities is central to the national debate on this issue.

What will be your level of involvement? There are numerous organizations that address environmental issues in health care (see Exhibit 1.5). Nurses can

EXHIBIT 1.5	**REPRESENTATIVE ORGANIZATIONS ADDRESSING ENVIRONMENTAL ISSUES IN HEALTH CARE**

Agency for Toxic Substances and Disease Registry (ASTDR), Environmental Health Nursing Initiative: http://www.atsdr.cdc.gov/ehn

American Nurses Association, Healthy Work Environment: http://www.nursingworld.org/MainMenuCategories/WorkplaceSafety/Healthy-Work-Environment

Alliance of Nurses for Healthy Environments: http://www.envirn.org

The Luminary Project: http://www.theluminaryproject.org

Healthcare Without Harm: http://www.noharm.org

National Environmental Health Foundation: http://www.neefusa.org

Practice Green Health (formerly Hospitals for a Healthy Environment [H2E]): http://www.practicegreenhealth.org

become part of these groups or access numerous resources available on their websites.

IMPLICATIONS FOR THE FUTURE

The aforementioned set of complex forces, workforce needs, quality and safety, health care reform, and environmental health reinforce the important role of leadership in health policy at the little "p" and the big "P" levels, whether one is advocating for government activities, institutional decisions, organizational positions, or professional standards. The pivotal role of leadership is supported with strong empirical data. Research has demonstrated that high-resonant leadership, where leaders are in tune with themselves, is significantly related to lower patient mortality (Cummings, Mododzi, Wong, & Estabrooks, 2010), as well as to better care environments that are associated with significantly lower risk of death and failure to rescue (Aiken et al., 2008). Magnet hospitals, which model transformational leadership, have significantly better work environments, lower mortality, and lower instances of failure to rescue (McHugh et al., 2013), and for very low birth weight babies, Magnet hospitals have significantly lower 7-day mortality, nosocomial infections, and severe intraventricular hemorrhage (Lake et al., 2012).

Another type of leadership that impacts policy that is now receiving much attention is the dearth of nurses serving on hospital governing boards. A 2005 study (Prybil et al., 2005) determined that only 2% of hospitals have nurses on their governing boards. The findings from a more recent study conducted in New York City indicated that physicians were found on boards in a large majority of the hospitals (over 90%), whereas nurses were only represented on 26% of the hospital boards (Mason, Keepnews, Holmberg, & Murray, 2013). If nurse input into the policy making of an organization is limited, then it makes it more difficult to fully operationalize safe quality care as employers of nurses lose a valuable frontline perspective when making policy.

Leadership is the focus in two of the eight recommendations of *The Future of Nursing* report: "expand opportunities for nurses to lead and diffuse collaborative improvement efforts" and "prepare and enable nurses to lead change to advance health" (IOM, 2011, pp. 11, 14). In fact, one can view the other *Future of Nursing* recommendations related to (a) education (bachelor of science in nursing [BSN]-prepared nurses, doctoral preparation, lifelong learning, and residencies), (b) practicing to full scope of education and training, and (c) workforce data infrastructure as providing support for the development of the leadership role of nurses in society. For to be a leader in nursing, one must be well versed in the strategies and tools of policy, and these recommendations, when achieved, will help provide the needed base structure for larger nurse involvement in policy from bedside to boardroom.

The American Academy of Nursing (AAN) has taken the initiative to publicize the impact of nursing on outcomes through its Edge Runners program. While this program is designed to highlight the impact of nursing through quantifiable outcomes, these really are stories of nursing leadership in action. These initiatives could not have been accomplished without dedicated, committed, knowledgeable, and savvy nurse leaders working to improve policy. Edge Runner Ruth Watson Lubic, a MacArthur Foundation "Genius" Award recipient, was known for creating a free-standing childbearing center in the southwest Bronx, an underserved community. She used her award to create a successful midwife/nurse practitioner-run program, the Family Health and Birth Center (FHBC), providing low-income women with cost-effective maternal/child care in Washington, DC. The FHBC lowered preterm births, reduced low birth weight, and decreased cesarean sections (AAN, 2013). Dr. Lubic's leadership in creating a successful nurse-midwife–led maternal and child care program provides not only the evidence that can be used by other organizations seeking to replicate her results, but also the financial savings that can be used to sway policy makers to obtain additional funding, as well as changes in reimbursement practices. These successful Edge Runner programs can and should be used as models for other organizations, and as springboards for nurses to develop essential leadership competencies.

The leadership of nurses in advocacy roles occurs not only through formal positions, but also in the daily routine activities of staff nurses. Nurses serve important roles as members of committees, councils, and workgroups where policy with a little "p," the policy that impacts nurses and their patients at the sharp end, is identified, planned, developed, and evaluated. We need to make sure that nurses work not only in nurse groups, but also in multidisciplinary groups. Substantive improvements in care will be hampered if interdisciplinary collaboration is not the norm. For example, a hospital may have a falls prevention committee, but if nurses do not interact with physicians, pharmacists, physical therapists, and other health care professionals, it may be difficult, if not impossible, to reduce fall rates, especially over time as rates are monitored and evaluated and drift from policy occurs. All that are impacted by policy must be involved in its development.

We know that being silent within an organization has repercussions for the safety and well-being of our patients (Henriksen & Dayton, 2006). Likewise, being silent within our society, our organizations, our associations, our community, and our government has repercussions for the advancement of our profession and the well-being of the patients entrusted to our care. Taking an active role in policy is every nurse's responsibility as a member of our profession.

Leadership in advocacy requires careful thought, preparation, and an ability to negotiate a complex set of relationships. As with many leadership roles, it is not a single action or single skill set that positions a nurse to assume a leadership role (see Chapter 12, "Serving the Public Through Policy and Leadership"). As we learned with the Policy Challenge, networking, being at the right place at the right time, education, experience, and competencies are all important for nurses in advancing to the next level of advocacy. See the previous Option for

Policy Challenge for recommendations for assuming the role of a board trustee. With some very slight modifications, these lessons can be applied to numerous other advocacy roles in one's organization and community, as well as at the state, federal, and international level.

KEY CONCEPTS

1. The policy process includes recognition and identification of a problem, formulation of the policy, implementing it, and then monitoring and evaluating the results.
2. Workforce issues including workforce development, workforce safety, adequacy of staffing and support services, respect and civility, and conditions of employment need to be addressed in order to enhance the quality and safety of patient care.
3. Nurses, by virtue of being at the sharp end of care and having intimate knowledge of the health care system, are critical to the development, monitoring, and evaluation of policy related to safety and quality.
4. Nurses are well prepared for interprofessional collaboration, which is increasingly taking on more significance in improving patient outcomes.
5. Passage of PPACA provides nurses with resources for education as well as opportunities for using nurses more effectively, and shaping policies for a reformed health care system.
6. Nurses have a long tradition of advocacy for our communities through the promotion of healthy environments.
7. Being a nurse means being a leader involved in policy regardless of the particular practice setting.
8. Nurses are ideally positioned to be leaders in their organizations, communities, and government, at the local, state, national, and international levels.

SUMMARY

Nurses are an essential part of health care delivery and, as such, they have an integral leadership role and responsibility in the development of health policy. Nurses have a myriad of opportunities for involvement in health policy on the continuum from bedside with the provision of direct care, to the boardroom with the formulation and implementation of policy at the top echelons of complex organizations, at the state, national, and even international levels. Forces influencing nursing practice and health care include nurse workforce needs, quality and safety, interprofessional collaboration, health care reform, and environmental health. Nurses are increasingly being called on to be leaders at the bedside and beyond. Being a leader means being involved in policy. Policy work is every nurse's work. Nurses are well positioned to lead the way in policy, from the bedside to the boardroom.

LEARNING ACTIVITIES

1. Compare and contrast current policy activities of the ANA and one specialty nursing organization.
2. Identify one or two policy activities that you will accomplish while in school and then determine what three to five goals related to policy you will accomplish within 3 years of graduation.
3. Discuss the rationale for your decisions and what strengths you have to accomplish these tasks.
4. On a daily basis for a week, read a paper and/or watch a news show and each day identify a political issue that is discussed. For every issue, discuss at least three reasons why the issue is important to nursing.
5. At your workplace or clinical practicum site, identify three policy issues that are currently under discussion. What is the impetus for those policies? Describe your role, or potential role, and the impact the policy will have on you.
6. Discuss the status of current workplace violence policies in your workplace, organization, and state.
7. Describe your goals for your policy involvement in the next 3 to 5 years and the steps necessary to achieve them.

E-RESOURCES

- Agency for Healthcare Quality and Research Patient Safety Organization .http://www.pso.ahrq.gov
- American Academy of Nursing Raise the Voice Edge Runner. http://www .aannet.org/edgerunners
- American Nurses Association: Shiftwork Sleep Disorders: The Role of the Nurse in Understanding SWSD for You and Your Patients. http://eo2 .commpartners.com/users/swsd
- American Nurses Association Policy and Advocacy. http://nursingworld .org/MainMenuCategories/Policy-Advocacy
- Florence Nightingale: Theory of Public Health Policy. http://www .uoguelph.ca/~cwfn/nursing/theory.html
- Food and Agriculture Organization: Basics in policy analysis: How governments should design and implement policies. http://www.fao.org/docs/ up/easypol/540/basics_in_policy_analysis_170en.pdf
- International Council of Nurses. (2008). *Promoting health: Advocacy guide for health professionals.* Geneva, Switzerland. http://www.whpa.org/ ppe_advocacy_guide.pdf
- World Health Organization. (2010). *Strategic directions for strengthening nursing and midwifery services 2011–2015.* Geneva: World Health Organization. http://whqlibdoc.who.int/hq/2010/WHO_HRH_HPN_10.1_eng.pdf

REFERENCES

Agency for Healthcare Research and Quality. (n.d.). *Defining the PCMH. Patient Centered Medical Home Resource Center.* Retrieved from http://pcmh.ahrq.gov/portal/server.pt/community/pcmh__home/1483/pcmh_defining_the_pcmh_v2

Aiken, L. H., Cimiotti, J. P., Sloane, D. M., Smith, H. L., Flynn, L., & Neff, D. F. (2012). Effects of nurse staffing and nurse education on patient deaths in hospitals with different nurse work environments. *Journal of Nursing Administration, 42*(Suppl 10), S10–S16.

Aiken, L. H., Clarke, S. P., Sloane, D. M., Lake, E. T., & Cheney, T. (2008). Effects of hospital care environment on patient mortality and nurse outcomes. *Journal of Nursing Administration, 38*(5), 223–229.

American Academy of Family Physicians. (2012). Independent practice authority for nurse practitioners could splinter care, undermine patient-centered medical home. *Annals of Family Medicine, 19*(6), 572–573. doi:10.1370/afm.1457

American Academy of Nursing (AAN). (2013). *Family health and birth center in the developing families center.* Retrieved from http://www.aannet.org/edgerunners

American Nurses Association. (2001). *Code of ethics for nurses with interpretive statements.* Silver Spring, MD: Nursesbooks.org

American Nurses Association. (2006, December 8). *Assuring patient safety: Registered nurses' responsibility in all roles and settings to guard against working when fatigued.* Retrieved from http://www.nursingworld.org/assurringsafetynurseps

American Nurses Association. (2010). *A nurse's duty to respond in a disaster.* Retrieved from http://www.nursingworld.org/MainMenuCategories/WorkplaceSafety/Healthy-Work-Environment/DPR/Disaster-Preparedness.pdf

American Nurses Association. (2011a). *Action issue: Home health.* Retrieved January 15, 2013, from http://www.rnaction.org

American Nurses Association. (2011b). *Health & safety survey report.* Silver Spring, MD: Author.

American Nurses Association. (2012). *The value of nursing care coordination. A white paper of the American Nurses Association.* Silver Spring, MD: Author.

American Nurses Association. (2014a). *Health care transformation: The Affordable Care Act and more.* Retrieved from http://www.nursingworld.org/MainMenuCategories/Policy-Advocacy/HealthSystemReform/AffordableCareAct.pdf

American Nurses Association. (2014b). *Workplace violence.* Retrieved from www.nursingworld.org/workplaceviolence

American Nurses Association. (n.d.). *Nurses currently serving in Congress.* Retrieved from http://www.nursingworld.org/MainMenuCategories/Policy-Advocacy/Federal/Nurses-in-Congress

Ballou, K. A. (2000). A historical-philosophical analysis of the professional nurse obligation to participate in sociopolitical activities. *Policy, Politics & Nursing Practice, 1*(3), 172–184.

Barabach, L. (2013, March 24). Now is the time to impact our children's mental health. *Cleveland Plain Dealer,* Retrieved from http://www.cleveland.com/opinion/index.ssf/2013/03/now_is_the_time_to_impact_our.html

Bekemeier, B. (2008). "Upstream" nursing practice and research. *Applied Nursing Research, 21*(1), 50–52. doi:10.1016/j.apnr.2007.11.002

Carthon, J. M., Kutney-Lee, A., Jarrin, O., Sloane, D., & Aiken, L. H. (2012). Nurse staffing and postsurgical outcomes in black adults. *Journal of the American Geriatrics Society, 60*(6), 1078–1084. doi:10.1111/j.1532-5415.2012.03990.x

Centers for Medicare and Medicaid Services (CMS). (2011). *Updated guidance on medication administration, Hospital Appendix A of the State Operations Manual.* Retrieved from http://www.cms.gov/Medicare/Provider-Enrollment-and-Certification/Survey-CertificationGenInfo/downloads/SCLetter12_05.pdf

Clark, J., & Lang, N. M. (1992). Nursing's next advance. An international classification of nursing practice. *International Nursing Review, 39*, 109–111.

Cook, E. T. (1913). *The life of Florence Nightingale* (Vol. I). (1820–1861). London, UK: MacMillan and Co. Retrieved from http://www.gutenberg.org/files/40057/40057-h/40057-h.htm

Cronenwett, L., Sherwood, G., Barnsteiner, J., Disch, J., Johnson, J., Mitchell, P., Sullivan, D. T., & Warren, J. (2007). Quality and safety education for nurses. *Nursing Outlook, 55*(3), 122–131.

Cummings, G. G., Mododzi, W. K., Wong, C. A., & Estabrooks, C. A. (2010). The contribution of nursing leadership styles to 30-day patient mortality. *Nursing Research, 59*(5), 331–339.

Economic Policy Unit: Office of the First Minister and Deputy Minister. (n.d.). *A practical guide to policy making in Northern Ireland.* http://www.ofmdfmni.gov.uk/practical-guide-policy-making.pdf

Emergency Nurses Association. (2010). *ENA toolkit: Workplace violence.* Retrieved from http://www.ena.org/practice-research/Practice/ViolenceToolKit/Documents/toolkitpg1.htm

Environmental Working Group. (2007). Nurses health. A survey on health and chemical exposures. Retrieved from http://www.ewg.org/sites/nurse_survey/analysis/summary.php

Falk-Rafael, A. (2005). Speaking truth to power: Nursing's legacy and moral imperative. ANS. *Advances in Nursing Science, 28*(3), 212–233.

Feldman, H. R., & Lewenson, S. B. (2000). *Nurses in the political arena: The public face of nursing.* New York, NY: Springer Publishing.

Gebbie, K. M. (2011, October 20). Laws are not the only barriers to scope of practice. Retrieved from http://www.rwjf.org/en/blogs/human-capital-blog/2011/10/laws-are-not-the-only-barriers-to-scope-of-practice.html

Gebbie, K. M., Wakefield, M., & Kerfoot, K. (2000). Nursing and health policy. *Journal of Nursing Scholarship, 32*(3), 307–315.

Gottlieb, L. N., Shamian, J., & Chan, S. (2004). Lessons from SARS: Challenges for the international nursing research community. *The Canadian Journal of Nursing Research, 36*(1), 3–7.

Greiner, A. C., & Knebel, E. and the (Eds.). Committee on the Health Professions Education Summit. (2003). *Health professions education: A bridge to quality.* Washington, DC: The National Academies Press.

Henriksen, K., & Dayton, E. (2006). Organizational silence and hidden threats to patient safety. *Health Services Research, 41*(4 Pt. 2), 1539–1554.

Institute of Medicine (IOM). (2011). *The future of nursing: Leading change, advancing health.* Washington, DC: The National Academies Press.

Institute for Safe Medication Practices (ISMP). (2010, September 9). CMS 30-minute rule for drug administration needs revision. *ISMP Medication Safety Alert®.* Retrieved from http://www.ismp.org/newsletters/acutecare/articles/20100909.asp

Khoury, C. M., Blizzard, R., Wright Moore, L., & Hassmiller, S. (2011). Nursing leadership from bedside to boardroom: A Gallup national survey of opinion leaders. *Journal of Nursing Administration, 41*(7–8), 299–305.

Koff, S. Z. (2004). *Nurse educators and politics.* Albany, NY: State University of New York Press.

Kohn, L. T., Corrigan, J., & Donaldson, M. S. (Eds.). (1999). *To err is human: Building a safer health system.* A report of the Committee on Quality of Health Care in America, Institute of Medicine. Washington, DC: National Academies Press.

Lake, E. T., Staiger, D., Horbar, J., Cheung, R., Kenny, M. J., & Rogowski, J. A. (2012). Association between hospital recognition for nursing excellence and outcomes of very low-birth weight infants. *JAMA, 307*(16), 1709–1716.

Lanier, J. (2012). Running for elective office: A different form of nursing advocacy. *Ohio Nurses Review, 87*(5), 8–9.

Leape, L. (2010). Who's to blame? *Joint Commission Journal on Quality and Patient Safety, 36*(4), 150–151.

Lucian Leape Institute. (2013). *Through the eyes of the workforce: Creating joy, meaning and safety health care.* Boston, MA: National Patient Safety Foundation.

Marx, D. (2003). How building a "just culture" helps an organization learn from errors. *OR Manager, 19*(5), 1, 14–15, 20.

Mason, D. J., Keepnews, D., Holmberg, J., & Murrary, E. (2013). Representation of health professionals on governing boards. *Journal of Urban Health, 90*(5), 888–901.

McDermott-Levy, R., Kaktins, N., & Sattler, B. (2013). Fracking, the environment, and health. *American Journal of Nursing, 113*(6), 45–51.

McHugh, M. D., Kelly, L. A., Smith, H. L., Wu, E. S., Vanak, J. M., & Aiken, L. H. (2013). Lower mortality in magnet hospitals. *Medical Care, 51*(5), 383–388.

McKinlay, J. B. (1986). A case for refocusing upstream: The political economy of illness. In P. Conrad & R. Kern (Eds.), *The sociology of health and illness: Critical perspectives* (pp. 484–498). New York, NY: Worth Publishers.

Newport, R. (2012, December 3). *Congress retains low honesty rating.* Gallup® Politics. Retrieved from http://www.gallup.com/poll/159035/congress-retains-low-honesty-rating.aspx

New York State Education Department. (2013). *Practice information: Working long hours.* Retrieved from http://www.op.nysed.gov/prof/nurse/nursevolovertime.htm

Nurse-led. (2013, January 14). *Nurse-led recycling initiative reduces OR waste at Hackensack.* Retrieved from http://news.nurse.com/article/20130114/NY02/301210006

O'Byrne, P., & Holmes, D. (2009). The politics of nursing care: Correcting deviance in accordance with the social contract. *Policy, Politics & Nursing Practice, 10*(2), 153–162.

Page, A. (Ed.) and The Committee on the Work Environment for Nurses and Patient Safety. (2004). *Keeping patients safe: Transforming the work environment of nurses.* Washington, DC: The National Academies Press.

Parsons, L. (2003*). Toronto: New SARS outbreak provokes nurses' protest.* Retrieved from http://www.wsws.org/en/articles/2003/06/sars-j10.html

Paynton, S. T. (2008, October, 27). The informal power of nurses for promoting patient care. *OJIN: The Online Journal of Issues in Nursing, 14*(1).

Prüss-Üstün, A., & Corvalán, C. F. (2006). *Preventing disease through healthy environments: Towards an estimate of the environmental burden of disease.* Geneva: World Health Organization.

Prybil, L., Peterson, R., Price, J., Levey, S., Kruempe, D., & Brezinski, P. (2005). *Governance in high-performing organizations: A comparative study of governing boards in not-for-profit hospitals.* Chicago: Health Research and Educational Trust.

Rains, J. W., & Barton-Kriese, P. (2001). Developing political competence: A comparative study across disciplines. *Public Health Nursing, 18*(4), 219–224.

Rogers, A. E., Hwang, W. T., Scott, L. D., Aiken, L. H., & Dinges, D. F. (2004). The working hours of hospital staff nurses and patient safety. *Health Affairs, 23*(4), 202–212.

SARS Commission. (2006). *The SARS Commission Final Report: Spring of Fear, 2,* 1–873. Retrieved from http://www.archives.gov.on.ca/en/e_records/sars/report/v2.html

Scott, L. D., Hwang, W. T., Rogers, A. E., Nysse, T., Dean, G. E., & Dinges, D. F. (2007). The relationships between nurse work schedules, sleep duration, and drowsy driving. *Sleep, 12,* 1801–1807.

Silk, E. (2010, September). Violence against nurses bill signed into law. *New York Nurse*.

Steinwachs, D. M., & Hinshaw, A. S. (2004). Preface. In A. Page (Ed.) and Committee on the Work Environment for Nurses and Patient Safety. *Keeping patients safe: Transforming the work environment of nurses* (pp. xi–xii). Washington, DC: The National Academies Press.

Trinkoff, A. M., Johantgen, M., Storr, C. L., Gurses, A. P., Liang, Y., & Han, K. (2011). Nurses' work schedule characteristics, nurse staffing, and patient mortality. *Nursing Research, 60*(1), 1–8. doi:10.1097/NNR.0b013e3181fff15d

Warner, J R. (2003). A phenomenological approach to political competence: Stories of nurse activists. *Policy, Politics & Nursing Practice, 4*(2), 135–143.

World Health Organization. (2013, April). *Diarrhoeal disease. Fact sheet No. 330.* Retrieved from http://www.who.int/mediacentre/factsheets/fs330/en/index.html

Zhou, X., Ferguson, S. A., Matthews, R. W., Sargent, C., Daruent, D., Kennaway D. J., & Roach, G. D. (2012). Mismatch between subjective alertness and objective performance under sleep restriction is greatest during the biological night. *Journal of Sleep Research, 21*(1), 40–49.

TWO

Advocating for Nurses and for Health

Debbie Dawson Hatmaker
Karen Tomajan

Our lives begin to end the day we become silent about things that matter.
—Martin Luther King Jr.

OBJECTIVES

1. Investigate advocacy as a means of improving the quality and safety of health care delivery.
2. Compare and contrast competencies needed to be an advocate in different health care settings.
3. Illustrate the relationship of social justice and ethics to the work of advocacy.
4. Describe the public's view of nursing in health care advocacy.
5. Verify barriers to patient advocacy that can impact success or failure.
6. Choose key resources to assist in developing the skill set to be an effective health care advocate.

Modern nursing's evolution from a vocation to a profession began in the late 1800s as Florence Nightingale published her views about how nurses should be educated and how patient care should be provided (Hegge, 2011). While Nightingale did not directly use the word *advocacy* in her writings, her work was consistently about advocating for change (Selanders & Crane, 2012). Her own words speak to the importance she put on change: "I think one's feelings waste themselves in words; they ought all to be distilled into actions and into actions which bring results" (Cook, 1913, p. 94).

The concept of advocacy is part of professional nursing. Advocacy includes a complex interaction among nurses, patients, professional colleagues, and the public at large (Selanders & Crane, 2012). To be an effective nursing professional, a nurse must understand and embrace the role of advocate—advocating for health and for the nursing profession. See the Policy Challenge, which describes how a recent graduate moves from advocacy for safe patient handling on an individual level to policy development in a health care facility.

POLICY CHALLENGE: Advocacy for Safe Patient Handling

Robert Cameron has just passed his first anniversary as a registered nurse (RN) and has learned a great deal in his staff nurse position on St. Joseph's Health System's orthopedic unit. While the hospital has a reputation for a positive work environment and has invested in some technology to move patients, Robert is concerned that the unit has fallen short with regard to developing a culture of safety and even lacks an organizational commitment to safe patient handling practices. He has spoken to the unit manager and she has suggested he bring this up for discussion at the unit's next staff meeting as well as consider sharing with the hospital's shared governance practice council. Robert remembers from his baccalaureate education program that the role of "nurse advocate" is foundational to practice. So he begins his research for the most current information on safe patient handling techniques in order to advocate on behalf of patients and nurses to promote safety and decrease injury while improving quality of care. He is looking for the answers to questions such as:

- What are the most effective ways to advocate for culture change on his unit?
- Which competencies are needed to be an advocate?
- What is the organization's philosophy about advocating for cultural change?
- What resources are available within the work setting to address work environment concerns?
- Are there advocacy organizations that can be helpful in promoting these changes?
- Are there standards, guidelines, or best practices available to provide evidence-based support to the advocacy process?

Answers to these questions can be found on health care organizations' websites, in the nursing and other health care literature, and from nurse educators. Robert decides to contact a colleague who works as a clinical nurse specialist at the hospital who has been instructive in the past about advocacy efforts and organizational culture. He also reaches out to a physical therapist colleague who has been talking about the "return on investment" that is possible when using safe patient handling technology. He discusses his concerns with the employee health nurse at his facility and has been asked to present his recommendations at the hospital safety committee. He was very interested in advocacy during his nursing education program and knows that it is a role he can develop more as he moves from beginner to expert nurse.

See Option for Policy Challenge.

This chapter provides an overview of the concept of advocacy, advocacy roles of nurses, and expectations of society and the profession regarding nurses' advocacy. The *Code of Ethics for Nurses* is used to describe the application of advocacy. In addition, competencies for advocacy, resources for becoming an advocate, and advocacy arenas will be identified. Advocacy exemplars are used to illustrate the various possible outcomes of nurses' advocacy efforts.

ADVOCACY DEFINITIONS

Advocacy is defined by the Merriam-Webster online dictionary (2013) as the act or process of supporting a cause or proposal. An *advocate* is one who pleads, defends, or supports a cause or the interest of another. Much of the literature related to advocacy comes from the legal profession and nonprofit and special interest groups that prepare advocates to influence legal proceedings or public policy. The strategies promoted by these groups are also useful for nurses and the nursing profession (Tomajan, 2012).

Multiple definitions of advocacy have been suggested, indicating that the role of the advocate is to work on behalf of self and/or others to raise awareness of a concern and to promote solutions to the issue (Tomajan, 2012). Amidei (2010) has described advocacy as "seeing a need and finding a way to address it" (p. 4). Family Care International (2008) defined advocacy as "the process of building support for an issue or cause and influencing others to take action" (p. 3). In speaking about advocating for change, Sharma (1997) stated, "Wherever change needs to occur, advocacy has a role to play" (p. 1). Advocacy can take many forms and may require working through formal decision-making bodies to achieve a positive result. This could include various committees, the administrative chain of command within a health care organization, a state commission, a regulatory body, and state or federal legislative entities.

The term *advocacy* was first included in the profession's codes by the International Council of Nurses (ICN) in 1973 (Vaartio & Leino-Kilpi, 2005). Nursing education documents prior to the mid-1970s did not reference advocacy as a clear expectation in nursing. In fact, early nursing education historically emphasized conformity, obedience, and authority (Selanders & Crane, 2012). Since this time, advocacy has increasingly been associated with the role of the professional nurse. This evolution of nursing practice from loyalty to advocacy has put forward a metaphor of the nurse as an advocate of patients' rights. However, there continue to be challenges associated with nursing's evolution toward a broader social justice advocacy model while retaining the individual patient–nurse advocacy model that continues to dominate in nursing practice today (Paquin, 2011).

In a review of empirical literature from 1990 to 2003, Vaartio and Leino-Kilpi (2005) identified three themes: advocacy motivated by the patient's right to information and self-determination, advocacy stemming from the patient's right to personal safety, and advocacy as a philosophical principle in nursing.

Bu and Jezewski (2007) discuss three core attributes of nursing advocacy: safe-guarding patient autonomy, acting on behalf of patients who are not able to act for themselves, and championing social justice.

PROFESSIONAL AND SOCIETAL EXPECTATIONS OF ADVOCACY

It has been noted that nurses readily accept the requirement of the professional nurses' advocacy role as it applies to their patients (Tomajan, 2012); however, advocacy activities on behalf of colleagues, the profession, or even oneself are often lacking. Two of the American Nurses Association's (ANA) core documents, the *Nursing: Scope and Standards of Practice* (2010a) and the *Code of Ethics for Nurses With Interpretative Statements* (2001), delineate the professional nurse's responsibility to work with colleagues to advocate for safe practice environments.

The ANA's *Nursing: Scope and Standards of Practice* (2010a) clearly iden-tifies "advocacy" within the scope of nursing practice, suggesting it is funda-mental to that practice. Advocacy for safe, effective practice environments is a key responsibility of the professional nurse. Standards competencies that speak directly to advocacy include the following (ANA, 2010a):

- Advocates for health care that is sensitive to the needs of health care consum-ers, with particular emphasis on the needs of diverse populations (p. 38)
- Advocates for the delivery of dignified and humane care by the interprofes-sional team (p. 40)
- Engages consumer alliances and advocacy groups, as appropriate, in health teaching and health promotion activities (p. 42)
- Advocates for equitable health care/consumer care (p. 47)
- Advocates for resources, including technology, that enhance nursing practice (p. 60)
- Advocates for the judicious and appropriate use of products in health care (p. 61)

The ANA's *Code of Ethics for Nurses With Interpretive Statements* (2001) identifies multiple advocacy expectations for the professional nurse. These include service to the profession through teaching, mentoring, peer review, involvement in professional associations, community service, and knowledge development/dissemination (Tomajan, 2012). These activities and skills are foundational for the advocacy role of the professional nurse.

Advocacy is based on a foundation of ethical principles that include auton-omy, beneficence, nonmaleficence, and fidelity. It is essential that advocates act in the interest of those they represent in the advocacy process and align their actions with these principles (ANA, 2011).

- *Autonomy*—Autonomy is respect for another's right to self-determine a course of action and to support independent decision making. Nurses should protect the autonomy of those for whom they are acting, which includes in-volvement in decision making.

- *Beneficence*—Beneficence is taking action to help others and to protect them from harm. The desire to do good and help others is a core principle of advocacy.
- *Nonmaleficence*—Nonmaleficence is the avoidance of harm or hurt. This principle is sometimes described as "do no harm" and is likewise an important role of the advocate.
- *Fidelity*—Keeping one's promises and being truthful and loyal to those being represented are unequivocal expectations of the advocate. Disclosing personal interests and being cognizant of one's own goals help to prevent conflict of interest when advocating on behalf of others.

AMERICAN NURSES ASSOCIATION *CODE OF ETHICS*

Advocacy carries with it a significant ethical dimension; therefore, principles of ethics can help to evaluate a nurse's effectiveness as an advocate. A code of ethics is fundamental for any profession. It provides a social contract with the population served, as well as offering ethical and legal guidance to members of the profession.

The ANA published its original *Code of Ethics* (http://www.nursingworld .org/codeofethics) in 1950. Through six revisions, the core value of service to others has remained consistent throughout the document (Fowler, 2008). Two significant changes have occurred since the Code's original publication: (1) the conceptualization of "patient" has expanded from that of an individual receiving treatment to include the individual's family and community; and (2) the provision that prompts nurses to recognize that, "the nurse owes the same duties to self as to others …" (ANA, 2001, p. 18).

Each of the nine Code provisions includes an aspect of advocacy:

Provision 1

The nurse, in all professional relationships, practices with compassion and respect for the inherent dignity, worth and uniqueness of every individual, unrestricted by considerations of social or economic status, personal attributes, or the nature of health problems (ANA, 2001, p. 7).

Respect for persons is identified as a core ethical principle in the Code, and this provision includes respect for autonomy. The nurse is expected to practice compassion and respect regardless of who is receiving care; this includes the nurse's colleagues as well. Although the nurse may not feel equally responsive to all humanity, he or she is expected to not let feelings of frustration or anger negatively impact care. Provision 1 maintains that nurses have a professional obligation to move beyond these feelings to provide the same level of care regardless of diagnosis, ethnicity, or economic status. Therefore, the nurse is ethically bound to care and advocate for all. Advocacy behaviors related to autonomy and self-determination may be exemplified by informed consent. "Patients have a moral and legal right to determine what will be done with their own person; to be given accurate, complete, and understandable information in a manner that facilitates an informed judgment; to be assisted with weighing the benefits, burdens, and available options in their treatment, including the choice of no treatment; to accept, refuse, or terminate treatment without deceit, undue influence, duress, coercion, or penalty; and to be given necessary support throughout the decision making and treatment process" (ANA, 2001, p. 8).

Provision 1 Exemplar—Right to Self-Determination

Mrs. Sadie Farmer is 83 years old and has recently been hospitalized with an acute myocardial infarction. She is mentally alert and lives alone, although two of her three grown children live in a town a few miles away. After initial testing, her cardiologist indicates that the results suggest this is not Mrs. Farmer's first heart attack and she admits to having had "spells" in the past and that she just "waited them out." Dr. Howard is recommending more intervention, but Mrs. Farmer does not want to undergo more procedures. Her brother-in-law died a few years ago after cardiac surgery and she indicates that she has "had a good life" and is "ready to go when the Lord calls me home." Dr. Howard has conceded to Mrs. Farmer's wishes, but her primary care physician is not quite ready to give in to her decision to abandon further intervention. Some of Mrs. Farmer's children and grandchildren are urging her to accept more treatment. Her nurse, Jean Evans, is becoming concerned that Mrs. Farmer seems to be more upset about her bickering family than about her treatment decisions. Nurse Evans calls a team meeting with Mrs. Farmer's health care providers and family members. Chaplain Jones has been asked to offer an ethics consult to the team in an effort to allow Mrs. Farmer to determine her own care.

Provision 2

The nurse's primary commitment is to the patient, whether an individual, family, group, or community (ANA, 2001, p. 9).

Ethical dilemmas will arise as the nurse attempts to balance a commitment to the patient, the family, and the community; however, this provision is clear that the nurse's primary obligation is to the patient. "Nurses strive to resolve such conflicts in ways that ensure patient safety, guard the patient's best interests and preserve the professional integrity of the nurse" (ANA, 2001, p. 10). Interpretation of this provision speaks to distributive justice when resources are limited, collaboration when caring for a patient in the complexity of the health care environment, and professional boundaries within the nurse–patient relationship (Lachman, 2009). Therefore, advocacy has its limits and limitations that must be observed.

Provision 2 Exemplar—Commitment to the Patient

Kathy Johnson, RN, works in the role of patient relations liaison. She receives a telephone call from a patient who had been cared for earlier that day in the emergency department for back pain. The patient was quite upset that during the visit the physician had been rude, called her a "drug seeker," and did not offer any pain relief treatment or medication. The patient explained that she has a chronic back injury and had just moved to the area and injured her back while unpacking boxes. Although she has an appointment with a local physician, she has not yet been seen, and the physician's office staff directed her to the emergency department. Nurse Johnson contacts the emergency department director and arranges for the patient to be reevaluated later that day.

Provision 3

The nurse promotes, advocates for, and strives to protect the health, safety, and rights of the patient (ANA, 2001, p. 12).

Provision 3 interpretive statements focus on the patient's right to privacy and confidentiality, as well as safeguarding research participants and addressing incompetent practice—whether it involves impairment or lack of knowledge or skill. The Health Information Portability and Accountability Act (HIPAA) demonstrates the complexity of confidentiality. HIPAA, like the *Code of Ethics for Nurses*, is intended to provide guidance to the health care professional, not absolutes (Lachman, 2009). The nurse must always weigh the patient's right to privacy with protection of the patient from harm. The latter sections of Provision 3 deal with the problem of incompetent practice. "The nurse has a responsibility to implement and maintain standards of professional nursing practice" (ANA, 2001, p. 13). Whether the incompetence is due to impairment or lack of knowledge, the nurse must report the issue to the appropriate person in the organization. If not acted on, the nurse must then take the next step in the organizational hierarchy or even consider reporting to an outside accrediting or regulatory body. Such advocacy skills as maintaining standards of care, advocating for impaired colleagues, or whistle-blowing may come into play with this provision.

Provision 3 Exemplar—Addressing Impaired Practice

John Smith, RN, has just completed his first year of practice on the telemetry unit. His nurse preceptor, Linda Johnson, has been a great support during his orientation and he is feeling very confident as he enters his second year. Linda has recently separated from her husband of 20 years and she's not seemed herself lately. John notices that she has been arriving late for work, is looking strained, and is disorganized. Linda has verbally blown up with a couple of coworkers in the past week. He's noticed alcohol on her breath the past 2 days she's come to work and he is really concerned about Linda and about her patients. When John points out that Linda almost administered an incorrect medication—a "near miss" error—he realizes he has to take his concerns to their nurse manager. Ethically he is bound to address his colleague's impaired practice and ensure the safety of patients.

Provision 4

The nurse is responsible and accountable for individual nursing practice and determines the appropriate delegation of tasks consistent with the nurse's obligation to provide optimum patient care (ANA, 2001, p. 16).

Accountability for actions is the cornerstone for a profession due to the implied social contract with the public (Fowler, 2008). Nursing has been identified repeatedly as the most trusted profession because its practitioners take the issue of accountability seriously. This accountability includes self-assessment of competency, seeking educational resources when less than competent to perform care, and appropriate delegation to other health care providers. This provision highlights the need for nurse's acceptance of accountability and self-assessment in order to be an effective advocate.

Provision 4 Exemplar —Accountability for Nursing Judgment and Action

Denise Lawrence, a pediatric faculty member in a baccalaureate school of nursing, works per diem in the summer on the pediatric or mother–baby units of a community hospital. One Saturday she reports to the pediatric unit only to learn that she has been assigned to float to the sixth-floor adult oncology unit due to low pediatric census and high census on the adult units. Denise has never been oriented to any of the other hospital nursing units and has not taken care of adult oncology patients since she graduated from nursing school more than a decade ago. She does not feel safe in providing nursing care to oncology patients. However, the house supervisor has not returned her call to address the issue so she goes to the sixth-floor nurses' station but tells the charge nurse that she will only agree to take patients' vital signs and do patients' personal care. When the supervisor makes rounds, Denise intends to inform her that she cannot ethically take accountability for complete care of these patients since she does not have the knowledge, competence, and experience to engage safely in their care.

Provision 5

The nurse owes the same duties to self as to others, including the responsibility to preserve integrity and safety, to maintain competence, and to continue personal and professional growth (ANA, 2001, p. 18).

Interpretative statements for Provision 5 focus on moral self-respect, professional growth, and maintenance of competence, as well as wholeness of character or integration of personal and professional values. Aspects of self-advocacy are inherent in this provision. Competency is seen as a self-regarding duty and not simply an instrumental good in service to others (Fowler, 2008). The preservation of integrity and moral self-respect can be challenged in our daily clinical practice. Nurses have an ethical obligation to disclose errors and neither falsify records nor tolerate verbal abuse from others (Lachman, 2009). Preservation of nurses' integrity under this provision would also allow for the concept of "conscientious objection," where a treatment, intervention, or activity is morally objectionable to the nurse. While nurses cannot abandon their patients, they must make it known to administration when situations place them in moral dilemmas that they find objectionable.

Provision 5 Exemplar—Wholeness of Character, Integration of Personal and

Professional Values

Mr. Wilson has just been diagnosed with lung cancer and his physician has explained treatment options that include surgery, chemotherapy, and radiation. After his family leaves the hospital, Mr. Wilson asks his nurse, Sarah Smith, her opinion about the best course of treatment. Sarah is an experienced RN and knows that while she could voice her opinion, ethically she should assist Mr. Wilson to clarify his own values in reaching an informed decision, thus avoiding unintentionally persuading him in one way or another (ANA, 2001). Sarah asks Mr. Wilson what he knows about his treatment options as they have been explained and what things are most important to him as he considers the treatment side effects and possible outcomes.

Provision 6

The nurse participates in establishing, maintaining, and improving health care environments and conditions of employment conducive to the provision of quality health care and consistent with the values of the profession through individual and collective action (ANA, 2001, p. 20).

While nurses often focus on ethics and advocacy as it relates to the individual patient, Provision 6 extends the nurse's obligation to advocate for change in unhealthy work environments that contribute to poor patient care and patient dissatisfaction. The nurse must advocate for an environment that will support the values central to the nursing profession. The reciprocal relationship between the nurse and the work environment is inherent in this provision. The work environment can either obstruct or support nursing values and ethical obligations. This Code provision sets forward an expectation of moral activism; the nurse should work to change the environment if it is obstructive. The goal is for nurses to work with administration to create an environment that supports safety and quality patient care (Lachman, 2009). Advocacy on a large scale is possible when nurses join with their professional associations and participate in collective action such as collective bargaining or workforce advocacy. When this is not possible and an organization refuses to support patient rights or put nurses in a position that violates professional standards of practice, nurses may have little choice but to leave the organization.

Provision 6 Exemplar—Improving the Health Care Environment

Patricia Brown is a staff nurse in a critical care unit. She is very committed to her colleagues and believes that maintaining a healthy work environment is the responsibility of every nurse. She overhears Jean Johnson, one of her colleagues, speaking condescendingly to a new nurse who has asked a question regarding the unit routine. After the conversation concludes, Patricia pulls Jean aside and relates what she heard between the two nurses. She shares her feelings that Jean was too harsh with the new nurse, and relays her concern that this is an example of lateral violence. She informs Jean that harsh communication with new staff is detrimental to the development of a positive unit environment and relays her belief that every staff member should feel comfortable asking questions of any colleague without fear of reprisal.

Provision 7

The nurse participates in the advancement of the profession through contributions to practice, education, administration, and knowledge development (ANA, 2001, p. 22).

Advancement of and advocacy for the nursing profession is the focus of Provision 7. Many activities are representative of this obligation: mentorship, service on organizational shared governance committees, and leadership in professional associations and civic activity at the local, state, national, or international levels. Nurses advocate via Provision 7 through many role-specific responsibilities: For example, nurse educators are responsible for nursing education standards; nurse researchers support clinical practice by providing practice-based evidence; and nurse administrators should create an environment that supports ethical integrity and empowerment (Lachman, 2009).

Provision 7 Exemplar—Advancing the Profession

State nurses associations routinely review new bills being presented in state legislatures to determine the impact on the health of citizens as well as the impact on the profession. A bill has been forwarded to the state legislature that allows clerical staff in the public schools to administer medications to students. The association's legislative committee believes that passing this bill could compromise the safety of school children, and that a better alternative would be to increase the number of school nurses employed within the state. They partner with school nurses, and involve their specialty organization, the National School Nurses Association, to jointly lobby against this bill in the legislature, citing potential risks to children.

Provision 8

The nurse collaborates with other health professionals and the public in promoting community, national, and international efforts to meet health needs (ANA, 2001, p. 23).

Advocacy for health concerns in the larger world is the focus of Provision 8. This is focused on the "broader health concerns such as world hunger, environmental pollution, lack of access to health care, violation of human rights, and inequitable distribution of nursing and health care resources" (ANA, 2001, p. 23). Many nurses work or volunteer their time with populations at risk: migrant farm workers, refugee centers, prisons, and homeless clinics. They offer direct care to those in need, educate the public to increase funds for care, and work to raise awareness in order to change policy and pass legislation to improve care to vulnerable populations. Included in this provision is the need for nurses to recognize their prejudices and demonstrate respect for the values and practices of others. Nurses must recognize their own biases in order to move beyond them, while advocating for culturally sensitive care on behalf of their patients.

Provision 8 Exemplar—Health Needs and Concerns

Soodabeh Joolaee is a recipient of the 2012 Human Rights & Nursing Award from the International Centre for Nursing Ethics (www.surrey.ac.uk/fhms/research/centres/ice). She has taught undergraduates and postgraduate nurses for over 20 years with a major focus on ethics. In her work to disseminate an ethical culture in clinical practice, she became aware that patients, physicians, and nurses were not consulted in the compilation of a patients' bill of rights that had been posted around the hospital; furthermore, none of them were fully aware of those rights. In 2010, she won the prestigious Avicenna Award of the Tehran University of Medical Sciences, given for outstanding education and research activities, for her PhD dissertation on the subject of patients' rights. These accomplishments gave her entry into health policy work and cooperation with the Iranian Ministry of Health and Medical Sciences. Since that time, she has been keenly focused on the rights of patients, negotiating with managers and leaders to educate nurses as patients' rights advocates, which is not an easy job for a nurse in a paternalistic health care context.

Provision 9

The profession of nursing, as represented by associations and their members, is responsible for articulating nursing values, for maintaining the integrity of the profession and its practice, and for shaping of social policy (ANA, 2001, p. 24).

Who advocates for the nursing profession? The focus of Provision 9 is on the profession through its associations, rather than toward the individual nurse, which is a dramatically new aspect of the Code. This version departs from previous codes by including all nurses in all nursing positions individually (i.e., not singling out nurses in direct care, nurse educators, nurse researchers) and all nurses collectively through their nursing associations (Fowler, 2008). A specific focus on social ethics reflects nursing's historical interest in how society affects health and illness. In addition to responsibilities related to social ethics, a nursing association works to maintain the integrity of the profession through a code of ethics, standards of nursing practice, educational requirements for practice, knowledge development, and continuing evaluation of professional nursing actions (Lachman, 2008).

Provision 9 Exemplar—Articulating Nursing Values and Maintaining Professional Integrity

Following the devastating hurricanes in Louisiana, Mississippi, Florida, and Texas in 2006, the ANA acted in concert with other professional associations and regulatory agencies to help define the responsibilities of nurses and other health care professionals in disaster situations. The ANA worked with state and national agencies and disaster relief organizations such as the American Red Cross to define the role of the RN in a disaster, establish structures to coordinate disaster response through the Medical Reserve Corps, and define potential legal protections for nurses acting in good faith in catastrophic situations (ANA, 2010c). These actions are examples of the association's advocacy for nursing as a profession, which impacts all nurses, not just the ANA members.

CLINICAL PRACTICE AND MORAL DISTRESS—THE REALITY OF PRACTICE ADVOCACY

Nurses in clinical practice encounter ethical issues that can lead to moral distress, negative feelings that result when one knows the ethically correct action to take but feels powerless to take that action (Epstein & Delgado, 2010). For nurses to be effective advocates, they must understand and accept their ethical responsibilities to the patient, family, community, and profession. But when nurses are unable to advocate due to practice barriers such as conflict between the nurse's responsibility to the patient and the nurse's duty to the employer, lack of colleague support, perceived lack of power, and even lack of education, moral distress may result, causing nurses to leave their jobs or the profession altogether (Epstein & Delgado, 2010; Hanks, 2007). When surveyed, nurses have identified ethical priorities to include the following (Pavlish et al., 2011):

- Patients' quality of life—an obligation to treat distressing symptoms, pain, and suffering
- Promoting patient autonomy—the notion that patient preferences should prevail over family wishes or health care team values
- Substandard health care—situations where the health care team either did not adhere to standards of care or was severely conflicted over treatment options

Many health care agencies have processes and policies that establish the chain of command to address ethical concerns, which may include an ethics committee tasked with addressing ethical dilemmas. Nurses increasingly have a voice in advocating for their patient within these organizations. However, the literature on moral distress indicates the processes available in many settings are inadequate in addressing the day-to-day issues confronting nurses in practice. Evidence-based nursing actions that address ethical conflicts are lacking; until further study is done, nurses will continue to be limited in their abilities to advocate for their patients who are experiencing complex ethical situations (Pavlish et al., 2011).

SOCIAL JUSTICE

Social justice speaks to how advantages and disadvantages are distributed to individuals in a society (Miller, 1999). While there are multiple and competing theories of social justice, all are based on the idea that justice is related to fairness of treatment and that similar cases should be treated in a similar manner (Butts & Rich, 2012). A community approach to social justice promotes the common good of the community rather than individual benefits and freedoms. Not being bound by borders promotes the consideration of how basic health care for all people can be provided and what can be done to prevent social injustice worldwide (Butts & Rich, 2012).

A strong commitment to social justice requires professional nurses to advocate for health for all persons. Advocacy activities are an expected outcome for a health profession that promotes the concept of social justice. Social justice advocacy is an inherent expectation of all nurses as expressed in the professional codes that guide nursing practice (Paquin, 2011).

EQUITY

One of the roles of the advocate is to promote equity and eliminate or mitigate the effects of health disparity at both the individual and system level. One of the features of health care reform has been to address disparities and promote equity in the health care system. Health disparity is defined as "substandard access, treatment or outcomes based on racial, ethnic or socioeconomic factors" (Hiles, 2010). Equity is defined as "the absence of systematic disparities in health (or its social determinants) between more or less advantaged social groups. Social advantage means wealth, power and/or prestige" (Braveman & Gruskin, 2003, p. 256). Equity is an ethical value based on social justice and is closely aligned with principles of human rights. The landmark 2003 Institute of Medicine (IOM) publication, *Unequal Treatment: Confronting Racial and Ethnic Disparities in Health Care*, revealed that significant racial and ethnic disparities in U.S. health care exist, even after controlling for factors such as insurance coverage, socioeconomic status, and other illnesses. These disparities contribute to infant mortality, disability, decreased life expectancy, and higher incidence of preventable hospitalizations (Robert Wood Johnson Foundation [RWJF], 2012). See Chapter 14, "Eliminating Health Inequities Through Policy, Nationally and Globally."

The principle of equity has been identified as one of the IOM's six aims for the future U.S. health system. These six aims are health care that is safe, effective, efficient, patient centered, timely, and equitable. In this context, *equitable* is defined as the provision of care that does not vary in quality because of personal characteristics such as gender, ethnicity, geographic location, and socioeconomic status (Corrigan, Donaldson, Kohn, Maguire, & Pike, 2001).

As a profession, nurses have led the way among health care professionals in their work to promote a health care system that is accessible to all and to address issues of disparity and inequality. In the advocacy role, nurses have worked to address equity needs of individual patients and patient populations and advance health policy at the health care system level.

The precautionary principle is a concept that impacts this discussion of advocacy, particularly as it relates to advocacy at the policy formation level. The precautionary principle advances the idea that if a product, action, or policy has a suspected risk of causing harm to the public or to the environment, the company, agency, or individuals responsible for the product or policy have a social responsibility to disclose the risk and act to protect the public even when the scientific evidence has not yet found a definitive causal relationship. The precautionary principle is based on the ethical principles of social justice and nonmaleficence ("first do no harm") and is aligned with the adage "better safe than sorry" (Science & Environmental Health Network [SEHN], 2011). Proponents of the precautionary principle assert that responsible entities should not wait for clear scientific cause-and-effect evidence between various actions or toxins and their harmful effect (Butts & Rich, 2012). Opponents of the precautionary principle believe that if science has not produced conclusive evidence that a particular activity or substance is harmful to humans and/or the environment, then the activity or substance is assumed to be safe until future evidence proves otherwise. Precautionary principle proponents would answer with the argument that by the time harmful causal relationships are established with certainty, irreparable damage may have already occurred. The harmful effect of cigarette smoking is one example of the precautionary principle. Long before scientific evidence was available showing a definitive causal link between cigarette smoking and lung cancer, advocates were encouraging smokers to quit.

Today there is evidence that the incidence of chronic diseases, birth defects, infertility, cancer, and Alzheimer's disease is increasing. While we do not have conclusive evidence of the causes, there are risk factors that have been identified. Proponents of the precautionary principle strongly advocate for communication of the risks to the public and action to limit exposure to potentially harmful substances when possible, despite the fact that causal evidence is not yet available (Butts & Rich, 2012).

PUBLIC EXPECTATION FOR ADVOCACY

You are traveling in a foreign country where you do not know the culture or language. How will you get your needs met? You may use nonverbal cues like gestures or pictures, but you are not certain you will be understood. What if you had an advocate, someone who knows the language, culture, and belief system? The U.S. health care system is foreign and challenging for many patients. There are lots of jargons, abbreviations, and euphemisms. Hospitals have hierarchies, policies and procedures, standards, routines, and rituals that are mysterious to patients, families, visitors, and students (Bosek & Savage, 2007). The public has come to expect nurses to serve in the role of advocate, assisting them to migrate through the "foreignness" of the health care system. While no single profession "owns" the role of advocate, nursing has traditionally seen this role as integral to good nursing care. The American public also sees the nurse in the role of advocate in that they have rated RNs as the most trusted profession for 14 of the past 15 years according to Gallup's annual survey (Gallup, 2013). RNs are increasingly recognized as leaders in transforming the health care system to meet the burgeoning demand for services with a focus on improving quality and managing costs. After 7 years without a permanent administrator, the U.S. Congress confirmed a nurse, Marilyn Tavenner, MHA, BSN, RN, as the permanent head of the Centers for Medicare and Medicaid Services (CMS). Tavenner had an early career as an intensive care unit (ICU) nurse, served as chief executive officer (CEO) of a large health system, and was Virginia's Secretary of Health and Human Resources. One might say that the CMS director serves as "chief advocate" in an agency that touches the lives of all Americans, through the Medicare, Medicaid, and children's health insurance programs.

While the public has come to know nurses' advocacy activities through their patient care experiences, they do not always see nurses in key leadership roles. A 2010 Gallup poll of 1,500 health opinion leaders said that they wanted nurses to have more influence in a variety of areas: reducing medical errors, increasing quality of care, and promoting wellness. They also believed that nurses should have more influence in planning policy development, as well as management (RWJF, 2010). However, those findings contrast with what is actually in place. A survey by the American Hospital Association of 1,000 U.S. hospitals found that nurses account for only 6% of hospital board members. This is in contrast to the number of physicians (20%) and other clinicians (about 5%) (Van Dyke, Combes, & Joshi, 2011). While nurses typically find advocacy for individual patients as integral to their nursing practice, they are less inclined to advance this advocacy role to larger systems and the public policy level. Nurses must see themselves as decision makers that influence health outcomes.

COMPETENCIES NEEDED TO BE AN ADVOCATE

Two of ANA's foundational documents, the *Code of Ethics for Nurses With Interpretative Statements* (2001) and the *Nursing: Scope and Standards of Practice* (2010a), address the professional nurse's responsibilities for advocacy. The documents cover required skills and activities, including service to the profession through teaching, mentoring, peer review, involvement in professional associations, community service, and knowledge development/dissemination (Tomajan, 2012). The skills of problem solving, communication, influence, collaboration, and resource identification can be used to support a cause on behalf of one's patient or oneself.

Problem Solving

Since advocacy is directed at problems in need of a solution, the problem-solving process is a necessary skill for the effective nurse advocate. Steps in problem solving and strategies to achieve each are illustrated in Figure 2.1.

Communication

Communication is key to an effective advocacy strategy. Verbal, written, and electronic forms of communication are used when advocates pull individuals to work collectively on a problem. It is important that all messages be based in fact and that messaging across time is consistent. While advocates are often "armed" with facts and figures when they attempt to influence decisions makers, it is equally important to "tell a story" of how the problem impacts patient care. Giving specific examples of patient care situations (without violating patient privacy) can demonstrate how the problem and suggested solution has a "real-world" impact (see Policy on the Scene 2.1).

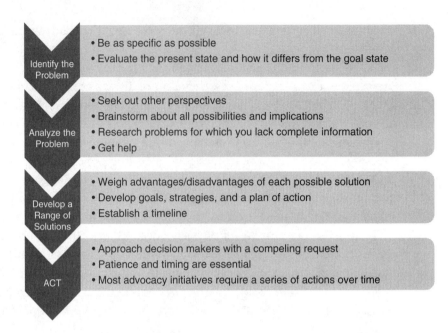

FIGURE 2.1 Problem-solving process.

POLICY ON THE SCENE 2.1: A Nurse-Managed Clinic

The story of Kelly Barnett, DNP, FNP-BC, and a nurse-managed clinic in the rural mountains of north Georgia communicates a strong message of advocacy and action. Ms. Barnett, a family nurse practitioner (NP), operates a nurse-managed clinic in the rural mountains of north Georgia. She received notice from her malpractice insurer that her contract was being canceled in 90 days because under her collaborative physician–nurse protocol, the physician was not "directly supervising" her practice. The insurer suggested that Ms. Barnett's clinic must be "under the same roof" as her supervision physician, despite this not being a requirement under current Georgia law. Kelly's panic set in as she was the sole provider for her family and now many of her patients would have to access their health care from clinics as much as 25 to 50 miles away from their community. She knew she needed help when her initial requests to the insurer were unheeded, and in her communication to the Georgia Nurses Association (GNA), Kelly said, "If I cannot bill the insurer, I will have to close my practice. There is no way I can financially make it otherwise. This means me and my other four employees will be out of our jobs. Where will my patients go if I close my doors?"

The GNA responded swiftly to assist Ms. Barrett and to save her north Georgia clinic. They worked closely with Kelly and acquired a memorandum of law on the actions of the insurer, which cited legal precedent, suggesting that as long as a collaborative agreement was in place, she is operating within what the current law allows. After reviewing the memorandum of law provided by the GNA, the insurer decided to rewrite their policy to allow NPs to be participating providers in their network. As long as her clinic meets the insurer's criteria and eligibility requirements, this nurse-managed clinic will continue to operate and provide much needed care to patients of rural Georgia.

"I couldn't have done this without the GNA's help and expert advice," Kelly stated in a recent message. "This is another step in the advancement of Georgia's NPs in health care practice."

Influence

To be effective, the nurse advocate must be able to influence others. Influencing an individual's or group's thoughts, beliefs, or actions is essential and built on competence, credibility, and trustworthiness (Tomajan, 2012). There are a number of ways that advocates attempt to use influence to effect change. Access to legislators may be gained through tactics such as letter writing campaigns, legislative testimony, and financial campaign contributions.

Using an influential leader or spokesperson can also bring attention to the issue. Celebrities are regularly tapped to bring their influence to important issues like Parkinson's disease research (Michael J. Fox) or pediatric cancer (Marlo Thomas).

To influence most effectively, the advocate must build a strong case for change—using facts, figures, and examples. Most importantly, the advocate must be able to influence with a strong delivery to decision makers. Developing an "elevator speech" is an important tool for the advocacy tool kit (see Exhibit 2.1; see also Chapter 10, "Working With the Media: Shaping the Health Policy Process").

Collaboration

In the complex world of health care, few changes are made in isolation. Collaboration and partnership are necessary to effect major changes. Collaboration is a process of working together for a common purpose. As opposed to cooperation (groups working together but focused on their own goals), collaborative ventures involve the development of common goals as well as common strategies and activities that will achieve that goal (Tomajan, 2012). Successful collaboration can be a time-intensive process requiring continuous communication with those involved, validating and reporting on progress toward the goal.

EXHIBIT 2.1   KEY ELEMENTS OF A GOOD ELEVATOR SPEECH

Follow these guidelines when preparing an elevator speech:

- *Keep it short.* After hearing a few sentences, your audience should know what you do and what you want. Limit your pitch to 60 seconds.
- *Have a "grabber"*—an opening line that grabs the person's attention and piques interest in hearing more.
- *Show your passion.* Your energy and dedication will help sell your proposal.
- *Make a request.* At the end of your speech, mention what you need. Do you want that person's business card? Do you want to schedule a meeting? Ask for a referral? Getting the person to take the next step is crucial. It's the reason you came up with your speech in the first place.
- *Practice.* Rehearse your elevator speech so that when the opportunity to use it comes up, you can do it well. Always be prepared to give your pitch so you can use it in a chance encounter. Memorize it. Revise as needed to keep it fresh and updated.

Reprinted with permission from Pagana (2013).

When collaborations are developed, it is helpful to consider all possible stakeholders to strengthen the advocacy efforts. Nurses may tend to partner with other nurses or nursing organizations when the issue is directly related to professional nursing practice, but collaborations with other health care providers can strengthen the advocacy efforts and message. An example of a coalition designed to address issues for advanced practice nurses and other health care providers is the Coalition for Patients' Rights (CPR). This coalition consists of over 35 health care organizations working to offset the efforts of the American Medical Association's Scope of Practice Partnership (SOPP) initiative that was developed to limit patients' choice of health care practitioners. CPR is predicated on the principle of patients having the right to choose their type of provider and having access to the right type of care at the right time (www.patientsrightscoalition.org).

Resource Identification

Another important skill for the nurse advocate is the ability to identify valuable resources. While this competency is necessary for any problem solving, searching for health policy information on the Internet can be seen as an essential skill when it comes to legislative advocacy (White et al., 2010). Searching the Internet for resources has become commonplace; however, with the explosion of web-based information, much of it lacking credibility validation, the task can be daunting. Steps to a successful health policy Internet search are illustrated in Figure 2.2.

Credible resources on the Internet that the nurse advocate should be utilizing include peer-reviewed and professional databases (PubMed, Cumulative Index to Nursing and Allied Health Literature [CINAHL]), organizations that focus on health policy (ANA, American Association of Colleges of Nursing,

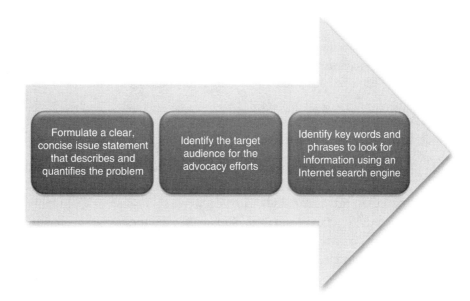

FIGURE 2.2 Steps for successful health policy searches on the Internet.

National League for Nursing, RWJF, Kaiser Family Foundation), and governmental entities (CMS, Centers for Disease Control, Department of Health and Human Services).

White and colleagues (2010) suggest the following criteria for evaluating websites:

- *Authority and Accuracy:* The author's identity, affiliation, and qualifications can serve to determine the credibility and reliability of the information presented. Scholarly references, well-maintained sites, and attention to detail add to credibility.

- *Purpose and Content:* Critically evaluate the website's information as to whether the author/organization presents a political agenda. Even non-profit organizations and government agencies have a particular "point of view."

- *Currency:* Unless seeking historical information, the website content should indicate how recently it has been updated. Broken URL links may indicate a poorly maintained site.

- *Organization and Ease of Use:* If the information is not easily obtainable, it has limited use for the searcher. Web pages, documents, and PDF files should load easily and quickly. Member-based organizations often place valuable information behind a locked "For Members Only" wall. This is another important reason that nurses should be members of their professional associations and other groups that support their advocacy work.

ARENAS FOR ADVOCACY

Nurses have numerous opportunities for advocacy. The one that most often comes to mind is the workplace. However, additional arenas for nurse advocacy include community, state, national, and international arenas.

Workplace

Nurses most commonly engage in advocacy on behalf of their patients in the clinical setting. Thus, the workplace, be it a hospital, public health clinic, long-term care facility, or primary care office, is often the location where nurses most frequently use their advocacy skills. Advocacy works best in environments that encourage its activity, where leaders are supportive and tools are available to make it happen.

The American Association of Critical-Care Nurses (AACN) has developed Standards for Establishing and Sustaining Healthy Work Environments (AACN, 2005) to address not only the physical environment but also less tangible barriers to staff and patient safety. The AACN highlights the ingredients for success as skilled communication, true collaboration, effective decision making, appropriate staffing, meaningful recognition, and authentic leadership. These standards are guidelines that the nurse as advocate can use to support a healthy work environment, an important factor in positive patient outcomes and professional satisfaction (Aiken, Clarke, Sloane, Lake, & Cheney, 2008).

The ANA, along with its partners and through its organizational relationships, is a leader in promoting improved work environments. The ANA protects, defends, and educates nurses about their rights as employees by addressing occupational hazards such as needlestick safety, back injuries, and violence. The ANA has developed a number of position statements and resources to support advocacy in the workplace (see Exhibit 2.2).

Community

When nurses are advocating in their community for increased access to care or other health care resources, the respect they have from the public strengthens their ability to persuade others to create the needed changes regarding patient care and services. The cost of health care continues to create barriers for patients. Patients and families often share with the nurse the difficulties they are experiencing in obtaining needed care due to the costs of treatments and medications. Nurses find themselves advocating for individual patients related to access issues and also at the community level specific to inadequate funding and its impact on patients' failure to receive appropriate health care services. Nurses have been engaged in identifying community resources for patients and establishing resources when they are inadequate. Due to the high expense of prescription drugs, many patients will forego treatment when they do not have the funds to obtain their needed medication. Nurses may be aware of community resources for drug discounts or even pharmaceutical companies' resources to allocate the needed treatment. Nurses have established many community-based clinics for those who do not have adequate access to health care (see Exhibit 2.3).

EXHIBIT 2.2 ANA POSITION STATEMENTS SUPPORTING ADVOCACY IN THE WORKPLACE

Assuring Patient Safety: The Employers' Role in Promoting Healthy Nursing Work Hours for Registered Nurses in All Roles and Settings (http://nursingworld.org/MainMenuCategories/WorkplaceSafety/Healthy-Work-Environment/Work-Environment)—12/8/06

Given the well-documented relationship between nurse fatigue and an increased risk of nurse error with the potential for compromising patient care and safety, it is the position of the ANA that all employers of registered nurses should ensure sufficient system resources to provide the individual registered nurse in all roles and settings with work schedules that provide for adequate rest and recuperation between scheduled shifts. In addition, sufficient compensation and appropriate staffing systems should be provided to foster a safe and healthful environment in which the registered nurse does not feel compelled to seek supplemental income through overtime, extra shifts, and other practices that contribute to worker fatigue.

Assuring Patient Safety: Registered Nurses' Responsibility in All Roles and Settings to Guard Against Working When Fatigued (http://nursingworld.org/MainMenuCategories/WorkplaceSafety/Healthy-Work-Environment/Work-Environment)—12/8/06

The ANA takes the position that, regardless of the number of hours worked, each registered nurse has an ethical responsibility to carefully consider her or his level of fatigue when deciding whether to accept any assignment extending beyond the regularly scheduled workday or -week, including a mandatory or voluntary overtime assignment.

Elimination of Manual Patient Handling to Prevent Work-Related Musculoskeletal Disorders—6/21/03, revised 3/14/08

In order to establish a safe environment of care for nurses and patients, the ANA supports actions and policies that result in the elimination of manual patient handling. Patient handling, such as lifting, repositioning, and transferring, has conventionally been performed by nurses. The performance of these tasks exposes nurses to increased risk for work-related musculoskeletal disorders. With the development of assistive equipment, such as lift and transfer devices, the risk of musculoskeletal injury can be significantly reduced. Effective use of assistive equipment and devices for patient handling creates a safe health care environment by separating the physical burden from the nurse and ensuring the safety, comfort, and dignity of the patient.

Just Culture—1/28/10

The ANA supports the Just Culture concept and its use in health care to improve patient safety. The ANA supports the collaboration of state boards of nursing, professional nursing associations, hospital associations, patient safety centers, and individual health care organizations in developing regional and statewide initiatives.

Patient Safety: Rights of Registered Nurses When Considering a Patient Assignment—3/12/09

The ANA upholds that registered nurses—based on their professional and ethical responsibilities—have the professional right to accept, reject, or object in writing to any patient assignment that puts patients, colleagues, or themselves at serious risk for harm. Registered nurses have the professional obligation to raise concerns regarding any patient assignment that puts patients or themselves at risk for harm. The professional obligations of the registered nurse to safeguard patients are grounded in

(continued)

EXHIBIT 2.2	ANA POSITION STATEMENTS SUPPORTING ADVOCACY IN THE WORKPLACE *(CONTINUED)*

Nursing's Social Policy Statement (ANA, 2010b), *Code of Ethics for Nurses With Interpretive Statements* (ANA, 2001), *Nursing: Scope and Standards of Practice* (ANA, 2010a), as well as state laws and rules and regulations governing nursing practice such as the Nurse Practice Act.

Registered Nurses' Rights and Responsibilities Related to Work Release During a Disaster (http://www.nursingworld.org/MainMenuCategories/WorkplaceSafety/ Healthy-Work-Environment/Work-Environment)—6/24/02

The ANA, which represents the 3.1 million RNs in the United States, recommends that registered nurses use the following guidelines to clarify the process of release from work for the purpose of addressing a disaster. A companion position statement titled "Work Release During a Disaster—Guidelines for Employers" offers guidance for health care employers in establishing work release policies and procedures during a disaster. The ANA strongly believes that nurses should be released as part of organized medical teams; however, individual nurses may still want to respond and should be given due consideration.

Sexual Harassment—4/2/93

ANA is deeply committed to the principles of civil rights and opposes any form of discrimination against individuals or groups of individuals based on sex, race, age, national origin, religion, disability, or sexual orientation. ANA believes that nurses and students of nursing have a right to and responsibility for a workplace free of sexual harassment. Sexual harassment has an adverse impact on the health care environment.

Work Release During a Disaster—Guidelines for Employers—6/24/02

The ANA, which represents the 3.1 million RNs in the United States, recommends that employers adopt the following work release policy to guide the process of releasing registered nurses from work for the purpose of addressing a disaster. A companion position statement titled: "'Registered Nurses' Rights and Responsibilities Related to Work Release During a Disaster" clarifies the role of the registered nurse who wishes to participate in disaster relief work. ANA strongly believes that registered nurses should be released as part of organized medical rescue teams during disasters; however, individual nurses may still want to respond and should be given due consideration.

Reprinted with permission from the American Nurses Association (n.d.).

State

While nurses may feel comfortable taking on the advocate role within their workplace or community, they may be hesitant to take it to the next level and use their advocacy skills at the state level. They may not feel confident about their presentation skills or believe that others know more about the issue than they do. However, they quickly find that their passion and health care knowledge will take them far in state advocacy. The ANA represents the

EXHIBIT 2.3 NURSE-MANAGED HEALTH CENTERS (NMHCs)

- NMHCs are community-based primary health care services, under the leadership of an advanced practice nurse. They emphasize health education, health promotion, and disease prevention, and their target population is usually the underserved. Unlike "minute clinics," which are also led by NPs, these centers are not-for-profit and usually have sliding scales for payment. A few NMHCs are federally qualified health centers.

- The National Nursing Centers Consortium is a member organization of NMHCs. Of the members, most (74%) are associated with academic nursing programs and, in addition to meeting the health care needs of under-served populations, these centers serve as training facilities for student nurses.

- There are at least 200 NMHCs currently operating in 37 states with an estimated 2 million patient encounters per year.

- About 60% of patients seen in these centers either are uninsured or have Medicaid.

- There is some evidence that if NMHCs operated at full capacity, the cost of care per visit would be less expensive than medical care in the same geographic area.

- There is some evidence that NMHCs had higher rates of generic medication fill and lower rates of hospitalizations than like providers such as community health centers.

- A major barrier to sustaining NMHCs is many managed care organizations' unwillingness to credential NPs as primary care providers, limiting the ability of these centers to get reimbursement from private insurers. In a recent study, only 53% of managed care responders (66% response rate) credentialed NPs; of these, only 56% reimburse primary care NPs at the rate as primary care physician.

Reprinted with permission from Kovner and Walani (n.d.).

interest of the 3.1 million RNs across the United States through its constituent and state nurses associations and its specialty nursing and affiliate organizations. With the implementation of the Patient Protection and Affordable Care Act (PPACA) and the ongoing state-level scope of practice issues that are barriers to advanced practice registered nurses (APRNs), there is much to be done at the state level. One important provision of the PPACA that highlights the need for effective state and national partnerships is the establishment of state insurance exchanges. These exchanges—online marketplaces where individuals are able to purchase health plans—have been established and much work has been done to set up the specifics as to how these will work for each state. The ANA works with CMS to use language that includes NPs and certified nurse midwives so as to ensure that patients have improved access to care.

Most of the barriers to APRN practice are at the state level as the result of state laws and regulations. It is vital for nurses to advocate within their state for removal of practice barriers such as requirements for physician supervision and prescriptive authority restrictions. The number one recommendation in the IOM report *The Future of Nursing* (IOM, 2011, p. 34) is "Remove scope-of-practice barriers. APRNs should be able to practice to the full extent of their education and training."

State nurses associations and state-based coalitions have been vital in moving advocacy activities and educating nurses to take on the additional responsibilities that are required at this level. State "Lobby Days" are one of the many activities that can be held to educate nurses about the important practice issues requiring focus and how they can make a difference when speaking to legislators, mayors and city council members, community activists, or the public at large. One state nurses association president reflected on her role as an advocate and leader:

Q: Over the years what has the Georgia Nurses Association (GNA) done for you?

A: [Fran Beall, GNA President 2009–2011] That is the wrong question! The question should be, "What have you done for yourself and your fellow nurses through your membership in GNA?" It always amazes me to think that any nurse would not understand that professional membership is a professional responsibility, and it is something you do for yourself and your profession. Period.

GNA has made me a better nurse! It turned me into a nurse activist early on, and my nursing career has been so much more interesting because of that! My patients have benefited from having a nurse with a clear sense of who I am and an awareness of my own responsibility and power to change things when they are not working.

On a more personal note, back in January of 1992, I experienced a ruptured AVM [arteriovenous malformation] over the right parietal lobe about 2 weeks before I was supposed to give the keynote address at the annual GNA Legislative Workshop. As the word got out, my husband Pat started receiving phone calls from GNA nurses he had never met who recommended rehab facilities and who told him to get me moved to rehab as quickly as possible after I was medically stable. You cannot imagine how comforting that was to have expert opinions during a time of great crisis.

During that period of time, I was vice chair of the GNA Cabinet on Governmental Affairs. [The chair of the Cabinet] suddenly had to back out of a scheduled meeting, necessitating that I, as vice chair, take over the meeting. So, the whole Cabinet came to the [rehab hospital], so that I could run the meeting. This became the "higher cognitive project" that my team of rehab specialists wanted me to do, in order to test my ability to eventually go back to work as an NP. Now what can you say about friends and colleagues like that? They never let me think for a minute that I would not be able to return to nursing, despite total left hemiplegia.

National

Moving advocacy to the national level typically takes nurses from their familiar practice settings to the unfamiliar world of policy and politics, a world in which many nurses do not feel prepared to effectively maneuver. Successful policy advocacy requires one to have the power, will, time, and energy, along with the political skills needed to "play the game" in the legislative arena (Abood, 2007). This move into national advocacy is challenging and time-consuming, but offers the nurse a unique opportunity to make a difference in patient care and the satisfaction of playing a role in improving the health care system.

Many nurses who are active in the national arena first honed their experiences at policy and legislative events sponsored by their state nurses association. There are also policy fellowships and workshops that can provide the needed opportunities to learn more about health care issues and the legislative process (see the e-resource section on the RWJF Policy Fellows program and the ANA's American Nurses Advocacy Institute Leadership Program). There are multiple ways to get actively involved: Write a letter or make a call to your representative in Congress, attend a state or national Lobby Day event, educate your colleagues on national aspects of health policy like the PPACA (U.S. Government Printing Office, 2010), and even run for elective office.

Many complex health policy issues require collaboration and sustained efforts to effect change. Organized nursing groups, the assistance of professional lobbyists, and sustained activity for months or even years are required when issues are as complex as health care reform or changing our models of care delivery. Nurses who participate in their state and national nurses associations have access to important resources and can strategize collaboratively to bring nursing's perspective to those legislative or regulatory decision makers. Professional nursing organizations, like the ANA, maintain as their core work the monitoring of public policy and educating their members as to the impact of policy issues. This is illustrated by the ANA's collaborative work conducted over many years in support of health care reform. When the U.S. Supreme Court was debating the constitutionality of President Obama's key legislation, PPACA, the ANA rallied its members once again for support (see Figure 2.3).

International

Advocacy on the international stage is quite daunting; fortunately, the International Council of Nurses (ICN) leads the profession in these efforts. The ICN launched a global vision for the 21st century in 1999 to "lead our societies to better health" (Benton, 2012, p. 1). The ICN, representing the interests of over 16 million nurses worldwide, works to shape health policy at the international level: publishing, disseminating, and updating position statements and educating nurses and the public at large about the issues. The ICN advocates for such policies that will contribute to the health of populations, sustainable development, and the security and just treatment of nurses and health care

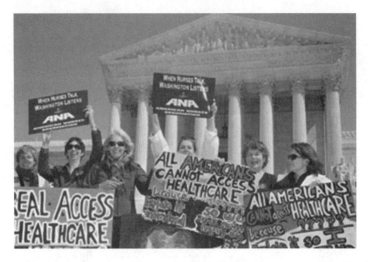

FIGURE 2.3 Nurses rally at the Supreme Court for the Patient Protection and Affordable Care Act.

professionals. As a federation of more than 130 national nurses associations, the ICN can work to affect change around the globe.

One of ICN's programs, Leadership for Change, is focused on developing strong nursing leaders to be more effective at their national level. Different leadership and advocacy approaches are needed in various countries based on their own issues, resources, and infrastructure. The ICN is responsive to taking different approaches such as working with Rwanda's national nursing association to introduce professional regulation, taking the Leadership for Change program to Papua New Guinea in an effort to increase public engagement with HIV testing, and using the visit of the ICN CEO in a public relations effort to join with the Paraguay Nursing Association to highlight the need for improved nurse staffing and nurses' greater policy influence (Benton, 2012).

Nurses across the globe are focused on the concept of advocacy as they provide care to their patients. Scandinavian nurse researchers examined how advocacy is defined by patients and nurses (Vaartio, Leino-Kilpi, Salanterä, & Suominen, 2006). Turkish nurses studied how intensive care unit nurses make decisions about distribution of scarce beds to their patients (Ersoy & Akpinar, 2010), and Iranian nurses developed their own patients' bill of rights and code of ethics while studying the extent of involvement in patient advocacy among their country's nurses (Negarandeh & Dehghan Nayeri, 2012; Salehi, Dehghan Nayeri, & Negarandeh, 2010).

WHEN ADVOCACY FAILS/WHEN ADVOCACY SUCCEEDS

One needs only to review the case example of U.S. health care reform to understand the arduous and complex nature of advocacy. From President Theodore Roosevelt's efforts toward national health insurance in the early 20th century, to the creation of Medicare and Medicaid in 1965 by President Lyndon Johnson, and finally to the 2010 passage of President Barack Obama's PPACA, the advocacy efforts of more than 100 years have brought us many improved programs but with many challenges left unresolved.

If advocacy is such an important aspect of nursing care, why do efforts sometimes fail? What are the barriers that prevent nurses from being effective advocates on behalf of their patients, themselves, or their profession? In a concept analysis on barriers to nursing advocacy, Hanks (2007) identified the most common barriers as conflict of interest between the nurse's responsibility to the patient and the nurse's duty to the employer, lack of support, lack of power, the nurse's lack of education, time constraints, threats of punishment, and the historical barrier of being a feminine profession with a tradition of subservience to the medical profession.

Institutional barriers to advocacy are challenging and often difficult to address. Nurses must know their legal scope of practice in their state and health care facility. Knowing the statutes and regulations will assist nurses in being more effective advocates. If more assistance is needed with the state nurse practice act or practice guidelines, nurses should contact their state nurses associations; however, it is important for nurses to understand that membership organizations can best support only those dues-paying members who contribute to their profession.

Clear, effective communication is central to overcoming advocacy barriers. The nurse's ideas and suggestions will be more effective when spoken clearly and without overt emotions like anger and frustration. Even body language makes a difference. Loud voices, leaning into another person's space, pointing fingers, or crossed arms will convey hostility and prevent the nurse's message from being received. Patient-centered language is the best approach when seeking to be an effective advocate. Written documentation may also prove important if the situation escalates or there are negative patient outcomes.

Understand and use the employer's chain of command. There are important organizational policies for reporting concerns and issues that arise. The employer may have an administrative structure that includes committees that support advocacy efforts (e.g., ethics committee, shared governance committee, and staffing committee).

Education has a major role to play in teaching effective advocacy. Faculty must teach the issues related to nursing advocacy as well as role model what it means to be an advocate—at the individual patient level and the political/policy level. The practicing nurse should seek a preceptor or mentor who demonstrates strong advocacy skills to assist in navigating difficult clinical issues and organizational processes. The following advocacy exemplars illustrate the range of issues, the different forms that an advocacy effort might take, and the different outcomes for the advocacy efforts.

Advocacy Exemplar: Understaffing

Labor and delivery nurse Mary Washington was tired, frustrated, and worried—her unit had been dealing with high census and low staffing for many months. The staff nurses had been complaining for a while and had met with the unit manager to voice their concerns. Mary had even presented her professional organization's staffing guidelines to nursing leadership in an effort to make the case for improved staffing. But it seemed that cost constraints were not allowing new staff to be hired and Mary knew it was just a matter of time before understaffing would cause a problem. Some signs of fetal distress might be missed and then a negative outcome would throw light on the consequences of the unit's staffing patterns. She was just a few years out of her undergraduate program so Mary consulted with one of her maternal–child health faculty members who gave her suggestions for advocacy efforts. She also consulted with her state nurses association to see if there were any regulations or other guidelines that might apply. She took all the suggestions to her unit manager, even the house supervisor, in an effort to advocate for safe patient care and protection of her own practice. Ultimately, Mary realized that she was being labeled a "troublemaker," so after discussing the situation with her colleagues she determined she had no recourse but to resign and take a position at a different hospital in the city.

Advocacy Exemplar: Removing Scope of Practice Barriers

Although Georgia was the last state to have APRN prescriptive authority in statute, the Georgia General Assembly passed legislation in 2006 that gave APRNs the authority to engage in written prescribing. A last-minute change in the bill included a push by the radiologists to limit APRNs from independently ordering certain radiological imaging tests except "in the case of an emergency." In subsequent years, APRNs in Georgia have provided data to support the removal of the radiological imaging language, demonstrating that it is unnecessary, leads to delays, and does not offer any needed patient protections. Despite efforts of the GNA, the Coalition of APRNs, many hospitals, and nurses across the state, the Medical Association of Georgia has fought the efforts and the Georgia General Assembly has yet to agree to remove this barrier to practice.

Advocacy Exemplar: The Whistle-Blowing Nurses From Winkler County, Texas

In 2009, two nurses, Anne Mitchell and Vickilyn Galle, anonymously reported Dr. Rolando Arafiles Jr. to the Texas Medical Board for unsafe care. Dr. Arafiles urged the county sheriff and county attorney to uncover who made the report and then struck back at the nurses who were charged with misuse of official information, a third-degree felony, and fired from their jobs. After their case was nationally publicized by the Texas Nurses Association and the ANA, Dr. Arafiles's attempts at retaliation against the two whistle-blower nurses were uncovered. Subsequently, Dr. Arafiles was charged with misuse of official information and retaliation, also *a third-degree felony. He was sentenced to 60 days in jail and fined $5,000. Three others involved in the case received jail sentences and lost their jobs as a result of the roles they played: Sheriff Robert Roberts Jr., Attorney Scott Tidwell, and Hospital Administrator Stan Wiley. Nurses Mitchell and Galle were completely exonerated and received a civil suit settlement of $375,000.*

ADVOCACY ORGANIZATIONS

Nurses advocate to support patient autonomy and rights; however, they are less effective when challenging problems such as inadequate staffing or patient access to care unless they collectively respond to such systemic issues. Within direct care clinical situations, individual nurses are staunch patient advocates, yet this focus of patient advocacy overlooks systemic problems that can cause harm to all patients (Mahlin, 2010). Although patient advocacy is most often framed in terms of an obligation to individual patients, it must include social and political activism in order to address the full spectrum of patient care issues. Collective activism for nurses is best accomplished through professional associations. In order for professional nurses associations to effectively advocate for their professionals, they must rely on their members to report instances of inadequate and substandard care as well as participate in the process of raising awareness.

Professional nurses organizations in the United States began two decades after formal education programs were established. The first training school for nurses in the United States opened in 1873 and, by 1893, nursing school administrators worked to form the American Society of Superintendents of Training Schools for Nurses (later becoming the National League for Nursing) in an effort to network, share best practices, and maintain a universal standard for training nurses (Matthews, 2012). When graduate nurses were seeking consistent standards in education and competency, they formed the Nurses Associated Alumnae of the United States and Canada (later renamed the ANA) in 1896 to elevate the standards of nursing education, establish a code of ethics, and promote the interests of nursing. Three documents developed by the ANA have served to form the foundation of nursing as a profession and establish the role of advocacy for the professional nurse: *The Code of Ethics for Nurses With Interpretative Statements* (2001), *Nursing: Scope and Standards of Practice* (2010a), and *Nursing's Social Policy Statement: The Essence of the Profession* (2010b).

Depending on the classification, there are approximately 100 national nurses associations in the United States. Most are specialty-focused, demonstrating the maturation, increased demands, and specialization that have occurred in nursing over the past 120 years. These organizations focus on their missions that include legislative and broad-scale advocacy, education, professional development, and support for the professional nurse and patients' rights. These organizations with differing strategic plans have identified the value of working collaboratively on a large number of issues. There are formal structures like the Nursing Organizations Alliance (www.nursing-alliance.org) and the ANA's Organizational Affiliates (nursingworld.org/FunctionalMenuCategories/AboutANA/WhoWeAre/AffiliatedOrganizations), as well as informal coalitions and groups that come together for a period of time to address a specific problem or issue. See the following Option for Policy Challenge for how an advocacy organization provides resources for nurses to address issues in their practice.

OPTION FOR POLICY CHALLENGE

Robert and his clinical nurse specialist colleague, Jane, have been gathering and appraising resources for safe patient handling in order to create change on his unit. They have discovered that the ANA (2013) had just published new guidelines titled: *Safe Patient Handling and Mobility: Interprofessional National Standards.* They review the new standards and ask to have this as an agenda item for the hospital's Nursing Practice Committee. In addition, they learned that the ANA has a comprehensive website for Safe Patient Handling and Mobility that includes tools and resources such as position statements, national resources from government agencies and other organizations, webinars, and continuing education (http://nursingworld.org/MainMenuCategories/WorkplaceSafety/Healthy-Work-Environment/SafePatient). They are pleased to learn that "Establish a Culture of Safety" is Standard 1, so they are excited to begin the advocacy journey to plan, implement, and evaluate needed changes on Robert's unit and throughout the hospital.

IMPLICATIONS FOR THE FUTURE

Advocacy at its best is about transformation. Wolf (2012) uses complexity science to understand how events, patterns, and system structures can be helpful in transforming an organization. Successful nurse advocates are able to look beyond the events of today, see patterns and trends that are occurring, and map the direction needed for tomorrow. Future orientation causes the nurse advocate to ask: What type of care will patients look for in the future? What patterns need to change to improve the care given today? What outcomes require focus now? How might our patient population be different in 5 years and in 10 years, and what must we do to prepare for that? What structures would support that difference? What policies need to change?

"The changes that are needed for patients will drive the changes that are needed for professional practice and become the source of advocacy" (Wolf, 2012, p. 309). The importance of transformational leaders to drive toward this future view of advocacy cannot be understated. The American Nurses

Credentialing Center's (ANCC) Magnet Recognition Program® recognizes organizations for quality patient care, nursing excellence, and innovations in professional nursing practice. Transformational leadership is a required element of Magnet recognition and these leaders convey a strong sense of advocacy, influence, and support on behalf of all staff and patients in a health care organization (American Nurses Credentialing Center, 2008). As nursing leaders explore the facts and observe how patterns fit together, they develop goals and objectives that will move the organization forward. They must use their influence in order to build collaboration and confidence, seeking staff input on how changes impact patient care, nurse satisfaction, and patient outcomes. When advocacy works best, all in the organization feel valued and engaged. Transformation in health care will only occur when advocacy is embraced by health care professionals and seen as an inherent part of their practice.

KEY CONCEPTS

1. The concept of advocacy is part of professional nursing.
2. Nurses readily accept the requirement of the professional nurses' advocacy role as it applies to their patients; however, advocacy activities on behalf of colleagues, the profession, or even oneself are often lacking.
3. The ANA *Code of Ethics for Nurses With Interpretive Statements* defines the expectations of advocacy in which the professional nurse is expected to be engaged.
4. A strong commitment to social justice requires professional nurses to advocate for health for all persons.
5. The American public sees the nurse in the role of advocate in that they have rated RNs as the most trusted profession for 14 of the past 15 years.
6. Nurse advocates need to have the competencies of problem solving, communication, influence, collaboration, and resource identification.
7. Advocacy works best in environments that encourage its activity, where leaders are supportive and tools are available to make it happen.
8. Moving advocacy to the state, national, and international levels typically takes nurses from their familiar practice settings to the unfamiliar world of policy and politics, a world in which many nurses do not feel prepared to effectively maneuver.
9. Common barriers to advocacy include conflict of interest between the nurse's responsibility to the patient and the nurse's duty to the employer, lack of support, lack of power, the nurse's lack of education, time constraints, threats of punishment, and the historical barrier of being a feminine profession with a tradition of subservience to the medical profession.

SUMMARY

Health care is undergoing dramatic changes and the role of the professional RN is evolving as well. The importance of nursing advocacy cannot be understated as more than 25 to 30 million uninsured in the United States will increasingly gain access to health care under the provisions of the PPACA. Nurses in direct care will continue their important role of advocating for individual patients. Collectively nurses must collaborate among themselves and other health care professionals to transform health care. Nurse managers and administrators advocate to obtain adequate resources for their staff and to promote positive work environments in which advocacy efforts can flourish. Nursing educators must prepare their students to take on the mantle of advocacy in order to strengthen the profession. Every nurse in every setting has the opportunity and responsibility to make a positive difference in the lives of their patients and the quality of their nursing care. Advocacy is the key.

LEARNING ACTIVITIES

1. Describe two specific actions you could employ to advocate for a "culture of safety"?
2. Explain how you would apply the precautionary principle to an issue in your practice or an issue that is of concern to you.
3. Describe one example of how you could infuse the *Code of Ethics for Nurses* into your daily practice.
4. Evaluate the resources available in your state for nurses who have been reported for impaired practice to the Board of Nursing in terms of addressing the nurses' needs.
5. Select an issue described in a *Code of Ethics Provision Exemplar* and describe the steps necessary to extend advocacy activities beyond a specific health care facility to the community, state, national, or international level.
6. What programs are available to assist with advocacy efforts in your workplace, or state? Identify three individuals you could consult to assist you with workplace concerns.
7. Identify a practice concern that you have experienced or read about and describe two potential solutions, one at the little "p" level and one at the big "P" level.

E-RESOURCES

- Advocacy Project. http://advocacynet.org
- Agency for Healthcare Research and Quality. http://www.ahrq.gov
- American Nurses Advocacy Institute (ANAI). http://www.capitolupdate.org/index.php/2009/12/the-first-american-nurses-advocacy-institute

- American Nurses Association. http://www.NursingWorld.org
- American Nurses Association. Code of Ethics for Nurses. http://www.nursingworld.org/codeofethics
- American Nurses Association. Policy & Advocacy. http://www.nursingworld.org/MainMenuCategories/Policy-Advocacy
- American Public Health Association. Advocacy & Policy. http://www.apha.org/advocacy/tips
- Amidei, N. (2002). *So you want to make a difference: advocacy is key.* http://www.foreffectivegov.org/node/169
- Centers for Medicare and Medicaid Services. http://www.cms.gov
- Child Health Advocacy Institute. http://www.childrensnational.org/advocacy
- Commonwealth Fund. http://www.commonwealthfund.org
- Department of Health and Human Services. http://www.dhhs.gov
- Institute for Healthcare Improvement (IHI). http://www.ihi.org
- Institute of Medicine (IOM). http://www.iom.edu
- Institute of Safe Medication Practice (ISMP). https://www.ismp.org
- International Council of Nurses (ICN). http://www.icn.ch
- Johnson & Johnson Discover Nursing/Nurse Advocate. http://www.discovernursing.com/specialty/nurse-advocate
- National Council of State Legislatures. http://www.ncsl.org
- National Patient Safety Foundation (NPSF). http://www.npsf.org
- Nurse-Family Partnership. http://www.nursefamilypartnership.org/public-policy/advocacy-resources
- Occupational Safety and Health Administration (OSHA). https://www.osha.gov
- RN Activist Tool Kit, ANA Governmental Affairs. http://www.nursingworld.org/MainMenuCategories/Policy-Advocacy
- Robert Wood Johnson Foundation (RWJF) Health Policy Fellows Program. http://www.healthpolicyfellows.org/aboutus.php
- Trust for America's Health. http://healthyamericans.org/policy
- United States House of Representatives. http://www.house.gov
- United States Senate. http://www.senate.gov

REFERENCES

Abood, S. (2007). Influencing health care in the legislative arena. *OJIN: The Online Journal of Issues in Nursing, 12*(1), Manuscript 2. Retrieved from |http://www.nursingworld.org/MainMenuCategories/ANAMarketplace/ANAPeriodicals/OJIN/TableofContents/Volume122007/No1Jan07/tpc32_216091.html

Aiken, L. H., Clarke, S. P., Sloane, D. M., Lake, E. T., & Cheney, T. (2008). Effects of hospital care environment on patient mortality and nurse outcomes. *Journal of Nursing Administration, 38*(5), 223–229.

American Association of Critical Care Nurses. (2005). *Standards for establishing and sustaining healthy work environments.* Retrieved from http://www.aacn.org/WD/HWE/Docs/HWEStandards.pdf

American Nurses Association. (2001). *Code of Ethics for nurses with interpretive statements.* Silver Spring, MD: Nursebooks.org.

American Nurses Association. (2008). *Adapting standards of care under extreme conditions: Guidance for professionals during disasters, pandemics and other extreme emergencies.* Retrieved from http://nursingworld.org/MainMenuCategories/WorkplaceSafety/Healthy-Work-Environment/DPR/TheLawEthicsofDisasterResponse/AdaptingStandardsofCare.pdf

American Nurses Association. (2010a). *Nursing: Scope and standards of practice.* (2nd ed.). Silver Spring, MD: Nursebooks.org.

American Nurses Association. (2010b). *Nursing's social policy statement: The essence of the profession* (2nd ed.). Silver Spring, MD: Nursebooks.org.

American Nurses Association. (2010c). *Who will be there? Ethics, the law and nurse's duty to respond in a disaster.* ANA Issue Brief. Retrieved from http://www.nursingworld.org/MainMenuCategories/WorkplaceSafety/DPR

American Nurses Association. (2011). *Short definitions of ethical principles and theories.* Retrieved from http://nursingworld.org/MainMenuCategories/EthicsStandards/Resources/Ethics-Definitions.pdf

American Nurses Association. (2013). *Safe patient handling and mobility: Interprofessional national standards.* Silver Spring, MD: Nursesbooks.org

American Nurses Association. (n.d.). *Workplace advocacy.* Retrieved from http://ana.nursingworld.org/MainMenuCategories/HealthcareandPolicyIssues/ANAPositionStatements/workplace.aspx

American Nurses Credentialing Center. (2008). *Magnet Recognition Program application manual.* Silver Spring, MD: Author.

Amidei, N. (2010). *So you want to make a difference: Advocacy is the key* (16th ed.). Washington, DC: OMB Watch.

Benton, D. (2012). Advocating globally to shape policy and strengthen nursing's influence. *OJIN: The Online Journal of Issues in Nursing, 17*(1), Manuscript 5. Retrieved from http://nursingworld.org/MainMenuCategories/ANAMarketplace/ANAPeriodicals/OJIN/TableofContents/Vol-17-2012/No1-Jan-2012/Advocating-Globally-to-Shape-Policy.html

Bosek, M. S. D., & Savage, T. A. (2007). *The ethical component of nursing education: Integrating ethics into clinical experiences.* Philadelphia, PA: Lippincott, Williams & Wilkins.

Braveman, P., & Gruskin, S. (2003). Defining equity in health. *Journal of Epidemiological Community Health, 57,* 254–258.

Bu, X., & Jezewski, M. A. (2007). Developing a mid-range theory of patient advocacy through concept analysis. *Journal of Advanced Nursing, 57*(1), 101–110.

Butts, J. B., & Rich, K. L. (2012). *Nursing ethics.* Sudbury, MA: Jones & Bartlett Learning.

Cook, E. T. (1913). *The life of Florence Nightingale. Vol. I. (1820–1861).* London: MacMillan and Co. Retrieved from http://www.gutenberg.org/files/40057/40057-h/40057-h.htm

Corrigan, J. M., Donaldson, M. S., Kohn, I. T., Maguire, S. K., & Pike, K. C. (2001). *Crossing the quality chasm: A new health system for the 21st century.* Washington, DC: National Academies Press.

Epstein, E.G., & Delgado, S. (2010). Understanding and addressing moral distress. *OJIN: The Online Journal of Issues in Nursing, 15*(3), Manuscript 1. http://www.nursingworld.org/MainMenuCategories/EthicsStandards/Courage-and-Distress/Understanding-Moral-Distress.html

Ersoy, N., & Akpinar, A. (2010). Turkish nurses' decision making in the distribution of intensive care beds. *Nursing Ethics, 17*(1), 87–98.

Family Care International. (2008). *Mobilising communities on young people's health and rights: An advocacy tool kit for programme managers.* Retrieved from http://www.familycareintl. org/UserFiles/File/Anglo_Toolkit_June2008.pdf

Fowler, M. D. (2008). *Guide to the Code of Ethics for Nurses: Interpretation and application.* Silver Spring, MD: Nursesbooks.org.

Gallup. (2013). *Nurses rated highest in honesty and ethical standards in 2013.* Retrieved from http://www.gallup.com/video/166502/nurses-rated-highest-honesty-ethical-standards-2013.aspx

Hanks, R. G. (2007). Barriers to nursing advocacy: A concept analysis. *Nursing Forum, 42*(4), 171–177.

Hegge, M. J. (2011). The lingering presence of the Nightingale legacy. *Nursing Science Quarterly, 24*(2), 152–162.

Hiles, A. (2010). *Culturally competent health care: A plan for employers to improve employee health and medical plan efficiency by eliminating disparities in care.* Retrieved from http://www.aon. com/attachments/culturally_competent_health_care.pdf

Institute of Medicine (IOM). (2011). *The future of nursing: Leading change advancing health.* Washington, DC: The National Academies Press.

Kovner, C., & Walani, S. (n.d.). *Nurse managed health centers (NMHCs).* Robert Wood Johnson Foundation Nursing Research Network. Retrieved from http://thefutureofnursing. org/sites/default/files/Research%20Brief-%20Nurse%20Managed%20Health%20Centers.pdf

Lachman, V. (2008). Practical use of the Nursing Code of Ethics: Part I. *MedSurg Nursing, 18*(1), 55–57.

Lachman, V. (2009). Practical use of the Nursing Code of Ethics: Part II. *MedSurg Nursing, 18*(3), 191–194.

Mahlin, M. (2010). Individual patient advocacy, collective responsibility and activism within professional nursing associations. *Nursing Ethics, 17*(2), 247–254.

Matthews, J. H. (2012). Role of professional organizations in advocating for the nursing profession. *OJIN: The Online Journal of Issues in Nursing, 17*(1). Retrieved from http:// www.nursingworld.org/MainMenuCategories/ANAMarketplace/ANAPeriodicals/ OJIN/TableofContents/Vol-17-2012/No1-Jan-2012/Professional-Organizations-and-Advocating.html

Merriam-Webster Online Dictionary. (2013). *Advocacy.* Retrieved from http://www.merriam-webster.com/dictionary/advocate

Miller, D. (1999). *Principles of social justice.* Cambridge, MA: Harvard University Press.

Negarandeh, R., & Dehghan Nayeri, N. (2012). Patient advocacy practice among Iranian nurses. *Indian Medical Ethics, 9*(3), 190–195.

Pagana, K. D. (2013). Ride to the top with a good elevator speech. *American Nurse Today, 8*(3), 14–16.

Paquin, S. O. (2011). Social justice advocacy in nursing: What is it? How do we get there? *Creative Nursing, 17*(2), 63–67.

Pavlish, C., Brown-Saltzman, K., Hersh, M., Shirk, M., & Rounkle, A. (2011). Nursing priorities, actions and regret for ethical situations in clinical practice. *Journal of Nursing Scholarship, 43*(4), 385–395.

Robert Wood Johnson Foundation. (2010). *Groundbreaking new survey finds that diverse opinion leaders say nurses should have more influence on health systems and services.* Retrieved from http://www.rwjf.org/en/about-rwjf/newsroom/newsroom-content/2010/01/groundbreaking-new-survey-finds-that-diverse-opinion-leaders-say. html

Robert Wood Johnson Foundation. (2012). *Reform in action: Equity in the context of health reform: Insights from aligning forces for quality and finding answers: Disparities research for change.* Retrieved from http://www.rwjf.org/en/research-publications/find-rwjf-research/2012/10/reform-in-action-equity-in-the-context-of-health-reform.html

Salehi, T., Dehghan Nayeri, N., & Negarandeh, R. (2010). Ethics: Patients' rights and the Code of Nursing Ethics in Iran. *OJIN: The Online Journal of Issues in Nursing, 15*(3). Retrieved from http://www.nursingworld.org/MainMenuCategories/ANAMarketplace/ANAPeriodicals/OJIN/TableofContents/Vol152010/No3-Sept-2010/Patients-Rights-and-the-Code-of-Nursing-Ethics-in-Iran.html

Science and Environmental Health Network. (2011). *Wingspread statement on precautionary principle.* Retrieved from http://www.sehn.org/precaution.html

Selanders, L., & Crane, P. (2012, January 31). The voice of Florence Nightingale on advocacy. *OJIN: The Online Journal of Issues in Nursing, 17*(1), Manuscript 1. Retrieved from http://nursingworld.org/MainMenuCategories/ANAMarketplace/ANAPeriodicals/OJIN/TableofContents/Vol-17-2012/No1-Jan-2012/Florence-Nightingale-on-Advocacy.html

Sharma, R. (1997). *An introduction to advocacy.* Retrieved from http://www.globalhealthcommunication.org/tool_docs/15/an_introduction_to_advocacy_-_training_guide_(full_document).pdf

Tomajan, K. (2012, January 31). Advocating for nurses and nursing. *OJIN: The Online Journal of Issues in Nursing, 17*(1), Manuscript 4. Retrieved from http://nursingworld.org/MainMenuCategories/ANAMarketplace/ANAPeriodicals/OJIN/TableofContents/Vol-17-2012/No1-Jan-2012/Florence-Nightingale-on-Advocacy.html

U.S. Government Printing Office. (2010). Public Law 111–148, *The Patient Protection and Affordable Care Act.* Retrieved from http://www.gpo.gov/fdsys/pkg/PLAW-111publ148/content-detail.html

Vaartio, H., & Leino-Kilpi, H. (2005). Nursing advocacy—A review of the empirical research 1990–2003. *International Journal of Nursing Studies, 42*(6), 282–292.

Vaartio, H., Leino-Kilpi, H., Salanterä, S., & Suominen, T. (2006). Nursing advocacy: How is it defined by patients and nurses, what does it involve and how is it experienced? *Scandinavian Journal of Caring Sciences, 20*(3), 282–292.

Van Dyke, K., Combes, J., & Joshi, M. (2011). *AHA health care governance survey report.* Chicago, IL: Center for Healthcare Governance.

White, P., Olsan, T. H., Bianchi, C., Glessner, T., & Mapstone, P. (2010). Legislative: Searching for health policy information on the Internet: An essential advocacy skill. *OJIN: The Online Journal of Issues in Nursing, 15*(2). Retrieved from http://www.nursingworld.org/MainMenuCategories/ANAMarketplace/ANAPeriodicals/OJIN/LetterstotheEditor/Response-to-the-Leg-Column-on-Advocacy.html

Wolf, G. (2012). Transformational leadership: The art of advocacy and influence. *Journal of Nursing Administration, 42*(6), 309–310.

THREE

Navigating the Political System

Eileen M. Sullivan-Marx

All politics is local.
—*Tip O'Neill, Jr., 55th Speaker of the U.S. House of Representatives*

OBJECTIVES

1. Compare and contrast the functions among the executive, legislative, and judicial government branches in the creation and implementation of policy.
2. Critique policy solutions obtained through regulatory and legislative processes.
3. Analyze strategies to create or influence policy during the regulatory rule-making processes.
4. Identify opportunities to provide testimony at local, state, and federal levels on policy issues.
5. Discuss how the public comment phase of policy can be used to influence its development.

In the United States, more than 200 years ago the founding fathers envisioned a country where democratic principles would govern the nation and create societal beliefs and expectations that have persisted and are lived out today. Some citizens take these principles and beliefs for granted. Whether through elected representatives or themselves, eligible citizens can participate in the identification, development, and creation of policies and laws. Basic to this participation are freedom of political expression, freedom of speech, and freedom of the press.

Historically, despite their distinctive body of knowledge, responsibilities, respect, and roles, nurses have not sufficiently acknowledged their power (Rafael, 1996). However, as described in Chapter 12, "Serving the Public Through Policy and Leadership," select nurses have exhibited exceptional records of accomplishments in policy making. They have made a difference in policy matters across legislative, regulatory, and judicial processes. These political activists have realized that clinical practice is not sufficient to meet the needs of patients. They have come to appreciate that nurses must be educated and engaged and advocate for patients through policy changes to successfully achieve quality, safe care; thus, nurses must exert their influence beyond the care of a small group of patients.

Nurses have a wide range of opportunities to be engaged with the full cycle of policy activities in a continuum of arenas, locally to internationally. Policy making, as alluded to in the previous quote by Tip O'Neil, often rests with a small group of individuals who engage in a variety of activities ranging from writing and editing language in a law or rule to more local activities like serving on a committee at work that changes practice through writing or updating new policies. Nurses are well recognized as a potent political force when they coalesce with their political power through organized campaigns to write letters, speak through nursing leadership, and represent themselves as a significant voting bloc. The sheer size of the nursing community (over 3 million U.S. nurses); the proximity of nurses in every one's life as neighbors, friends, or family; and the trust that society holds in nursing certainly are recognized by politicians who are always concerned with voters and voting communities.

In spite of these abilities and strides, nurses remain relatively invisible in the policy process. Few nurses run for elected office, hold a political appointment, work as a staff member for a legislator, or work on a candidate or issue campaign. They are more commonly employed in staff positions within government administrative agencies where they are responsible for implementing administrative policies and clarifying and informing their respective employing agency regarding health and nursing issues. But these positions are not widely known in nursing.

Thus, the opportunities for nurses to engage in the policy process that are not as widely known or visible are discussed in this chapter, including activities such as engaging in development of proposed legislation, testifying, or writing comments on federal or state regulatory rule making, serving on local boards, chairing committees, working on campaigns, and vetting local politicians for endorsement by organizations. Before details of these activities are examined, the key features of governmental processes are discussed, as understanding these processes is vital to undertaking policy opportunities. Equally important is appreciating the long view of policy; creation and implementation can take years with many different stakeholders. This chapter's Policy Challenge, APRN Practice: Forging a Sustainable Pathway, illustrates several aspects of policy making and how long the process can take. The exemplar further illustrates how professional groups set goals for policy making related to the licensure, appropriate credentials, accreditation, certification, and education. All elements are important to those seeking to teach in nursing programs, those looking to hire high-value advanced practice registered nurses (APRNs), and those interested in title protection and minimum requirements for licensure and to practice safely.

POLICY CHALLENGE: APRN Practice: Forging a Sustainable Pathway

Mary Jean Schumann, DNP, MBA, RN, CPNP, FAAN
Assistant Professor of Nursing, Interim Senior Associate Dean for Academic Affairs, George Washington University School of Nursing Washington, DC

Imagine nurse practitioner (NP) programs graduating students who are ineligible to take certification examinations and therefore unable to practice. Imagine an acute care world where the title clinical nurse specialist (CNS) is not recognized by boards of nursing (BONs). Imagine a country where psych NPs are APRNs but psych CNSs are not. Imagine a practice world in which new advanced practice specialties are not allowed to emerge or be recognized. Imagine as an NP graduate you are required to complete an additional year in a residency (probably unpaid) before being granted an APRN license. And imagine an Institute of Medicine (IOM) report on the future of nursing where no consensus model existed to explicitly state how all APRNs are educated, certified, and regulated. Without the 2008 APRN Consensus Model, our imaginings would be reality today.

For decades, APRNs worked to meet the needs of underserved, uninsured, and geographically rural Americans. Demonstrating effectiveness in providing safe reliable care, nurses sought additional education and work experiences, participated in voluntary national certifications, and acquired advanced specialty knowledge in order to become APRNs.

Equally important in APRN policy work is the work of the National Council of the State Boards of Nursing (NCSBN). In the mid-1990s, acting to fulfill its mission to protect the public's general welfare and responding to external pressures about the safety of APRNs, the NCSBN announced a plan to certify all NPs across all care populations (e.g., neonatal and geriatric) regardless of their population focus to practice upon passing one single core examination. NP certifiers and NPs joined together to successfully stop development of this examination. By 1998, certifiers and educators had put in place master's degree requirements for NP education, accreditation standards for NP educational programs, and accreditation of certifiers.

In 2002, BONs surfaced further issues, focusing on NPs prepared in specialty practice and as CNSs. NCSBN proposed recognition of only a limited number of advanced practice specialties, targeting palliative care NP programs and examinations as an example. Simultaneously, the value of CNS education was questioned, in part because of BON pressure for all NPs to have an advanced practice license in the state in which they practiced, while CNS leadership insisted that they did not need this secondary APRN license. In 2004, the Texas Board of Nurse Examiners (TBNE)

(*continued*)

declared that it would no longer recognize CNS practice and that schools of nursing in Texas might as well stop educating and preparing CNSs since they would not be able to work in this role. However, in December 2004, the American Nurses Association (ANA) and the American Association of Critical-Care Nurses (AACN), in agreement that a single BON, like TBNE, could not be allowed to set precedent by making decisions that would effectively change the shape of advanced practice for many years, jointly convened the larger nursing stakeholder community to address these issues.

See Option for Policy Challenge.

This Policy Challenge illustrates the numerous ways that regulations and laws can be developed that complement the needs of nursing practice. Further, it illustrates how complex policies often take years to evolve and develop into sustainable and agreed-upon regulations and legislation.

Often numerous stakeholders, years of work, and various political solutions are needed for effective long-term defensible solutions. The evolution and current status of the doctor of nursing practice (DNP) followed a typical policy creation course. The dramatic changes in health care and prominent reports (PEW Health Professions Commission, *Competencies for the 21st Century* [1998]; IOM, *Crossing the Quality Chasm* [2001]; and IOM, *Health Professions Education* [2003]) cited the need for a better and differently educated workforce. Identified was the need to develop advanced competencies for increasingly complex clinical, faculty, and leadership roles along with the need for enhanced knowledge to improve nursing practice and patient outcomes.

Nursing doctorate (ND) programs were introduced in 1979 as an innovative entry-level program at Case Western Reserve University in Cleveland, Ohio (Patzek, 2010). This was as the first clinical doctoral program in nursing. With the increasing need for and growth of nursing research, doctor of philosophy (PhD) and doctor of nursing science (DNS) programs continued the focus on development of researchers to create the evidence base for nursing. The changing perspectives on nursing education called for visionary leadership to guide future policy discussion and decisions and to create parity with other health professions. Stakeholders were convened and they recommended AACN create a standard set of assumptions and guidelines for the terminal practice degree programs. Over time, the clinical doctorate, the DNP, was established with core content and core competencies.

Today the DNP is the terminal graduate degree for many and, in particular, for advanced nursing practice preparation, including but not limited to the four current APRN roles: CNS, nurse anesthetist, nurse midwife, and NP.

This Policy Challenge illustrates how policy making is often an amalgamation of processes that can span a combination of policy activities. It may not be one piece of legislation, but several that are required to effect the desired policy outcome, or it may be a combination of an executive order and subsequent legislation that is needed. No one strategy fits across all health care policy making. Further, the process is often evolutionary, taking time, a commitment to the long-term policy goal, and an ongoing understanding of the policy-making process at both the little "p" and the big "P" levels.

POLICY-MAKING STRATEGIES AND JURISDICTION

Frequently, as one considers policy solutions, legislation is often seen as the most obvious one. However, as is discussed, judicial and/or regulatory options can be considered. The approach to use is often determined when the policy agenda is being set. At that time, after the problem is clearly identified, the most appropriate jurisdiction (e.g., legislative and executive) for advancing the policy agenda is set. See Chapter 6, "Setting the Agenda."

Professional associations have a vital role in each of these options. As discussed in Chapter 7, "Building Capital: Intellectual, Social, Political, and Financial," selective associations have strong roles in lobbying for legislation and, equally as important, they are also key to monitoring implementation of newly passed legislation to examine for opportunities to help craft rule-making language and options after laws are passed.

The Patient Protection and Affordable Care Act (PPACA) is an example of legislation that has been impacted by legislative, regulatory, and judicial processes. During the PPACA 8-year implementation timeline (2010–2018), a focused nursing community remained engaged to achieve the intention of the legislation. At times, monitoring the Federal Register (www.access.gpo.gov/su_docs/aces/aces140.html) resulted in a call to action for the profession to react or suggest draft language for regulation and implementation of hundreds of the provisions. For example, as agencies determine who can be eligible health care providers in new, patient-centered, team-based models of care, such as "medical homes" and "accountable care organizations," draft language was submitted urging that APRNs be specifically identified as primary care providers. At other times, the judicial processes are essential to uphold interpretation and intention of the legislation. In 2012, the ANA joined five other health care groups (nursingworld .org/FunctionalMenuCategories/MediaResources/PressReleases/2012-PR/IndividualMandate-HealthCareReform.pdf) representing millions of health care professionals in filing an amicus brief with the U.S. Supreme Court in support of the Affordable Care Act's (ACA) "minimum coverage provision." As frontline witnesses to those who are uninsured and defer needed care, nurses have a unique perspective to share and guide the Court regarding the consequences of removing or delaying the provision. While not all legislation calls for intervention in the judicial system, an engaged nursing community can make a difference in the outcome when the situation warrants this level of action, as in this case.

LEGISLATION

Like many policy issues, legislative solutions usually occur over time and with representation from many stakeholders representing a variety of special interest groups. While considered complex, the legislative process (Figure 3.1) is a series of well-documented steps in which a bill can become a law. The process is essentially the same for both state and federal legislation. However, it is very common that a bill, once introduced, never becomes law. During 2011 through 2013, in the 112th Congress, only 2% of proposed bills (284) were enacted into law (Govtrack.us, n.d.). See Exhibit 3.1 for websites that provide an up-to-date status of proposed bills.

Knowing the status and progress of proposed legislation is critical to determine the numerous opportunities for input and to influence the progression, the delay, or even the overturning of a bill. This input can occur as early as when the proposed legislation is developed and drafted to the day it is passed by both the House of Representatives and the Senate. In the following sections, several examples of these opportunities are examined.

Giving Spark to Legislation and Ongoing Support

The journey from an idea, to its introduction as a bill, to passage, and then to enactment of legislation is indeed a lengthy and circuitous process. In state legislation, nurses have most commonly been involved in the introduction, support,

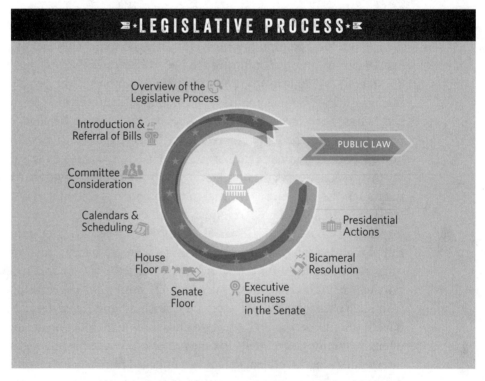

FIGURE 3.1 Legislative process.

From Congress.gov (n.d.)

EXHIBIT 3.1 SELECT LEGISLATIVE WEBSITE RESOURCES

Bill status	Congress.gov (formerly Thomas.gov) and www.govtrack.us. Updated daily. Legislative activity appears the next business day.
Member votes	The Senate (www.senate.gov), House (www.house.gov), and www.govtrack.us websites. Updated hourly.
Bill text	Congress.gov. Updated daily, but text typically only becomes available one to three business days after a bill is filed or engrossed.
Upcoming bills	The Senate and House websites. Updated daily.
Upcoming Committee meetings	The Senate and House websites. Updated daily.
State legislative information	National Conference of State Legislatures (www.ncls.org). Provides links to individual state legislature websites.

and enactment of legislation regarding regulation of scope of nursing practice and other nurse-centric issues. Increasingly though, nurses are engaged in issues of importance to the general health of the public and supporting, as an organized group, legislation regarding access to care, support for preventive health services, and other health issues such as driving safety or reducing exposure to toxins. Bringing an idea to a legislator at the state or federal level may be welcomed by the legislator and staff. They may have an interest in the issue, or the idea may spark their attention. Once a bill is identified, an early step often includes issuing of a request for a "Dear Colleague" letter. This involves the legislator who introduced the bill issuing a request for letters of support for the legislation. "Dear Colleague" letters can also be issued to obtain cosponsorship of a bill or even to oppose a bill. Nurses can be instrumental in engaging with a legislator's office to work with other legislators' offices, asking them for support and to sign off on a "Dear Colleague" letter. This step in support of a "Dear Colleague" letter can often be overlooked by nurses who are at the grassroots level, but with engagement, particularly through association works, it can be critical to move a bill from legislation to committee.

Thus, support of legislation can be immediate and relatively simple, but the support for a piece of legislation often involves ongoing work. It is necessary to keep nurses engaged over extended periods of time and over varying permutations of legislation. It involves strategizing. Policy on the Scene 3.1 demonstrates how nurse-managed care legislation has evolved and how data on effectiveness were used to support this legislation.

POLICY ON THE SCENE 3.1: Nurse-Managed Centers: Going Beyond Letter Writing

During the enactment of PPACA, many nurses supported the inclusion of nurse-managed centers as a safety net provider in this Act. As in most situations, usually an organization or several organizations collaborating together will work with legislators to draft legislation or suggest revisions to existing bills. In this situation, the National Nursing Center Consortium (NNCC) provided leadership and promoted the inclusion of nurse-managed centers in several pieces of legislation prior to the introduction of the ACA. Nurses and supporters of the PPACA revision language visited and contacted federal legislators and their staff by e-mails, letters, and phone calls. The NNCC website promoted ways that nurses could get involved and support strategies for nurse-managed centers as safety net providers (capwiz.com/healthaction/home).

Throughout the process of the PPACA, the NNCC and others suggested language that fit their intention to bring nurse-managed centers to the forefront as a distinct provider among community health centers that are part of funded centers in the U.S. Department of Health and Human Services. Nurse-managed centers are "safety net providers" that deliver care by nurses who focus on wellness, patients, families, and non-traditional community-based services. To move away from predominantly grant funding to support services provided at nurse-managed centers, nurses and NPs in nurse-managed centers were gradually able to directly bill insurance, Medicaid, and Medicare but not fully enough to cover all services. In addition, since many nurse-managed centers are associated with universities and schools of nursing, they are not eligible for federally qualified health center (FQHC) funding. Therefore, creating language in legislation to support nurse-managed health centers separately from community health centers and FQHCs was critical for their continuation.

Essential to successful inclusion of this provision was accumulated outcome data. Ten years or so prior to the PPACA, NNCC and nurse-managed centers' databases demonstrated clinical and financial outcomes, showing that nurse-managed centers made important differences in health and cost for those individuals and families who might otherwise not receive health care (Pohl, Tanner, Pilon, & Benkert, 2011). Consolidating messages about nurse-managed centers and the data enabled a clear, concise message to policy makers and legislators. The NNCC website highlights these messages (www.nncc.us/site/index.php/about-nurse-managed-care). These efforts led to the successful inclusion of funding to support nurse-managed centers in the PPACA. In March 2013, following the enactment of PPACA, testimony before the House Ways and Means Committee for appropriation of funding for nurse-managed centers continues (www.nncc.us/site/images/pdf/testimonyhouselhhs_2013.pdf).

The strategy to have nurses working in nurse-managed centers work directly with the NNCC to provide the language was critical. They were able to describe and speak to legislators about the meaning of their work in nurse-managed centers compared with other community health centers. Nurses' voices were much stronger writing about their work and outcomes than had they only written letters in support of funding. The authenticity of these nurses who spoke about their centers and the communities made a difference in legislative support.

Paying Attention to Reenactment Laws

Laws may be written in such a way that they are funded for limited periods of time and then must come back to a legislative body for reenactment. Anticipating laws that are due for reenactment legislation and expressing opinion early on why a particular program or piece of legislation remains important or how it can be updated and renewed for current health issues are very important.

The well-known Ryan White HIV/AIDS Program (kff.org/hivaids/factsheet/the-ryan-white-program and hab.hrsa.gov/abouthab/aboutprogram.html) was slated for reauthorization in September 2013 and is pending action. It has been amended and reauthorized four times: in 1996, 2000, 2006, and 2009. Each reauthorization was adjusted to accommodate new and emerging needs. The program fills the gaps in care for those with the HIV disease who do not have sufficient health care coverage and financial resources. For 20 years, nurses have been engaged in services provided in Ryan White programs for those with HIV/AIDS, their families, and their communities. In January 2014, many aspects of the PPACA took hold and addressed some issues covered by the Ryan White HIV/AIDS Program. However, nurses are in a good position to speak authoritatively on the benefits of reauthorization and the breadth of services still needed for those with HIV/AIDS, regardless of the PPACA provisions.

One example of vigilance that is important to understand is in states with "sunset" clauses in their legislation and regulations for governmental agencies and boards. These clauses require intermittent review as they require periodic legislative action to reauthorize or extend the law. Agencies, like BONs in some states, are susceptible to these regulations and may possibly change or be eliminated if action is not taken. Some states have witnessed their BON come precipitously close to being dissolved and eliminated. Without renewed legislation, these BONs would not exist or have authority to regulate nursing. The unintended consequence is that anyone would be allowed to practice

EXHIBIT 3.2 LEGISLATIVE STEPS IN WHICH NURSES HAVE INFLUENCE

- Electing legislators who share common views and values
- Drafting legislation language
- Participating in congressional committees' hearings
- Informing congressional offices before voting on legislation
- Informing the White House before the president signs or vetos passed legislation
- Providing comments to agency-proposed regulations
- Alerting and informing stakeholders about common legislative issues

nursing, that newly graduated nurses would not be able to obtain licensure and/or employment, and that no one would investigate nurse practice violations. Typically, it is nurses (through state nurses associations) who monitor these activities to ensure any sunset legislation is managed through review and reauthorization to protect the practice of nursing within their states. Most laws and BONs do not have sunset clauses and therefore remain in force indefinitely. However, it is the responsibility of nurses to be aware of such legislation and to make sure that such processes go smoothly. Another example is the funding for nursing education, which needs annual reauthorization (see Chapter 7). Exhibit 3.2 summarizes key legislative steps in which nurses have been successful in influencing.

In most incidents, addressing these steps requires involvement and support through organizations and professional associations in order to be successful.

Educating Through Testimony: Public Hearings

Legislation, once it is introduced, often calls for public hearings held by congressional committees. Public hearings are not only held on a variety of topics for legislation but are also routinely held by congressional committees, appointed commissions, and federal or state agencies seeking information (Figure 3.2).

Hearings as a part of a formal process provide a distinct opportunity to provide detailed reports and answer questions. Hearings are often a major step toward enactment of legislation and symbolize its importance. Legislative committees use this method to assemble information and solicit opinions from officials of the executive branch, other members of Congress, representatives of interest groups, experts, and concerned citizens. Hearings usually include written testimony that can be submitted alone or with an oral presentation and questioning by members of Congress. Presenters usually represent organizations, but individuals can provide both written and oral testimony (see www .rnaction.org/site/PageNavigator/nstat_congressional_testimony.html for selective testimony presented by ANA or see the Law Library of Congress for a collaborative collection of the Library's entire collection of printed hearings at www .loc.gov/law/find/hearings.php).

Processes for hearings are typically well established with common expectations. Exhibit 3.3 lists commonsense approaches to preparing for and presenting at hearings.

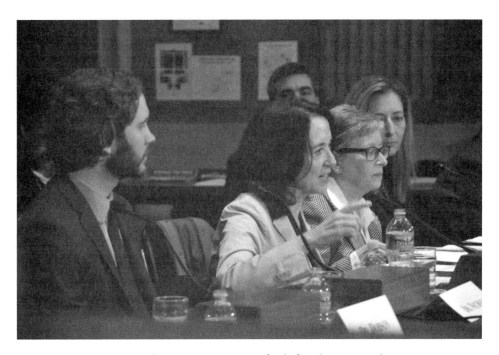

FIGURE 3.2 Dr. Margaret Flinter, ARPN, c-FNP, testifies before the Senate Subcommittee on Primary Care and Aging on the importance of nurse practitioners as primary care providers in the nation's community health centers.

The chair of the committee or host of the hearing selects the number and timing of oral presenters. Nurses can participate several important ways in the testimony process: they can (a) provide contextual information on the topic, (b) provide examples that emphasize the critical nature of the topic, or (c) give oral testimony, including answering questions at the hearing. Individual nurse clinicians and researchers who present as members of their organization who have close working knowledge of the topic are often able to bring a sense of proportion and reality to the discussion. Exhibit 3.4 lists a number of congressional committees that more often play a role in issues that impact nursing and health care and often conduct hearings.

EXHIBIT 3.3 DO's OF PROVIDING TESTIMONY

- Review hearing guidelines ahead of time and be compliant
- Talk ahead of time with the staff member assigned to the hearing chairperson
- Dress well—professional business attire
- Come early, be on time, and be prepared to spend the entire day
- Rehearse your spoken testimony before the hearing. Keep it under time limits
- Address legislators politely and answer questions if asked. Say "thank-you" for the opportunity to speak
- Be courteous and respectful of the legislators, regardless of their opinion, as well as respectful and courteous to all who testify
- "PASS" when called to speak if you are uncomfortable or answer simply "representative/senator, I will have to look into your question and get back to you"
- Realize there will be elected and/or appointed officials coming in and out during the hearing

Committees are the heart of the legislative process where the nuts and bolts of work are done. Committees have enormous power. They are important for review not only for their importance to health care but also because it is important to identify if representatives from your district serve on these committees. As a constituent and as a nurse, you may have a role to advocate to your representative as laws are drafted, debated, and voted upon that impact nursing or your patients.

Because nurses are a trusted body by the public and also represent a large number of potential voters, they are valued participants during hearings. It is

EXHIBIT 3.4 KEY CONGRESSIONAL COMMITTEES FOR NURSES AND HEALTH CARE ISSUES

SENATE	HOUSE OF REPRESENTATIVES
Appropriations Committee The committee that controls the federal purse strings and determines federal funding for all government functions, from defense to biomedical research	**Appropriations Committee** The committee that controls the federal purse strings and determines federal funding for all government functions, from defense to biomedical research
Labor, Health, and Human Services (LHHS)-Education Appropriations Subcommittee The specialized subcommittee that determines federal funding for federal agencies, including the Health and Human Services (HHS), National Institutes of Health (NIH), Centers for Disease Control and Prevention (CDC), and Health Resources and Services Administration (HRSA), which administers the nursing workforce development programs	**LHHS-Education Appropriations Subcommittee** The specialized subcommittee that determines federal funding for federal agencies, including the HHS, NIH, CDC, and HRSA, which administers the nursing workforce development programs
Health, Education, Labor, and Pensions The authorizing committee with jurisdiction over all non-Medicare and non-Medicaid health care policy issues	**Energy and Commerce Committee and Its Health Subcommittee** The authorizing committee with policy jurisdiction over the Medicaid program, Part B of the Medicare program, and all non-Medicare/Medicaid health care issues
Finance Committee and Its Health Care Subcommittee The authorizing committee with policy jurisdiction over Medicare and Medicaid	**Ways and Means Committee and Its Health Subcommittee** The authorizing committee with policy jurisdiction over the Medicare program (shares jurisdiction over certain parts of Medicare with the House Energy & Commerce Committee)

(continued)

| EXHIBIT 3.4 | KEY CONGRESSIONAL COMMITTEES FOR NURSES AND HEALTH CARE ISSUES (*CONTINUED*) |

SENATE	HOUSE OF REPRESENTATIVES
Committee on Veterans Affairs Provides oversight of U. S. veterans' issues	**Veterans Affairs Committee** The committee has oversight responsibility; it also monitors and evaluates the operations of the VA
Special Committee on Aging Serves as a focal point for discussion and debate on matters relating to older Americans; reviews Medicare's performance, pension coverage, and employment opportunities for older Americans	

Adapted from American Nurses Association (n.d.).

critical that their presentation be accurate and consistent with other nurses when appropriate. Working and coordinating with nursing associations that you hold membership in is a benefit. The association can help support individuals participating in hearing by providing collaboration and background information that can further enhance talking points. This additional help with preparation for testimony and the presence of a representative of the association at the hearing to supplement responses can help bring confidence and assurance to nurses presenting.

Numerous federal and state agencies appreciate the working relationship with professional nursing associations and special topics of interest that are part of the agencies' core missions. Some agencies that nurses can contribute to might include the Environmental Protection Agency on lead exposure among children, U.S. Department of Agriculture on food safety and healthy eating, and the Federal Housing Agency's affordable housing, which align with nursing's core concerns. Examples of other relevant shared concerns would include the U.S. Department of Health and Human Services Administration for Community Living's focus on disability and aging home care and the U.S. Department of Defense emphasis on brain injuries, post-traumatic stress disorder, and family health. Nurses in practice, research, and education can provide data and context for these agencies as they prepare testimony to give at congressional hearings or in public statements. Exhibit 3.5 lists a number of congressional committees and governmental agencies that more often play a role in issues that impact nursing and health care and often conduct hearings.

Attending public hearings as a visitor or an observer at local, state, and federal levels can be strategic as well. Those who attend demonstrate interest to the host and often are acknowledged by the host committee to thank all those attending. Moreover, attending hearings provides an excellent opportunity to network with staff and other interested stakeholders. Exchanging contact information, discussing an issue, or commenting on presentations can lead to future opportunities. Building relationships is an invaluable task in policy making, and sharing an interest or assisting someone in his or her job will be greatly appreciated and lead to future contact on other issues of mutual interest that could lead to further opportunities. Federal hearing schedules are published in advance and can be viewed in the Federal Register. Tracking hearing schedules requires regular review of the Federal Register (www.federalregister.gov), committees and agencies' websites, or local publications for schedule announcements. Typically, state governments also have established mechanisms to review hearing schedules and can be acquired by contacting your state legislator for assistance. State nurses associations often publish state hearing schedules and identify individuals to deliver comments. Some associations have created databases of experts to provide critical presentations.

REGULATIONS

After a bill is passed and signed into law, it is sent to the agency responsible for proposing rules and regulations to implement the law. This phase at the federal or state level is a great opportunity to influence policy. Each rule in the regulation has the potential to be an effective, powerful policy. At the federal level, the executive branch is responsible for developing final regulations. Relevant federal agencies are responsible for this process of creating rules. As part of this rule making, they publish the proposed rules in the Federal Register for public comment. The public has an important role in the comment phase of the process as these remarks and notes help finalize the regulations and rules that make the law have impact. Resources have been created to encourage public comments; one such resource is found at the Department of Health and Human Services' (DHHS) HHS Regulations Tool Kit (www.hhs.gov/regulations/rulemaking-tool-kit.pdf).

Prior to the publication of proposed rules, however, interested parties can recommend language and meet with agency staff responsible for rule making to express points of view. Hence, even if nurses did not fully support a newly formed law, they can work to influence the rules on that law to address specific issues or mitigate action that may be a detriment to nursing's position. This process is painstaking yet the impact is great. Simple phrasing can emphasize or deemphasize points. Terminology is critical; for example, the term mid-level provider, an erroneously misleading term referring to NPs and physician assistants, is often used informally by those who adhere to hierarchical principles when viewing health care professionals. Yet the term mid-level provider does not exist in any regulation or rule in the federal registry because nursing and physician assistant organizations have

EXHIBIT 3.5 KEY GOVERNMENTAL AGENCIES

Agency for Healthcare Research and Quality (AHRQ)	Sponsors and conducts research that provides evidence-based information on health care outcomes; quality; and cost, use, and access. The information helps health care decision makers—patients and clinicians, health system leaders, purchasers, and policy makers—make more informed decisions and improve the quality of health care services.
Centers for Disease Control and Prevention (CDC)	Is the lead federal agency for protecting the health and safety of people—at home and abroad—providing credible information to enhance health decisions, as well as promoting health through strong partnerships. The CDC serves as the national focus for developing and applying disease prevention and control, environmental health, and health promotion and education activities designed to improve the health of the people of the United States.
Centers for Medicare and Medicaid Services (CMS)	HHS agency responsible for administering the Medicare program and parts of the Medicaid program. CMS has historically maintained specifications for various certifications and authorizations used by the Medicare and Medicaid programs. Responsible for oversight of HIPAA administrative simplification transaction and code sets, health identifiers, and security standards.
Department of Health and Human Services (HHS)	Principal agency for protecting the health of all Americans and providing essential human services through more than 300 programs that are administered by 11 HHS operating divisions, including eight agencies in the U.S. Public Health Service and three human services agencies.
Department of Justice (DOJ) Antitrust Division	Promotes and protects the competitive process—and the American economy—through the enforcement of the antitrust laws. The antitrust laws apply to virtually all industries and to every level of business, including manufacturing, transportation, distribution, and marketing. It prohibits a variety of practices that restrain trade, such as price-fixing conspiracies and corporate mergers—likely to reduce the competitive vigor of particular markets—as well as predatory acts designed to achieve or maintain monopoly power.
Department of Labor (DOL)	Charged with issues relating to workplace safety and health, pensions and benefit plans, employment, and other issues related to the American workplace.

(continued)

EXHIBIT 3.5   KEY GOVERNMENTAL AGENCIES (CONTINUED)

Department of Veterans Affairs (VA)	Responsible for providing veterans benefits and services and operating the nation's largest integrated health care system.
Drug Enforcement Agency (DEA)	Enforces the controlled substances laws and regulations of the United States.
Food and Drug Administration (FDA)	Ensures that foods are safe, wholesome, and sanitary; human and veterinary drugs, biological products, and medical devices are safe and effective; cosmetics are safe; and electronic products that emit radiation are safe.
Health Resources and Services Administration (HRSA)	Improves and expands access to quality health care for all by eliminating barriers to care, eliminating health disparities, ensuring quality of care, and improving public health and health care systems.
National Institute for Occupational Safety and Health (NIOSH)	Conducts research and makes recommendations for the prevention of work-related disease and injury. The institute is part of the CDC.
National Institute of Nursing Research (NINR)	Supports clinical and basic research to establish a scientific basis for the care of individuals across the life span, from management of patients during illness and recovery to the reduction of risks for disease and disability, the promotion of healthy lifestyles, promoting quality of life in those with chronic illness, and care for individuals at the end of life.
Occupational Safety and Health Administration (OSHA)	Establishes protective standards, enforces those standards, and reaches out to employers and employees through technical assistance and consultation programs.
Substance Abuse and Mental Health Administration (SAMHSA)	Charged with improving the quality and availability of prevention, treatment, and rehabilitative services in order to reduce illness, death, disability, and cost to society resulting from substance abuse and mental illnesses.
Bureau of Citizenship and Immigration Services (BCIS)	Responsible for the administration of immigration and naturalization adjudication functions and establishing immigration services policies and priorities. BCIS is an agency of the Department of Homeland Security.

Adapted from American Nurses Association (n.d.).

ensured that the correct professional terminology (health care provider) is used in statute and regulations. Reminding administrators and insurance companies of correct terminology is important in enforcing regulations at the organizational level.

Another important area for having input on rules is through state BONs. Similar to federal agencies, state BONs publish all proposed rule changes in various public sources. For example, in Texas, the *Texas Register* is a weekly publication that serves as the notice bulletin of state agency rule making. The Texas Register contains emergency, proposed, and adopted rules; notices of withdrawn and repealed rules; notices of rule review; and other information submitted by state agencies for publication. Often dates and agenda for the Board's regular meeting are published on its website along with meeting minutes. It is essential that BON hearings are monitored by individual nurses and by state nurses and specialty nurse associations.

Of course, the Centers for Medicare and Medicaid Services (CMS) is perhaps the most influential administrative agency in health care. Regulations on payment, procedures for programs, and approval of services for Medicare beneficiaries are first proposed and published in the Federal Register. Proposed rules and proposed rule making present an opportunity for comment by the public, including individuals and organizations. The CMS and federal agencies that proposed the rules must respond to comments from the public and publish the comments. The period between proposed rule making and final rule is limited and may require the technical assistance of policy experts for a cogent and significant response from nurses or nursing organizations; nonetheless, the relevance of a rule to nursing practice and the impact on the nursing profession are regarded as critical by the federal agency, which must respond to the comments. This time period between proposed rule making and final comments is also a time to contact agencies and agency staff regarding positions in addition to submitting public comment.

No matter whether your comments are for federal or state review, Exhibit 3.6 illustrates the key components of writing a public comment. It outlines the goal, objective, scope, and product for a position paper along with a suggested strategy for writing a public comment.

EXECUTIVE OPPORTUNITIES

The executive branches of federal and state governments are responsible for implementation of laws and, consequently, oversee the agencies that are responsible for programs and services supported by legislation. Vast opportunities exist for nurses to influence the implementation of services and programs. All agencies need to hear from those with real information or expertise, presentation of research, or how it affects patients or their local areas.

Executive Branch Policy Influence Through Executive Orders

Under the power granted in the U.S. Constitution, the president can issue executive orders to officials and federal agencies. Executive orders have the full authority under the law and are made in pursuance of certain congressional actions that explicitly delegate discretionary power to the agency and the president. Executive orders can have significant influence over internal government operations and focus of federal agencies. In essence, as an option, the president can issue executive orders that create policy where and when legislation fails or does not exist.

Executive orders have been issued by every president since George Washington. Some presidents have been accused of abusing executive orders and using them to make laws without congressional approval or impacting existing laws from their original mandates. Similar to legislation and regulations promulgated, executive orders are subject to judicial review, and may be struck down if deemed by the courts to be unsupported by statute or the Constitution (U.S. courts have overturned only two executive orders). President Franklin D. Roosevelt had over 3,500 executive orders, while recent presidents had fewer than 400 each. The entire listing of executive orders can be viewed online at the American Presidency Project (americanpresidency.org).

Executive Branch Policy Influence by Federal Agency Appointment Selection

In any given presidential term, several thousand individuals are appointed. A publication known as the *United States Government Policy and Supporting Positions* (available from the Government Printing Office) and more commonly referred to as the Plum Book lists over 7,000 federal civil service support and leadership positions in the legislative and executive branches of the federal government that may be subject to noncompetitive appointment. Such positions include justices in federal courts, presidential cabinet, members of boards, heads of agencies and their immediate subordinates, policy executives and advisors, and aides who report to these officials. As described in Chapter 7 and Chapter 11, "Applying a Nursing Lens to Shape Policy." The ANA and other nursing organizations have the opportunity to make recommendations for appointments to key policy positions in governmental agencies. As evident with recent presidents, nursing efforts were successful in lobbying for appointments. President Clinton appointed nurses to key senior leadership positions. Beverly Malone, PhD, RN, FAAN, was appointed to serve as a deputy assistant secretary for health within the DHHS, while Virginia Trotter Betts, MSN, JD, RN, FAAN, was appointed a member of President Clinton's Health Care Reform Task Force, and senior advisor on Nursing and Policy to the secretary and assistant secretary in the DHHS. President Obama appointed Mary Wakefield, PhD, RN, FAAN, as administrator of the Health Resources and Services Administration (HRSA), and Marilyn Tavenner, MHA, RN, as administrator of the CMS. These individuals and other nurses who have been selected in presidential or governor appointment processes are in ideal positions to influence health policy.

EXHIBIT 3.6   HOW TO WRITE A PUBLIC COMMENT

Goal

Share knowledge of actual or proposed procedures to implement new law or regulations, and either state your support, and why, or offer draft alternatives; explain which alternative you desire, and state why.

Scope

Limit comments to the specific proposed administrative action

Format

- Keep it short and to the point; offer further information if requested
- Format your comments with a beginning, middle, and end
- Be respectful and format comments as a letter
- Avoid negative language or attacking as you will diminish your credibility and undermine your message

Do

- Share comments on your knowledge and authority to respond
- If you have a personal story, share it; refer to your personal skills and experience with phrases like, "As a nurse in the emergency room ..."
- Hit the key points
- Offer alternative you want and what you're against
- Be realistic
- Provide your full contact info, but at the minimum provide your city and state as this will be tallied

Don't

- Spend a lot of time thanking for the opportunity to comment
- Directly copy and paste bullets and paragraphs from action alerts
- Get distracted and miss deadlines for submission

When you are finished

- Send it in a timely manner
- Share your public comments with appropriate nursing associations and copy friends and colleagues to show them how easy it is to comment

JUDICIAL OPTIONS

The third governmental branch is the judicial system; it is less well known and less involved in the nursing profession policy efforts. Historically, the ANA has participated in U.S. Supreme Court proceedings with cases of broad implications and interest to the profession. Typically, these cases have dealt with nurses' rights, workplace issues, and human right issues involving individual patient rights and access to health care.

At the federal judicial level, the Supreme Court is well known for its powers that include interpreting the Constitution and reviewing laws. Unlike the criminal court system, the Supreme Court usually does not hold trials but rather interprets the meaning of a law, decides whether a law is relevant to a particular set of facts, determines how a law should be applied, and, most importantly, determines whether a law or regulation is permitted under the Constitution or is unconstitutional. The Supreme Court may hear an appeal from lower courts on any question of law, provided it has jurisdiction. Once a decision is made, the lower courts are obligated to follow the precedent set by the Supreme Court when rendering decisions.

The justices on the Supreme Court are appointed by the president of the United States and confirmed by the U.S. Senate. Justices in lower courts can be appointed or elected depending on the jurisdiction and purpose of the court. Unlike the legislative and executive branches, one's ability to influence judicial decisions is greatly limited. The only opportunity to influence judicial decisions is prior to justices being elected or appointed. Supporting and electing candidates running for judicial positions or judicial nominees is an acceptable mechanism to have potential justices that represent and align with your values and views. Lobbying justices or members of juries is considered inappropriate and would not be tolerated outside the legal proceedings.

It is critical that advantageous information to the situation be presented in testimony or legal briefs from the involved parties, as well as from *amici curiae*, or "friends of the court." Amici curiae are most often advocacy groups such as professional associations and unions that will file a brief known as an amicus brief to advocate for or against a particular legal change or interpretation. Amicus briefs can introduce concerns or support about the broader implications and effects in the court rulings. Whether to admit the information is at the discretion of the court.

In prominent cases, amicus briefs are generally provided by organizations with available content expertise, legal, and financial resources to produce strong documents that present convincing information and argument to support their position. Over the years, the ANA has filed several amicus briefs either as a single association or with others on common causes. For example, the ANA, along with a diverse group of health care providers (American Academy of Pediatrics; American Medical Student Association; Doctors for America; National Hispanic Medical Association; and the National Physicians Alliance), banded together in support of a provision in the ACA as it was being implemented.

While the judicial branch plays a significant role in making policy through the interpretation of laws and rules, they do not make the laws nor do they have the power to enforce laws and rules. It is essential that legislation and rules that are clear, appropriate, constitutional, and "respecting rights be written up front to avoid long, lengthy legal challenges. An example is the situation in California,

American Nurses Association v. Torlakson, which is further described along with other legal strategies in Chapter 6. A controversial ruling allowed unlicensed personnel to administer insulin in the school system. Years later, the policy matter has not resolved and complexity of interests of various stakeholders remains engaged to find a better solution.

INFLUENCE OF YOUR VOICE AND YOUR VOTE

Exercising your rights to express your opinion and to vote are some of the most influential actions a nurse can perform. As will be discussed throughout the book, nurses have earned the respect of many and are in a position to influence others with their thoughtful comments. For example, working on political campaigns and educating candidates about issues can be invaluable in the long run. If elected, the candidate, now legislator, will remember your support during the campaign but more importantly will be potentially influenced about issues discussed. Other activities related to navigating campaigns can be found in Chapter 7.

OPTION FOR POLICY CHALLENGE: APRN Practice:
Forging a Sustainable Pathway
Mary Jean Schumann

In 2004, probably no one predicted that the Robert Wood Johnson Foundation would shortly fund the IOM to complete its study on the future of nursing. Without the 2008 APRN Consensus Model, endorsed by over 40 national nursing organizations, and its accompanying Model Rules, unanimously approved by every state BON, the 2010 report might have had far different consequences. With the profession demonstrating complete agreement regarding its system of licensure, accreditation, credentialing, and education (LACE) of APRNs, the task force was able to focus on other more appropriate areas of debate. The findings of the IOM Task Force and *The Future of Nursing* report have heavily contributed to APRNs' importance in the ACA, breakthroughs in the recognition of nurse-led health care homes, and further funding for APRN education.

There is much that one could say about the 4 years of conflict over thorny issues by APRN stakeholders, consensus-building efforts, national stakeholder meetings, and futuristic brainstorming that occurred from 2004 to 2008. Three factors were critical to success. First, when the APRN Consensus Work Group and the stakeholder community gained a view of the whole professional landscape, it was clear that BONs, educators, accreditors, certifiers, professional associations, and those in practice had the same goal—to ensure safe competent care. With that, all things were possible. Second, when stakeholders agreed to put aside the past, focus

(continued)

on the future, and acknowledge that what was done was done, the work moved forward rapidly. Discussions became less guarded in the belief that ethically, for the sake of the greater good, everything was fair game for change.

Ethical considerations led to the third factor, embracing of a philosophy that all stakeholder groups, in order to achieve the goal, would likely have to relinquish something they personally held dear. Sacrosanct had been provisions such as single licensure, narrow specialization without broad population expertise, abbreviated knowledge in advanced pharmacology, control over specialization, direct care versus population-focused care, and definitions of APRN practice versus advanced nursing practice. Those dearly held beliefs required all members of the consensus group to challenge their own constituencies' leaders repeatedly to analyze why the element was so important. Key discussions focused on whether the belief was critical for practice and safety reasons, for historical reasons, or for financial reasons. Stakeholder representatives reported back to the consensus group not only regarding new-found clarity on the endearing quality, but whether the entity's leadership was willing to acknowledge that its importance was second to the greater good.

The ongoing implementation of the consensus model through LACE continues. Stakeholder representatives change, some rationale for why certain decisions were made may be difficult to recall, but higher level views of what was needed to achieve the agreed-upon goal remain.

IMPLICATIONS FOR THE FUTURE

The current environment for health care and the implementation of the PPACA will provide nurses with opportunities to address issues related to health as well as regulatory issues that impact the delivery of nursing care. Modifications to health care reform legislation, adjustments, or "cleanups" will enable nurses to move forward with legislative and regulatory proposals that promote full practice authority for APRNs. No legislation is perfect, nor are all the provisions that nurses and health care professionals deem to be essential usually included in a single piece of legislation or set of regulations. Therefore, nurses will need to be proactive to introduce new legislation or be at the table during the process of writing and revising regulations. However, as nurses and APRNs are increasingly employed by large health care organizations, this may result in changing legislative political interests and policy positions. As health care organizations increase in size through acquisitions and mergers, they will play an increasingly important role in attempting to influence the development of health care policy.

Nurses will have the opportunity to be involved in policy and political action as debates about specific issues come to the forefront of the public's attention in the legislative and regulatory arena. These may include providing health care services to the swelling ranks of veterans and aging veterans, the use of telehealth services, the expansion of Medicaid under the PPACA, and an aging population using Medicare. Advances in telehealth might provide the opportunity to remove practice barriers for APRNs. While the goal will be to expand access to health care for all, and ensure the safety of the public, financial pressures will be a part of these debates. Greater consumer transparency will increasingly drive the disclosure of costs and medical errors while calling for additional public reporting.

Legislative polarization at the national level will of necessity drive legislative initiatives to the state level. This will create additional opportunities for savvy nurses to develop close relationships with their legislators in order to advance specific initiatives. Increasingly, consumer groups may take a judicial approach to advance policy, and these approaches may have an impact on health or how nursing is practiced. Consequently, nurses will need to partner with consumer groups and also be aware of specific claims in order to provide their expertise in support or opposing a particular issue.

KEY CONCEPTS

1. There are numerous opportunities for nurses to be involved across a variety of policy strategies.
2. Passing legislation has many steps in which the nurses' voice should and can be heard.
3. All types of legislation should be monitored, but in particular any reauthorization can be an opportunity to improve existing legislation and implementation.
4. Rule making is a critical step after legislation has been passed and is an opportunity to influence the legislation implementation.
5. While not often recognized, action through judicial processes has been utilized by nurses' associations.
6. Judge elections and appointments are crucial since the normal lobbying activities in the judicial processes would be considered inappropriate.
7. Executive orders and appointments can be effective mechanisms to create policies when legislation is not an option or likely to occur.

SUMMARY

The range of contributions and impact that nurses can have in policy areas is limitless. Nurses have unique perspectives on the health care of individuals, families, and communities that are characterized by advocacy, trust, action, accountability, and authenticity. To fully actualize the voice of nurses, engagement with stakeholders and policy activity requires individual and organized action. Broadening policy action for nurses beyond letter writing to include key strategies such as testimony at public hearings, legislative engagement with staff writing language for bills, and public comment on proposed technical rules following enactment of laws will amplify the nursing voice as an advocate for all.

LEARNING ACTIVITIES

1. Identify your local government leaders (e.g., mayor, councils, or boards) and your legislative representatives at the state and federal governments. For three of these representatives, identify at least one stance they have taken on a health care issue.
2. Identify one nursing issue that has been adjudicated in the state and the federal court system. Discuss highlights of the decision and how it has impacted nursing. Are there ongoing efforts to appeal these decisions?
3. Locate testimony provided at the federal, state, or local level on an issue that is important to nurses or health in general. Critique the testimony. Identify what should be included to influence the opinions of the group holding the hearing.
4. Determine whether your state has received Tobacco Settlement Funds, who decides how these funds are spent, and whether there are future opportunities to influence the process to promote the health of your state's citizens.
5. Locate proposed rules and regulations pertaining to a nursing or health issue. Identify the appropriate mechanism for providing comments. Critique the proposed rules and regulations for their support of nursing and/or how an important health care issue is addressed.
6. Plan strategies to successfully gain support for a policy proposal at a mock city council meeting.
7. Prepare a 3-minute testimony that will be presented at a BON hearing in regard to proposed nursing regulations that require an NCLEX-type of examination every 5 years for license renewal.
8. A great follow-up to this section would be discussion of how to make an impact at a town hall meeting or school board meeting. This would provide the opportunity to discuss local activities.
9. Identify all departments and administrators in your state government that hold a responsibility and authority over matters of interest to the nursing profession.

E-RESOURCES

- Congress. http://beta.congress.gov
- Government Accountability Office. http://www.gao.gov
- GPO Access (Government Printing Office). http://www.gpoaccess.gov/index.html
- Guide to Rulemaking. http://www.federalregister.gov/uploads/2011/01/the_rulemaking_process.pdf

- Health Resources and Services Administration. http://www.hrsa.gov
- House of Representatives. http://www.house.gov
- House: How Our Laws Are Made (by House of Representatives Parliamentarian). http://thomas.loc.gov/home/lawsmade.toc.html
- Judges as Policy Makers. http://www.youtube.com/watch?v=qhsO4L5LezU
- National Council of State Legislatures. http://www.ncsl.org
- National Council State Board of Nursing Contact Information. https://www.ncsbn.org/contactbon.htm
- Senate. http://www.senate.gov
- Senate: Enactment of a Law (by Senate Parliamentarian). http://thomas.loc.gov/home/enactment/enactlawtoc.html
- The Legislative Processes. http://beta.congress.gov/legislative-process
- Thomas (Library of Congress). https://beta.congress.gov
- Tracking the United States Congress. https://www.govtrack.us
- U.S. Congress and Health Policy Tutorial. http://kff.org/interactive/the-u-s-congress-and-health-policy-tutorial
- White House. http://www.whitehouse.gov

REFERENCES

American Nurses Association. (n.d.) *Agencies & regulations*. Retrieved from http://nursingworld.org/Agencies-RegulatoryAffairs

Congress.gov. (n.d.). The legislative process. Retrieved from https://beta.congress.gov/content/legprocess/legislative-process-poster.jpg

Govtrack.us. (n.d.) *Statistics and historical comparison*. Retrieved from https://www.govtrack.us/congress/bills/statistics

Institute of Medicine. (2001). *Crossing the quality chasm: A new health system for the 21st century*. Washington, DC: The National Academies Press.

Institute of Medicine. (2003). *Health professions education: A bridge to quality*. Washington, DC: The National Academies Press.

Patzek, M. J. (2010). Understanding the DNP degree. *American Nurse Today*, 5(5), 49–50. Retrieved from http://www.americannursetoday.com/Article.aspx?id=6656&fid=6592

PEW Health Professions Commission. (1998). *Competencies for the 21st century*. San Francisco, CA: Author.

Pohl, J. M., Tanner, C., Pilon, B., & Benkert, R. (2011). Comparison of nurse managed health centers with community health centers as safety net providers. *Policy, Politics, & Nursing Practice*, 12(2) 90–99.

Rafael, A. R. (1996). Power and caring: A dialectic in nursing. *Advances in Nursing Science*, 19(1), 3–17.

II

Analyzing Policy

FOUR

Identifying a Policy Issue

Rose Iris Gonzalez
Sheila A. Abood

Problems are only opportunities in work clothes.—Henry J. Kaiser

OBJECTIVES

1. Discuss the critical nature of problem identification in the policy process.
2. Explore sources of problems for policy development in nursing.
3. Investigate types of groups that may be used to identify policy problems.
4. Examine the use of an environmental scan for identifying a nursing policy issue.
5. Demonstrate the use of a SWOT (strengths, weaknesses, opportunities, and threats) analysis in examining an issue in nursing.

Problems abound in today's health care system. We, as nurses, observe and experience problems every day in our practice settings and in the communities. The problems we see most often relate to patients under our care and our environments in which we work and live. These problems, whether clinical, managerial, or environmental, require an alignment of the problem with a workable solution or solutions and favorable political conditions. This confluence of factors when aligned is often referred to as the opening of a window of opportunity (Kingdon, 2011). Solving challenging problems encountered in the health care arena requires an appreciation and recognition of the alignment of necessary variables that are prerequisite to opening a window of opportunity. Without this appreciation and skill, it is likely that any expenditure of time, resources, and energy may not yield the desired policy change.

Not all problems are created equal and not all problems lend themselves to a policy solution. It is easy to become frustrated, but this chapter assists in developing skills to identify issues that need a policy solution. The Policy Challenge illustrates the political activism of a nurse practitioner (NP) in writing a letter on a problem. Hear her frustration about a federal ruling that impacts the patients in her practice.

Writing a letter such as this is an important activity for nurses and is often a first step for many as they begin their involvement in policy. To begin to make

POLICY CHALLENGE: Asking American Nurses Association's (ANA) Government Affairs (GOVA) Department for Assistance

Dear GOVA

I am an NP who has an independent practice providing primary care services in a rural community. In 2009, I worked really hard to support the Affordable Care Act legislation and to educate my patients of the benefits it will provide related to increased access to care and preventative services. I was excited to learn that there were many provisions that worked to support community-based care and the role of advanced practice nurses including NPs, but recently I received communication that concerns me about a recent change in the process used for ordering durable medical equipment (DME) for patients. It's communication from the Centers for Medicare and Medicaid (CMS), which says there are new rules that could negatively impact my practice.

The notice further went on to say that in November 2012, CMS released its Medicare Physician Fee Schedule Final Rule, issued on November 1, and effective on January 1, 2013, that included the DME Face-to-Face Encounters rule. Related to DME Face-to-Face Encounters, the CMS clarified that NPs, clinical nurse specialists (CNSs), and physician assistants (PAs) can conduct face-to-face encounters required for DME, but the statute, Section 6407 of the Affordable Care Act, requires a physician to document that encounter.

Beginning with orders for DME made on or after July 1, 2013, for an item of DME that is included on the list that the CMS has established for this purpose: a physician must document that the physician, or an NP, a CNS, or a PA, has had a face-to-face encounter. The encounter with the beneficiary must occur within 6 months before delivery of DME. I have provided a link for a detailed explanation of the requirements of the rule and a complete list of items for your review (DHHS, 2013; http://www.nursingworld.org/MLN-Matters-DocumentationDME.pdf).

This recent rule will greatly restrict the access of my patients to the care and services they require and it can be viewed as an unjustified restriction of my legal scope of practice. I prescribe one of these items at least daily and having to arrange for a physician to cosign these notes is simply impractical and will negatively impact my current practice. I need help to get this changed.

Sincerely yours,

Frustrated nurse practitioner, DNP, CRNP

See Option for Policy Challenge.

sustained contributions to problems like these, however, a necessary skill is the ability to define problems. Once problems are defined, then you can determine the agenda you will pursue in tackling the policy issue (see Chapter 6, "Setting the Agenda") and move from frustration to activation.

PROBLEM IDENTIFICATION: MORE THAN MEETS THE EYE

To effectively address the most challenging problems in the strongest and most efficient manner requires thoughtful preparation including a systematic examination of the problem, collection of relevant data, and conduction of concurrent analysis. Once this preparation is completed, it is then possible to think about the problem in a systemic way.

Patient falls, a common issue across all settings, illustrates an unfolding approach to this problem. If a patient falls on a cardiac unit, for example, this would be considered an adverse event. Responding by helping the patient back to bed is appropriate, but nothing has been done to prevent future patient falls. If a nurse attends to the fallen patient and then proceeds to collect data by studying the number of falls on the unit during the past month, the age of the patients who have fallen, and the time of day or night during which the majority of falls have taken place, then data are used to identify patterns. These more detailed data provide additional information for closer analysis of the problem. It might be observed that more falls take place in the early evening when some staff are taking a break. After analysis, the staff break schedule might be adjusted to provide better coverage during that time period. The unit staff are adapting to the problem but it remains uncertain whether the root causes of the problem causing an unacceptable number of patient falls on the unit are actually being addressed.

Now, suppose the lens is widened to examine what is happening in relation to falls on other units in the hospital. This requires examining existing patient safety standards and policies, the number of patient and family complaints, modifiable risk factors, and what other hospitals in the area are doing. The search may be expanded to include both national and international data (see Chapter 13, "Evaluating Policy Structures, Processes, and Outcomes") for benchmarking against other health care systems. These data provide more information about the size and impact of the problem and the data required for the next steps. An interprofessional task force could be formed to analyze the data, collect additional information, and make recommendations for possible short-term solutions, which could eventually be applied more globally. Follow-up evaluations may generate long-term solutions or may indicate that new patient safety policies may need to be developed and implemented.

Examining a particular problem beyond a single incident can offer a broader perspective that helps one see events, as well as patterns that in turn help to answer a critical question: When does a problem become more than an isolated event and when does solving a problem require the time, effort, and resources necessary for a successful policy solution?

The number of patient falls example shows a common local organizational policy change, but health care policy occurs at all levels throughout the health care system. Start at the local level with policies and regulations designed to meet goals, and allocate resources to accomplish the work at the unit level or, more broadly, to meet the organization's mission and purpose. Moving on, there are also policies that govern health care at the community-wide level, policies that guide public and private health care at the state level, and finally at the national level where enacted and implemented policy decisions can impact large segments of the entire U.S. health care system.

To introduce a new health care policy or to modify existing policy is a challenging endeavor that does not happen in a vacuum and is not the work of one individual. It takes more than an idea to move a proposal through the policy process. It takes resources, energy, persistence, patience, time, and the ability to compromise in order to achieve the desired results.

Policy changes at the national level to address problems typically begin with a vision. This vision may have its genesis in one individual or a group of dedicated individuals concerned about something they observe or experience in their current environment. Trends identified in the larger health care environment may also generate ideas related to the anticipated need for increased resources to meet national health care goals. Rich complex exemplars of problems in nursing are found in the daily practice of frontline clinicians. Common sources of problems are those surrounding the issues related to the removal of practice barriers and reimbursement for APRNs.

OPENING A WINDOW: ELEMENTS FOR SUCCESS

The policy-making process is a complex and cyclical process that takes knowledge, relationships, human and fiscal resources, and a willingness to negotiate and compromise to reach one's vision and goal. Changing policy at the macro level or the big "P" level requires one to understand that change is an incremental process that requires stamina and patience, as well as always keeping the long-term goal in sight. Even at the little "p" level the process can be slow, as change is often hard work no matter at what level it occurs (see Chapter 8, "Changing Organizations, Institutions, and Government").

If the problem is within a hospital setting, it could be that a simple change can be made at the unit level or perhaps a new hospital-wide policy must be implemented. At the macro level, or the big "P" level, the change could require drafting of legislation with the goal of creating a new law or adding language to clarify an existing regulation. The success and failure of any of these policies will eventually depend on the political environment in place at the time the change is proposed. Thus, within complex environments, how does an issue come to the forefront? How does one recognize that a problem exists?

Problem Identification

Problem identification is a crucial and basic, but often complex, stage of the policy-making process. It often not only involves clearly identifying the problem, as well as identifying related policies that are needed or existing policies that are problematic, but also involves determining how aware the public is of the problem and the surrounding issues, deciding who will participate in fixing it, and considering what means are available to accomplish a solution. The answer to these deliberations will help determine which, if any, policy changes are requisite to address the identified problem or if an existing policy needs to be changed or eliminated.

These steps may be initially asked individually or as part of a group process. Identifying a problem and then clearly defining it are not only critical to making a problem known, but also essential to having the right people at the table (stakeholders) and to forming a solution. Problem identification is a necessary component for all policy work and is often embedded in agenda setting (see Chapter 6). It is not, however, a simple step. While it is often discussed as part of agenda setting, it is examined as a necessary skill in detail in this chapter, as a poorly defined problem minimally wastes time and resources; however, poor definition can lead to innumerable harms such as disengaged nurses, loss of the window of opportunity, and/or failure to change policy. Albert Einstein captures the importance of clearly thinking about the problem and identifying it, "If I had an hour to solve a problem I'd spend 55 minutes thinking about the problem and 5 minutes thinking about solutions."

Nurses know from firsthand experience that there are times when even defining a single patient problem or clearly stating an evidence-based question can be difficult. Problem identification in policy work is no less complex. As nurses working in a range of settings, problems in the little "p" arena can involve not only clinical problems but also a variety of issues depending on settings and/or roles, for example, educational, managerial, and workplace. Further complicating policy problem identification, like in patient care work, may involve intraprofessional and interprofessional collaboration.

To begin clarifying the problem, start by making a short statement about what the best situation is compared to what is current and what are the consequences if the situation is not corrected. Clarity and conciseness are the watchwords of problem identification. You might start by writing down the current state (e.g., falls are increasing, restraint use has resulted in a complaint, and nurses are verbalizing there is not enough time to complete tasks). It is not important at this juncture to worry about wording; the point is to commit to an issue and to get something in writing so that you and others can react to it. Sometimes it is easier to start with the goal or a description of the best or ideal situation. Thus, another way to start may be to write that the ideal is "zero falls," "a restraint-free environment," "improved nurse satisfaction scores," or "providing access care to a vulnerable population in a rural area." Then, write the consequences that may result if the current situation is not changed. Consider the current and possible future effects of the problem. Often at the little "p" level, those impacts are on the nurses' work environment, the patients, or both. The problem statement should be two to three sentences long. Once these components are drafted, it is easier to refine them and to get help and feedback. Policy is, as will be discussed shortly, a team sport that requires input from a group of people.

Nurses are crucial to identifying problems. In everyday work, there are numerous opportunities to see problems as a result of contact with patients, experience with equipment, and the centrality of safety in nurses' work. Therefore, problems will come to the attention of nurses in various ways. Sometimes the problem seems obvious. An event happens that has an impact on a clinician. The event may be at the little "p" level while caring for a patient or working with a colleague. A fall on a unit or a readmission of an elderly clinic patient might be an example of how a problem comes to one's attention. Sometimes the problem is one that arises from the big "P" arena. Large-scale disasters are an example of one way that big "P" problems can come to your attention. Often nurses are so embroiled in day-to-day work that they fail to see problems that have policy implications (see Exhibit 4.1).

Once a problem is reasonably stated, it is important to carefully consider what can be done about the problem and who has the responsibility and authority to address the problem as a policy issue. These aspects are more thoroughly discussed in Chapter 6, but deserve some caveats here. While defining the problem is necessary to determine who has the responsibility and authority to address the problem and the policy that follows, not all problems require

---

EXHIBIT 4.1 ACTIONS FOR IDENTIFYING LITTLE "P" PROBLEMS

Reflect about the work environment:
- Identify complaints about daily routines and procedures
- Observe colleagues interacting with each other about an issue
- Observe patients affected by the problem and their responses
- Consider workflow breakdowns
- Review and write about a work-related critical incident
- Attend presentations about successful work changes
- Review nurse satisfaction surveys
- Examine exit interviews
- Participate in meetings where issues related to the problem can be raised

Reflect about a clinical issue:
- Examine the most common patient complaints
- Review the newest treatments for the most commonly encountered clinical problems
- Monitor for new accreditation requirements and recommendations
- Visualize going through patient experiences (e.g., admission and treatments)
- Review unusual and unplanned clinical events

policy and not all policy needs input from nursing (see Chapter 8, "Changing Organizations, Institutions, and Government," and Chapter 11, "Applying a Nursing Lens to Shape Policy"). The effort of moving a problem from its definition to determining what can be done about it and who is responsible is a dynamic process with back-and-forth movement. Even seemingly straightforward problems like patient falls may be refined over and over again, depending on factors such as who is involved in defining the problem. An example of this work was done in Canada that recast falls in the issue of injury. They proposed testing whether a "policy of publicly funded provision of hip protectors to all elderly Ontario nursing home residents could result in cost savings due to decreased spending on initial acute hospitalization for hip fracture in this population" (Sawka et al., 2007, p. 820).

Often, many problems that are of concern to nurses and nursing can be framed in numerous ways. The nursing shortage may be cast as an issue of recruitment and retention, an aging workforce, job dissatisfaction, increased demand, faculty shortage, or a combination of these factors. Advanced practice nurses may wish to frame issues in terms of access to care, quality, cost, or practice barriers. As the problem is refined and discussed more widely, words matter. Even the language is an issue of framing, for example, whether *nursing shortage* or *nurse shortage* is used. How the problem is framed can be instrumental in providing direction for a policy solution.

The Patient Protection and Affordable Care Act (PPACA) of 2010 is a complex piece of legislation that will be debated for many years to come, much as Medicare legislation introduced in 1965 is still being debated. Policy solutions of this magnitude often result in debate from many perspectives, including the identification or definition of the problem at the time of the development of the policy. Then, after enactment, questions will be raised about whether the definition of the problem remains relevant over time or was originally well identified. Medicare and PPACA are examples of legislation designed to address the problem of health care financing. Framing the problem of health care reform as an issue of health care financing is a less controversial or more neutral approach to opening the discussion of the problem. This is an example where the choice of words matters. While analysis of health care financing legislation is beyond the scope of this chapter, it is relevant in demonstrating how nursing can play a role in problem identification. The American Nurses Association (ANA) backed both the enactment of Medicare legislation in 1965 and, more recently, the PPACA. Since 1958, the ANA, in particular, has identified health care financing as an issue; at its website, numerous resources are available about its involvement in health care financing (Woods, 1996). Policy on the Scene 4.1, however, describes what it was like for one nurse who was involved in helping to define the problems of health care financing during the Clinton administration.

A problem becomes a policy issue when there is a lack of policy to address it or there is an existing policy that does not effectively address the problem.

**POLICY ON THE SCENE 4.1: Identifying Problems While
on Assignment at the White House**
**Kay Ball, PhD, RN, CNOR, FAAN, Associate Professor, Nursing
Otterbein University, Westerville, OH**

During the Clinton administration, I was thrilled to get a call inviting me to work at the White House to represent nurses in specialty practice as problems with health care in the United States were being examined for reform. This work at that time was being led by Hillary Clinton. This unique opportunity came to me because I was a nurse in specialty practice (Association of periOperative Registered Nurses [AORN], and vice chair of the Nursing Organization Liaison Forum [NOLF]). This gave me outreach to over a million nurses and access to their opinions about health care problems and their solutions.

While at the White House, I contributed to problem identification by participating in planning and conducting rallies and events about our health care system's status. A special project, the "Health Security Express," involved buses traveling across the United States to converge in Independence, Missouri, and then in Washington, DC. These buses transported patients and health care providers who had powerful stories about health care problems. As a nurse, I listened to their experiences, helped them find the words to tell their stories to the news media, and advocated for quality patient care. Many of these stories were heartbreaking and tragic, but these concerned citizens and health care professionals appeared hopeful that their voices would be heard about the problems and that something could be done to promote some sort of reform in our health care system. These stories resonated with the people in the communities we visited and helped identify other related problems.

Getting the message out was extremely important so the public could understand the problems in health care and the issue of improved health care for all. At one stop, protestors wrongly thought that the bus trip was in support of abortions and limiting access to providers. The protestors physically rocked a bus full of patients and providers. They soon realized their mistake. Health care and the need for a fair and equitable health care system for all was the core mission of this very visible and engaging bus trip.

While working on the health care reform agenda, I listened to countless stories of how the health care system was failing individuals. I was asked to deliver testimonials and presentations advocating for safe patient care. I was invited to speak on national television with Senator Jay Rockefeller and then Secretary of Health and Human Services (HHS) Donna Shalala. The mid-1990s was a peak period for nurse involvement in congressional testimony, a key strategy for problem identification and the generation of solutions. This hunch is corroborated by a recent analysis of nurse testimony between 1993 and 2011. The narrow 1993 to 1994 time frame accounted for 90 of 434 (20.7%) nurse testimonies (Cohen & Muench, 2012) and illustrates the extent of nurse involvement in political action. While the Clinton years focused on problem identification for health care reform, testimony can be and has been used at a number of points in the policy process.

My experiences with health care reform efforts at the White House may have been brief, but it left a powerful imprint on my life as a nurse and patient advocate. Strong relationships and positive attitudes are the core traits for success. Listening closely to others who may represent a competitive or controversial perspective helps to comprehend the enormity of a problem and its pervasiveness in society. Discussing advantages or limitations of multiple solutions leads to clearer problem definition. Learning from these experiences enabled me to easily use these tools both locally and statewide for other compelling problems as I continue my active involvement in health care policies and legislation.

Developing or modifying a policy assumes that some collective good will result and that codifying actions will lead to better patterns of behavior or improved conditions; if not, then the problem is not likely to be "fixed" by policy. Unfortunately, the wrong policy solution may be applied to a particularly vexing problem, yielding unintended consequences. Being involved on the ground floor of problem identification can go a long way toward the development of more effective policy solutions.

Problem identification takes refinement and, often, ongoing rework. Once preliminary ideas are committed to writing the next step in seizing the window of opportunity for policy, action involves formation of a stakeholder work group (see Chapter 6). These groups often at first are composed of interested individuals who can help you further refine the problem. In all likelihood, the formation of a working group will result in some modification of the problem definition. As with any problem solving, the process is not static or linear.

Formation of a Core Working Group

Who are the interested parties currently willing and able to invest in the work of moving a problem/issue along through the policy process? Who are the stakeholders or interested parties who will likely oppose your ideas? These are the stakeholders who may have their own solutions to propose or they may be satisfied with the status quo (see Chapter 6).

When dealing with changes in health care policy, representatives of nursing organizations, physician groups, employers, consumers, hospital organizations, and other coalition groups are all possible participants. These are the identifiable stakeholders who may or may not benefit from a change in the status quo. Formation of a core working group of supportive stakeholders typically takes place at the organization or the coalition level. Participation, commitment, and support by recognized organizations at this level add credibility, expertise, and resources as efforts move forward. At this early policy development stage, nurses organizations need and frequently seek out member volunteers with appropriate expertise to serve on these types of policy groups. Opportunities for participation as part of this core group may be one of the most desirable direct benefits of membership as it provides unique opportunities for active engagement in the problem identification and policy agenda-setting phase. This is illustrated by the process used by the American Association of Colleges of Nursing leadership in developing the doctorate of nursing practice (ANA, 2011).

Committees, councils, task forces, subcommittees, and boards are examples of groups where policy is often born—that is, defined—and solutions identified. Membership in these groups can be voluntary, appointed, or elected. Some groups like boards and/or policy committees are understood to have overt or frank policy responsibilities; in reality, however, most formal group efforts at the little "p" and the big "P" levels involve some policy work.

A recent approach to involving patients as key stakeholders in their care is the development of patient advisory councils. These councils may serve a department or a hospital and provide feedback on services, programs, and policy. This type of a council can be instrumental in defining problems and then subsequently helping determine solutions. This is not unlike the approach used in participatory action research where key stakeholders drawn from the community of interest participate and are actively engaged in advancing knowledge.

As the core working group for any policy, the initial task is defining and clarifying the problem to be addressed. This step also includes accurate documentation of the problem events and patterns of occurrences. What is the history associated with this problem? Has it been addressed previously? What was the response? Does this problem meet the criteria for a policy solution? Then, possible solutions are identified and the final projected desired outcomes are determined. Have all alternative solutions been considered? Are all the internal stakeholders on the same page regarding perceptions of how the problem should be defined, and the desired outcomes? Are there acceptable and agreeable compromise positions that could be negotiated? These types of answers often come from group work, especially for major problems.

Numerous groups and panels have helped to identify health care problems. One example is the report by Surgeon General Luther Terry whose office issued the first Surgeon General's Report on Smoking and Health in 1964 (U.S. Department of Health Education and Welfare [USDHEW], 1964). This example is mentioned not merely because of its historic 50th anniversary but also to demonstrate the level of formality that a work group can encompass. Since 1964, there have been over 50 Surgeon General Reports. About half of these are about smoking, as the Public Health Cigarette Smoking Act of 1969 (a legislative response to the 1964 report) mandates an annual review of research on smoking. These formal work groups vary with the project and surgeon general, but they illustrate the central role of group work in policy processes. It also shows that it is often not the work of one group but sometimes many groups, especially when the problem is so widespread and embedded in society. While nurses were not consulted in the first surgeon general report, this has changed over the years. Ellen Feathery, MS, RN, associate director, International Research, Campaign for Tobacco-Free Kids, Washington, DC, was a contributing author for the recent report, *Preventing Tobacco Use Among Youth and Young Adults* (U.S. Department of Health and Human Services [USDHHS], 2012).

Many professional and specialty nursing associations have opportunities for group work on policy-related matters, as outlined in Chapter 7, "Building Capital: Intellectual, Social, Political, and Financial." These groups may have standing committees or task forces to work on policy matters. The ANA, for example, always revises the scope and practice standards they produce with the efforts of members in a group format. The APRN Consensus Model (2008) is another example of group work (see Chapter 3, "Navigating the Political System") in identifying a problem and proposing solutions that have far-reaching implications for removing scope-of-practice barriers. These barriers impact the problem of access to care and the ability of our country to provide primary care in an efficient and cost-effective manner (Pohl, Hanson, Newland, & Cronenwett, 2010). Policy on the Scene 4.2 illustrates the power of group process in the identification of a problem and advancing the policy process in relation to disaster preparedness.

Bringing key stakeholders together takes time, and also depends upon having and sustaining long-standing relationships. A broad range of viewpoints is essential in identifying policy issues. The use of a policy conference is an example of how nurses took advantage of a window of opportunity presented by heightened professional and public interest.

TOOLS

To effectively plan for policy and fully take advantage of a window of opportunity requires data about the environment and the contextual factors impacting the situation. Often an environmental scan is conducted through an analysis of the SWOT associated with an issue. It is a necessary step in identifying a problem. In this section, we discuss the elements of an environmental scan and then demonstrate a SWOT analysis using needle safety as an exemplar.

POLICY ON THE SCENE 4.2: ANA Making the Problem of Disaster Preparedness Visible
Linda J. Stierle, MSN, RN, Brigadier General
USAF, Nurse Corps (Retired)

In the mid-2000s, the ANA board decided to hold a policy conference to better support one of its primary missions: creating policy to advance the nursing profession and protect the public. The purpose of the policy conference was to create a vehicle to provide more nurses with the opportunity to become engaged in policy creation. This would not only increase the policy expertise of nurses across the nation, but would also increase the commitment of the nursing community to the policy generated from the conference due to the personal involvement of individual nurses and participating organizations.

Then, in August 2005, Hurricane Katrina wreaked havoc on the Gulf coast. The ANA played an integral role in keeping the larger nursing community informed of how it could be involved in a variety of disaster relief activities. The ANA has a long history of being engaged with nurses' disaster preparedness. The ANA also supported organizations providing relief and services in Alabama, Louisiana, and Mississippi, the three states most impacted by Hurricane Katrina, with contact information for nurses with specialized skills and expertise.

The Department of Health and Human Services (DHHS) invited the ANA to participate in the Lessons Learned Presentation in 2006 with the ANA chief executive officer (CEO), and the ANA director of practice and policy attending. Based on the problems encountered as a result of Hurricane Katrina, the presentation identified the need for improved policy and direction across the health care system to increase our nation's readiness for disasters.

During the same time frame, the ANA participated in an Institute of Medicine (IOM) Roundtable convened to identify ways of increasing disaster preparedness among all health care professionals. These two events, the DHHS debriefing and the IOM Roundtable, coupled with the ANA's own experiences with Hurricane Katrina all contributed to the decision that disaster preparedness would be a very timely and appropriate topic for ANA's first policy conference in 2007. As part of the process, a multidisciplinary expert panel was convened prior to the conference to advise the ANA and to develop strategies for health professions in challenging circumstances like Hurricane Katrina. Conference attendees evaluated the expert panel's (drawn from the larger health care community) recommendation that ultimately resulted in seminal national nursing policy, *Adapting Standards of Care Under Extreme Conditions* (ANA, 2008) (nursingworld. org/MainMenuCategories/WorkplaceSafety/Healthy-Work-Environment/ DPR/TheLawEthicsofDisasterResponse/AdaptingStandardsofCare.pdf).

The conference and policy document was a success that became a significant resource for the IOM Roundtable and other organizations addressing this critical policy issue for future disasters.

Disaster preparedness in the health care system, like many problems, involves a confluence of issues that are a microcosm of the larger issues facing the profession. These include the primary issue addressed at the policy conference most important to patients and their frontline clinicians, standards of care under extreme conditions, as well as issues surrounding credentialing, interstate practice, scope of practice, collaboration, access, quality, employer response, employee responsibilities, health care disparities, and personal readiness for disasters. Identifying the problems related to disaster preparedness and working them through have the potential to foster the relationships necessary for addressing similar issues that occur in nondisaster situations.

The Environmental Scan

Part of the preparatory work essential in identifying a problem with a policy solution is conducting an environmental scan of external and internal factors related to the particular problem/issue. An environmental scan is a systematic way to examine an issue within the context of current events and situations. Environmental scans are commonplace in all planning across settings, from business to education to health care. The setting and purpose will help define the environmental scan that is carried out. The American Hospital Association (AHA), for example, regularly publishes an annual environmental scan of market forces that are anticipated to impact health care (O'Dell, Aspy, Jarousse, & AHA, 2013).

Health care policies do not exist in isolation, so taking the necessary time to conduct and analyze an environmental scan can pay off by identifying both positive and negative factors, which may impact the problem. The scan also should indicate the following: the stakeholders involved and the resources available, which of these factors will or will not influence the successful outcome, which factors can be influenced, and which factors are outside your scope of influence. The results of the scan and analysis of those results should help to identify important trends and events in the larger external environment, which provide a basis for developing strategies to move the issue toward the policy agenda.

Environmental scanning is typically conducted through a group process. The stakeholder group proposing a legislative solution to an identified problem may form a small task force or an ad hoc committee to carry out the environmental scan or, depending on available resources, may hire an outside consultant to do this important work. There are no hard and fast rules for conducting an environmental scan and it is only one component of an external analysis.

The environmental scan can be informal, mainly observational, and consist of identifying and gathering existing information, or it can take on a more formal aspect where new data are collected through surveys or other research methods. Information may be gathered through review of relevant publications, media resources, Internet sites, statements or opinions by social critics, experts, and activists as well as other existing data.

Although determining what is important to scan or examine is usually specific to the problem being addressed, there are some common methods and considerations to help organize the environmental scan. It is usual to start with an internal scan to identify the strengths within one's own interest group that can be leveraged to advantage efforts and also to identify any weaknesses associated with the group that will need adaptation or neutralization as the group moves the issue through the legislative process. This internal scan, discussed in more detail later in this chapter, is often examined using a SWOT analysis. Some questions to consider when gathering information about the relevant components of the external environmental scan are as follows (MDF Training and Consultancy, 2005):

- Political environment: What is happening in the political/legislative arena? Is there the political will to support or alter the change you are proposing? Understanding the political dimensions of health policy is essential to better anticipate opportunities as well as constraints and helps individuals and groups design more effective policies.
- Economic environment: Are there critical economic factors that most affect the issue? What are the dynamics of the general national economic climate? Are there serious fiscal constraints?
- Sociocultural environment: Are there demographic trends or changes? What is the status of public health programs? Are there underserved and/or vulnerable populations that will be impacted by the proposed health policy? Are there ethical considerations?
- Technological environment: What is the pace of technological advancement? How will technology impact the knowledge base, skills, and talents of the workforce? How will social media impact development and dissemination of the issue message?

The aforementioned external environment factors are sometimes referred to as a PEST (political, economic, sociocultural, technological) analysis. The use of PEST is a suggested strategy to help explore more fully external factors that can be easily missed in a traditional SWOT analysis. In some circumstances, legal and environmental factors may also need to be examined; hence, PEST is sometimes referred to as PESTLE. The interaction between SWOT and PEST(LE) is thought to reflect a more encompassing analysis.

Exhibit 4.2 provides some preliminary questions to ask and consider about the political environment before executing a strategic plan to advance an issue.

These questions are often thought to relate to public policy, but in reality, they have applicability to all policy.

EXHIBIT 4.2 CONSIDERATIONS WHEN SCANNING THE POLITICAL ENVIRONMENT

Determine leadership	• Assess who has the ability or desire to lead the policy change. • Recognize what individual or group has the capacity, expertise, reputation, and established relationships. • Determine if this is an interprofessional issue.
Consider relationships/reputation	• Anticipate how stakeholders will be impacted. • Determine stakeholders' engagement with each other. • Determine stakeholders' level of support and/or opposition for the issue.
Identify possible stakeholders	• Assess what organizations or groups have a vested interest in the issue. • Identify who will be impacted whether status quo is maintained or a change is implemented. • Determine those who hold supportive and unsupportive positions.
Examine relationships	• Assess whether a relationship exists between the groups (like the nurses association) and identified stakeholders. • Determine if a relationship exists among the branches of government and the association or between the group and the administration at the organizational work level. • Evaluate if the group leading the policy forward is viewed as credible and speaking for all involved. • Review whether other groups (e.g., organizations) wield strong policy influence. Further determine what is the association's relationship with the organization(s). • Establish if the group participates in any coalitions. If yes, what is their reputation?

Define and assess adequacy of resources needed to advance an issue	• Identify resources needed to help clarify the problem— "carry the water."
	  – Human: in terms of staff, contract lobbyist (if appropriate) and volunteers.
	  – Financial: depending upon the campaign needed, do you have a political action committee (PAC)?
	  – Physical: such as a grassroots system. If not, with what group(s) can the association partner?

Consider timing: determine if a history is associated with the issue/initiative	• Investigate whether the issue had been addressed previously and by whom.
	  – What was the response?
	  – If not favorable, what were the barriers?
	• How much time has elapsed since last attempted?
	• Analyze unintended consequences of the timing.
	• Plan for the best time to act.

(continued)

EXHIBIT 4.2	CONSIDERATIONS WHEN SCANNING THE POLITICAL ENVIRONMENT (*CONTINUED*)
Identify bases of power	• Which party dominates in the legislative/executive branch leadership? • Is it an election year and will the power change as a result?
Determine relevancy	• Anticipate if the issue will be reflected in the legislature's/regulatory agency's agenda or is likely to be. • Determine the possible competing policy issues. • Identify the level of public awareness. Has the issue been in the news? • Identify what will influence relevancy. • Assess if this initiative costs money.

Adapted from the American Nurses Association (2013).

Following data collection for each of the selected environmental sectors, some analysis is necessary to assess the external opportunities and threats. Information gathered should be shared with the larger working group. Activities in some identified sectors may need to be tracked over a period of time to monitor changes in the environment and to clarify their importance for the proposed health policy change. Environmental scans are recognized as valuable tools in health care decision making as they can identify the problem, the affected population, and the responsibility for the problem. All these factors influence the responses of policy makers.

SWOT Analysis

A SWOT analysis is a tool to help one assess the viability of a project. It is a logical means of examining an issue strategically in order to better identify a pathway to success. Online tools such as Mind Tools (2007–2011) for a SWOT analysis are readily available. The following provides an example of a real-world issue—needle safety, a topic that nurses across the country are continuing to address. Examining the strengths, weaknesses, opportunities, and threats using a SWOT analysis approach, we demonstrate how the ANA and other stakeholders seized a window of opportunity and successfully addressed this issue at the national level.

A postmortem SWOT analysis exemplar shown in Exhibit 4.3 on a needle-stick injury issue gauges its viability for advancement in the federal legislative arena. This illustrates some of the preliminary work that was completed prior to introduction of federal legislation to address this issue. This analysis is helpful to see the history of a problem that resulted in federal legislation being passed in the United States in 2000 (Needlestick Safety and Prevention Act). This legislation has resulted in good outcomes, but needlestick and sharps safety still remains an ongoing issue. (For an update on the status of needle safety and future directions, see Chapter 13.)

EXHIBIT 4.3 EXEMPLAR: SWOT ANALYSIS FOR NEEDLESTICK SAFETY

INTERNAL

Strengths
- Nurses and health care workers had compelling stories of needlestick and sharps injuries.
- Prominent nurses started to speak out publicly and push the issue to the forefront.
- Data were available describing the extent and pervasiveness of needlestick injuries.
- Costs available for workers' compensation cases opened due to needlestick injuries.
- Nurses acknowledged by the Gallup poll as the most trusted health professional.
- ANA has a strong communications department with experience in developing similar issue campaigns.

Weaknesses
- Lack of media attention and lack of communication outlets and resources to share these stories of life-altering injuries.
- Competing agendas: staffing, mandatory overtime, funding for nursing education, direct Medicare reimbursement for advanced practice nurses. Too many issues for the ANA to address. What was the priority?
- Lack of sufficient association resources (staff, financial) to address the issue.
- Strong need to build an economic case on the issue in order to build a compelling message for those not familiar with this industry issue.

EXTERNAL

Opportunities
- Nurses, state nurses associations, unions, and individual collective bargaining units were organized and supportive of advancing legislative initiatives. The issue also served as a good organizing vehicle.
- Collaboration among important stakeholders led the push for the adoption of state legislation; increased momentum developed.
- Increased calls for action as result of the impact of increased incidence of HIV and hepatitis C infections from a reported 800,000 to 1 million injuries, as well as increased workers' compensation cases.
- New safer technology (e.g., needleless systems) development.
- Manufacturers in support of advancing the issue helped develop the economic case.
- In 1999, legislation was adopted in three states and introduced in another 18, building momentum.
- Stakeholders endorsed the ANA to take the lead on this issue.

Threats
- Opposition claimed the burden of costs was prohibitive.
- New safer technology was more expensive and would require workflow redesign.
- American Hospital Association (AHA) was a strong opponent, and a powerbroker with financial and political resources.
- Opposition argued about the impact on patient care costs.
- Data on workers' compensation were held by employers.
- Reluctance to collect and disclose sharps injuries data.

This SWOT analysis on needlestick safety clearly outlines the strengths and weaknesses identified by the ANA that could impact its ability to advance this issue in the federal legislative arena. It also identified the potential threats that could be encountered while outlining the opportunities. With this information in hand, the ANA contacted its state nurses associations and other stakeholders in an attempt to identify the best way to address this issue. By this time, it was understood that there was movement at the state level and the momentum was increasing. This allowed the ANA to then explore whether it should shift its efforts from advancing this issue in the state legislative arenas to move toward a more national approach. At this point in time, 16 states had passed legislation related to needlestick injuries. At times, a critical mass of states acting on an issue is needed to move an issue forward. This analysis of factors revealed that the time was right to move this issue from the state houses to Congress.

Scenario Analysis

Scenario analysis, sometimes called scenario framing or planning, is a strategy used to identify potential future problems and policy solutions. It was first used in World War II to analyze the consequences of nuclear proliferation, and then popularized by the Dutch Shell company and other businesses that used it for strategic planning (Swart, Raskin, & Robinson, 2004). Scenario analysis is a qualitative approach designed to address a wide range of possible outcomes. Its use in health care has been most often for the identification of problems that may occur as a result of public health policies or crisis situations. The process usually involves various stakeholders, who are presented with a futuristic, but plausible scenario. The problem usually requires broad input from multiple constituencies. Those present are divided into small groups and each analyzes strategies to address the scenario that are then presented to the larger group.

A scenario example is an outbreak of pandemic flu with limited supplies of a vaccine for the flu. This policy problem was used throughout the Veterans Affairs system in their community planning process (Lurie et al., 2008). The ANA also used this scenario topic in preparation for discussions with stakeholders in the larger health care community. Challenges presented by this example are policies related to who should get scarce vaccine flu first to prevent the spread of disease and maintain essential public services. The topic selected is usually one that has high impact. This process helps to identify problems with different versions of policy solutions. Scenarios can be developed for different purposes with descriptive scenarios using what is known about a situation that leads to certain outcomes to examine intended and unintended consequences. In addition, normative scenarios that lead to a specific view of the future are used to examine the possibilities for the achievement of outcomes (Swart et al., 2004). This process allows for the analysis of policy problems within the context of a constantly changing environment.

The systematic selection and use of tools for the identification of a policy problem provides direction for subsequent steps in the policy-making process.

The choice of a tool and the extent of preparatory work completed as part of an environmental scan are dependent upon the interplay of numerous factors and the current political environment, be it within an organization or the governmental arena.

The efforts to provide a safe working environment for nurses are an ongoing process, as are efforts to remove practice barriers, eliminate health care inequities, and other policy issues in health care. Policies often are not perfected on the first attempt. Sometimes, there are trade-offs on what will be included in a particular piece of legislation or regulation, and sometimes, new problems emerge because of changes in practice that move ahead of the policy process. See the Option for Policy Challenge: Turning Frustration Into Action.

OPTION FOR POLICY CHALLENGE: Turning Frustration Into Action

Dear frustrated nurse practitioner:

While we recognize the PPACA was a significant accomplishment for patients and providers alike, broadening the health care arena to increase access and services in diverse communities as well as a step forward toward comprehensive health care, it is not a perfect law. It's not surprising that during implementation, some issues will arise that will need to be addressed. An early example of a section of the law that requires modification is Section 6407(b) of the PPACA, which addresses APRNs ordering and signing for DME.

The ANA, as well as the nursing community, submitted comments in a letter dated August 30, 2012, to CMS acting administrator Marilyn Tavenner addressing this rule (click here to view the ANA's and the nursing community's comments: www.nursingworld.org/physfeesched2012). Initially, implementation of this rule was delayed and rescheduled to go into effect on July 1, 2013. Stakeholder advocacy accomplished an additional delay until October 2013.

What are the options for action by an individual NP, such as yourself, to address this issue? There are several:

- Gather data and facts to build the case regarding how this will impact the individual patient and your practice.
- Contact your professional and specialty organizations to support their advocacy efforts. Multiple voices with a unified message are more likely to be heard.
- Create a list of items most frequently ordered that should be minimally controversial to include in your potential communication with the secretary of Health and Human Services (HHS) to request that he or she

(continued)

consider placing these items on an opt-out list related to the requirement for a physician signature.

- Write a letter to the secretary of the HHS with a copy to the administrator for the CMS to share your data and how this regulation would negatively impact the quality of patient care and access to needed services.
- Contact your member of Congress with your concerns and educate him
or her about the impact of the issue using the data gathered. Emphasize
its impact to patient care delivery and his or her constituents. Request a
legislative option to address the issue. Report back to your professional
organization with information gleaned.
- Write to HHS and the CMS and urge them to indefinitely delay the
implementation of this rule.

As an individual provider, your most valuable resource is your professional organization. Working with them to address this issue, providing
them with your real-life experience, and knowing how these changes are
impacting patients serve as a valuable resource and can help to move the
policy challenge in your direction.

You can rest assured that organized nursing will continue to work on
this and we hope we can continue to count on you to share your real-life
experience with decision makers to help us make a difference.

IMPLICATIONS FOR THE FUTURE

Nursing has to be vigilant in identifying problems and taking responsibility for creating favorable political circumstances by voting and electing individuals who share nursing's philosophy. Nursing can no longer expect to exist
in a silo using disparate voices to demand change. As the health care system
moves toward models of care that require interprofessional education and
practice environments, nursing will need to position itself so that, as a profession, it is able to be viable and integral to this changing health care system, as
called for in *The Future of Nursing: Leading Change, Advancing Health* report
(IOM, 2011). This changing environment will become even more competitive as
players vie to carve out their niche and protect their existing status, while others try to enhance/expand/control their roles. To be effective, nursing needs to
be aware of the internal strengths and external opportunities that exist related
to their advocacy initiatives, activities, or goals in order to determine whether
these variables outweigh the internal weaknesses and the external threats. Only
then will nurses be able to determine their ability to move forward in identifying
and tackling problems or issues in any system. Nurses need to cultivate allies to
support and champion issues. Nursing can be a major stakeholder if we unite on
common goals. Joining professional nursing organizations enables us to build our
diversity and strength of numbers in order to participate in advocacy activities,

as well as shape favorable political circumstances. Nurses who become informed citizens engaged in the full participation of the electoral process can better position themselves in boardrooms, as well as political and administrative leadership positions at the local, state, and federal level. As you can see, opportunities for policy change occur at many levels, and nurses need to be ready to seize positions of power and influence to effect change. In those roles we know nurses can work to realize more favorable circumstances to create change and advance their vision for nurses and patients alike from the bedside to the boardroom.

KEY CONCEPTS

1. Not every problem requires a legislative solution, and not every problem requires a policy solution.
2. Problem identification is a critical initial step in moving forward with the policy process.
3. Words matter when describing the policy problem to stakeholders and members of the external environment.
4. A confluence of aligned factors creates a window of opportunity for advancing a policy solution for an identified problem.
5. Identifying key stakeholders and understanding their positions is critical because policy work is most often carried out by groups.
6. Change is possible at every level and changes at one level often impact other levels.
7. Careful preparation and the systematic examination of a problem from a broad perspective within the context of current events and situations are essential for the effective evaluation of policy direction.
8. An encompassing analysis of the environment can include using the SWOT and PESTLE tools.
9. It takes an ability to compromise in order to achieve results.
10. It is important to have an ear to the ground, listening and gathering information from individuals impacted by the problem.
11. Policy making is cyclical; nothing is perfect.
12. Modification and refinement are part of the ongoing process.
13. Uniting on common goals and participating in the advocacy work of associations can shape favorable political outcomes.
14. Persistence and patience are necessary components for success.

SUMMARY

Learning the steps necessary to identify and analyze problems, developing possible solutions, building stakeholder support, and evaluating the existing political circumstances are essential components in the process of identifying policies proposed for action. Engaging in SWOT and PESTLE analyses can be used to conduct a thorough environmental scan. Moving through these steps is preparatory for the recognition of the confluence of factors that create a favorable window of opportunity. Several key examples demonstrate the challenges encountered when one advances a vision through the policy.

LEARNING ACTIVITIES

1. Identify a health care issue that, in your opinion, is a problem that calls for a policy solution. Explain how you would begin to gather data about the issue and to develop a plan to address the problem. Discuss the tools that will help you in gathering the data.
2. Discuss some of the factors that indicate that a window of opportunity is opening, making it possible to move a proposed problem solution forward in the policy process. Use an example from a policy at work, school, or the community where you live to illustrate when a window of opportunity might open.
3. Robert Wood Johnson Foundation, Heritage Foundation, Urban Institute, Kaiser Family Foundation, and the Commonwealth Fund are all examples of research/policy organizations. Investigate the websites of at least three research/policy organizations to identify their organizational health care priorities.
4. Identify a current health story in the news that has potential policy implications. List the political institutions that are germane to the discussion about this health news issue. Brainstorm some possible policies that address this issue and then identify one policy from the list where a nursing voice can have the greatest impact.
5. Select one of the following e-resources to share with a work or school colleague or someone you supervise. Prepare a short summary of its purpose and applicability for policy that is tailored to the audience.
6. Link to C-SPAN at http://www.c-span.org and select a topic that has implications for nursing. Discuss the problem identified and what contributions nursing can make to the definition of the problem.
7. Investigate the use of an advisory council where you work or go to school. Summarize its purpose, when it was developed, and current problems and solutions for which the group is being asked to provide advice or investigate.
8. Identify a practice barrier for an advanced practice nurse and identify a policy solution to address the barrier.

E-RESOURCES

- Agency for Healthcare Research and Quality (AHRQ): Building Relationships Between Clinical Practices and the Community to Improve Care, Literature Review, and Environmental Scan. http://innovations.ahrq.gov/linkages/report2.aspx

- American Nurses Association: Advocacy-Becoming More Effective. http://www.nursingworld.org/AdvocacyResourcesTools
- *An Environmental Scan of Self-Direction in Behavioral Health: Summary of Major Findings.* Chestnut Hill, MA: National Resource Center for Participant-Directed Services, 2013. http://www.bc.edu/content/dam/files/schools/gssw_sites/nrcpds/BH%20Scan/Summary_Scan%20of%20SD%20in%20BH_May2013.pdf
- National Highway Traffic Safety Administration (NHTSA) Community How to Guide: Needs Assessment and Strategic Planning for Underage Drinking Prevention. http://www.nhtsa.gov/people/injury/alcohol/Community%20Guides%20HTML/Book2_NeedsAssess.html

REFERENCES

American Nurses Association. (2008). *Adapting standards of care under extreme conditions: Guidance for professionals during disaster, pandemics, and other extreme emergencies.* Silver Spring, MD: Author.

American Nurses Association. (2011). The *doctor of nursing practice: Advancing the nursing profession.* [Position Statement]. Silver Spring, MD: Author.

American Nurses Association. (2013). *Conducting a political environmental scan.* Silver Spring, MD: Author.

APRN Consensus Work Group & the National Council of State Boards of Nursing APRN Advisory Committee. (2008, July 7). Consensus model for APRN regulation: Licensure, accreditation, certification & education. Retrieved from https://www.ncsbn.org/Consensus_Model_for_APRN_Regulation_July_2008.pdf

Cohen, S., & Muench, U. (2012). Nursing testimony before Congress, 1993-2011. *Policy Politics Nursing Practice, 13*(3), 170-178.

Institute of Medicine. (2011). *The future of nursing: Leading change, advancing health, report recommendations.* Washington, DC: National Academies Press.

Kingdon, J. W. (2011). *Agendas, alternatives, and public policies* (Update 2nd ed.). Glenview, IL: Pearson.

Lurie, N., Dausey, D. J., Knighton, T., Moore, M., Zakowski, S., & Deyton, L. (2008). Community planning for pandemic influenza: Lessons from the VA health care system. *Disaster Medicine and Public Health Preparedness, 2*(4), 251–257.

MDF Training and Consultancy. (2005). *MDF Tool. Environmental scan.* Retrieved from http://assets.sportanddev.org/downloads/environmental_scan.pdf

Mind Tools Ltd. (2007–2011). *SWOT analysis worksheet.* Retrieved from http://www.mindtools.com/pages/article/worksheets/SWOTAnalysisWorksheet.pdf

Needlestick Safety and Prevention Act of 2000. Pub. L. 106-430.

O'Dell, G. J., Aspy, D. J., Jarousse, L. A., & American Hospital Association (AHA). (2013). 2014 American Hospital Association environmental scan. *Trustee, 66*(8), 15–17, 19–22, 24–25 passim.

Patient Protection and Affordable Care Act (PPACA) of 2010. Pub. L. 111-148, 124 Stat. 119.

Pohl, J. M., Hanson, C., Newland, J. A., & Cronenwett, L. (2010). Unleashing nurse practitioners' potential to deliver primary care and lead teams. *Health Affairs, 29*(5), 900–905.

Public Health Cigarette Smoking Act of 1969. Pub. L. 91-222 (1970).

Sawka, A. M., Gafni, A., Boulos, P., Beattie, K., Papaioannou, A., Cranney, A., Hanley, D. A., Adachi, J. D., Cheung, A., Papdimitropoulos, E. A., & Thabane, L. (2007). Could a policy provision of hip protectors to elderly nursing home residents result in cost saving in acute hip fracture care? The case of Ontario, Canada. *Osteoporosis International, 18*(6), 819-827.

Swart, R. J., Raskin, P., & Robinson, J. (2004). The problem of the future sustainability science and scenario analysis. *Global Environmental Change, 14*, 137–146.

U.S. Department of Health and Human Services. (2012). *Preventing tobacco use among youth and young adults: A report of the Surgeon General.* Atlanta, GA: U.S. Department of Health and Human Services, Centers for Disease Control and Prevention, National Center for Chronic Disease Prevention and Health Promotion, Office on Smoking and Health. 2012. Retrieved from http://www.surgeongeneral.gov/library/reports/preventing-youth-tobacco-use/full-report.pdf

U.S. Department of Health and Human Services (DHHS), Centers for Medicare and Medicaid Services. (2013). The *Durable Medical Equipment, Prosthetics, Orthotics, and Supplies (DMEPOS) Competitive Bidding Program: Traveling Beneficiary* (MLM Matters Fact Sheet, ICN 904484). Retrieved from http://www.nursingworld.org/MLN-Matters-DocumentationDME.pdf

U.S. Department of Health Education and Welfare (USDHEW). (1964). *Smoking and health. Report of the Advisory Committee of the Surgeon General of the Public Health Service. Official Report.* Retrieved from http://profiles.nlm.nih.gov/ps/access/NNBBMQ.pdf

Woods, C. Q. (1996). Evolution of the American Nurses Association's position on health insurance for the aged: 1933–1965. *Nursing Research, 45*(5), 304–310.

FIVE

Harnessing Evidence in the Policy Process

Kathleen M. White

The acquisition of knowledge is the mission of research, the transmission of knowledge is the mission of teaching and the application of knowledge is the mission of public service. —James A. Perkins

OBJECTIVES

1. Describe issues and resources that impact translation of evidence into policy.
2. Analyze the types of evidence that have the potential to influence health policy.
3. Compare and contrast how evidence can be used at both the local level and beyond to influence policy.
4. Advocate for the implementation of policy initiatives based on evidence at different levels of policy making.

The power of harnessing evidence for public policy can be easily traced in nursing from the data collected and analyzed by Florence Nightingale during the Crimean War and her advocacy efforts in the years that followed. Harnessing evidence, in this chapter, implies finding evidence and coupling it at the right times and places in the policy-making process. As illustrated in the lifelong work of Nightingale, the role of finding evidence and using it to make policy change does not always follow a steady course in nursing or in health care in general.

Shortly after Florence Nightingale began her work, President Abraham Lincoln established the National Academy of Sciences (NAS) in 1863 to gather scientific information. It was not until 1930 that the Ransdell Act formalized the establishment of the National Institute of Health (NIH) as a single agency whose research focus was biological and medical issues. In 1948, the singular NIH was renamed to the plural name, the National Institutes of Health we recognize today (Harden, 1998). In 1986, the National Center for Nursing Research (NCNR) was created and then, in 1993, the National Institute of

Nursing Research (NINR) was transitioned to institute status, 130 years after the NAS was established.

Institutionalization of research has not, however, ensured a clear path to policy making. Currently, there is much discussion on policies that were developed and are still operational that did not look at, or in some cases seemed to ignore, strong evidence contrary to the policies. Phrases heard at the big "P" level like "when policy trumps science" and at the little "p" level like "putting sacred cows to pasture" are testimony in common vernacular that attest to the disputes about the use of evidence in policy making. The spectrum of policy making has myriad examples where evidence can be put to better use.

At the big "P" level, policy makers often need help to make sense of evidence and its practical relevance to policy. In response to this need, the Robert Wood Johnson Foundation (RWJF) began a project called the Synthesis Project with the aim of succinctly critiquing and summarizing research findings around health policy questions as opposed to synthesizing evidence on clinical issues. These findings are reported through briefs, podcasts, and/or reports (Colby, Quinn, Williams, Bilheimer, & Goodell, 2008).

At the little "p" level, strict fasting policies prior to surgery like "NPO after 12MN" (Sendelbach, 2010) and restriction in visiting policies in adult intensive care units (Ciufo, Hader, & Holly, 2011) are examples of practice policies that most nurses have experienced firsthand. These clinically focused policies demonstrate the often-found disconnect between research and policy at the local level and the life of their own that policies can develop.

The Policy Challenge illustrates an example of a practice policy that was changed using evidence-based practice (EBP) and outlines how policy can be further evaluated using quality improvement. This voiding before discharge project had guidance from nurses with advanced degrees, showing the potential role of masters- and doctoral-prepared nurses in assisting staff at the local level to connect practice policy to the best evidence. In spite of the seeming simplicity of the example, policy changes of this nature are not always "simple." As discussed next, controversy often surrounds harnessing the evidence.

CONTROVERSY

The tremendous emphasis on use of evidence to inform practice in health care has changed the health care practice environment. Clinicians at all levels and points of care are held accountable to ensure that health care practices are based on the best available evidence. Those involved with policy question why the same attention has not been paid to using health services research to develop policies. Many articles have been written over the past 15 years addressing this question. The titles or phrases in some of those articles indicate the conundrum we face: "The Paradox of Health Services Research: If It Is Not Used, Why Do We Produce So Much of It?" (Lavis et al., 2002), and "How Research Influences Policy Makers: Still Hazy After All These Years" (Green & Seifert, 2005) and,

POLICY CHALLENGE: Changing Practice Using Evidence—Voiding Before Discharge

The nurses in the postanesthesia care units (PACUs) at Johns Hopkins Hospital questioned the long-held policy of routinely requiring patients to void prior to discharge from the PACU. This is a common problem faced by nurses across the country who find that, regardless of the type of surgery or anesthesia delivery, they must hold patients in the PACU until they void. This delay can minimally create backups, extra hours of nonproductive time, increased lengths of stay, and decreased patient satisfaction. Thus, a team with PACU nurses at the center and with support of administration, management, and researchers developed an EBP project based on the questions, "For adult ambulatory surgery patients, does discharge from the PACU prior to voiding versus discharge from the PACU after voiding result in increased urinary retention?" (p. 174).

After settling on the question, the team moved to reviewing the evidence on voiding expectations for adult ambulatory surgery patients. They started looking at the American Society of PeriAnesthesia Nurses (ASPAN) Standards, and when they found no clear guidance they carried out a literature search. Of 100 articles found, 59 articles were examined and 26 were determined to be appropriate for closer examination and review. In addition, the team also checked with PACUs across the country. The policy was changed so that a patient would be assigned a risk level for retention based on the patient's history and type of surgery and anesthesia and then discharged based on the level of risk. Staff education and patient education were rolled out accordingly. Added to the routine follow-up phone calls to patients postdischarge from the PACU was assessment of voiding.

Adapted from Krenzischek, Ares, Lewis, Tanseco, and Newhouse (2007).
See Option for Policy Challenge.

---

finally, a favorite, "Translation of Research to Practice, Why We Can't Just Do It" (Lewis, 2011). These articles and many others suggest that the challenge to evidence-based policy is the gap that exists among the research, policy, and practice worlds.

More recently, the notion of whether evidence-based policy is achievable has been questioned. As noted in earlier chapters as well as in chapters that follow, there are numerous influences on policy, and evidence is not always the most definitive determinant of public health policy (Anderson et al., 2005). Hewison (2008) argues well that EBP cannot and should not be the sole determinant of policy and that too much emphasis on EBP as a basis for policy may detract from nurses developing the full range of competencies needed for policy activism.

Evidence-informed policy has gained considerable attention and the realm of evidence has been greatly expanded to include preferences, political contingencies, and behavioral theory (Lavis, Oxman, Lewin, & Fretheim, 2009; Lewis, 2011). Likewise, the World Health Organization (WHO, 2009) formed an Evidence-Informed Policy Network (EVIPNet) that promotes the use of health research evidence for better decision making and health policy making. EVIPNet defines evidence-informed health policy making as an approach to policy decisions that aims to ensure that decision making is well informed by the best available research evidence. It is characterized by the systematic and transparent access to, and appraisal of, evidence as an input into the policy-making process (WHO, n.d.; www.who.int/evidence/about/en). This assumes that once a policy problem is identified, evidence is obtained, and thus, the relationship between evidence and policy making is linear. Often, policy making is not linear (see Chapter 1, "Leading the Way in Policy"). The complexity of the policy-making process is well documented in the national unfolding of the passage, subsequent debate, and implementation of the Patient Protection and Affordable Care Act (PPACA).

CHALLENGES IN MOVING EVIDENCE INTO POLICY

The important role that research, in particular, plays in improving health care and the development of health care policies has been recognized for some time. Brownson, Royer, Ewing, and McBride (2006) summarily note, "If it was easy, it would have been done by now," referring to the use of research by policy makers. They stated that researchers and policy makers are "travelers in parallel universes." Why are researchers and policy makers thought to be traveling in parallel universes? What are the issues? Policy makers, whether at the big "P" or little "p" level, and researchers often have conflicting roles and needs.

As early as 1979, Caplan sought to explain the issue by suggesting that there are cultural differences between researchers and policy makers, noting these groups have different views of the world. Gaps exist between the two in values, language, reward systems, and professional affiliations; researchers are mainly concerned with pure science and esoteric issues, whereas policy makers are more interested in immediate relevance and have an action orientation.

Another issue is where the responsibility for ensuring the use of or translation of new research into policy and practice lies. The difficulty in identifying or assigning responsibility is explained using technology transfer theory. It is postulated that there is a unidirectional responsibility. There is either a science push or knowledge-driven model where the information flows from researchers to policy makers, resulting in specific policy decisions, or a demand pull or problem-solving model whereby there is a commissioning of information from researchers by policy makers with the intent of addressing a well-defined policy problem.

Published systematic reviews provide strong evidence of numerous barriers in translating research into practice. As a result of these gaps in translating research into practice, researchers have tried to determine (a) what barriers make the gap so hard to bridge and (b) the most effective strategies that help close the gap. To identify the barriers and facilitators to using research in policy making, Innvaer, Vist, Trommald, and Oxman (2002) examined 24 studies, finding that barriers and facilitators to using research for policy making were very similar, but often on different ends of the continuum. For example, personal contact between those carrying out the research and policy makers was found in 13 of 24 studies to facilitate research evidence uptake in designing policy, while the lack of personal contact between these two groups was shown in 11 (of 24) studies to impede the use of research.

A more recent systematic review of the gap between public health policy and evidence, examining 15 qualitative studies and three surveys, found that research evidence was used, but the specificity of its use was unclear (Orton, Lloyd-Williams, Taylor-Robinson, O'Flaherty, & Capewell, 2011). The barriers were similar to some of those found by Innvaer and colleagues (2002); recommendations for strategies to reduce barriers were less clear, and they were not tested. However, the important role of communication between researchers and those using the research was noted in four of the studies (Orton et al., 2011).

In a systematic search of "model" public health laws (i.e., a public health law or private policy that is publicly recommended by at least one organization for adoption by government bodies or by specified private entities), Hartsfield, Moulton, and McKie (2007) identified 107 model public health laws, addressing 16 areas. The most common model laws were for tobacco control, injury prevention, and school health, whereas the least commonly covered topics included hearing, heart disease prevention, public health infrastructure, and rabies control. In only 6.5% of the model laws did the sponsors provide details demonstrating that the law was based on scientific information (e.g., research-based guidelines).

Several initiatives have been developed because of the lack of use of evidence in practice and policy making. In 2002, the NIH initiated a series of consultations with the research community to define major scientific trends that led to the development of the NIH Road Map for Medical Research (Zerhouni, 2003). One of the major themes that emerged from these consultations was the complaint that clinical research was becoming more difficult to conduct and less attractive to new investigators, and that clinician–scientists were moving away from patient-oriented research. This led the NIH Road Map to include the theme, "Re-engineering the Clinical Research Enterprise," in order to initiate the funding of Clinical and Translational Science Awards (CTSAs) for the conduct of original clinical and translational research as part of a full-spectrum biomedical research enterprise (Zerhouni, 2005).

Another major initiative to help "bridge the gap" was developed by the RWJF. This ongoing Synthesis Project focuses on producing briefs, podcasts, and reports that condense complex research for policy makers based on data that showed policy makers had three criteria for research use in policy making: "... translation, accessible and easy-to-use information, and relevance to the policy context" (Colby et al., 2008, p. 1178).

In 2010, the PPACA established the Patient-Centered Outcomes Research Institute (PCORI) within the Centers for Medicare and Medicaid Services (CMS) to evaluate the best available evidence to help people make more informed decisions about their health care (PCORI, n.d.). While each of these initiatives has a different focus, they illustrate the value of evidence and efforts to move it into practice and policy.

TERMINOLOGY

Another key piece in the puzzle to understanding the harnessing of evidence for policy making is that there can be variation in how terminology is used. Different terms have been used to explain the complex process of moving evidence to both practice and policy, with perhaps more attention given to practice. But both practice and policy have their own barriers in moving research and some authors have used the term *valley of death* to illustrate how difficult it may be to cross these gaps between research and practice, as well as research and policy (Meslin, Blasimme, & Cambon-Thomsen, 2013).

One of the most common buzzwords used today is *translational research*, a term originally designed for use in the medical world. It emerged in response to concern over the long time lag between scientific discoveries and changes in treatments, practices, and health policies that incorporate the new discoveries. Rubio and her colleagues (2010), in a search of Medline for an answer as to why research is not used to inform the development of policy practice, found that the term *translational research* appeared as early as 1993, but that there were few references to the term in the 1990s and most were in reference to research about cancer.

However, translational research has different definitions, means different things to different people, and is interpreted differently, but it seems important to almost everyone (Levine, 2007; Naylor, Bowles, McCauley, Maccoy, Maislin, Pauly, Newby, & Webb, 2010; Woolf, 2008). For instance, Woolf (2008) comments that some researchers define it as what occurs from bench to bedside in the development of new drugs, devices, and treatment options for patients, while others view it as "translating research into practice." As seen in this one example, one definition is product driven and the other community and policy focused.

Translational research is further explained in several ways: using new knowledge produced as part of the science of discovery and applying that knowledge to improve health and health care, or the application of new and unproven laboratory discoveries to improve health, or research that explores and develops potential treatments and tests the safety and efficacy of those treatments in randomized controlled trials (RCTs). These definitions of translational research are referred to as T1 translation (White, 2011; Woolf, 2008).

Nursing has also developed definitions associated with translational work. In 2003, the University of Iowa held an invitational conference focused on translation science and nursing's role in translation. A definition of translation research was generated that is widely used in nursing research today. Translation research is "the scientific investigation of methods, interventions, and variables that influence adoption of EBPs by individuals and organizations to improve clinical and operational decision making in health care. This includes testing the effect of interventions on *promoting* and *sustaining* the adoption of EBPs" (Titler, 2004 p. S1).

Because the issue of translation is so important, the NIH established the National Center for Advancing Translational Sciences (NCATS) in 2011. NCATS is not disease or discipline focused. Its purpose, as implied in its name, is the translation of research. Of major interest to the work of this center is policy work. To that end, NCATS has developed the Office of Policy, Communications and Strategic Alliances (OPCSA; www.ncats.nih.gov/about/org/divs-offices/divisions-offices.html), which has dedicated time and resources for this arena. This center and the research agencies mentioned in the chapter's introduction are described in Exhibit 5.1.

Further complicating use of terminology is the confusion existing about the meaning of research, EBP, and quality improvement, and the interplay among them. Many practitioners use these three terms incorrectly. Many nurses in practice today may have had little formal education in all of these processes, and nurses who have had such education may not have adequate opportunity to practice each of these separate but overlapping processes.

EXHIBIT 5.1 SELECTED U.S. HEALTH RESEARCH ENTITIES

AGENCY AND YEAR ESTABLISHED	DESCRIPTION
Agency for Healthcare Research and Quality (AHRQ); 1999	An agency of the U.S. Department of Health and Human Services that oversees health services research. It is complementary to the research mission of the National Institutes of Health. Originally known and established as the Agency for Health Care Policy and Research (AHCPR), it was reauthorized as AHRQ in 1999.
Institute of Medicine (IOM); 1970	Last of four federally authorized independent, nonprofit institutions called the National Academies established to provide expert, unbiased scientific information for health decisions. The other agencies include the National Academy of Sciences, National Academy of Engineering, and the National Research Council.

(continued)

EXHIBIT 5.1 SELECTED U.S. HEALTH RESEARCH ENTITIES *(CONTINUED)*	
National Institutes of Health (NIH); 1948	An agency of the U.S. Department of Health and Human Services that oversees 27 institutes and centers that conduct research to improve health and life including length and decreasing both illness and disability. Link to mission: http://nih.gov/about/mission.htm
National Institute of Nursing Research (NINR); 1993	Originally established as a center in 1986, the mission of this institute is specifically research that increases the health of individuals, families, communities, and populations across the life span.
National Center for Advancing Translational Sciences (NCATS); 2011	This is one of the six centers of the NIH. The center's aims stress novel approaches and outcomes, and using evidence and technology to advance, establish, and publicize improvements in translational science. Its work is meant to complement the research of other NIH institutes and centers.
Office of Policy Communications and Strategic Alliances (OPCSA); 2011	Office within NCATS. Established to analyze translational science issues and work with stakeholders to develop and implement policy solutions based on science. Includes strategic planning, legislative issues, and evaluation for NCATS.
Patient-Centered Outcomes Research Institute (PCORI); 2010	Established as an independent nonprofit organization to conduct research to help patients and their health care providers make decisions based upon the best available evidence about prevention, treatment, and care options that is derived from research guided by patients, caregivers, and the broader health care community.

Evidence-Based Practice

The EBP approach is credited in medicine to Archie Cochrane in the early 1970s and so the term *evidence-based medicine* is often heard. The more generic term EBP is useful as it is not discipline specific. EBP is a problem-solving approach that was designed for practice that includes three major components: the incorporation of best evidence with clinical knowledge and patient preferences and values (Melnyk & Fineout-Overholt, 2005).

To ensure a practice based upon evidence, health care providers are encouraged to use a framework or model to approach the search, critique, and translation of evidence for implementation into practice policy. Many nursing models of EBP are available for guiding practice. The Johns Hopkins Nursing EBP model is defined as "… a problem-solving approach to clinical decision-making within a health care organization that integrates the best available scientific evidence with the best available experiential (patient and practitioner) evidence, considers internal and external influences on practice, and encourages critical thinking in the judicious application of such evidence to care of the individual patient, patient population, or system" (Newhouse, Dearholt, Poe, Pugh, & White, 2007). Three key goals in having an EBP are the following: (a) to ensure that the highest quality of care is provided to achieve the best outcomes for patients; (b) to support rational decision making (including structural changes) that reduces inappropriate variation in care; and (c) to create a culture of critical thinking and ongoing learning that grows a practice environment where evidence supports clinical and administrative decisions (Newhouse, Dearholt, Poe, Pugh, & White, 2005). The highest quality is often assumed to be the biggest and latest finding, but that might not necessarily be the case. And it is just as important to eliminate practices that are no longer valid as it is to institute new practices based on evidence.

An EBP inquiry is performed for many different reasons, but most often it is because nurses are questioning their practices and are concerned about practice outcomes. Some typical reasons why an EBP inquiry is performed include needing improvement for a high-risk, high-cost, and/or high-volume patient problem; negative outcomes are being reported; variations in care are noticeable; policy reviews are being completed; and/or health care team members are aware of new evidence or that their practice is different from the professional or community standard.

The EBP inquiry process, while designed for practice, has more recently been examined as an approach to policy making. Some of the key steps in the EBP movement (searching, critiquing, appraising, and synthesizing evidence) may be helpful to policy makers who are faced with how to find, evaluate, use, or discard scientific information in areas foreign to their background like health care. This problem is aptly called a "research glut and information famine" (Colby et al., 2008). Nurses who are well acquainted with EBP could use its steps to provide policy makers with usable data to guide policy questions and subsequent policy development.

Research

Research is conducted to discover and generate evidence, the generation of knowledge. The need to conduct research can result from an EBP inquiry when the search for evidence has found poor-quality evidence, conflicting evidence, or no evidence to support a practice change. Research as defined by the Office for Human Research Protections (OHRP) at the U.S. Department of Health and Human Services (DHHS 2009) is a systematic investigation, including research development, testing, and evaluation, designed to develop new knowledge or contribute to generalizable knowledge (www.hhs.gov/ohrp/humansubjects/guidance/45cfr46.html). Researchers must complete formal educational training to meet OHRP standards for protection of human subjects and have their research protocols reviewed and approved by their organization's institutional review board (IRB). Report of the research results must include specific protections for confidentiality.

There are generally three types of research that can influence policy: disciplinary research, policy research, and policy analysis (Hinshaw, 2011). Disciplinary research and policy research are particularly important to harnessing evidence. Each is discussed briefly here.

Disciplinary research in nursing, which is often applied in nature, is the type of research most nurses know. Disciplinary research is carried out to provide new knowledge specific to any number of health care fields including but not restricted to nursing. Indeed, many times nurses will draw on other disciplinary research to inform their own work. A strong emphasis is placed nationally and often locally on collaborative research among disciplines. In the Policy Challenge that introduced the chapter, postoperative voiding policies might be informed by disciplinary research from general surgery, anesthesia, or nursing. In the area of disciplinary research there is often a large disconnect with policy and why critiquers of research ask the question, "So what?" Likewise, journal or presentation requirements may ask for "policy implications."

Policy research is conducted with the purpose of appraising policy translation and use in particular settings or situations to determine effectiveness and usefulness. Nursing policy research has not reached its potential. The body of policy research is small in comparison to applied disciplinary research. Policy research is often guided by priorities developed by professional and specialty associations and government agencies. Policy research in nursing is often guided by the priorities. The NINR, for example, has laid out its strategic plan and the themes that will guide the projects they fund. Similarly, associations such as the National Pressure Ulcer Advisory Panel (NPUAP) have made their research priorities for pressure ulcer prevention, treatment, and policy public. These can be found at www.npuap.org/research-priorities-identified-for-pressure-ulcer-prevention-treatment-policy.

Today, leading nurse researchers are having a profound effect on policy development. The research evidence provided by nurses in many arenas is being used to direct management solutions and policy development that benefit patients, nurses, and the employers of nurses. Dorothy Brooten, PhD, RN, FAAN, was an early pioneer in policy research. She examined the impact of advanced practice nurses (APNs) in providing transitional care for very low birth weight (VLBW) infants. Her Quality Cost Model of Advanced Practice Nurses Transitional Care, developed in 1980, was expanded to include other high-risk and high-cost patient groups (women with unplanned cesarean births, high-risk pregnancies, hysterectomy surgery, and elders) to have their care managed by APNs (Brooten et al., 2002).

Policy analysis is carried out to determine how well a policy has realized its intended outcomes and whether it has resulted in unintended outcomes (see Chapter 13, "Evaluating Policy Structures, Processes, and Outcomes"). Policy analysis is often carried out by staff or commissioned by government agencies, organizations, or associations. Policy analysis is a systematic and formal approach that includes using specific criteria to examine and evaluate a policy problem. It involves developing policy alternatives or options, assessing the potential outcomes of each, and making a selection of a preferred alternative from among the proposed choices. The policy analysis process includes specific steps quite familiar to nurses: define the problem, establish evaluation criteria, identify policy choices among alternative solutions, formulate the chosen policy, implement the policy solution, and evaluate the policy. One of the challenges in policy analysis is that it tends to be issue specific, which makes it difficult to identify the nursing contribution. This complexity also makes it more challenging for nurses to understand how they can contribute to policy analysis.

In Policy on the Scene 5.1, a research project was carried out in a community hospital and arose from an everyday clinical question. It involved a clinically based policy that required research to determine the best direction for policy formulation. The example is illustrative as it demonstrates where nurses returning to school for advanced degrees can use their new skills in leading teams investigating these little "p" issues. These little "p" initiatives are often carried out based on the immediacy of a clinical problem.

Quality Improvement

Quality improvement is a process designed to evaluate systems and clinical processes with the primary purpose of improving health care quality and health

---

POLICY ON THE SCENE 5.1: Evidence Lacking for Policy Change: Doing Research in a Community Hospital

The nursing staff at a community hospital questioned a manufacturer's new recommendation that bedside blood glucose testing did not have to follow the two-drop method previously used in practice. The two-drop method for testing blood glucose required the first drop of blood obtained by fingerstick to be wiped away; a second drop of blood was to be used for the blood glucose test. When the nurses were informed that this was no longer necessary, they wanted to search the evidence to see why the long-held procedure had been changed. After an exhaustive search, no evidence was found in support for or against making this practice change, so a research study was designed to determine whether there is a clinically significant difference in the blood glucose value between the first and second drop of blood obtained by fingerstick in the hospital setting. One hundred bedside glucose tests were performed using both the first drop and the second drop obtained. The data supported using the one-drop method. The policy was changed and the nurses embraced the policy change.

care outcomes for a specific health care organization and its client population. Evaluating these processes usually involves small tests of local changes to the organization's health care delivery. The intent of quality improvement work is to describe and share lessons learned rather than demonstrating a cause and effect to create generalizable knowledge. In quality improvement efforts, the patient is expected to benefit directly (Newhouse, Pettit, Poe, & Rocco, 2006; Reinhardt & Ray, 2003; Shirey et al., 2011).

One final comment should be made here. There are types of quality improvement efforts that are considered to be research and become subject to OHRP standards and regulations. When quality improvement projects involve introducing an untested clinical intervention for the purposes of improving the quality of care or also collecting information about patient outcomes for the purpose of establishing scientific evidence to determine how well the intervention achieves its intended results, it is considered research. For example, if a multihospital system implements a medication reconciliation procedure with the expressed purpose of reducing medical prescription errors and then collects prescription drug information from the medical record, this would constitute quality improvement that would be subject to OHRP standards and regulations because the system is trying to determine if medication prescription errors have decreased as predicted because of the new procedure. While there may be overlap or lack of clarity in what constitutes research, EBP, or quality improvement, it is important that clinicians have human subjects protection training so that they are familiar with OHRP standards and their own organization's policies. Furthermore, IRBs at different facilities may view protocols and the application of regulations differently. Therefore, it is best to address issues of human subjects protection early in the planning process, well in advance of any data collection procedures. This is particularly important when collaborating across several institutions.

As can be seen in several of these definitions, the connection to policy is not overt, so the term *implementation science* has come into use. This is the study of approaches that support the incorporation of evidence and research findings into both health care policy and practice. Implementation science involves addressing the "complexity and systems of care, individual practitioners, senior leadership, and ultimately changing health care cultures to promote an evidence-based practice environment" (Titler, 2010). Implementing evidence-based policies involves understanding what strategies work and are most effective in a particular care setting.

EVERY NURSE'S ROLE IN TRANSLATING EVIDENCE INTO POLICY

Translating evidence into policy (and practice) involves communicating the new evidence to decision makers in a way that is both understandable and useful. But once again, differing terms are often encountered in describing the process of translation. The term *knowledge transfer* is also used. Knowledge transfer is defined as a systematic approach to capture, collect, and share tacit knowledge in order for it to become explicit knowledge so that individuals and/ or organizations can access and utilize essential information, which previously was known intrinsically to only one person or a small group of people (Graham et al., 2006). Another term, *diffusion*, refers to a broad process whereby knowledge or evidence is communicated throughout an organization or a larger system. Finally, the term *dissemination*, which is used frequently in the translation literature, refers to communicating knowledge or evidence in journals, at conferences, or through some other media. The discussion of the nurses' role in translation will refer to multiple avenues of communication.

The translation of evidence into health care practice and policy faces multiple challenges. Those challenges are found throughout the health care system with individual providers, or teams of providers, at the organizational level and both public and private organizations at the local, state, and national levels, such as professional organizations and governmental agencies.

It is important for all health care professionals to use evidence to make informed decisions about practice and policy, and yet we know this does not happen consistently. An often-cited study by McGlynn and colleagues (2003) found that adults in the United States received less than 55% of recommended care; children receive 46.5% of recommended care in ambulatory settings (Mangione-Smith et al., 2007). Brownson, Chriqui, and Stamatakis (2009) found that of the 10 great public health achievements of the 20th century, only 6.5% of the sponsors of these achievements cited research evidence to promote their value. Other studies have shown that policy makers infrequently use evidence from research or synthesized evidence in systematic reviews (Lavis et al., 2002; Oxman, Lavis, & Fretheim, 2007). In many organizations (e.g., health departments, clinics, hospitals, and educational programs) internal data and benchmarks are only used when data may be available at a regional, state, or national level. Using internal data may, however, result in false reassurance about the effectiveness of a program. Internal data from a project, while useful, may not necessarily be subject to the rigor of external peer review.

Translation of evidence to practice and policy requires that attention be directed toward decreasing barriers to evidence adoption and that the factors that facilitate adoption are enhanced. For instance, consideration needs to focus on communicating evidence in a timely and relevant manner, responding to needs of the health care profession or organization, and presenting findings in a user-friendly manner easily understandable to decision makers.

Good examples of translation of evidence to policy do exist. Seat belt laws that have been proven to save lives are present in 49 states, the District of Columbia, and many U.S. territories. New Hampshire is the only state without such legislation. Strong evidence exists for wearing motorcycle and bicycle helmets to decrease injuries from accidents. Legislation for motorcycle helmets has been passed in 47 states, but not always with the same requirements.

Nineteen states require helmets for all riders and the other 28 require helmets for only certain riders. Bicycle helmet legislation has only been passed in 21 states; however, many localities have passed bicycle helmet legislation for their communities. Tobacco control legislation is similar in that legislation continues to be passed in many U.S. jurisdictions, but the uptake or passage of this legislation takes different formats due to local social, cultural, and economic factors. In many of these areas, nurses have made substantial contributions to the research evidence.

Translation of injury prevention guidelines for health care workers in the United States has also shown widespread uptake, as both state and organizational policy known as Safe Patient Handling and Mobility. Similarly, with the increased focus on quality and safety in health care organizations, high-quality research has shown that preoperative shaving increases postoperative infections in surgical patients. Health care organizations have widely accepted and adopted no preoperative shaving policies, and it has become a reportable measure of quality for health care organizations, at both the state level and nationally.

Professional organizations have also participated in the translation of evidence to policy through promulgation of position statements and clinical practice guidelines (CPGs). The professional organizations bring together panels of experts to review, appraise, and synthesize evidence about a professional issue or a disease condition or symptom management in order to make current practice recommendations to their membership and the health care community at large. These recommendations may be published in journals or posted on websites, and have been adopted at all levels of policy making (organizational, state, and national). They may also be submitted to the National Guideline Clearinghouse, a searchable website hosted by AHRQ (www.guideline. gov). Safe Patient Handling and Mobility is an example of how organizations are promoting policies based upon evidence (see Chapter 2, "Advocating for Nurses and for Health"). The identification of this problem started with professional organizations and moved through other levels of policy development at the organizational, state, and national levels, involving both the private sector (e.g., businesses, nongovernmental organizations [NGOs]) and government agencies. Let us now look more in depth at examples of the translation of research at the federal, state, local, and organizational policy levels.

Federal Level

A widely cited example of the translation of nursing research to policy can be found in the PPACA. There is strong evidence showing that hospital readmissions can be significantly reduced and the quality of care for patients can be improved by implementing a program that targets transitions of care. The Community-Based Care Transitions Program (CCTP) under the auspices of the CMS (CMS, n.d.), created by Section 3026 of the

PPACA, tests models for improving care transitions from the hospital to other settings and reducing readmissions for high-risk Medicare beneficiaries. The goals of the CCTP are to improve transitions of beneficiaries from the inpatient hospital setting to other care settings, to improve quality of care, to reduce readmissions for high-risk beneficiaries, and to document measurable savings to the Medicare program (innovation.cms.gov/initiatives/CCTP/?itemID=CMS1239313; Naylor, Bowles, McCauley, Maccoy, Maislin, Pauly, & Krakauer, 2013).

Nurse researcher Dr. Mary Naylor worked with Dorothy Brooten, mentioned earlier in this chapter, and developed one of the CCTP models. Naylor's Transitional Care Model (TCM), a translation of an evidence-based strategy into a practice delivery model, uses APNs with specialized training to care for older adults with multiple chronic conditions and support their family caregivers (Naylor et al., 2013).

Testing the TCM has demonstrated significant and sustained outcomes including avoiding hospital readmissions and emergency room visits for primary and coexisting conditions, improvements in health outcomes after discharge, enhancement in patient and family caregiver satisfaction, and reductions in total health care costs (Naylor et al., 2013). The outcomes of transitional care interventions have been evaluated with the goal of providing guidance for the implementation of transitional care programs under the PPACA (Naylor, Aiken, Kurtzman, Olds, & Hirschman, 2011). In addition to the TCM being included in the PPACA, Aetna has adopted the TCM to achieve better outcomes for its older adult enrollees with multiple chronic problems, AARP has recommended expansion of the services of the TCM to its members, and the National Quality Forum endorsed deployment of evidence-based transitional care such as the TCM as one of 25 national preferred practices for care coordination.

State Level

States are pursuing a variety of strategies for getting the research and analytical assistance they need, including expanding their relationships with university-based health services research and policy analysis programs. These collaborations raise a number of questions about the fit between states' analytic needs and universities' interests and capacity, as well as the appropriate role of the university research organization in the often highly politicized state environment (Coburn, 1998). The Maryland Hospital Hand Hygiene Collaborative and the Michigan Keystone ICU Project are examples of two successful collaborative efforts.

The Maryland Health Quality and Cost Council (2013), created in 2007 by executive order and subsequent legislation, focuses on implementing evidence-based strategies to improve health outcomes. The Maryland Hospital Hand Hygiene Collaborative began in 2010 with the goal of reducing preventable infections through better hand hygiene. The Collaborative is a voluntary, statewide effort led by the Maryland Patient Safety Center (MPSC) with support from the Maryland Hospital Association and the Delmarva Foundation, in partnership with the Maryland Health Quality and Cost Council and the Maryland Department of Health and Mental Hygiene. The Collaborative involves the use of trained observers to collect hand hygiene compliance observations for health care providers on entry and/or exit from the patient environment for adult and pediatric inpatient units and critical care units. To fully participate in the Collaborative, "hospitals must have 80% of their required units reporting with 30 or more observations; this is known as the 80/30 rule" (Maryland Health Quality and Cost Council, 2013). After three years of intensive monitoring and improvement campaigns, the MPSC reported in June 2014 that they have reached an average compliance rate of 90% for all Maryland hospitals (MPSC, personal communication, June 30, 2014). They continue to monitor and hope to better that mark.

Another well-known and published translation of evidence to practice and policy at the state level was established by the Michigan Health and Hospital Association Keystone Center for Patient Safety and Quality. This Michigan statewide safety initiative is known as the Michigan Keystone ICU Project. Michigan hospitals with adult ICU beds were asked to implement an evidence-based intervention to reduce the incidence of catheter-related bloodstream infections (CRBSIs). Data were obtained from 67 hospitals, representing 1,625 beds or 85% of all ICU beds in Michigan. The statewide initiative resulted in a large and sustained reduction (up to 66%) in CRBSI rates that were maintained throughout the 18-month study period (Pronovost et al., 2006). Similar statewide evidence-based safety collaboratives have been implemented in over 40 states.

Local Level

On a local level and a public–private collaborative, the city of Baltimore has an initiative called B'more for Healthy Babies (BHB) that was designed to improve the quality of care provided by physicians, nurses, social workers, and others who work with pregnant and postpartum women and has helped all home visiting programs in Baltimore to transition to evidence-based models of care. The BHB Initiative is sponsored by the Office of the Mayor of Baltimore, the Baltimore City Health Department, and the Family League of Baltimore City, Inc., with catalytic funding from CareFirst BlueCross BlueShield and other donors. One major program is an evidence-based strategy called the BHB sleep initiative: Alone. Back. Crib. (www.healthybabiesbaltimore. com). The BHB sleep initiative has distributed culturally sensitive video materials to more than 120 sites to educate families on proper evidence to prevent crib deaths. The initiative has developed a poster that features one of the Baltimore Ravens football players providing the evidence for Alone. Back. Crib. (see Figure 5.1).

Although a direct correlation between the initiation of BHB and the drop in the infant mortality rate (IMR) cannot be made, the Baltimore IMR has dropped 3 years in a row following the initiation of the BHB sleep initiative in 2009; in 2012 the rate dropped to 9.7, the first time Baltimore's IMR dropped below 10.0 (Office of Governor Martin O'Malley, 2013). However, the African American IMR rate, while declining from 14.5 in 2011 to 12.6 in 2012, indicates that additional work needs to be done in this community (Office of Governor Martin O'Malley, 2013) (see Chapter 14, "Eliminating Health Inequities Through Policy, Nationally and Globally").

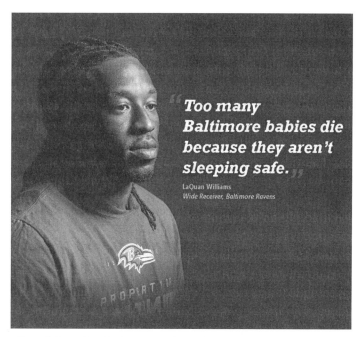

Most infant deaths happen when a baby sleeps with someone else in a bed or on a sofa.

As a dad, it's my job to protect my child. The safest way for your baby to sleep is alone, on his or her back, in an empty crib. Babies can suffocate if they sleep with an adult or another child, or if they sleep with blankets or pillows. Tell everyone who takes care of your baby that you want your baby to

SLEEP SAFE—Alone. Back. Crib. No exceptions.

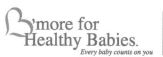

For more information, visit
www.HealthyBabiesBaltimore.com
www.facebook.com/bmoreforhealthybabies

FIGURE 5.1 Alone. Back. Crib. No exceptions.

Reprinted with permission from Baltimore City Health Department.

Organizational Level

At the organizational level, there are many examples of translation of evidence into practice and policy, and often these are different types of translations because of the origins of their evidence. Two of these are illustrated in the Policy Challenge and Policy on the Scene 5.1 that appear on the preceding pages. Strong evidence exists on the health hazards of smoking. Translating that evidence in organizations has offered specific challenges and great opportunities to an organization. The University of Arkansas for Medical Sciences, Healthy Arkansas, and the Arkansas Department of Health developed an evidence-based approach to creating a Smoke-Free Workplace and a Smoke-Free Hospital Tool Kit: A Guide for Implementing Smoke-Free Policies aimed at three audiences: employers, health care providers, and community members (Sheffer, n.d.). The tool kit recommends that a comprehensive smoke-free workplace implementation needs to include a policy, a timeline, training, a communication plan for a smoke-free message, assistance with smoking cessation for employees and patients, and a plan for ongoing support of the implementation (www.uams.edu/coph/reports/smokefree_toolkit/Hospital%20Toolkit%20Text.pdf). The guide suggests that smoke-free policies should include purpose, definition, facilities and areas affected, use of those facilities by outside parties, patient and visitor smoking, tobacco sales on campus, progressive counseling and enforcement, available smoking cessation programs, breaks, and smokeless tobacco use.

Another example of an organization-wide translation, resulting from strong, high-quality evidence, is the implementation of policies regarding the wearing of artificial nails for direct caregivers in the hospital setting. In 2002, the Centers for Disease Control and Prevention (CDC, 2002) published *Guideline for Hand Hygiene in Healthcare Settings*, recommending that health care workers not wear artificial fingernails or extenders when having direct contact with patients at high risk, such as in intensive care units, transplant units, or operating rooms. It should be noted that Elaine Larson, PhD, RN, FAAN, CIC, who has conducted extensive research on hand hygiene, was a member of the two major committees (CDC Hospital Infection Control Practices Advisory Committee and the Hand Hygiene Task Force) that authored the hand hygiene. Each year since 2007, The Joint Commission (TJC, 2014) has published National Patient Safety Goals that include a goal to reduce the risk of health care–associated infection and with specification that health care organizations must comply with current CDC or WHO hand hygiene guidelines. Additionally, many nursing specialty organizations have also endorsed the utilization and translation of the evidence in the form of CPGs. The Association of Operating Room Nurses recommends that acrylic (artificial) nails should not be worn, providing rationale that numerous studies validate the increased number of bacteria cultured from the fingertips of persons wearing artificial nails, both before and after hand washing.

Another opportunity for translation at the organizational level is to ensure that policies and procedures are based on the best available evidence. This opportunity to question current evidence or seek out new evidence arises frequently when there is a need to develop a new policy or procedure or during the annual review of current policies and procedures. Not all policies will need to be reviewed with an extensive evidence-based protocol; it is necessary to consider other influencing factors, like other initiatives that may be taking place, along with an assessment of the priority of policy needing to be changed. This assessment may come from a number of sources; for example, quality data, new knowledge, or staffing issues in implementing a policy.

Knowing how to find evidence is a vital skill set. It is important for nurses with advanced education to have these skills in order to guide and mentor others in finding evidence resources. Finding evidence can be a daunting experience regardless of your background. While there are numerous resources available, all policy issues will not have adequate data to inform policy, and access to resources may be limited. When working in a clinical agency with electronic health records, access to the evidence used for the clinical decision-making tools provided with the software may be available. A nursing program's library resources may vary from those where you have been employed. Listing these resources is beyond the scope of this book, but a good overview of resources can be found at many academic and hospital library home pages. A medical librarian is an invaluable member of a team when searching for evidence. The library at the University of Rochester provides an example of resources and explanation of resources that can be found online (see Tools for Nursing Research—Finding the Evidence at www.urmc.rochester.edu/libraries/williams/electronic_resources/NursingResearchEBP.cfm).

However, there are many other examples when health care practices are questioned in organizations and the quality, quantity, and consistency of evidence is not available to make a practice change. In these cases and many others, it is necessary for the organization to generate its own evidence to support practice decisions in the form of quality improvement or research. Policy on the Scene 5.2 shows interprofessional collaboration and how answering one question on policy may lead to another.

STRATEGIES FOR DISSEMINATION OF EVIDENCE

Carrying out evidence-based research or quality improvement is not complete if the work is not disseminated and the policy implications explicated. Often, however, dissemination is not given consideration, especially at the level of the little "p," until someone outside of the project hears about it and encourages dissemination. Dissemination should be part of the early planning of projects. Seasoned researchers in particular know the value of developing

> ## POLICY ON THE SCENE 5.2: What Are the Risks and Benefits of Frenotomy Performed on Newborns to Treat Ankyloglossia?
>
> This is an example of an EBP question raised by the nursing staff and was a practice question of concern to their physician colleagues. Ankyloglossia or tongue tie occurs in about 4.6% of newborns who are usually unable to breastfeed properly due to severe nipple discomfort and failure to latch on adequately. Frenotomy can be performed before discharge to improve breastfeeding outcomes. The interprofessional team reviewed the literature and found that there was limited strong research evidence to promote performing frenotomy. However, the review raised the awareness of treatment options for ankyloglossia when it is diagnosed in the newborn. This provides an example of nurses questioning practice, generation of limited evidence (quality and quantity), inability to implement clear practice change, and the need for a research study to assess the effects of early ankyloglossia detection, early frenotomy, and how this affects the infant's breastfeeding.
>
> Adapted from Dixon and White (2012).

dissemination plans from the earliest planning of a project and being cognizant of dissemination opportunities that may develop as a project develops. To effectively harness evidence for policy, there must be some method of dissemination.

Over time, authors have identified key determinants and strategies that can guide translation of evidence to policy makers (Grimshaw, Eccles, Lavis, Hill, & Squires, 2012; Jacobson et al., 2003; Lavis, Posada, Haines, & Osei, 2004). Four major elements that are basic to messaging in general and to researchers conveying messages about evidence they have harnessed are knowing and selecting your audience, selecting dissemination techniques, understanding that context matters, and providing communication that is timely, relevant, understandable, and practical. Although listed as separate elements, there is overlap. The type of audience you select will influence what method you use to communicate your evidence. The immediacy of the evidence to a problem at hand is likely to influence how quickly and widespread you will want to convey your work.

Know Your Audience

Choosing dissemination strategies involves identifying and knowing the audience who needs to be involved in the translation. Identifying those with something to gain and something to lose is critical to the planning (Weston, White,

& Peterson, 2013). Also see Chapter 7, "Building Capital: Intellectual, Social, Political, and Financial," and Chapter 10, "Working With the Media: Shaping the Health Policy Process."

At a minimum, evidence from projects needs to be shared across an organization, and wider audiences should be routinely sought out. As you strategically plan for dissemination, consider who within your organization should be informed about the project: patients, professional colleagues, staff, managers, and/or administration. Outside the organization, consider if your audience is local, national, and/or international; you will also need to consider who you should target. It may be that your results have bearing across a number of audiences including lay audiences.

Often you choose to disseminate your evidence to predetermined stakeholders who are decision makers or who are strongly influential in the issue at hand. Clinicians, administrators, researchers, and lay audiences may all be important stakeholders. In policy analysis and later during the translation of evidence to policy, it is important to perform a stakeholder analysis. A stakeholder analysis identifies those that may influence success of your project either positively or negatively, allows you to anticipate their influence, and provides you the opportunity to get the most effective support for the project and address barriers to implementation early on in the translation. There are key steps in any stakeholder analysis (see Chapter 6, "Setting the Agenda").

Early research into understanding audiences and targeting interventions to them focused on the appropriateness and efficacy of specific interventions showed there was considerable lack of knowledge about which strategies work best for different audiences. Research on the translation of research into practice initiatives funded by the AHRQ indicates that the most commonly used intervention to translate evidence to the relevant audience was educational (Farquhar, Stryer, & Slutsky, 2002). However, educational materials (distribution of recommendations for clinical care, CPGs, audiovisual materials, and electronic publications) and didactic educational meetings (such as lectures) have been shown to be the least effective ways to reach an audience (Bero et al., 1998).

More recently, Yuan and colleagues (2010) reviewed four national campaigns designed to disseminate evidence for practice policy improvement and developed a *Blueprint for Effective Strategies in the Dissemination of Evidence-Based Practice Through a National Quality Campaign* (see Exhibit 5.2). In proposing these strategies, the authors stated that the existing literature was not able to evaluate which of these eight strategies are most important and if any subset is sufficient. This supports previous work suggesting that dissemination strategies for uptake of evidence should be multifaceted even when aimed at a single audience.

EXHIBIT 5.2	BLUEPRINT FOR EFFECTIVE STRATEGIES IN THE DISSEMINATION OF EVIDENCE-BASED PRACTICE THROUGH A NATIONAL QUALITY CAMPAIGN

Strategy 1: Highlight evidence base and relative simplicity of recommended practices

Strategy 2: Align the campaign with the strategic goals of the adopting organizations

Strategy 3: Increase recruitment by integrating opinion leaders into the enrollment process and employing a nodal organizational structure

Strategy 4: Form a coalition of credible campaign sponsors

Strategy 5: Generate a threshold of participating organizations that maximizes network exchanges

Strategy 6: Develop practical implementation tools and guides for key stakeholder groups

Strategy 7: Create networks to foster learning opportunities

Strategy 8: Incorporate monitoring and evaluation of milestones and goals

Reprinted with permission from Yuan et al. (2010).

Select Dissemination Techniques

Once you have determined who your audience will be, then it is also important to consider what method or methods of communication will be used to disseminate your evidence. The audience and purpose will be vital to knowing how you disseminate your evidence. There are numerous other types of dissemination that should be considered and several of these (e.g., press releases and white papers) are discussed in Chapter 10. Often dissemination is not a singular act. If, for example, you have an article selected for a major publication or a premier research conference, you may want to consider a press release for the local newsletter of an association or for work, as well as submitting the release to the local paper or even a letter to the congressional representative.

Researchers may only think of journal articles and peer-reviewed presentations for purposes of dissemination. However, venues do not often reach policy makers and often the policy implications are not often called for or discussed in articles. Thus, a caveat to consider is how you can meaningfully discuss policy implications in the venue you have selected, or consider using venues that routinely consider policy implications of research as a requirement for the work, or consider writing a policy article with the research findings providing the evidence. Finally, consider whether the professional dissemination you have planned (e.g., poster or article) lends itself to its own publicity. Consider working with your marketing department to highlight work that has received acclaim by being accepted or by being published in a major venue.

To help in the consideration of avenues for disseminating one's work, consider whether the evidence lends itself to the written or oral format or both. Often, a combination of dissemination modalities may be considered and often it is helpful to convey your findings. Besides formal posters at professional organizations, consider displaying a poster exhibited at a conference in a public spot at work so that colleagues and administrators or lay audiences

EXHIBIT 5.3 DISSEMINATION BEYOND ARTICLES

- Classroom presentations
- Fact sheets
- Newsletters
- Pamphlets
- Posters
- Public meetings; for example, school board meetings and support groups
- Reports (technical or research)
- Social media sites
- Town halls
- Webpages
- Workshops

or students may be exposed to it. Exhibit 5.3 lists some examples of venues to consider for presenting evidence.

A unique way of dissemination was used by a small 100-bed community hospital. The shared governance council for research suggested that a continuing education program be offered based on the numerous presentations that had been done internally at annual research days and externally at peer-reviewed conferences to share the peer-reviewed presentations that the RNs of the hospital made (R. Ludwick, personal communication, November 24, 2013). With the efforts of organizational development and the director of nursing research, a PowerPoint presentation was developed and posted on the Internet that was freely accessible to all staff. Completing the continuing education program embedded in the PowerPoint presentation provided the nurses with one continuing education contact hour. The PowerPoint presentation provided an introduction to research, EBP projects, and quality, and then was followed by 17 abstracts and electronic poster versions of each project. Many of these projects were carried out on one unit, but had the potential to be incorporated across several others. Bedside shift report, for example, was an EBP project that was piloted in the step-down unit, but it spread to other units. The exposure to nurses and the managers across units can help spread policy uptake as well as recognize nurses' work.

Context Matters

It is critical to recognize and understand the social, political, economic, historical, ethical, and legal contexts and other forces in the environment, both facilitating and constraining, that are present in any effort to integrate evidence into policy and practice. How do we increase the use of evidence for policy making among health care professionals and nurses specifically? There are several strategies. First is attempting to understand how nurses and other health professionals receive, critique, and adopt evidence for practice and policy change. Research into how adoption occurs, known as diffusion of innovations, is manifested in different ways because of organizational and individual factors and how decisions to adopt are made. Researchers have identified five categories of adopters differentiated by their speed and acceptance of change: innovators, early adopters, early majority, late majority, and laggards (Greenhalgh, Robert, Macfarlane, Bate, & Kyriakidou 2004; Rogers, 2003).

Likewise, identify which organizational factors that play a role in facilitating translating evidence and innovations into practice and policy are present and can be counted on to assist in the translation process. These factors include an organizational structure that facilitates communication and relationships, strong involvement by senior leadership; effective clinical leadership and interprofessional team practice; organizational culture supportive of learning and inquiry; and resources, expertise, and infrastructure to support evidence acquisition, appraisal, change implementation, and management.

Another strategy to identify the barriers for the uptake of evidence to change practice and create policies is based on evidence. Murthy and colleagues (2012) listed obstacles that health systems face when dealing with a large volume of research evidence and the difficulties they have adapting evidence to the local setting. They suggest that a practical intervention might be to develop an organization's summaries of systematic reviews to improve the accessibility of findings. In addition, on the local level, organizations should consider employing a specialist to synthesize evidence to inform local decision making. The authors concluded that if the message is relatively clear and simple that passive dissemination of the evidence can work.

Context also matters at the big "P" level. Policy makers want to know research findings that have policy implications for their constituents. When providing information about new evidence that supports a policy change, the communication should be in plain language and include how many constituents may be affected by the change.

Communicating Research Should Not Be Rocket Science

When asked what they needed in order to use evidence for decision making, policy makers identified three needs for use of research evidence in the development of policy: a clear translation of the information that is relevant to their needs, information that is available and accessible when needed, and information that is presented in user-friendly format (Colby et al., 2008; Innvaer et al., 2002). Thus, like many of us in everyday life, we want material that tells us what we need to know and makes the information easy to obtain. Because the language of research itself can be complex and researchers talk among themselves using research language, it is easy to forget about other audiences and talk in research terms that are not well understood outside of research communities. A similar phenomenon can be seen in our overuse and complexity of "medical speak" with patients.

The evidence message must be clearly stated, timely, relevant, and responsive. Frequently, when evidence is needed, it is not readily accessible or available to those who need it. Or, if the information is available, the evidence message is not described in a way that resonates with those targeted to receive the message.

Data supporting the importance of adopting new evidence into practice and policy can help propel decision makers to act (Bradley et al., 2004). Select data points or "killer numbers" for use in the messaging as appropriate. Today's dynamic environment requires that effectiveness data are included whenever possible. As many have experienced, if new evidence is going to be adopted, something else might have to be given up, such as an old way of doing things. Making the "business case" for the translation of evidence to practice and policy, such as any financial or administrative data to accompany the clinical evidence, might motivate an otherwise complacent decision maker.

In order to convey the message, it is critical to have a well-thought-out and comprehensive communication plan that allows you to "tell your story." What communication media will be used? Will there be different messages for different media presentations? To increase the success of the translation, know what is newsworthy in the environment (organizational, local, state, or national) (see Chapter 10).

The plan should design messages that fit the audience or different audiences. For example, presentation to a large audience might include a Power-Point presentation or a video. Equally important is the 30-second sound bite or elevator speech that is designed to be given in the 30 seconds that you have as you run into an essential stakeholder in the hallway or at a meeting.

In summary, when considering the development of the message, a challenge arises to identify the key messages for different audiences and to present them in the appropriate understandable format. Unfortunately, journal articles and research reports are written for researchers, not decision makers. However, there are several formats that are used to communicate evidence depending on the needs of the audience. As the message is crafted, it is important to inform, not inundate.

Too often the dissemination of evidence into practice and policy is hampered by inadequate presentation of the new information. The goal of translating evidence into practice and policy requires first that the new evidence is synthesized into usable information in a readable format for decision makers. There are several understandable and reader-friendly formats that are used to communicate new research evidence to decision makers, health care practitioners, and the public. At a local level, one method of conveying information that many across clinical systems are familiar is an SBAR (situation, background, assessment, and recommendation). The same approach can be used to show why a policy change is needed and what evidence exists for the change.

Decision makers are often besieged with information and have very little time to stay abreast of changes in current research or emerging evidence that could be of great use. They are interested in short, easily skimmed, and policy-focused information that focuses on the evidence findings, rather than all the research methods. Up-to-date systematic reviews, or other syntheses of research findings, facilitate the communication of evidence to inform decision makers. A systematic review is used to identify, select, appraise, and synthesize existing research on a specific topic. Systematic reviews can be found in the peer-reviewed literature indexed in familiar databases such as the Cumulative Index to Nursing and Allied Health Literature (CINAHL) or Medline, or at repositories developed for evidence such as the Cochrane Library (2013) or the Joanna Briggs Institute. The purpose of writing a systematic review is to identify, judge, and synthesize all the observed evidence that meets prespecified criteria in order to answer a given research question. The author of the review uses explicit methods aimed at minimizing bias in order to produce more reliable findings that can be used to inform decision making. However, even systematic reviews are criticized because the content of evidence resources is often not enough for the needs of the decision makers as many of these reviews focus on the strength and validity of evidence rather than its applicability. To be useful, the systematic review must clearly state its research question and not only describe the synthesis methods, but also include a discussion of the intervention and any recommendations made. However, in a systematic review on how to improve use of systematic reviews by policy makers, it was concluded from eight studies that there was not strong evidence to support using a singular best approach to develop awareness and knowledge of the new evidence (Murthy et al., 2012). Thus, while systematic reviews can play a role in policy making, their potential use needs further exploration and development for wider adoption by policy makers.

OPTION FOR POLICY CHALLENGE

The policy about voiding was successful. No problems of retention were identified in the routine follow-up phone calls and no patients were found who had been seen in the emergency department for distention. Like many projects of this nature that are successful, further options could be considered. An additional approach to consider after a policy change of this nature is to establish a quality improvement project to measure if the change in policy had any effect on outcomes. Quality data could also be collected. Administrative data could be requested and examined to detect changes in PACU length of stay or cost of care. Additionally, patient satisfaction data could be used to detect any increase or decrease in satisfaction among patients, family, and providers caring for these patients.

This case was then disseminated as noted in the citation (Krenzischek et al., 2007). This account of evidence on voiding for policy was presented as an illustration to ASPAN. It served as an example for ASPAN as it established its EBP model (Krenzischek).

A common dissemination tool specific to policy is a "policy brief." A policy brief is a succinct presentation of an issue with policy options (usually includes the new evidence) geared to a particular audience. It is usually written for decision makers and is often referred to as a two-pager. It attempts to create understandable information by presenting information on the problem or issue, delineating policy options to deal with the issue, and usually making a recommendation on the best option. The details of a policy brief and an example can be found in Chapter 10. For some decision makers, the policy brief on the topic may be the first and only thing they read on the subject; for others, it may be the first effective compilation of evidence in a single accessible format; and for others, it may be entirely redundant.

IMPLICATIONS FOR THE FUTURE

While harnessing evidence is not without controversy, it is expected that evidence use for all levels of policy making will continue to be emphasized. As we move to the near future when more nurses are prepared with the skills to advance research and better understand the processes of quality and EBP, as well as the potential interplay among all three, nurses can produce better-quality evidence with the purpose of impacting policy. Involving all nurses, in all positions, in monitoring evidence related to policy is essential. It is not sufficient for us to defer quality improvement to the "quality nurses," or EBP to nurses who are members of an EBP internship or academy, or research to academics in nursing or to projects done while in school that are never applied to a real practice setting. A challenge that will remain is to integrate and use the evidence from these three processes more effectively and efficiently. Harnessing evidence is important at the big "P" level as well; therefore, nurses who are carrying out disciplinary or interprofessional research must consider the policy implications of research they undertake as they design their work. We must be thoughtful and explicit when translating research for policy not only in how we present evidence, but also to whom we present the evidence.

In the future, more attention will be given to the difficult job of eliminating long-standing policies based on outdated information that could potentially harm patients. We have many policies based on evidence that may not be synthesized, evidence that is ignored because of cultural beliefs, outdated evidence carried over from outdated education, or the competition's adoption of a policy.

Furthermore, we need to be poised with the range of policy skills to make use of evidence; research evidence alone will not change policy. Communicating and disseminating evidence more quickly and more efficiently are critical to moving good practice from isolated practices and organizations to systems and regions and beyond. Lag time from evidence to viable policy must be decreased.

KEY CONCEPTS

1. Harnessing evidence involves locating evidence and using it at the right times and places in the policy-making process.
2. Institutionalization of research does not create a clear path to policy making as illustrated by the disconnect between research evidence and policies found in clinical settings.
3. Evidence-informed policy has been expanded to include preferences contingencies and behavioral theory.
4. Efforts have been instituted globally to ensure that decision making in policy is informed by evidence.
5. Cultural differences between researchers and policy makers create challenges in translating evidence into practice.
6. The responsibility for ensuring transfer of new research into policy and practice tends to be viewed as a unidirectional flow from researchers to policy makers.
7. Communication between researchers and policy makers has an important role in translating research into policy.
8. Efforts to enhance the translation of research into policy include the NIH's Road Map, the RWJF's Synthesis Project, and the establishment of the PCORI.
9. Differences in the understanding and use of research, EBP, quality improvement, and translation research illustrate the complexity of harnessing evidence for practice and policy.
10. Translating research into policy involves communicating information about research in a useful and understandable manner.
11. Challenges in translating evidence into policy include decreasing barriers and enhancing facilitators of evidence adoption.
12. Translation of evidence into policy has been successful at the federal, state, local, and organizational levels.
13. Opportunities within organizations for translating evidence into policy include ensuring that current practices and policies are based on the best available evidence.
14. Carrying out research, EBP, or quality improvement requires a comprehensive dissemination plan in order to harness evidence for policy.
15. Nurses need to be prepared in a wide range of skills to make use of data that have implications for policy.

SUMMARY

The term *evidence-based policy* is used in the literature, yet generally relates to one type of evidence—that of scientific research. The literature and some organizations, including the WHO, are using the term *evidence influenced* or *evidence informed* to reflect the need to consider different types of evidence

EXHIBIT 5.4	**KEY STEPS TO ENHANCE USE OF EVIDENCE IN THE FORMULATION AND IMPLEMENTATION OF POLICIES**

1. Familiarize yourself with the evidence related to practice issues
2. Understand the difference between research, EBP, and quality improvement
3. Build relationships with policy makers at all levels (organizational, local, state, and national)
4. Raise questions about the evidence used in policies
5. Lead the development of a research, EBP, or quality-improvement project
6. Develop an action plan for the dissemination of evidence
7. Disseminate evidence in a variety of outlets pertinent to the policy issue
8. Use implementation science principles to carry out policy changes

and use of the best available evidence when dealing with everyday problems and issues in the health care environment. Research and nonresearch evidence both play an important role in translation of evidence to practice and policy. This chapter has presented the importance of context as critical to translation. When new evidence is generated or discovered, it is essential that not only the new evidence is evaluated on the quality and strength of that evidence, but also an organization must consider the "fit and feasibility" of the uptake and adoption of that evidence in that environment (organizational, professional, local, state, and national). The fit and feasibility test will take into account things in the environmental context such as values, beliefs, norms, history, resources, infrastructure, legislation and regulation, politics, and the competency, skills, and knowledge of those involved. See Exhibit 5.4 for a summary of key steps to enhance use of evidence for policy.

Translation of evidence is not a linear process and attention needs to be given to actively coordinating the dissemination to ensure that the evidence is implemented according to the plan.

LEARNING ACTIVITIES

1. Ask nurses employed in clinical positions in various settings about their knowledge and use of clinical guidelines available from specialty organizations and government agencies, such as the AHRQ or the CDC.
2. Locate resources for EBP at your place of employment and compare them to the resources for EBP at an academic institution.
3. Visit the NPUAP website: *Research Priorities Identified for Pressure Ulcer Prevention, Treatment & Policy* (www.npuap.org/research-priorities-ident ified-for-pressure-ulcer-prevention-treatment-policy). Compare and contrast the 11 areas of policy identified as a priority against what is being done at a clinical agency with regard to education, research, administration, or practice about pressure ulcers.
4. Visit the websites of your federal and state legislators and identify one bill that they support or do not support that has health care implications. Write a

letter to a legislator citing evidence for support or nonsupport of this particular piece of legislation.

5. Identify a policy in your organization (work or school) related to health or nursing education. Discuss the level of evidence that is available to support the change.

6. Locate three research articles on a topic of interest to you and your organization. Evaluate the degree to which policy implications are discussed in each article. For each, briefly summarize policy implications that need further explication.

7. Discuss two to three policies needing change in a health care organization. Describe the approach or combination of approaches (research, EBP, or quality improvement) to change one of the identified policies.

E-RESOURCES

- AARP Public Policy Institute. http://www.aarp.org/research/ppi
- Academy Health. http://www.academyhealth.org
- Agency for Healthcare Research and Quality (AHRQ). http://www.ahrq.gov
- Center for Economic and Policy Research (CEPR). http://www.cepr.net
- Cochrane Collaboration. http://www.cochrane.org
- The Commonwealth Fund. http://www.commonwealthfund.org
- The Dartmouth Institute for Health Policy and Clinical Research. http://www.tdi.dartmouth.edu
- Evidence-Informed Policy Network (EVIPNet). http://www.who.int/evidence/about/en
- Health Research and Policy Systems. http://www.health-policy-systems.com
- Institute for Women's Policy Research (IWPR). http://www.iwpr.org
- The Joanna Briggs Institute. http://joannabriggs.org
- Kaiser Family Foundation. http://kff.org
- RAND Corporation. http://www.rand.org/about/glance.html
- Robert Wood Johnson Foundation (RWJF). http://www.rwjf.org

REFERENCES

Anderson, L. M., Brownson, R. C., Fullilove, M. T., Teutsch, S. M., Novick, L. F., Fielding, J., & Land, G. H. (2005). Evidence-based public health policy and practice: Promises and limits. *American Journal of Preventive Medicine, 28*(5 Suppl), 226–230.

Bero, L. A., Grilli, R., Grimshaw, J. M., Harvey, E., Oxman, A. D., & Thomson, M. A. (1998). Closing the gap between research and practice: An overview of systematic reviews of interventions to promote the implementation of research findings. *British Medical Journal, 317*(7156), 465–468.

Bradley, E. H., Webster, T. R., Baker, D., Schlesinger, M., Inouye, S. K., Barth, M. C., & Koren, M. J. (2004). Translating research into practice: Speeding the adoption of innovative health care programs. *Issue Brief (Commonwealth Fund), 724*, 1–12.

Brooten, D., Naylor, M. D., York, R., Brown, L. P., Munro, B. H., Hollingsworth, A., … Youngblut, J. M. (2002). Lessons learned from testing the quality cost model of advanced practice nursing (APN) transitional care. *Journal of Nursing Scholarship, 34*(4), 369–375.

Brownson, R. C., Chriqui, J. F., & Stamatakis, K. A. (2009). Understanding evidence-based public health policy. *American Journal of Public Health, 99*(9), 1576–1583.

Brownson, R. C., Royer, C., Ewing, R., & McBride, T. D. (2006). Researchers and policy-makers: Travelers in parallel universes. *American Journal of Preventive Medicine, 30*(2), 164–172.

Caplan, N. (1979). The two-communities theory and knowledge utilization. *American Behavioral Scientist, 22*(3), 459–470.

Centers for Disease Control and Prevention (CDC). (2002). Guideline for hand hygiene in healthcare settings: Recommendations of the Healthcare Infection Control Practices Advisory Committee and the HICPAC/SHEA/APIC/IDSA hand hygiene task force. *MMWR Morbidity and Mortality Weekly Report, 51*(RR16), 1–45.

Centers for Medicare and Medicaid Services (CMS). (n.d.). Community-Based Care Transitions Program. Retrieved from http://innovation.cms.gov/initiatives/CCTP

Ciufo, D., Hader, R., & Holly, C. (2011). A comprehensive systematic review of visitation models in adult critical care units within the context of patient- and family-centered care. *International Journal of Evidence-Based Healthcare, 9*(4), 362–387.

Coburn, A. F. (1998). The role of health services research in developing state health policy. *Health Affairs, 17*(1), 139–151.

Cochrane Library. (2013). *About Cochrane systematic reviews and protocols.* Retrieved from http://www.thecochranelibrary.com/view/0/AboutCochraneSystematicReviews.html

Colby, D. C., Quinn, B. C., Williams, C. H., Bilheimer, L. T., & Goodell, S. (2008). Research glut and information famine: Making research evidence more useful for policymakers. *Health Affairs, 27*(4), 1177–1182.

Department of Health and Human Services (DHHS). (2009). *Code of Federal Regulations Title 45 Public Welfare Part 46 Protection of Human Subjects Subpart A Basic HHS Policy for protection of Human Research Subjects.* Retrieved from http://www.hhs.gov/ohrp/humansubjects/guidance/45cfr46.html

Dixon, D., & White, K. (2012). Ankyloglossia, frenotomy, and breast-feeding. [Exemplar]. In S. L. Dearholt & Dang, D. (Eds.), *Johns Hopkins nursing evidence-based practice: Model and guidelines* (pp. 219–222). Indianapolis, IN: Sigma Theta Tau International.

Farquhar, C. M., Stryer, D., & Slutsky, J. (2002). Translating research into practice: The future ahead. *International Journal of Quality in Health Care, 14*(3), 233–249.

Graham, I. D., Logan, J., Harrison, M. B., Straus, S. E., Tetroe, J., Casswell, W., & Robinson, N. (2006). Lost in knowledge translation: Time for a map? *Journal of Continuing Education in the Health Professions, 26*(1), 13–24.

Green, L. A., & Seifert, C. M. (2005). Translation of research to practice: Why we can't just do it. *Journal of the American Board of Family Practice, 18*(6), 541–545.

Greenhalgh, T., Robert, G., Macfarlane, F., Bate, P., & Kyriakidou, O. (2004). Diffusion of innovations in service organizations: Systematic review and recommendations. *Milbank Quarterly, 82*(4), 581–629.

Grimshaw, J. M., Eccles, M. P., Lavis, J. N., Hill, S. J., & Squires, J. E. (2012). Knowledge translation of research findings. *Implementation Science, 7*, 50.

Harden, V. A. (1998). *A short history of the National Institutes of Health.* Retrieved from http://history.nih.gov/exhibits/history/index.html

Hartsfield, D., Moulton, A. D., & McKie, K. L. (2007). A review of model public health laws. *American Journal of Public Health, 97*(Suppl 1), S56–S61.

Hewison, A. (2008). Evidence-based policy: Implications for nursing and policy involvement. *Policy, Politics & Nursing Practice, 9*(4), 288–298.

Hinshaw, A. S. (2011). Science shaping health policy: How is nursing research evident in such policy changes? In A. S. Hinshaw & P. A. Grady (Eds.), *Shaping health policy through nursing research* (pp. 1–15). New York, NY: Springer.

Innvaer, S., Vist, G., Trommald, M., & Oxman, A. (2002). Health policy-makers' perceptions of their use of evidence: A systematic review. *Journal of Health Services Research & Policy, 7*(4), 239–244.

Jacobson, N., Butterill, D., & Goering, P. (2003). Development of a framework for knowledge translation: Understanding user context. *Journal of Health Services Research & Policy, 8*(2), 94–99.

Joint Commission. (2014). *Hospital: 2014 National Patient Safety Goals.* Retrieved from http://www.jointcommission.org/2014_national_patient_safety_goals_slide_presentation

Krenzischek, D. A., Ares, M., Lewis, R., Tanseco, M., & Newhouse, R. P. (2007). To void or not void? [Exemplar]. In R. P. Newhouse, S. L. Dearholt, S. S. Poe, L. C. Pugh, & K. M. White (Eds.), *Johns Hopkins nursing evidence-based practice model and guidelines* (pp. 173–175). Indianapolis, IN: Sigma Theta Tau International.

Lavis, J. N., Oxman, A. D., Lewin, S., & Fretheim, A. (2009). SUPPORT Tools for evidence-informed health policymaking (STP) 3: Setting priorities for evidence-informed policymaking. *Health Research Policy and Systems, 7*(Suppl 1), S3.

Lavis, J. N., Posada, F. B., Haines, A., & Osei, E. (2004). Use of research to inform public policymaking. *Lancet, 364*(9445), 1615–1621.

Lavis, J. N., Ross, S. E., Hurley, J. E., Hohenadel, J. M., Stoddart, G. L., Woodward, C. A., & Abelson, J. (2002). Examining the role of health services research in public policymaking. *Milbank Quarterly, 80*(1), 125–154.

Levine, J. (2007). Lost in translation: Facing up to translational research. *Diabetes, 56*(12), 2841.

Lewis, S. (2011). How research influences policy makers: Still hazy after all these years. *Journal of the National Cancer Institute, 103*(4), 286–287.

Mangione-Smith, R., DeCristofaro, A. H., Setodji, C. M., Keesey, J., Klein, D. J., Adams, J. L., ... McGlynn, E. A. (2007). The quality of ambulatory care delivered to children in the United States. *New England Journal of Medicine, 357*(15), 1515–1523.

Maryland Health Quality and Cost Council. (2013). *Annual report to the Governor and General Assembly.* Retrieved from http://msa.maryland.gov/megafile/msa/speccol/sc5300/sc5339/000113/018000/018508/unrestricted/20132526e.pdf

McGlynn, E. A., Asch, S. M., Adams, J., Keesey, J., Hicks, J., DeCristofaro, A., & Kerr, E. A. (2003). The quality of health care delivered to adults in the United States. *New England Journal of Medicine, 348*(26), 2635–2645.

Melnyk, B. M., & Fineout-Overholt, E. (2005). *Evidence-based practice in nursing and health care: A guide to best practice.* Philadelphia, PA: Lippincott, Williams & Wilkins.

Meslin, E. M., Blasimme, A., & Cambon-Thomsen, A. (2013). Mapping the translational science policy "valley of death". *Clinical and Translational Medicine, 2*(1), 14.

Murthy, L., Shepperd, S., Clarke, M. J., Garner, S. E., Lavis, J. N., Perrier, L., ... Straus, S. E. (2012, September 12). Interventions to improve the use of systematic reviews in decision-making by health system managers, policy makers and clinicians. *Cochrane Database of Systematic Reviews, 9*, CD009401.

Naylor, M. D., Aiken, L. H., Kurtzman, E. T., Olds, D. M., & Hirschman, K. B. (2011). The care span: The importance of transitional care in achieving health outcomes. *Health Affairs, 30*(4), 746–754.

Naylor, M. D., Bowles, K. H., McCauley, K, M., Maccoy, M. C., Maislin, G., Pauly, M. V., & Krakauer, R. (2013). High-value transitional care: Translation of research into practice. *Journal of Evaluation in Clinical Practice, 19*(5), 727–733.

Naylor, M. D., Bowles, K. H., McCauley, K. M., Maccoy, M. C., Maislin, G., Pauly, M. V., Newby, D. E., & Webb, D. J. (2010). Translational research: A priority for health and wealth. *Heart, 96*(11), 815–816.

Newhouse, R. P., Dearholt, S., Poe, S., Pugh, L. C., & White K. M. (2005). *The Johns Hopkins nursing evidence-based practice model.* Baltimore, MD: Johns Hopkins Hospital & Johns Hopkins University School of Nursing.

Newhouse, R. P., Dearholt, S. L., Poe, S. S., Pugh, L. C., & White, K. M. (2007). *Johns Hopkins nursing evidence-based practice model and guidelines.* Indianapolis, IN: Sigma Theta Tau International.

Newhouse, R. P., Pettit, J. C., Poe, S., & Rocco, L. (2006). The slippery slope: Differentiating between quality improvement and research. *Journal of Nursing Administration, 36*(4), 211–219.

Office of Governor Martin O'Malley. (2013, August 29). *Governor Martin O'Malley announces Maryland infant mortality driven down to new record low in 2012.* Retrieved from http://www.governor.maryland.gov/blog/?p=9124

Orton, L., Lloyd-Williams, F., Taylor-Robinson, D., O'Flaherty, M., & Capewell, S. (2011). The use of research evidence in public health decision making processes: Systematic review. *PLoS One, 6*(7), e21704.

Oxman, A. D., Lavis, J. N., & Fretheim, A. (2007). Use of evidence in WHO recommendations. *Lancet, 369*(9576), 1883–1889.

Patient-Centered Outcomes Research Institute (PCORI). (n.d.). *PCORI 101.* Retrieved from http://www.pcori.org/assets/articulate_uploads/PCORI_1018/story.html

Pronovost, P., Needham, D., Berenholtz, S., Sinopoli, D., Chu, H., Cosgrove, S., … Goeschel, C. (2006). An intervention to decrease catheter-related bloodstream infections. *New England Journal of Medicine, 355*(26), 2725–2732.

Reinhardt, A. C., & Ray, L. N. (2003). Differentiating quality improvement from research. *Applied Nursing Research, 16*(1), 2–8.

Rogers, E. M. (2003). *Diffusion of innovations* (5th ed.). New York, NY: Free Press.

Rubio, D. M., Schoenbaum, E. E., Lee, L. S., Schteingart, D. E., Marantz, P. R., Anderson, K. E., … Esposito, K. (2010). Defining translational research: Implications for training. *Academic Medicine, 85*(3), 470–475.

Sendelbach, S. (2010). Preoperative fasting doesn't mean nothing after midnight. *American Journal of Nursing, 110*(9), 64–65.

Sheffer, C. (n.d.). *Smoke free hospital toolkit: A guide for implementing smoke-free policies.* Retrieved from http://www.uams.edu/coph/reports/smokefree_toolkit/Hospital%20Toolkit%20Text.pdf

Shirey, M. R., Hauck, S. L., Embree, J. L., Kinner, T. J., Schaar, G. L., Phillips, L. A., Ashby, S., … McCool, I. A. (2011). Showcasing differences between quality improvement, evidence-based practice, and research. *Journal of Continuing Education in Nursing, 42*(2), 57–68; quiz 69–70.

Titler, M. (2004). Overview of the U.S. Invitational Conference: Advancing quality care through on translational research. *Worldviews on Evidence-Based Nursing, 1*(Suppl 1), S1–S5.

Titler, M. (2010). Translation science: Theory and context. *Research and Theory for Nursing Practice, 24*(1), 35–55.

Weston, M., White, K., & Peterson, C. (2013). Creating nursing's future: Translating research into evidence-based policy. Communicating Nursing Research Conference Proceedings: Creating a Shared Future of Nursing: *Research, Practice, and Education, 46,* 47–54.

White, K. M. (2011). Translational research. In J. F. Fitzpatrick & M. W. Kazer (Eds.), *Encyclopedia of nursing research* (3rd ed., pp. 517–520). New York, NY: Springer.

Woolf, S. (2008). The meaning of translational research and why it matters. *Journal of the American Medical Association, 299*(2), 211–213.

World Health Organization. (2009). *WHO guidelines on hand hygiene in health care. First global patient safety challenge clean care is safer care.* Geneva, Switzerland: WHO Press. Retrieved from http://www.who.int/gpsc/5may/tools/9789241597906/en

World Health Organization. (n.d.). Evidence-informed policy-making. Retrieved from http://www.who.int/evidence/en

Yuan, C. T., Nembhard, I. M., Stern, A. F., Brush, J. E. Jr., Krumholz, H. M., & Bradley, E. H. (2010). Blueprint for the dissemination of evidence-based practices in health care. *Issue Brief (The Commonwealth Fund), 86,* 1–16.

Zerhouni, E. (2003). Medicine: The NIH Road Map. *Science, 302,* 63–64, 72.

Zerhouni, E. (2005). Translational and clinical sciences—Time for a new vision. *New England Journal of Medicine, 353*(15), 1621–1623.

SIX

Setting the Agenda

Linda K. Groah
Amy L. Hader

Things do not happen. Things are made to happen.—John F. Kennedy (1963)

OBJECTIVES

1. Explain the importance of effective agenda setting in the policy process.
2. Discuss critical components of agenda setting.
3. Analyze effective strategies for advancing a policy agenda.
4. Describe methods to overcome barriers to advancing a policy agenda.
5. Compare and contrast options for agenda setting at the organizational, local, state, and national levels.
6. Identify nonlegislative strategies to move an organizational, local, state, or national agenda forward.

Agenda setting is the first step, and some would argue the most important step, in the policy process. It is your navigation tool in your policy journey. It is an extension of the problem identification and prerequisite to successful policy development at all levels. Agenda setting is critical whether you are working on big "P" or little "p" issues. Agenda setting can seem a simple process; however, if you consider setting an agenda for a meeting and reflect on meetings that have gone in less than desirable directions, you can start to envision that agenda setting is an iceberg and only the tip is visible. Consider the complexities of agenda setting related to health care reform at the national and state levels in the United States. Thus, once you have identified a policy issue (see Chapter 4, "Identifying a Policy Issue") and evaluated the available research (Chapter 5, "Harnessing Evidence in the Policy Process"), it is time to set the agenda.

This chapter discusses the importance of policy agendas and strategies for controlling and influencing the agenda-setting process. You are guided through the processes of agenda setting and the pivotal role that nursing plays in agenda setting. Consideration is given to variations in the agendas. The agenda-setting process is based on a variety of intersecting factors such as the policy problem, scope of the issue, stakeholders, timing, personal agendas, and public agendas. Agenda setting at the federal level, within key nursing organizations, and for key clinical issues are highlighted to showcase the critical role nurses must play in agenda setting. Nurses' full understanding and control of agenda setting are foundational to nurses achieving sustained power in policy. Knowing the basic concepts related to agenda setting is prerequisite to appreciating the power of agenda setting. The Policy Challenge illustrates a turning point for agenda setting for advancing baccalaureate education.

POLICY CHALLENGE: Advancing the BSN Requirement in Nursing—The New York Experience
Barbara Zittel, PhD, RN, Formerly Executive Secretary of the New York State Board for Nursing, Delmar, NY

On Friday, December 8, 2003, the New York State Board of Nursing (the Board) had an extensive discussion of the following motion:

Statutory change be sought permitting future RN applicants who have completed an associate degree or diploma in nursing to continue to receive licensure as an RN, but requiring such persons to obtain a baccalaureate degree in nursing within 10 years of initial licensure.

The motion was unanimously approved by the nurse practitioners (NPs), registered nurses (RNs), licensed practical nurses (LPNs), and public members, who comprise the Board's membership, amid moans of anguish from several of the observers at the public meeting.

Within 2 days, letters of opposition began to arrive, primarily from presidents of community colleges with associate degree nursing programs—presidents with long-term collegial relationships with the regents and the commissioner (with authority over the Board). Although the Board was able to counter the opposition with twice as many letters of support from such inspirational nursing leaders as Margaret McClure, Marjory Gordon, and Claire Fagin, their comments did not have the same political impact as letters from known colleagues. As the executive secretary, I was summoned to the deputy commissioner's office to justify the Board's position. Despite the fact that my job security was tenuous, the Board and I persisted in strategizing ways to decrease opposition and increase support. Our initial emphasis focused on garnering support from nursing faculty, primarily from associate degree programs (New York has only one diploma-based nursing program). We had taken a momentous step for nursing by embarking upon a path to advance nursing education in our state. There was no turning back from this historical moment.

See Option for Policy Challenge.

AGENDA IDENTIFICATION

A problem or issue must get the attention of those who want to help make a change before the policy process starts. On any given day, numerous problems command and compete for our attention. The repetition of a problem (e.g., frequency of nurse musculoskeletal injuries or number of patient falls with injuries) or the magnitude of a problem (e.g., the number of Americans without health insurance) are often seen as instrumental in shaping the agenda-setting process, but repetition and magnitude are not guarantees that an issue will make it to an agenda. Understanding the definition of an agenda, the importance of an agenda, who sets and defines an agenda, and levels of agendas are interrelated but key concepts that are basic to getting an issue for an agenda identified.

What Is an Agenda?

An agenda is a complex process that involves laying out issues and solutions: "An agenda is a collection of problems, understandings of causes, symbols, solutions, and other elements of public problems that come to the attention of members of the public and their governmental officials" (Birkland, 2007, p. 63). This definition can be reworked more generically as follows, to encompass both the big "P" and the little "p" of policy: An agenda is a collection of difficulties or issues and their causes, representations (privately and publicly), and their suggested resolutions that get the attention and consideration of policy makers locally, nationally, or internationally within or across institutions, organizations, or governments. Thus, agenda setting is not solely applicable to government policy. In fact, nurses can and must be active in policy where they work, in their communities, and in their profession.

The purpose of an agenda is to influence events, news, and understanding. An agenda can be as simple as an identified issue and the proposed solution, or as comprehensive as a descriptive series of problems that require solutions from varying vested individuals or groups (e.g., stakeholders in government, private sector, individuals, and communities). For example, for a state nurses association, an agenda might include a list of legislation that has been introduced that has an impact on nursing. It could also include a more comprehensive analysis of legislative and regulatory changes that need to take place within a state in order to remove barriers to advanced nursing practice. Kingdon (2011) conducted hundreds of interviews with government officials and policy makers, yielding a comprehensive review of research on agenda setting. His findings indicated that context was important—timing, political climate, and other political realities—in the policy-making and agenda-setting process. For nurses considering or already engaged in policy work, it is important to know that our current context includes a strong focus and continuing emphasis on improvements in health care.

The Importance of the Agenda

Many writers and speakers intent on urging readers and listeners to become more involved in the political process have employed the saying, "*If you are not at the table, you're on the menu.*" This is an old saying in Washington, which bears repeating here. Individuals and organizations whose priority issues are not on the agenda stand little chance of influencing policy regarding their priorities; at worst, they may experience backward progress and lose ground on their issues. Agenda setting is about power. Power is exercised by determining what gets on the agenda and what is blocked from getting on the agenda. Groups compete not only to gain access to the agenda, but also to deny access to the agenda (Birkland, 2011).

Nursing issues at the big "P" level almost always lie within the policy issue category of health care. Given the plentiful debate over the Patient Protection and Affordable Care Act (PPACA) and President Obama's continued inclusion of health care on the White House's published agenda, we know that patient safety and health care remain prominent on the national agenda as well as on local agendas within institutions and within professional organizations.

More specifically, the PPACA contains a comprehensive approach to health insurance market and health care delivery system reforms designed to improve the quality of care, decrease the cost of that care, and expand access to care for millions of Americans. The Act sets forth a rollout structure for many of its key provisions. Some key provisions are already in effect—in 2010, many Americans began receiving cost-free preventive services; in 2011, Medicare beneficiaries began receiving many preventive services at no cost; and in 2012, accountable care organizations began to take shape. Also in 2012, the Medicare hospital value-based purchasing program began tying payment to performance on certain quality measures, and a separate penalty for hospitals with comparatively high readmission rates went into effect. In subsequent years, the law seeks to improve quality and lower costs by improving preventive health coverage, expanding authority to bundle payments, and increasing funding for primary care under Medicaid and the Children's Health Insurance Program. Consumer protections such as prohibiting discrimination based on preexisting conditions or gender, eliminating annual insurance coverage limit caps, and ensuring coverage for individuals participating in clinical trials went into effect in 2014. We can expect to see a shift away from fee-for-service payments with a new emphasis on value and quality instead of volume (U.S. Department of Health and Human Services [DHHS], n.d.).

Your goals and action plan may vary from seeking legislative or regulatory changes to increased public awareness of a public health issue, or even incremental policy changes within your health care facility. The national political climate, as well as interest groups and individual connections, will all coalesce to inform your policy agenda and action plan. "Agenda setting is crucial because if an issue cannot be placed on the agenda, it cannot be considered, and nothing can possibly happen in government" (Peters, 2013, p. 65).

Who Sets and Defines Agendas?

All organizations and state and federal agencies and their subdivisions have mission statements and strategic plans that are routinely reviewed and updated. Agendas are defined by missions and strategic plans. The mission and strategic plans guide agenda setting at all levels and determine priorities for action. If an agenda is not linked to the mission and strategic plan, then it is difficult if not impossible for the agenda to gain traction among key stakeholders. Understanding these connections among missions, strategic plans, and agendas is vital for nurses to move an agenda forward. Too often the assumption is made that money, media, and power control agendas. Acceptance of this assumption can feed a sense of powerlessness that often leads to nurses' disillusionment about their ability to change policies, legislation, and regulation that have an impact on their practice environment.

One example of a government institution's role in leading policy changes can be seen in the approach to safe patient handling taken by the U.S. Department of Veterans Affairs (VA). The VA health facilities use the latest specialized devices and proven methods to keep patients and health care workers safe when moving patients. Many health systems look to the VA model for safe patient handling guidance when seeking to implement best practices at their facilities. The VA's close attention to the issue lends weight to the importance of the issue and can be referenced as an example by unit peer leaders looking to implement best practices or to purchase new devices and equipment.

Nurses associations have well-established procedures for formulating their agendas. Some associations routinely seek and include members' ideas and concerns when developing their agendas. As membership organizations, they follow a democratic process that includes mechanisms to collect suggestions or mandates from the membership. Many associations' annual meetings include a process where topics are debated and voted to determine future actions. These topics often end up in policy agendas. Exhibit 6.1 provides links to the policy agendas of several professional associations. Agendas may focus on specific policy. Sometimes organizations may have a separate research agenda to address priorities for research. Sometimes landmark reports serve an agenda-setting function. This is illustrated by two seminal reports, the Institute of Medicine's (IOM) *To Err Is Human* (Kohn, Corrigan, & Donaldson, 2000), which brought focus to the problem of safety by publicizing the statistic of 98,000 annual deaths due to medical errors, and the IOM/Robert Wood Johnson Foundation (RWJF) report on *The Future of Nursing* (IOM, 2011). Similarly, the Consensus Model for APRN Regulation serves an agenda-setting function for standardization of advanced practice licensure, accreditation, certification, and education across the states (Advanced Practice Registered Nurse [APRN] Consensus Work Group, 2008).

Levels of the Agenda

Prior to Kingdon's (2011) extensive examination of political agendas and the policy-making process, Roger Cobb and Charles Elder (1972)

EXHIBIT 6.1	POLICY AGENDAS OF SELECTED SPECIALTY NURSING ORGANIZATIONS	
ORGANIZATION	**TYPE OF AGENDA**	**WEBSITE**
American Association of Colleges of Nursing (AACN)	Federal Policy Agenda	http://www.aacn.nche.edu/government-affairs/legislative-goals
American College of Nurse-Midwives (ACNM)	Federal and State Policy Agendas	http://www.midwife.org/Federal-State-Policy-Agendas
Association of periOperative Registered Nurses (AORN)	Legislative Priorities	http://www.aorn.org/LegislativePriorities
Emergency Nurses Association (ENA)	Public Policy Agenda 2011–2012	http://www.ena.org/government/Documents/2011PublicPolicyAgenda.pdf
National Association of Clinical Nurse Specialists (NACNS)	Legislative and Regulatory Agenda 2013–2015	http://www.nacns.org/docs/LegReg-Agenda2013-2015.pdf
National Association of Pediatric Nurse Practitioners (NAPNAP)	Health Policy Agenda 2013	http://www.napnap.org/NAPNAPAdvocacy/HealthPolicyAgenda.aspx
Oncology Nursing Society (ONS)	Health Policy Agenda, 113th Congress, 2nd Session	http://www2.ons.org/LAC/media/ons/docs/LAC/pdf/HealthPolicyAgendaJan2014.pdf

examined the importance of the political agenda. Their work showcased the difference between issues or problems under discussion in society—which can be thought of as systemic agenda or public problems—and institutional or organizational agendas. Birkland (2011) expands this concept to include four levels of increasing specificity: the agenda universe, the systemic agenda, the institutional or organizational agenda, and the decision agenda. The agenda universe consists of all the possible problems related to the issue. The systemic agenda or public problems are those that are worthy of the public's attention and are within the scope of authority of a government. The institutional agenda includes those problems that are up for active consideration by officials. The decision agenda includes those items that are ready for action. Without prominence on the institutional or organizational agenda, an issue is unlikely to make any meaningful headway through the political system (see Figure 6.1). While any number of issues may be important components of a nurses association agenda, the goal would be to move an issue closer to the decision agenda so that desirable actions can be taken.

Often not discussed is the importance of an agenda in one's local environment, and in particular the importance of nurses owning the policy agenda for their practice. For example, rather than becoming frustrated with the failure to move forward with a policy that implements an evidence-based practice (e.g., fasting times before surgery, postoperative urinary retention prevention strategies, meal tray delivery, and insulin administration times), nurses need to examine how to get their issue on the policy agenda of the group or groups that can best help implement the practice. It is vital to show how the practice issue fits with the mission or strategic plan related to safety and/or cost. This is illustrated by the efforts to implement practices designed to improve breastfeeding rates and other practices associated with Baby-Friendly designation (see Policy on the Scene 6.1). Regardless of whether an issue requires attention at the legislative or regulatory level, within your health care institution, or even within a municipality or local civic group, an issue's prominence often directly correlates to the level of attention it receives from decision makers and stakeholders. Identifying the systemic and, more importantly, the institutional agendas of the decision makers you are trying to influence provides the foundation for the development and refinement of your agenda.

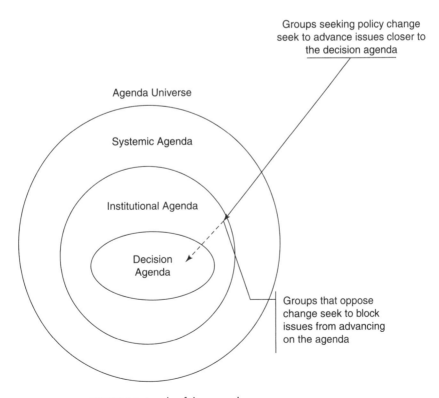

FIGURE 6.1 Levels of the agenda.
Reprinted with permission from Birkland (2011).

POLICY ON THE SCENE 6.1: Setting the Agenda to Achieve Baby-Friendly Designation
Kate Salmon, MSN, RNC, IBCLC, Lynn Barabach, MSN, RNC
Lakewood Hospital, a Cleveland Clinic Hospital, Lakewood, OH

Hospitals and other health care agencies in an increasingly competitive market are always looking for strategies to improve the quality of their care as well as the achievement of external benchmarks demonstrating excellence. Achieving Baby-Friendly designation is an example of such a process as illustrated here.

Several years ago, a clinical educator (KS), who was an international board certified lactation consultant (IBCLC), decided that the hospital where she was employed, Lakewood, needed to be designated as a Baby-Friendly hospital. To obtain a Baby-Friendly designation, the hospital needed to demonstrate that it was meeting the *Ten Steps to Successful Breastfeeding* (World Health Organization [WHO], 1989). The designation would ultimately show the hospital's commitment to breastfeeding mothers and their newborns from early pregnancy through the infant's first year of life.

The clinical educator used a variety of strategies to set an agenda in order to achieve the goal of Baby-Friendly designation. Initially, she gathered information about Baby-Friendly and the designation process, and began to formulate a plan. Then, she began to lobby the birthing center leadership by presenting information about the impact being a Baby-Friendly hospital would have on families, nurses, providers, and the hospital. Nursing leadership agreed that working toward a Baby-Friendly designation was the right thing to do for the families. The clinical educator, with the nursing leadership team, began to lobby hospital administration to secure support for the birthing center's journey toward Baby-Friendly designation. Hospital administration provided full support for the journey toward the designation, including annual funding to cover the expenses of staff education and designation fees. The clinical educator also lobbied individual providers to ensure their support for the journey to Baby-Friendly designation.

The next step in the process was the formation of a committee by the birthing center leadership that began to plan the journey. The clinical educator chaired the hospital's committee, which included several stakeholders: nurse manager, assistant nurse managers, lactation consultants, an obstetrician, and a certified nurse midwife. As often occurs with agenda setting, the need for additional changes was identified: (a) staff, provider, and patient education; (b) hospital policy development; and (c) implementation of new models of care including skin-to-skin care and rooming in. The committee worked for several years to plan, to ensure that the appropriate changes occurred, and to monitor data for success. The committee worked with nurses as a group and individually to ensure that education was provided, including a 4-hour class on skin-to-skin care, an online educational program, and one-on-one time with a lactation consultant. The committee worked to develop materials that were used to educate providers as well as information for prenatal office visits.

Early in the birthing center's journey, the other birthing hospitals within the Cleveland clinic system also decided to begin their journeys toward Baby-Friendly designation. The clinical educator and her committee joined forces with other hospital groups, bringing on additional stakeholders to create a system-wide interprofessional committee to develop policies related to breastfeeding and a plan to educate staff throughout the system. Policies were developed for the hospital system, as well as breastfeeding guidelines. Additionally, the system committee worked to develop standardized patient education, system-wide formula purchase agreements, standardized equipment, and a "ban the bag" campaign to eliminate the distribution of free diaper bags from formula companies.

During the journey to Baby-Friendly, the birthing center staff and providers began to change as well. The birthing center began to embrace the unit's policy to follow the *Ten Steps of Successful Breastfeeding*. The activity surrounding Baby-Friendly was not only about being designated, but was about confirming who they were to themselves and the outside world. The nurses began to advocate for keeping mothers and babies together by not having infants routinely returned to the nursery for examinations and procedures (much to the dismay of some pediatricians). Providers agreed that infants should be placed skin-to-skin right from birth, including in the operating room.

Ultimately, the birthing center was awarded designation as a Baby-Friendly hospital in March 2012. What started out as a desire by one nurse to influence her hospital's policy to support breastfeeding and advocating for new mothers resulted in a transformation.

DEVELOPING AN AGENDA

Agenda development includes defining the problem and establishing the agenda. These are two intertwined and evolving processes. Articulating the problem provides the launching pad for establishing the agenda.

Defining the Problem

A problem clearly stated is a problem half solved.—Dorothea Brande

Conditions and problems can become agenda items, but there is a difference between them. Weather, illnesses, and poverty are conditions. Conditions become problems when someone decides to do something about them (Kingdon, 2011). Agenda setting is a process. Issues gain and lose attention in the spotlight every day. Widely accepted policy agenda items in the United States are the problem of poverty and the quality of our public education system; policy issues that have had enthusiastic and then waning interest are environmental concerns and drug enforcement issues (Peters, 2013).

A large part of agenda setting is defining the problem. For example, after the mass tragedies of September 11, 2001, in our country, security for airline travel became a pressing issue. Everyone agreed on the importance of the issue of airline travel security. However, the finer points of how to actually increase travelers' security while balancing travelers' privacy were the subject of much disagreement. Whether to allow body scans, pat downs, profiling, and even liquids on airplanes became the subject of national debate. The next steps on the nation's agenda were framed largely by perceptions of the root of the problem. Did the problem lie in a failure to enforce existing rules, or were additional rules necessary to ensure nothing like September 11 could ever happen again in our country and to our citizens? Should existing or new security measures for airline travel now be applied to other mass transit such as trains, subway systems, and buses? A person's reaction to and support for the agenda would depend in large part on the answer to these questions.

Another example of defining the problem can be seen in drug enforcement policy. Drug abuse is part of the national systemic agenda, but whether one views it as an education, public health, or poverty-related problem will influence the remedies likely to be chosen (Peters, 2013).

A group must define its problem with the objective of swaying the right policy makers at the right time in the group's favor. Thus, it is important to have the right problem on the agenda. Individual and organizational or institutional stakeholders, including government agencies, will be affected differently, depending on how a problem is defined. For example, a state nurses association may be successful in getting a legislator to introduce a bill on nurse title protection so that non-nurses are not allowed to call themselves nurses. However, the ultimate passage of the bill will depend on the committee to which it has been referred (see Chapter 3, "Navigating the Political System"). Some committees may provide a more favorable context for the passage of a particular piece of legislation than others (see Project Vote Smart: votesmart.org/education/how-a-bill-becomes-law#).

An example of an ongoing policy problem for nurses and their patients is nurse staffing. Weston, Brewer, and Peterson (2012) confirm not only that nurse staffing is a very complex issue but also that it has been an issue for decades. In 1981, the DHHS defined the problem as "perennial and universal" (as cited in Weston et al., 2012, p. 247). Weston, Brewer, and Peterson concede that an absolute solution is elusive, but not without first offering explanations for why the problem has been difficult to solve. Proffered explanations include unexpected occurrences, rapid changes in patient acuity, and erratic flow of patients through the hospital.

Because nurse staffing has long been a persistent yet elusive problem, the American Nurses Association (ANA)—the national professional association representing the interests of the nation's 3.1 million RNs—maintains safe nurse staffing as one of its federal legislative priorities and dedicates its government affairs resources toward solving the problem. A great example of the importance of defining the problem is illustrated by the association's fact sheet for legislators, legislative staff, and stakeholders on the safe staffing (ANA, n.d.). The safe staffing fact sheet from the ANA presents the association's position on and support for a federal Registered Nurse Safe Staffing Act, which would require hospitals to establish and publicly report unit-by-unit staffing plans that must be developed by a committee composed of at least 55% direct care nurses or their representatives. The ANA fact sheet begins by defining the problem for the reader:

> Massive reductions in nursing budgets, combined with the challenges presented by a growing nursing shortage have resulted in fewer nurses working longer hours and caring for sicker patients. This situation compromises care and contributes to the nursing shortage by creating an environment that drives nurses from the bedside. (ANA, n.d., para. 1; http://www.nursingworld.org/SafeStaffingFactsheet.aspx)

The fact sheet then presents the solutions that are set forth in the proposed federal legislation. It connects the dots between data and practice related to the problem for policy makers. The fact sheet also includes applicable research and evidence and then continues on to address and dispense with alternative proposals that have been advanced by different interest groups on the same topic of nurse staffing on the second page. This ANA fact sheet gives us a great working example of how a policy interest group such as a membership organization of professionals can work to define a problem for policy makers and then showcase how the group's proposed solutions would solve the problem.

Nurses can also work on identifying similar problems at the state and local levels. Strategically, agenda setting evaluates the best approach and in what venue the issue should be first attempted. Some problems get addressed on a state-by-state basis first, before its impact is recognized at the national level. The support of an issue at the local and state levels is often strategically planned before introduction at the federal level. The process can vary significantly, however. Sometimes a problem is identified by numerous organizations within and beyond nursing. Sometimes problems repeatedly fail to gain traction at the state level only to be recognized at the federal level.

Establishing the Agenda

There will always be competition among groups for policy makers' attention to their problem. Issues with ramifications for greater numbers of people or important institutions may take precedence over issues with lessened societal impact, but not necessarily and not as often as the public might like. Issues that may seem perfectly rational to some may not resonate as clearly with others. Immigration and gun control may be important one year, only to slide off the radar the next year without any solution to the problems that thrust them onto the agenda in the first place.

The Gallup company has been routinely surveying Americans on the "most important problem facing this country today" for years (Gallup, 2012). In November 2012, the majority of respondents (64%) cited economic problems—such as unemployment, the deficit, and taxes—as the most important problem. Other answers provided with varying frequency include dissatisfaction with government, health care, ethics/moral/religious decline, poverty/hunger/homelessness, foreign aid/focus overseas, education, judicial system/courts/laws, and unifying the country (Gallup, 2012). Such polls can lend insight into groups looking to launch their issue onto policy makers' agendas. At any given time, people may be more or less receptive to proposed policy changes, depending on the nation's and policy makers' mood and preoccupation with other issues perceived to be more pressing.

Kingdon (2011) posits that, in general, there are two categories of factors affecting agenda setting: the participants who are active and the processes by which the issues presented come into prominence. Another policy scholar, Birkland (2007, p. 77), writes of agenda setting in public policy, "The likelihood that an issue will rise on the agenda is a function of the issue itself, the actors that get involved, institutional relationships, and, often, random social and political factors that can be explained but cannot be replicated or predicted."

Key influencers can work in favor of a policy issue gaining prominence on the agenda, but they can also work against a policy issue. A new government administration, new nursing leadership on your unit or at your health care facility, and even a planned accreditation visit can create new opportunities for issues to be presented to the decision makers and potentially be placed on the agenda. Unpredictable events such as weather-related disasters, a mass accident, or other local or regional tragedy may also focus the public and decision makers' attention on or off an issue without warning. Natural disasters have elevated America's concern for preparedness and response to catastrophes (Peters, 2013). After Hurricane Katrina, the ANA (2008) significantly engaged the nursing profession in policy development, resulting in the policy document, *Adapting Standards of Care Under Extreme Conditions: Guidance for Professionals During Disasters, Pandemics, and Other Extreme Emergencies.* Some issues of seemingly public importance may not rise on the agenda "because of the financial cost, the lack of acceptance by the public, the opposition of powerful interests, or simply because they are less pressing than other items in the competition for attention" (Kingdon, 2011). It is not uncommon to have many issues of national importance in our country, or even many issues in our own communities, take a backseat as budgets wax and wane.

Implementing public policies requires a budget and institutional infrastructure. A prominent national example at the legislative level was the budget and tax issue of 2012 that became known as the "fiscal cliff." The term *fiscal cliff* refers to over $500 billion in tax increases and government spending cuts that were set to automatically take effect on January 1, 2013, unless Congress passed a law altering both future tax rates and the slated government spending cuts. Because of the importance of the fiscal cliff for the nation's economy, little else was accomplished in Washington in late 2012.

At the federal level, resources are allocated among competing federal agencies for their programs, the decisions of which are necessarily informed by the president's economic beliefs and policy goals (Peters, 2013). At the institutional level, budgets and financial constraints are similarly a leverage point with key executives and decision makers. Obtaining funding for quality improvement projects within a health care institution can be as long and complex a process as seeking policy changes at the state and federal levels.

At the local level, nurses' agendas are expected to address cost effectiveness with their practice and policy development. One strategy in helping overcome this potential challenge is to provide data with sound cost–benefit ratio rationales when working for policies that have financial implications. Although it may not be readily apparent, most policies and agendas have financial implications. For example, in creating an agenda to begin work on improving patient flow in the emergency department (ED), you must consider not only the financial impact of the changes, but also patient, employee, and physician satisfaction in offsetting costs.

STAKEHOLDERS

Careful consideration is necessary to determine whose interests and welfare should be considered in the agenda-setting process. Identification and inclusion of stakeholders are crucial in advancing a policy agenda. Stakeholders can be for an issue, against it, and even neutral. Inclusion of those who are for an issue, against an issue, or neutral—in fact, all stakeholders, regardless of their position—facilitates the broadest discussion and development of policy solutions. Stakeholders are the people, groups, and/or entities that are vested in the issue you are exploring or promulgating. Knowing the stakeholders is essential in helping to define the problem and in setting the agenda. Stakeholders may include political parties, interest groups, the media, and the public and will vary depending on the issue itself, the level, and the timing of the issue.

An example of stakeholders can be seen in the recent (2013) California Supreme Court decision, *American Nurses Association v. Tom Torlakson*. The ANA filed an amicus brief in support of California school nurses (Balestra, 2012). This controversial ruling allows trained school personnel to administer insulin in the California school system. Exhibit 6.2 illustrates the diversity and complexity of interests of various stakeholders related to this policy agenda.

As seen earlier, identifying the list of stakeholders can be lengthy. A complete analysis of who the stakeholders are and their positions is necessary for setting effective policy agendas. Identifying the stakeholders is about not only knowing who your allies and opponents are, but also strategizing about effective ways to capitalize on both. In the following sections, we describe how to

EXHIBIT 6.2 STAKEHOLDERS AND INSULIN ADMINISTRATION IN SCHOOLS

STAKEHOLDER	INTEREST
Children with diabetes and their parents	Strong interest to have their health care needs addressed
Nurses in the school district	School nurses are affected but some may not want to get involved
Teachers and staff in each school	Those impacted with new duties will have great interest, while those whose duties remain the same have less interest
Principal and administrative staff in each school	Strong interest having been told to implement the plan with some potential ability to give input to the plan; interest in hiring fewer school nurses
State Department of Education	Strong interest to resolve issues to reduce costs to school districts
National Association of School Nurses	Strong interest and expertise
American Nurses Association	Strong interest and concern about implications for other practice arenas
American Diabetes Association	Strong interest to address their focused special interest
Local community	Strong interest but not a formed, cohesive group prepared to be involved
Local and state media	Not much interest, but if given the right information at the right time they could be very interested
Local politician	Indifferent, but may change in election year

use interest groups to advance your agenda and how to assess your opposition to overcome the obstacles they may present.

The inclusion of stakeholders can be strategic in terms of advancing the agenda. Sometimes key stakeholders are included in the initial development of an agenda. Initially, for more controversial issues, groups may choose to start by including those who are primarily supportive of an agenda direction. This provides the group with the opportunity to examine its strategies, refine its arguments, and gain support for an issue, and to be sure that "everyone is on the same page." Subsequently, others may be invited to join when the initial group has gained a core sense of direction. This might be illustrated with any of a number of the regional action coalitions (RACs) established around the country in support of *The Future of Nursing* recommendations. The leaders of a RAC might believe that its region would be best served by clarifying the focus and direction of their agenda before inviting potential supporters and funders to join in the process. While some need to be in on the development from the ground up, others don't want to expend their resources unless there is a clear expectation and direction. Each RAC needs to determine what is best depending on its unique circumstances and political landscape.

The Importance of Interest Groups

Interest groups are often formed for common interests or purposes and to promote a cause. They may at some point decide that their mission and their needs will be met by influencing policy. Research has demonstrated that interest groups "often play a central role in setting the government agenda, defining options, influencing decisions and directing implementation" (Grossman, 2012, p. 172). Interest groups are credited with policy accomplishments in all three branches of government—influencing not only legislative changes, but also court rulings, executive orders, and agency administrative decisions. Nurses can become part of an interest group by joining one. Types of interest groups include advocacy groups, consumer groups, community groups, business interest groups (e.g., chambers of commerce and corporations), academic groups, professional associations, unions, think tanks, and foundations.

Interest Groups Aligned With Your Agenda

State nurse and specialty nurses associations are professional interest groups typically open to RNs and occasionally to other health care providers who support the association's mission. These associations can be a wise choice for enlisting support of a policy agenda. Partnering with your state nurses and specialty associations is an important initial step in becoming an active and effective participant in setting the policy agenda. See Policy on the Scene 6.2, which illustrates how registered nurse first assistants (RNFAs) in Minnesota partnered with their state nurses association in establishing reimbursement for RNFAs as a component of the Minnesota Nurses Association (MNA) policy agenda.

Partnering with MNA provided RNFAs with a number of advantages as well as challenges in setting their policy agenda.

The RNFA story highlights the importance of a state nurses association's involvement in legislative movements initiated by a smaller and informal specialty nurse group and individual nurses. The RNFAs' success was facilitated by a number of strategic decisions. The RNFAs recognized that in order to achieve greater political clout, they needed to partner with an organization (MNA) that had visibility and credibility in their statehouse. With MNA's mission to represent all nurses, the partnership would appear to be logical to external constituencies, such as legislative bodies. Diversity in interest group support along with

---

POLICY ON THE SCENE 6.2: Partnering to Advance a Policy Agenda
Mary K. Weis, MSN, RN, CNOR, CRNFA

In the fall of 1993, RNFAs in Minnesota began discussing strategies for passing legislation for RNFAs reimbursement in our state. We were encouraged to seek the assistance of our state nurses association and other partners. By spring 1994, we were holding regular statewide RNFA meetings. We continued developing communications with key interest groups, including legislators, hospital medical directors, and the medical and nursing associations. A key strategy was educating these stakeholders about the RNFA role.

We collected examples of how and why RNFAs are the best surgical assistants for providing total patient care. Included were stories of barriers to RNFA employment, and cost-effectiveness of RNFA services. Our team implemented a campaign to educate MNA members about the RNFA role that included attendance at district meetings, the statewide meeting, and the distribution of fact sheets, brochures, and cost comparisons.

The culmination of our efforts resulted in RNFA reimbursement being placed on the multiple stakeholders' agendas, including the MNA's legislative agenda. This action meant that we would have additional resources available. The MNA helped craft our bill, broaden our language, lobby, and shepherd it through the legislative process. A legislative stakeholder, who subsequently became lieutenant governor, advanced our agenda by holding discussions with the state health committee. We engaged in traditional lobbying tactics of correspondence, phone calls and meetings with legislators, a lobby day, and providing testimony. Our legislative success in achieving state-mandated reimbursement for RNs assisting in surgery was clearly attributable to the involvement of multiple stakeholders.

Adapted with permission from Association of periOperative Registered Nurses (AORN) (2007).

the traditional grassroots strategies demonstrate the success of this approach. Expanding interest group support for your policy agenda involves not only determining who would naturally be aligned with your position, but also identifying the advantages for interest groups with seemingly divergent goals. However, as we have seen with the RNFA and MNA experience, keeping the issue on the agenda involves building and sustaining the relationship in order to keep the agenda item from stalling and to realize success. Since Minnesota passed their RNFA reimbursement bill in 1996, legislation has been introduced in 20 states and passed in 15.

Professional associations can bring credibility and prominence to an agenda, and enhance the potential for a policy agenda's success. Other kinds of interest groups where nurses can have an impact include business and industry groups. For example, a nurse responsible for directing an ambulatory surgery center might join, as a representative of the ambulatory surgery center, her local chamber of commerce in order to elevate the ambulatory surgery center's opportunity to have a voice in local business regulation that might affect the ambulatory surgery center. Nurses in certain areas and specialties may also join other groups such as unions in order to advance their policy agendas.

Consumer groups may also have an impact on policy agendas. Consumer groups are often formed to champion causes framed as "in the public interest," such as consumer-protection groups and "good government" organizations. Other examples of public interest groups also include groups formed to speak for populations that cannot speak for themselves, such as children. These kinds of groups are often called upon to respond to others' agendas on behalf of their constituents and intended beneficiaries. Consumer groups are often portrayed as counterpoints to the self-interested business, labor, and professional groups, but consumer groups do not exist solely to respond to the agendas of others. At times consumer groups may have their own issue agendas.

Knowing the Opposition

Knowing groups that may be aligned with your policy agenda is not enough. It is equally important to consider your possible opposition as you advance your policy agenda. It is vital to try to understand early on what obstacles your group faces or may face in response to your policy initiatives. Early identification of barriers will help you determine how best to work toward your objectives and to keep your goals realistically attainable. Knowing the opposition involves identifying those who would oppose your agenda as well as the specifics of their positions. Points to consider in determining the opposition and their positions are illustrated in Exhibit 6.3.

Knowing and understanding the opposition allows you to identify competing interests. The information allows you to frame the issue, develop your arguments, and formulate strategies that are part of framing the issue (see Chapter 10, "Working With the Media: Shaping the Health Policy Process").

EXHIBIT 6.3 ASSESSMENT OF THE OPPOSITION

- What is the nature of the opposition (e.g. finances, values, and/or stereotypes)?
- Is the opposition proposing an alternative?
- Is the opposition from within your organization?
- Is the opposition coming from an individual or a group of individuals?
- Can you identify common ground with the opposition?
- Does the opposition answer to a constituency?
- How does the public view the opposition?
- Will swaying the opposition to a neutral position help your agenda?
- What are the financial resources of the opposition?
- To what extent is your agenda item important to the opposition?

Unaligned Interest Groups

Some stakeholder or special interest groups may be unaligned with your policy agenda. It is just as important to identify groups that potentially have an interest in your policy agenda, but either are uninvolved or have taken a neutral position, as it is to identify the opposition. Key decision makers will be interested in the positions of other organizations in relation to your agenda. When a nurse visits a legislator, he or she may be asked about the position of other groups. A legislator may want to gauge constituent interest in the issue. While nurses can't answer for other groups, nor should they, they should be aware of these positions in order to be prepared. In fact, it is generally wise to avoid answering questions about the positions of other organizations.

Unaligned groups may be indicative (a) of internal disagreement about an issue, (b) of private support for an issue when public expression of support may be politically incorrect for the organization, or (c) that the issue is too far removed from the mission or focus of the group. Just because a stakeholder group is unaligned does not necessarily mean the group will stay unaligned. Likewise, it may be considered a victory when a stakeholder group moves from a position of active opposition to neutrality. Sometimes large coalitions will encourage a member organization that can't fully support the focus of a coalition's policy initiative to remain silent on the issue.

Networking and Coalition Building

Influence is basic to agenda setting and should be taken into consideration, whether you are trying to influence others or others are trying to influence you. A number of factors are associated with success and/or failure of influence when setting an agenda. A person's status, for example, may play a role in others granting unconditional support and following; a well-respected nurse leader may get more support for an idea based on status. Three ways to build influence in support of your agenda are networking, building coalitions, and raising awareness of your issue.

Networking

Nurses seeking to advance a policy agenda should use a network. Building relationships is important so that they are in place when they are needed. You want to involve your network early in helping to create an agenda, foster engagement, and plan for the resources needed. Nurses can practice the art of networking every day in many ways—at work, at their children's schools and sporting events, at church, and even at the gym. Networking takes practice. Many nurses may have entered the profession when there were many employment choices available. That reality has changed for new nurse graduates who are being quickly thrust into the realities of today's job market where networking might be the only strategy for securing an interview. So, networking may be uncomfortable initially, but it really is just transferring communication skills into advocacy.

Networking certainly includes connecting with your legislators. Effective networking begins with simple steps. For example, legislators and their staff appreciate brief communications. This may include a note of thanks for a legislative position or a success attributable to their office. Legislators and their staff also may appreciate informational notes. For example, AORN, the Association of periOperative Registered Nurses, and others similarly dedicated to advancing safety and quality agendas promote a National Time-Out Day annually to highlight the importance of the "time out" in preventing wrong site, wrong side, wrong patient, wrong procedure surgeries. As part of this campaign, AORN asks its nurse members to write letters to the editor of their local newspapers explaining the key role perioperative nurses play in implementing the time out and advancing patient safety in the operating room. When a nurse's letter is published in his or her local paper, AORN urges the nurse to send a copy of the published letter to his or her elected legislators with a personal note, as shown in Exhibit 6.4. Even simple notes like this will be remembered, thus increasing the likelihood that a legislator and his or her staff will remember an individual's name when that constituent later asks the legislator for support.

Persistence is often the key to success in networking with all contacts. Success does not happen with only one e-mail or phone call. Networking needs to be a habit, a way of interacting with people and using opportunities for putting forward an agenda. Having a wider network allows you to share your policy agenda with more people. A network takes time to build, but the reward is the expansion of your influence. Networking does not only involve legislators, but also involve nurses, community leaders, and members of the business community, as well as members of other professions. See Exhibit 6.5 for tips on networking. See Chapter 11, "Applying a Nursing Lens to Shape Policy."

EXHIBIT 6.4 SAMPLE LETTER TO LEGISLATOR OFFERING EXPERTISE

Dear [Senator or Representative name], I thought you might be interested in this letter to the editor of [newspaper name] as an example of how complex health care has become and what perioperative nurses in your district are doing to improve patient safety in our surgical invasive environments such as operating rooms, ambulatory surgery centers, and catheterization labs. As a registered nurse with many years of experience, I am available to assist and offer my expertise in these times of complex health care issues. I look forward to working with you and having ongoing conversations. Thank you for your service to our district and our country.

Sincerely, NAME, CREDENTIALS, CONTACT INFORMATION

EXHIBIT 6.5 TIPS ON NETWORKING

1. Learn the person's name and repeat later in the conversation
2. Listen to the concerns of the individual and learn what is important to him or her
3. Arrive early and stay late for meetings
4. Volunteer for community or charitable events, legislative days
5. Supplement your networking with an online professional network
6. Introduce people to others who have common interests
7. Follow up with a note, e-mail, or phone call
8. Keep messages about your policy agenda brief and to the point.
9. Share why your issue is important from your networking contact's perspective
10. Be prepared with a description of your organization and its accomplishments
11. Demonstrate knowledge and enthusiasm for your issue
12. As appropriate, thank the individual for the meeting

Coalition Building

Coalition building can be an effective tool for setting an agenda to influence a target audience. Coalitions can be official (formal) or unofficial (informal). Coalitions are alliances of organizations supporting a common policy goal, such as the Future of Nursing State Action Coalitions that have formed to advance nursing issues. Coalitions marshal the energy of large numbers of people through organizations. The impact is greater when a coalition of several organizations supports a formal agenda than when separate organizations work alone. This partnership demonstrates that the organizations are not speaking from a narrow position of self-interest (Smith, Bucklin, & Associates, 2000). The Future of Nursing Campaign for Action (n.d.) has evidence-based indicators of success for building successful coalitions developed by the California Endowment (available at campaignforaction.org/effective-coalition-tcc).

Nurse groups looking for other stakeholders not only should look to other nursing groups such as state nurses associations and other specialty nurses associations, but can also look to business groups, patient safety groups, and other groups in the community whose agendas align. Nurses need to reach beyond the usual partners to develop coalitions. Just because a group has opposed a nursing initiative in the past does not mean that same group may not support a different initiative proposed by your nursing group. Credible organizations will take policy positions by issue, less often by "group." As consensus builds on your agenda, the merits of your solution should spread through the policy community (see Chapter 7, "Building Capital: Intellectual, Social, Political, and Financial," for more details).

Raising Awareness of the Agenda

Creating public awareness can also increase your group's chances at getting on a legislative agenda. Increasing public understanding of the scope of a problem will increase your group's chances of regulatory, legislative, and other success. There are numerous junctures and outlets for raising awareness of your agenda. Research studies, posters, protests, media campaigns, fundraising events, educational speeches, and informational flyers are all tactics that can be used to raise awareness or your interest group's policy agenda. Raising awareness of your identified policy agenda and your proposed solution can motivate people to support your cause or to actively join your interest group. This can cause a ripple effect so that others contact policy makers on your behalf, and spread the word, creating an even greater awareness, and in turn increasing the likelihood that your agenda will receive support from key policy makers (see Chapter 10). While your organization may wish to increase the visibility of an issue, the level of attention that is received by an issue is dependent on a number of factors including the issue's political attractiveness with regard to vote-seeking (Green-Pederson & Wilkerson, 2006). Similarly, the strategies used at any given time for agenda setting depend upon the issue's stage of development, as well as the extent to which key stakeholders have knowledge and understanding of an issue (Kozel et al., 2006).

Highlighting how your group's solution fits within the existing health care policy agendas to improve quality and safety while increasing access and cost-efficiencies is another media tip. Nurses who are formulating issues, defining problems, and preparing their agendas must also remember to promote and capitalize on the nursing profession's high esteem in America per the Gallup poll (Newport, 2012). As the most trusted health profession, when presented thoughtfully and with an eye toward the nation's current temperature and health care priorities, nursing's voice should be clearly heard in the offices of legislators and administrators.

An important caveat about raising awareness is the need to speak with one unified voice. Cohesion among the group provides a distinct advantage in getting buy-in for an agenda. With numerous associations representing nurses, it is vital to speak with one voice in order to convince policy makers that an issue has support. An often-heard lament in the past is that nurses did not always speak with one voice. It does not take much to imagine the importance and power of 3 million nurses speaking with a single, united voice.

FOCUSING THE AGENDA

An important step in agenda setting is focusing the agenda to maximize the influence of policy decisions. This includes assessing the most appropriate jurisdiction and determining whether legislative, regulatory, or judicial approaches would be most beneficial in advancing the agenda.

Jurisdiction

An important concrete step is determining who has jurisdiction over your identified issue. In other words, who is the decision-making body with power to implement your agenda? Is legislative action necessary, or can the issue be remedied more expeditiously through a rule-making process at an agency level?

At the state level, health policy issues may fall within the purview of the state's department of health. Issues relating to hospitals, ambulatory surgery centers, and other health care facilities often fall within the state agency responsible for licensing, certification, and/or oversight of such facilities. Scope of practice issues and other issues specific to licensed health care professionals fall under the state board with licensing authority, such as the board of nursing (BON) for RNs and APRNs, and the board of medicine for physicians and often physician assistants. An effective way for nurses to influence health care policy and delivery in their state is to get to know their state BON. Many state boards rely on practicing nurses as clinical experts; when an issue comes before a board that relates to a certain specialty, board members will reach out to their nursing friends and colleagues in that field for advice and guidance. Some nurses may find that they want to influence policy more directly by actually serving as a member of the BON or a state agency's advisory committee. As state health departments tend to regulate hospitals and ambulatory surgery centers (ASCs), another way for nurses to influence health care policy in their state is to get to know the department staff responsible for the agency's policy decisions in their area of practice.

While we generally think of jurisdiction in relation to government entities, it is just as important to consider jurisdiction in relation to a health care organization, community group, or association. The goal is the same—to advance the agenda with the individuals or groups who have the power to make the decision. For example, nurses may complain to the materials management department about the ineffectiveness of a product rather than taking the issue to a nurse practice council, which might examine policy and safety related to the product's use and gather relevant data and evidence to make a change. Sometimes nurses in frustration and without investigation of available channels and resources will ask a favorite physician or involve a patient to "complain" and hopefully get the intended change, as well as to champion an issue when the nursing department clearly has the primary jurisdiction. This "work-around" in effect may create anger, stall progress on the agenda item, foster the status quo, and create significant unintended consequences. Going through others who don't have authority to handle the problem may backfire and is not often recommended.

Once you have an understanding of the jurisdictional issue for your agenda, the next step in the process is venue shopping. "Venue shopping refers to the activities of advocacy groups and policymakers who seek out a decision setting where they can air their grievances with current policy and present alternative policy proposals" (Pralle, 2002, p. 1). Venue shopping is a legitimate strategy to ensure success. For example, for nearly 25 years, NPs in Pennsylvania fought to obtain prescriptive privileges. When the first regulations were passed, they only applied to NPs collaborating with medical physicians, not osteopaths. This created a different set of practice requirements based upon which type of physician the NP was working with in his or her practice setting; very often, it was both in the same setting. The NPs were gearing up to go through the entire rule-making process again with the osteopathic board, but instead a legal ruling was made applying the regulations to collaboration with osteopaths as well. In this instance, changing the focus from creating the regulation to interpreting the regulation resulted in success for the NPs. Now the agenda will focus on removing other practice barriers and gaining full practice authority for NPs, and the likely venue will be legislation.

Legislation

The first assumption that typically comes to mind when people think of policy and advocacy work by an interest group is often that the group is working to pass a new law. Not all agendas involve legislative activities. Legislation is often viewed as an ideal solution to a problem and passage of laws can be a very effective way to achieve the group's goals for the agenda. Legislation is often preferred because once a proposed solution is passed into law, it is less likely that the legislature or administration will later act to reverse the action, particularly as individuals and stakeholders begin their compliance efforts and the effect of the law becomes visible to society.

Other decisions that need to be made about setting an agenda are determining which legislative body is the most appropriate for advancing your agenda. Consideration needs to be given to the likelihood of success in one legislative arena or another and the long-term implications for success. A critical mass of successes at the local or state level may be necessary before other jurisdictions will consider an agenda item. Smoke-free environments began with success in local jurisdictions before success could be achieved at the state level. For example, Chicago adopted a smoke-free policy before it was adopted by Illinois. Likewise, when working with national organizations, deciding where to advance an agenda first can be strategic in terms of subsequent successes.

Regulations

Regulations made by state and federal agencies with rule-making authority present opportunities for policy gains for interest groups. Agencies with directors who are appointed by the president or a governor will be more accountable to the current executive administration's policy agenda, while agencies created by statute with staffing decisions made further outside the purview of a current administration might be more likely to attend to an issue not prominently on the current administration's agenda.

These appointed positions can be opportunities for nurses. For example, Mary Wakefield, PhD, RN, FAAN, who has a long history as a health policy activist, was named administrator of the Health Resources and Services Administration (HRSA) by President Barack Obama on February 20, 2009. HRSA is a critical agency of the DHHS. In this position, Dr. Wakefield's expertise has been instrumental in expanding the utilization of RNs and improving services for the uninsured or underserved population while addressing severe provider shortages across the country. The nursing community supported Dr. Wakefield for the HRSA position and was pleased to see this major milestone for nursing.

Some legislation designates an agency to implement regulations to enforce the law. Laws governing nursing—state Nurse Practice Acts—designate the state BON in most states as the implementing authority. Often, laws governing hospitals and other health care facilities designate the state department of health or an other licensing body as the regulatory authority. The DHHS, within which the Centers for Medicare and Medicaid Services, the Agency for Healthcare Research and Quality, the Food and Drug Administration, and the Centers for Disease Control and Prevention reside, is often the federal regulatory authority for implementing federal health care laws.

The regulatory process is intended as a way for agencies with more expertise than legislators to add specificity to laws by providing implementation, interpretations, definitions, and compliance and enforcement provisions. For example, a nurse overtime law in a state may generally prohibit mandatory nurse overtime in hospitals. Further explanation of the prohibition and important definitions, such as definitions of "overtime" or "on call," might then be provided by the state agency charged with oversight responsibilities for hospitals. Such rules and regulations can only be adopted by state agencies after a specific rule-making process, typically set forth in a state's administrative procedure law. The specifics will vary by state but, generally, state agencies are required to publish proposed rules in advance and allow a specified time period for public comment and possibly a hearing. Agencies are to consider all comments before issuing final regulations or rules.

Agencies can also take action that falls shy of regulation but still may have enormous impact. Some agencies have the power to issue advisory opinions, reports, and other guidance that is outside the rule-making process. For example, state boards of nursing offer position statements, advisory opinions, and other guidance for the RNs licensed under its Nurse Practice Act. This guidance is less formal than regulation but is nevertheless intended to guide the practice of nursing in a particular state and often does in fact have the same effect as regulation.

Another example is when a state agency is charged with studying an issue and then publishing a report, either for the legislature or for another government body. For example, after a failed legislative initiative in Washington State to mandate certification for surgical technologists in Washington hospitals and ambulatory surgery centers, the Washington State Department of Health was asked to conduct a thorough review to examine the public policy impact of changing the surgical technology profession's scope of practice. In September 2012, after collecting written comments and holding a 4-hour hearing on the issue of whether the state should require surgical technologists working in Washington hospitals and ambulatory surgery centers to hold and maintain national certification, the Department of Health issued a 216-page comprehensive report that included the presentations from those who submitted comments and testified at the hearing. The report recommended against mandatory certification of surgical technologists with a detailed recommendation and its rationale for the Washington legislature (Washington State Department of Health, 2012). This report does not have the force of law or even regulation, and legislators are not bound to follow it. However, given the breadth of the research and the deference traditionally given by lawmakers to agency expertise, it is unlikely that the Washington legislature will pass a law requiring certification of surgical technologists without the support of the Washington State Department of Health.

Another less formal way to affect and influence health care policy is at the institutional level. How a hospital interprets and implements a practice, a state regulation, or standard from The Joint Commission can vary. Nurses must establish channels to provide their expertise as institutions adopt and revise health care policies and directives. Even items such as continuing education programs, hospital newsletters, and staff development initiatives offer opportunities for nurses to shape and influence health care delivery within their institutions.

One example of hospitals leading policy changes is in the area of healthy and sustainable food. Many hospitals across the nation are taking part in healthy food initiatives focusing on both nutrition and food sustainability in response to a Healthy Food in Health Care program, an initiative of the Health Care Without Harm organization (Knudson, 2013). Hospitals are leading changes in communities by using their enormous purchasing power to favor local organic fruits and vegetables and healthy food from sustainable sources. Examples of baseline policy actions facilities in the program might initially include taking a pledge or formally adopting a policy. Hospitals that have been successful in implementing change have used interprofessional teams with nurses heavily involved and often leading the efforts.

Litigation

Using the legal system is another policy strategy that is used by interest groups to advance a cause or seek an intended outcome. In addition to resolving claims and disputes between individuals and corporations and adjudicating the innocence or guilt of persons accused of violating criminal laws, our American judicial system is used to establish, affirm, or clarify constitutional and statutory rights. Litigation initiated to accomplish policy outcomes is known as "impact" litigation. Most recently, in June 2012, in response to a challenge brought by many states' attorneys general, the U.S. Supreme Court upheld President Barack Obama's landmark health care reform legislation, the Affordable Care Act (*National Federation of Independent Business v. Sebelius,* 2012). However, using litigation as a means to enforce existing legislation or regulations can be very expensive. The American Civil Liberties Union (ACLU) is a well-known example of a funded interest group that uses impact litigation to accomplish its policy goals. The ACLU has over 500,000 members who financially support its work; its litigation efforts are paid for by member dues, contributions from individuals, and grants from private foundations.

The ANA, state, and national specialty associations have impacted litigation that is important to the profession's agenda while protecting RNs and patients' rights and well-being.

Another way to use the legal system is to file amicus briefs in cases of interest to the group, but in which the group is not actually a party. *Amicus curiae* means "friend of the court" in Latin. Interest groups may file amicus briefs with a court to provide information on the possible legal effects of a court decision and its potential impact on others who are not party to the litigation. For example, the ANA, Louisiana State Nurses Association (LSNA), and the Louisiana Alliance of Nursing Organizations (LANO) filed an amicus brief as a friend of the court in the Louisiana First Circuit Court of Appeal supporting the full scope of practice for certified registered nurse anesthetists (CRNAs). The focus of the brief was specific to CRNAs' interventional pain management (e.g., injection of local anesthetics).

While the options for venues may vary with the issue and the particular locale, agenda setting is an important part of the policy process. The Option for Policy Challenge illustrates one route taken in New York for advancing baccalaureate education. Other options or combinations of options may work better in other settings and may include different groups of stakeholders. It is to our advantage to think "outside of the box" in considering possibilities for setting the agenda.

OPTION FOR POLICY CHALLENGE: Advancing the BSN Requirement in Nursing: The New York Experience
Barbara Zittel

Our journey for advancing the BSN requirement in New York involved systematic and strategic actions to garner support for our plan. In 2004, during three all-day meetings, the Board and nursing faculty members utilized a collaborative, constructive decision-making process to clarify the intent and misunderstandings of the Board's 2003 motion, and to obtain feedback and further recommendations. Early in 2005, an official letter of support arrived from the New York State Associate Degree Nursing Council. The Council's change of position was a decisive moment for the Board and demonstrated that opinions could be altered with discussions that respectfully acknowledged concerns and sought collaboration.

Our priorities were adjusted to advancing our agenda forward instead of merely defending it. Revitalized, the BON strategized to find a partner who would spearhead the legislative initiative. The perfect collaborator was found in the New York Organization of Nurse Executives (NYONE), an organization of nurse leaders that includes major employers of RNs throughout the state. The New York State Nurses Association (NYSNA) also provided support and guidance with expertise in the legislative process. By the end of 2005, legislative language was developed and sponsors were identified in the State Assembly and Senate.

Strategic outreach achieved results while state and national groups announced their support. Organizations included the ANA, the Black Nurses Association of Manhattan, the Indian American Nurses Association, the Philippine Nurses Association of New York, Inc., the New York Chapter of the Association of Hispanic Nurses, and the Pharmacists Society of the State of New York.

The Board met with groups that, despite the best arguments, maintained their opposition (1199 Service Employees International Union, Public Employees Federation, and the NYS Union of Teachers). The Healthcare Association of New York State (HANYS), formerly the Hospital Association, also opposed, based mainly on the same opinion held by the aforementioned labor unions, that such a mandate would significantly increase their costs for educating RNs to the BS degree.

Nonetheless, our advocacy efforts continued and expanded to include a paid lobbyist. The number of legislators sponsoring the bill increased steadily each legislative session. NYONE developed an executive summary focusing on economic benefits. Support was strengthened

(continued)

and opposition dampened when the American Nurses Credentialing Center's Magnet Recognition Program® emphasized the need to increase the number of staff nurses with BSN in acute care facilities.

The economic environment slowed and altered hiring practices. Large health care systems such as North Shore/Long Island Jewish Health System publicized their position that new RN graduates without a BS degree would be hired on the condition that their continued employment would be contingent on conferral of a BS degree in nursing within 5 years. Other facilities began to preferentially hire RNs with a BSN. Then in 2010 the prestigious IOM report, *The Future of Nursing: Leading Change, Advancing Health,* included among its recommendations that to meet the future health care needs, the proportion of nurses with a BS needed to increase to 80% by 2020. Based on expert analysis, we concluded that this target is not achievable in the near future without passage of our legislative proposal.

By 2013, continued support developed with HANYS voting to support the legislation. This alliance, with its strong political connections in the legislature, will do much to turn the tide of opposition. Legislative sponsors now reflect members of the majority in both the Senate and House—a situation that did not occur until after the 2013 legislative session. The time is now; the strategic efforts decreased opposition while improving support as our desire for change remains strong.

One of my heroines is Elizabeth Cady Stanton, a New York social activist and leading figure of the 19th-century women's rights movement. She worked unceasingly for 50 years, died before passage of the 19th amendment, and her story is now overshadowed by the contributions of Susan B. Anthony, her lifelong friend. Stanton writes, "I never forget that we are sowing winter wheat, which the coming spring will see sprout and other hands than ours will reap and enjoy."

Change takes time. It requires people with tenacity and persistence, people who are willing to persevere even in the face of overwhelming opposition, people who respect opposing thoughts and the willingness to find common ground, people with creativity. But given these conditions, change does occur.

We found that in order to maintain interest and enthusiasm, a group e-mail termed *Friday's Update* would apprise persons about weekly progress made and actions to take and permit them to ask questions, make suggestions, and relay information from the "front." That publication is now sent out each week of the legislative session to over 500 persons. It will soon enter its sixth year of distribution. When we were willing to compromise and accept a 10-year as opposed to a 6-year time frame for future RNs to obtain their BS degree after licensure, our willingness to yield on this matter gained us the support of associate degree nursing educators. We found that multiple requests were required in order to obtain letters of support from most organizations.

The economic benefits for passage of this bill changed more minds than most other points.

Employing a lobbyist made a significant difference in having our positions and presence felt by legislators. While other states express interest in the essence of the bill, they await its passage in New York before actively pursuing a course of action in their own jurisdiction

This legislation needs to be passed. Standardization in nursing's educational system is imperative. Patient outcomes are dependent upon it. I am hopeful that I will be present when it is enacted ... in the meantime, however, I rest in the assurance that the seed has been sown and our plan has been activated.

IMPLICATIONS FOR THE FUTURE

As you take steps to implement your agenda, you will begin to see political ramifications and responses. Nurses should capitalize on their unique professional talents to establish and advance their agenda. Nurses are excellent negotiators, communicators, problem solvers, and team players (Boswell, Cannon, & Miller, 2005). These skills are used by nurses every day to manage conflict, cope with challenging personalities, and diffuse potentially explosive situations, all in the name of patient care and safety. It is well established that teamwork is essential for patient safety (Kalisch, Weaver, & Salas, 2009). Nurse advocates must draw on these same talents and skills as they engage in policy discussions at both individual and institutional levels. "Once a nurse is motivated to try to change or develop policy, and becomes engaged in the process, many of the basic approaches to work and problem solving developed in nursing education and practice prove useful" (Gebbie et al., 2000, p. 314).

KEY CONCEPTS

1. Agenda setting is a complex process involving the laying out of problems and solutions so that the issue comes to the attention of the public and governmental officials.
2. Agendas are designed to influence events, news, and understandings.
3. The context of an agenda, timing, political climate, and political realities are important in the agenda-setting process.
4. Organizations, or groups within an organization, work to get their priority issue on the agenda in order to influence policy.

5. An organization's agenda needs to be linked to its mission and strategic plan in order to gain traction with key stakeholders.
6. Agendas have levels of increasing specificity: the agenda universe, the systemic agenda, the institutional or organizational agenda, and the decision agenda. Issues need to reach the institutional agenda in order to achieve progress toward a decision.
7. Nurses need to own the agenda for their practice, within their organizations, and the profession.
8. Agenda development includes defining the problem and establishing the agenda.
9. Numerous internal and external factors influence whether an issue gains prominence on the agenda such as a new administration, new leadership, unpredictable events, finances, public acceptance, opposition of powerful interests, or competing issues.
10. Knowing the numerous stakeholders and their varying degrees of support are invaluable in planning strategies for moving an agenda forward.
11. Interest groups, including associations, corporations, and consumer groups, may be supportive, neutral, or opposed to an agenda.
12. Understanding obstacles to an agenda will facilitate designing a strategy to move an agenda forward.
13. Networking provides opportunities to build relationships with legislators, regulators, and key organizational and community leaders.
14. Coalitions provide an opportunity to expand influence in support of a common policy goal.
15. Raising awareness of an agenda either in the public arena or within an organization increases the chance of moving an agenda forward.
16. Speaking with a unified voice is important to the success of an agenda.
17. Focusing an agenda on a specific venue such as legislative, regulatory, or judicial can be strategic in maximizing successes.
18. Agenda setting is a process that can be used both in the public arena and within organizations in order to achieve important policy goals.

SUMMARY

Setting the agenda is a process that is in constant flux and the strategies need to change to reflect the dynamics of the situation. Policy changes rarely happen quickly. Advocates must be prepared, persistent, and patient in their approach to changes. Windows of opportunity may open and close over years or shorter periods of time. Just when your group is about to close in on a regulatory success, a key agency personnel or elected official change may derail your efforts. Maintaining a long view is helpful and healthy. During times when your legislature is not in session, or executives sensitive to your issue are not in office, do not sit idle.

Remain focused and monitor your policy makers' agenda. Seize opportunities to raise your issue on that agenda. Keep your group and grassroots advocates engaged and prepared. Review and refine your messaging. Meet with public officials and legislators and their staff to educate on your issue, even if you know this is not the year your issue will advance on the policy agenda. Stay committed to your group's mission and goals while continuing to redefine your policy issue as needed. Work to identify a solution in ways that stand the best chance of resonating with the largest number of policy makers and stakeholders.

LEARNING ACTIVITIES

1. Determine the policy issues important to the governor in your state, your local representative, and one professional nursing organization. Describe the methods you used to obtain the information and critique ease of access among the three sources.
2. Talk to a nurse leader or identify for yourself how a new agenda in management or in shared governance has been successfully or unsuccessfully introduced.
3. Identify the details of your state governor's agenda items that relate to health care. Compare those agenda items to the agenda of the nursing organizations with which you are involved and describe how you could frame your nursing organization's issues within the state executive's agenda.
4. Find fact sheets from various organizations, including a national organization, a state organization, and a consumer group, and identify strengths and weaknesses. Try to find fact sheets from opposing groups on the same issue and compare how the groups define the problem.
5. Find examples of press releases and other materials designed to increase public awareness of an issue. For example, the Coalition for Patients' Rights issues press releases and media stories are designed to educate the public about the importance of the patient's right to choose providers. Can you find others?
6. Which groups comprise the IOM state action coalition in your state? What groups could be included in your state's action coalition? In your state and others, can you find examples of successes and policy changes accomplished by the IOM state action coalitions?
7. Locate the mission statement and/or strategic plan and identify how a practice issue that you believe needs to be on the agenda fits with the statement or plan.

E-RESOURCES

- Agency for Healthcare Research and Quality Setting the Agenda for Research on Cultural Competence in Health Care. http://www.ahrq .gov/research/findings/factsheets/literacy/cultural/index.html

- American Nurses Association. http://www.nursingworld.org
- American Nurses Association. Health System Reform Agenda. http://www.nursingworld.org/Content/HealthcareandPolicyIssues/Agenda/ANAsHealthSystemReformAgenda.pdf
- American Nurses Association. Nursing's Agenda for the Future. http://ana.nursingworld.org/MainMenuCategories/HealthcareandPolicyIssues/HealthSystemReform/Agenda/Principles/AgendafortheFuture.aspx; http://infoassist.panpha.org/docushare/dsweb/Get/Document-1884/PP-2002-APR-Nsgagenda.pdf
- Canadian Nurses Association, Nursing and the Political Agenda. http://www.cna-aiic.ca/en/advocacy/nursing-and-the-political-agenda
- National Council on Research for Women. http://www.ncrw.org
- Oncology Nursing Society (ONS) Research Agenda. http://www2.ons.org/media/ons/docs/research/research-agenda-executive-summary-2009-2013.pdf
- World Health Organization. *Health Service Planning and Policy-Making: A Tool kit for Nurses and Midwives, WHO Module 2: Identifying and analyzing the stakeholders and establishing networks.* http://www.wpro.who.int/publications/docs/hsp_mod2_BB2D.pdf

REFERENCES

American Nurses Association. (2008). *Adapting standards of care under extreme conditions: Guidance for professionals during pandemics, and other extreme emergencies.* Retrieved from http://nursingworld.org/MainMenuCategories/WorkplaceSafety/Healthy-Work-Environment/DPR/TheLawEthicsofDisasterResponse/AdaptingStandardsofCare.pdf

American Nurses Association. (n.d.). *Safe staffing: The registered nurse safe staffing act: H.R. 1821.* Retrieved from http://www.rnaction.org/site/DocServer/Safe_Staffing_Fact_Sheet.pdf?docID=1621

American Nurses Association v. Tom Torlakson. 2013, s184583 Ct.App C061150 Sacramento County Super. Ct. No. 07AS04631. http://www.cde.ca.gov/ls/he/hn/documents/anav-torlakson2013.pdf

AORN. (2007). *RN first assistant guide to practice* (3rd ed.). Denver, CO: AORN.

APRN Consensus Work Group & the National Council of State Boards of Nursing APRN Advisory Committee. (2008, July 7). *Consensus model for APRN regulation: Licensure, accreditation, certification & education.* Retrieved from https://www.ncsbn.org/Consensus_Model_for_APRN_Regulation_July_2008.pdf

Balestra, M. (2012). Amicus brief supports administration of insulin to students only by licensed nurses. *Journal of Nursing Law, 15*(1), 27–32.

Birkland, T. A. (2007). Agenda setting in public policy. In F. Fischer, G. J. Miller, & M. S. Sidney (Eds.), *Handbook of public policy analysis: Theory, politics, and methods* (pp. 63–78). Boca Raton, FL: CRC Press.

Birkland, T. A. (2011). *An introduction to the policy process: Theories, concepts, and models of public policy making* (3rd ed.). Armonk, NY: ME Sharpe.

Boswell, C., Cannon, S., & Miller, J. (2005). Nurses' political involvement: Responsibility versus privilege. *Journal of Professional Nursing, 21*(1), 5–8.

Cobb, R. W., & Elder, C. D. (1972). *Participation in American politics: The dynamics of agenda-building.* Boston, MA: Allyn & Bacon.

Future of Nursing Campaign for Action. (n.d.). *What makes an effective coalition?* Retrieved from http://campaignforaction.org/effective-coalition-tcc

Gallup. (2012). Most important problem. Retrieved from http://www.gallup.com/poll/1675/most-important-problem.aspx

Gebbie, K. M., Wakefield, M., & Kerfoot, K. (2000). Nursing and health policy. *Journal of Nursing Scholarship, 32*(3), 307–315.

Green-Pederson, C., & Wilkerson, J. (2006). How agenda-setting attributes shape politics; basic dilemmas, problem attention and health politics developments in Denmark and the US. *Journal of European Public Policy, 13*(7), 1039–1052.

Grossman, M. (2012). Interest group influence on US policy change: An assessment based on policy history. *Interest Groups & Advocacy, 1*(2), 171–192.

Institute of Medicine (IOM). (2011). *The future of nursing: Leading change, advancing health.* Washington, DC: National Academies Press.

Kalisch, B. J., Weaver, S. J., & Salas, E. (2009). What does nursing teamwork look like? A qualitative study. *Journal of Nursing Care Quality, 24*(4), 298–307.

Kingdon, J. W. (2011). *Agendas, alternatives, and public policies* (update 2nd ed.). Glenview, IL: Pearson Education.

Knudson, L. (2013). Healthier hospital food can affect health of patients and the planet. *AORN Journal, 97*(6), C1, C9–C10.

Kohn, L. T., Corrigan, J. M., & Donaldson, M. S. (Eds.). (2000). *To err is human: Building a safer health system.* Washington, DC: National Academies Press.

Kozel, C. T., Kane, W. M., Hatcher, M. T., Hubbell, A, P., Dearing, J. W., Forster-Cox, S., … Goodman, M. (2006). Introducing health promotion agenda-setting for health education practitioners. *Californian Journal of Health Promotion, 4*(1), 32–40.

National Federation of Independent Business v. Sebelius. 567 U.S.; 132 S.Ct. 2566 (2012). Retrieved from http://www.scotusblog.com/case-files/cases/national-federation-of-independent-business-v-sebelius

Newport, F. (2012). *Congress retains low honesty rating.* Retrieved from http://www.gallup.com/poll/159035/congress-retains-low-honesty-rating.aspx

Peters, B. G. (2013). *American public policy: Promise and performance* (9th ed.). Thousand Oaks, CA: CQ Press.

Pralle, S. B. (2002). *Venue shopping as political strategy. Conference Papers—American Political Science Association*, 1–32.

Project Vote Smart. (n.d.). *Government 101: How a bill becomes law.* Retrieved from http://votesmart.org/education/how-a-bill-becomes-law#.Uh98yX92kkh

Smith, Bucklin & Associates, Inc. (2000). *The complete guide to nonprofit management* (2nd ed.). New York, NY: John Wiley & Sons.

U.S. Department of Health & Human Services. (n.d.). *Key features of the Affordable Care Act by year.* Retrieved from http://www.healthcare.gov/law/timeline/full.html

Washington State Department of Health. (2012). *Surgical technologist certification.* Retrieved from http://www.doh.wa.gov/Portals/1/Documents/2000/SurgTechCert.pdf

Weston, M. J., Brewer, K. C., & Peterson, C. A. (2012). ANA principles: The framework for nurse staffing to positively impact outcomes. *Nursing Economics, 30*(5), 247–252.

World Health Organization. (1989). Protecting, promoting and supporting breastfeeding: The special role of maternity service. A joint WHO/UNICEF statement. Geneva: Author. Retrieved from http://whqlibdoc.who.int/publications/9241561300.pdf?ua=1

III

Strategizing and Creating Change

SEVEN

Building Capital: Intellectual, Social, Political, and Financial

Suzanne Miyamoto

My dad used to have an expression—don't tell me what you value; show me your budget.
—Vice President Joe Biden

OBJECTIVES

1. Compare and contrast the types of capital used in policy and advocacy.
2. Relate the concept of capital to its policy impacts.
3. Explore competencies to successfully build capital, given an advocate's resources.
4. Examine the contributions and challenges of coalitions in developing political capital.
5. Discuss the critical role of lobbying and its impact for nursing.
6. Compare the phenomena of the "free rider syndrome" and grassroots in relation to the impact to the profession.

What does building capital truly mean, how does it shape policy, and to what extent is it important for nurses to engage in developing capital? At its core, capital is a necessary tool that can shape status, power, and reputation; in other words, influence. Capital can be developed in intellectual, social, political, and financial forms. For the individual, capital has ramifications on one's personal and professional life. For example, capital could be used to win the school board election or secure the promotion at work. Capital is necessary for state and national organizations to be effective in their mission. National organizations seeking to be leaders in health policy development and implementation may use all four forms of capital to their advantage. Essentially, the more capital an individual, group, or institution controls, the more effective it is in influencing and shaping policy.

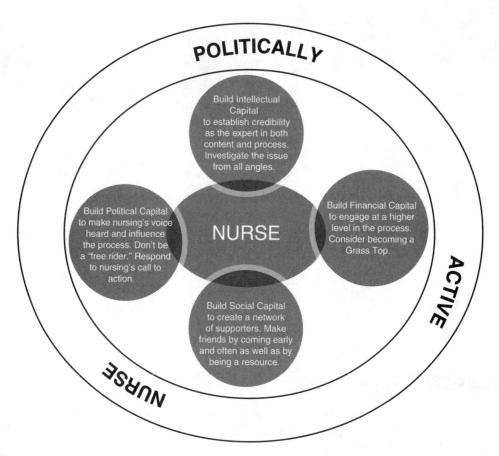

FIGURE 7.1 Creating capital for nurses' political engagement.

It is critical to understand not only the importance of building capital, but also how to amplify the resources necessary to do so. Therefore, this chapter explores the individual nurse's role in developing personal capital, as well as how the individual nurse supports the growth of the profession's capital. Figure 7.1 illustrates the centrality of the nurse to the policy-making process.

Each type of capital will be examined for its role in policy making at the big "P" (e.g., congressional agenda) and little "p" (e.g., policies where you work and live) levels. Nurses and the nursing profession have all of the essential resources to maximize the four forms of capital to engage policy makers at the local, state, and national levels. The Policy Challenge highlighted here demonstrates the use of capital at the national level.

As we see in this Policy Challenge, there was an opportunity for nurses to maximize their political capital to achieve a set of united health care priorities during the debates that would consume Congress for nearly 2 years. This chapter explores the four types of capital (intellectual, social, political, and financial), their interdependency, and how they can be maximized to advance health care policy.

INTELLECTUAL CAPITAL

Intellectual capital for nursing is the knowledge of an individual or the collective knowledge of a group that can be expended to influence policy makers to use or adopt suggestions, viewpoints, and solutions about health care and the health care environment. Nurses have the brainpower to effectively influence policy at both the big "P" and little "p" levels.

The Big "P"

In 2010, the Robert Wood Johnson Foundation (RWJF), in collaboration with Gallup, conducted a survey of over 1,500 health care thought leaders (e.g., from government and the health care sector) to ask their opinions about the

---

POLICY CHALLENGE: Are Nurses at the Health Care Reform Table?

The year is 2008. Congress, the administration, industry, and the public are all focused on health care reform. President Obama established health care reform as his top priority with the growing expectation that new legislation would happen. Nursing's expertise was critical to insert feasible policy solutions to achieve health care reform but was the capital available? That year, nursing's capital rose as three RWJF Health Policy Fellows were situated in key positions on Capitol Hill. Susan Hinck, PhD, RN, was in Senator Rockefeller's (D-WV) office; Senator Rockefeller also sat on the Senate Finance Committee[1]; Nancy Ridenour, PhD, RN, APRN, BC, FAAN, was staff to the House Ways and Means Committee[2]; and Dr. Deborah Trautman, PhD, RN, was in Speaker Nancy Pelosi's[3] (D-CA) office. These nurses were able to leverage their capital and contribute to the health care debates of Congress's most powerful committees and to Congress's most powerful leaders. But they could not do it alone.

The nursing profession needed to come together and find a unified voice to advance a health care reform agenda that placed the patient at the center. The RWJF Health Policy Fellows shared with the national nursing associations that they were hearing from physician colleagues, pharmaceutical companies, and the insurance industry concerning their health care reform platforms. They urged the national nursing representatives to move quickly and in concert with each other in order to have a seat at the table. Nursing's next steps were crucial to determining not only if its voice would be heard but also if the profession has an influence on the outcomes of the health care reform legislation discussions at the White House and on Capitol Hill.

See Option for Policy Challenge.

role nurses play and can play in policy. The large majority reported that nurses should have a greater part in policy. Few nurses today, however, would argue that nursing's full intellectual power has been capitalized on in the policy arena. In fact, the thought leaders were asked to state how they believed that nursing could take on more leadership in the health care delivery system. The top response was to increase their input and make their voices heard (RWJF, 2012).

Nursing and other leaders across the country believe that the science, experience, and skills that are unique to the nursing profession can drive positive system reforms. However, policy can seem an elusive process to many individual nurses. So, first, this section discusses some ways individual nurses have capitalized on their unique skills at the level of the federal government.

The nursing profession is not in short supply of experts. From nationally and internationally renowned nurse researchers to the nurse practicing at the bedside, every nurse in his or her own right is an expert and can drive change from his or her knowledge. A textbook example of a nurse using intellectual capital to inform policy change is Mary Naylor, PhD, RN, FAAN, professor and director of the NewCourtland Center for Transitions and Health at the University of Pennsylvania. For years, Dr. Naylor demonstrated the successful use of advanced practice registered nurses (APRNs) to reduce readmission rates, known as the transitional care model. This model was valued and a similar approach was included in the Patient Protection and Affordable Care Act (PPACA) [Pub. L. No. 111-148] in Section 3026, or the Community-Based Care Transitions Program. According to the Centers for Medicare and Medicaid Innovation (CMMI), this program "... tests models for improving care transitions from the hospital to other settings and reducing readmissions for high-risk Medicare beneficiaries" (CMMI, 2013, p. 1). This example illustrates how a nurse's expertise was used to shape national policy, but it may not be clear that vital to her success was her understanding of the policy process. Earlier in her career, Mary had a W. K. Kellogg Foundation leadership fellowship with the Senate Committee on Aging. Many nurses carry out research, but they fail to tie their work to policy or are not savvy about the political process; thus, their research and expertise never bears full fruition.

Therefore, it is important to understand that while expertise in a particular area is necessary, intellectual capital also refers to understanding the policy process and keeping abreast of policy issues. Congressional staff, nurse lobbyists, and medical lobbyists as groups have identified understanding of the process as an essential strategy to move an issue forward (Begeny, 2009). Understanding the intricacies of policy making, like timing of an issue, is vital to success. For example, if an intended goal is to increase funding for nursing education, knowing when to ask for increased funding or knowing when to support a request that has been made is vital. The request for additional appropriations must come during the time Congress is developing its spending bills. A strong place to start learning this process and what is happening on the national agenda is through nursing associations (for examples, see Exhibit 7.1).

EXHIBIT 7.1   SELECTED RESOURCES FOR BUILDING INTELLECTUAL CAPITAL

Examples of Policy News From Nursing Organizations
American Association of Colleges of Nursing's Policy Beat: http://www.aacn.nche.edu/government-affairs/policy-beat
American Association of Nurse Practitioner's Federal and State News: http://www.aanp.org/legislation-regulation/news
American Nurses Association's Capital Update: http://www.capitolupdate.org
American Organization of Nurse Executive's Washington Report: http://www.aone.org/advocacy/washrpt.shtml
Examples of Federal Agencies
White House's HealthCare.gov: https://www.healthcare.gov
Department of Health and Human Services: http://www.hhs.gov
Agency for Healthcare Research and Quality: http://www.ahrq.gov
Centers for Medicare and Medicaid Services: http://www.cms.gov
Health Resources and Services Administration: http://www.hrsa.gov/index.html
National Institutes of Health: http://www.nih.gov
Examples of National Journals, Nonprofit Organizations, and Think Tanks
Center for American Progress: http://www.americanprogress.org
Health Affairs: http://www.healthaffairs.org
Henry J. Kaiser Family Foundation: http://kff.org
Heritage Foundation: http://www.heritage.org
Institute of Medicine: http://www.iom.edu
The Robert Wood Johnson Foundation: http://www.rwjf.org
National Governors Association: http://www.nga.org/cms/home.html
Examples of Political Newspapers
Politico: http://www.politico.com
Examples of Association Tool Kits
American Association of Critical-Care Nurses Advocacy 101: http://www.aacn.org/wd/practice/content/publicpolicy/advocacy101.pcms?menu=practice
American Association of Nurse Practitioners Policy Toolbox: http://www.aanp.org/legislation-regulation/policy-toolbox

(continued)

EXHIBIT 7.1 SELECTED RESOURCES FOR BUILDING INTELLECTUAL CAPITAL *(CONTINUED)*

American Nurses Association Activist Toolkit: http://www.rnaction.org/site/ PageServer?pagename=nstat_take_action_activist_tool_kit&ct=1&ct=1
Association of periOperative Registered Nurses Advocacy Tools and Resources: http://www.aorn.org/ToolsAndResources
National Association of Clinical Nurse Specialist: Starter Kit for Impacting Change at the Government Level: http://www.nacns.org/html/toolkit.php
National Association of Neonatal Nurses Federal Health Policy Advocacy Tool-kit: http://www.nann.org/uploads/files/Federal_Health_Policy__Advocacy_Tool-kit.pdf

Nurses associations are rich with resources such as tool kits, newsletters, and web pages. Many associations send out monthly policy electronic newsletters that provide the most current policy actions occurring at the state and federal levels. Federal agencies, national journals, think tanks, and policy newspapers are all resources a nurse can use to build his or her intellectual capital. These organizations and media sources report on what Congress is addressing and what health care topics are gaining or losing support.

Many state and specialty nurses associations also offer workshops in conjunction with what are referred to as "advocacy days" to learn the policy process. Advocacy days are events, usually 1 day long, held in a capital and are sponsored by the nurses association. The event is educational and incorporates meeting with legislators and members of the governor's office. The goal is helping nurses understand the legislative process and providing them with proactive steps to advocate for their patients and practice. These events are open to nurses and nursing students and provide nurses associations the opportunity to brief their members and nursing students on the political climate and legislative requests.

A number of short-term programs are available for nurses and nursing students to develop their policy skills (see Exhibit 7.2). The American Nurses Association (ANA) created the American Nurses Advocacy Institute (ANAI), "a year-long mentored program for the purpose of developing nurses into stronger political leaders and expanding the grassroots capacity for the nursing profession and health care" (J. Haebler, personal communication, July 19, 2013). For nursing students, the American Association of Colleges of Nursing (AACN) hosts an annual Student Policy Summit (SPS), which is a 3-day immersion program in policy and politics (see Figure 7.2). For nursing faculty, AACN also offers a short intensive program.

Attending a policy and advocacy conference such as the Nurse in Washington Internship (NIWI) opens the doors to endless possibilities (see Policy on the Scene 7.1). Aside from gaining information about the legislative processes that drive our federal government, the chance to network with other

---

EXHIBIT 7.2 OPPORTUNITIES TO BUILD INTELLECTUAL CAPITAL

For Registered Nurses:

American Nurses Advocacy Institute (ANAI)

The American Nurses Association (ANA) created the ANAI, which is a year-long mentored program designed to develop nurses into stronger political leaders and expand grassroots capacity for the nursing profession and health care. To be considered, the nurse must belong to both ANA and a state nurses association (SNA). Upon completion, each Fellow counsels the SNA in establishing legislative/regulatory priorities, recommends strategies for execution of the advancement of a policy issue, and educates members about the political realities, as well as assists in advancing the ANA's agenda.
http://www.nursingworld.org/AdvocacyResourcesTools

The Alliance: Nursing Organization Alliance's Nurse in Washington Internship (NIWI)

Open to any registered nurse (RN) or nursing student (all levels of education) who is interested in learning about the current issues in nursing and the legislative process. Each participant spends time meeting with his or her members of Congress while participating in the NIWI Annual Advocacy Days.
http://www.nursing-alliance.org/content.cfm/id/niwi

For Nursing Students:

American Association of Colleges of Nurses (AACN) Student Policy Summit (SPS)

The SPS is a 3-day conference held in Washington, DC, and is open to baccalaureate and graduate nursing students enrolled at an AACN member institution. It is a didactic immersion program focused on the nurse's role in professional advocacy and the federal policy process.
http://www.aacn.nche.edu/government-affairs/student-policy-summit

For Nurse Faculty:

AACN's Faculty Policy Intensive (FPI)

The FPI is a 4-day immersion program designed for faculty of AACN member schools interested in actively pursuing a health care and nursing policy role. It offers the opportunity to enhance existing knowledge of policy and advocacy by strengthening understanding of the legislative process and the dynamic relationships between federal departments and agencies, national nursing associations, and the individual advocate.
http://www.aacn.nche.edu/government-affairs/fpi

---

nurses and health care leaders is invaluable (social capital). It is important for nurses and nursing students wanting to become further involved in policy and advocacy to participate in opportunities that help build their knowledge base and professional experience like conferences such as NIWI. Nurses are true experts of their profession and have the ability to make true and lasting impact.

Nurses derive their expertise from the knowledge gained in their specialized education, from their work experience, and from research and evidence-based practice. The challenge is how to effectively communicate this expertise to a policy maker. When it comes to nursing science, there

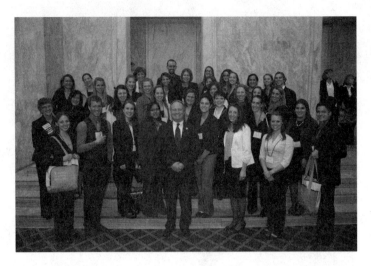

FIGURE 7.2 AACN Student Policy Summit attendees, taking part in the association's advocacy day, are featured with co-chair of the House Nursing Caucus, Representative David Joyce (R-OH).

are concrete factors that make research relevant to policy makers. Hinshaw and Grady (2011) interviewed policy influencers who provided the specific characteristics of science and research that are most useful in shaping health care policy. These are outlined in Exhibit 7.3.

Legislators are not trained as scientists; therefore, the information that is presented to them and their congressional staff must be easily understood and the findings framed in the policy context (i.e., how do the findings save health care dollars, increase access, save lives, or improve quality). Likewise, clinical experience and knowledge must be communicated clearly and in a manner that is understandable. The intellectual capital that comes from experience and knowledge can often be seen as "real world" to a policy maker and stories are often one way to help an issue be seen more clearly (see Chapter 10, "Working With the Media: Shaping the Health Policy Process").

To better hone both your intellectual and political capital, consider getting help that lobbyists from nurses associations or a university can provide. Both of these types of lobbyists have an understanding about intellectual capital and will often have relationships with congressional staff members and can help arrange a meeting to discuss the findings of a particular study. They can assist in putting the nursing research into context for the legislator. Further, when nurses' expertise is shared with their national or state associations, those organization may use them as expert witnesses for a congressional or state legislative hearing.

Intellectual capital is critical for nurses in every type of position. Think about it this way: Although there are federal and state legislators who are RNs, the majority of appointed officials and their staff members are not. They have

POLICY ON THE SCENE 7.1: Capitalizing on Capital
Lauren Inouye, MPP, RN, Associate Director of Government Affairs
AACN, Washington, DC

As a new graduate nurse practicing in the intensive care unit (ICU), I found tremendous satisfaction in my role as patient advocate. I was inspired by my coworkers' ability to serve as tireless advocates and their inherent ability to collaborate with an interprofessional care team, effectively shape an appropriate care plan, and connect with their patients by synthesizing and translating health information in a way the patient would be able to understand (intellectual capital). But, I was also puzzled why more nurses were not utilizing these strong advocacy skills in policy and political arenas. I realized that my advocacy skills used for my patients could also be directed toward serving my profession through a career in policy and advocacy.

I was fortunate to attend the NIWI 3-day conference, which opened new horizons in my pursuit of this career goal. NIWI was instrumental in my path toward becoming a professional nurse advocate. In addition to learning about legislative procedures and how advocacy influences decisions of policy makers, we exercised our advocacy skills during Capitol Hill office visits. For many of us, this was our first experience meeting with federal legislators and their staff. What I will always remember about my first experience with "The Hill" was being in awe. Awe, because I had only 2 years of practice, and yet had the opportunity to discuss nursing issues with highly influential, readily recognizable individuals who were some of the leaders of the profession that I love. And yet to the staff who worked on Capitol Hill, I was the expert.

The second day of the conference marked the turning point in my nursing career. I decided then to pursue my passion in earnest and make the transition from ICU to policy. It was on this day I met a well-known nurse policy leader, Dr. Suzanne Miyamoto (née Begeny). As I listened to a panel of nurse lobbyists who represented national nurses associations at the federal level, I was struck by Dr. Miyamoto's passion and enthusiasm as she described her path from nursing practice to professional advocacy. Her words resonated deeply as she encouraged all of us to become the leaders of our profession.

I introduced myself after the panel (building social capital) at which time she suggested I interview for an internship with the AACN's Government Affairs Department. I received the internship and began to learn the ropes of the policy process and professional lobbying. I continued working full time in critical care and came into AACN's office 1 to 2 days per week. Subsequently, I became the Government Affairs manager for AACN and began a public policy graduate program. Today, I have finished my masters in public policy and was promoted to AACN's associate director of Government Affairs.

EXHIBIT 7.3 FIVE CHARACTERISTICS OF USEFUL SCIENCE AND RESEARCH

- Research is credible
- Information is clearly presented in understandable lay terms
- Data are provided in a quantitative mode
- Results give clear suggestions for actions to be considered
- Findings are framed in a policy context

Source: Hinshaw and Grady (2011).

---

no practical context for what it is like to provide care to a patient, run a nurse-managed health clinic, or educate the next generation of nurses. Only nurses have this expertise. Therefore, the individual nurse has more experience and expertise in a particular area of health care than the legislator or staff. They rely on their expert constituents to provide them with the background for varying health care policies. But the critical piece for nurses to understand is that members of Congress, the vast majority of the time, will not reach out to an individual constituent for advice unless they have an established relationship, as discussed later in the chapter.

The Little "p"

A nurse's individual expertise is vital to shaping policy change at every level, but nurses must be diligent to share this expertise. From the unit level to the hospital system level, the observation of one nurse could improve quality of care, save the health care system hundreds of thousands of dollars, improve the efficiency of care delivery, or develop a national policy standard. Yet, an exceptional idea will never come to fruition if it is not heard.

Empowered nurses can use their expertise to enact change in their organization (Bradbury-Jones, Sambrook, & Irvine, 2008). On the contrary, if nurses do not feel empowered, feelings of frustration and failure emerge (Laschinger & Havens, 1996; Manojlovich, 2007). A thorough literature review conducted by Rao (2012) examined the concept of nurse empowerment over time. This analysis revealed that nurses have viewed empowerment through a lens that focuses on organizational structure. According to Rao (2012), nurses rely "too heavily on rigid bureaucratic structures rather than their own professional power to guide practice. Limiting nurses in this way denies the professional power their role affords them and constrains their ability to achieve extraordinary outcomes" (p. 401). According to Des Jardin (2001), nurses may not believe that they have a role to "challenge the structure of the health care system or the rules guiding that system" (p. 614). Since policy is change, this can cause tension for nurses (Des Jardin, 2001). Therefore, the first steps in many cases are recognizing one's intellectual capital and then overcoming the inertia and speaking out. At work, this process starts by regularly attending meetings and bringing forth issues that have policy implications and that your expertise can help guide. Substantive policy changes often start when people see problems as they carry out their jobs. The policy may relate to an array of practice or clinical issues.

A simple life example about a hospital's policy on the use and filling of water pitchers illustrates the nurse's role at the little "p" level. In a small community hospital, a nurse who saw that using water pitchers was time-consuming for staff, often awkward for patients, and not eco-friendly presented the issue at a shared governance meeting and gained support to lead a 6-week trial of using water bottles instead of water pitchers. Staff and patients answered three questions about the use of the water bottles. The staff (99%) and patients (93%) overwhelmingly supported the conversion to water bottles. Nurses' insights included: "able to keep better track of intakes and outputs, less clean up when patients drop the bottles, and used at home after discharged" (J. Williard, personal communication, August 15, 2013). This nurse used knowledge (gained from working nights when pitchers were routinely filled) and the shared governance process to implement a change in policy that was adopted hospital wide.

In summary, nursing's expertise is a commanding form of capital and needed across the spectrum from the big "P" to the little "p" (see Chapter 5, "Harnessing Evidence in the Policy Process").

SOCIAL CAPITAL

As noted, intellectual capital has to be expended to be of benefit; it needs to be shared. Thus, the second interdependent capital to discuss is social. Developing social capital is essentially relationship building. More specifically, relationships are built and nurtured with key decision makers at the state and national levels to influence policy change. For the nursing profession, social capital should be the most basic, intuitive, and strongest form of capital. Nurses create relationships with their patients, their patients' families, fellow nurses, managers, and so on. Contextually, it relates to the key elements that are necessary for a positive relationship, namely, honesty and trust. As is often repeated in this book, but not capitalized on by nursing, the nursing profession consistently ranks highest among all others as being the most honest profession (Gallup, 2009, 2010, 2011, 2012, 2013).

The Big "P"

Social capital at the big "P" level involves the development of relationships with appointed and elected officials. Members of Congress will listen to the voices of their constituents. This is a reality that every lobbyist inherently knows well. It is constituents who will reelect legislators to serve another term, not the registered lobbyist. Therefore, opinions of constituents are tremendously more relevant than any political wonk in the nation's capital. So even though many believe, and there is evidence that wealth plays an influential role in swaying policy, the value of constituents' opinions and support cannot be dismissed; however, constituents must make their opinions known.

To simply be a nurse constituent in the district of a member of Congress does not mean your voice will be heard among the other hundreds of thousands of constituents. You must be savvy. One of the best ways to accomplish this is to gain guidance from national or state nurses associations. If a nurse has the opportunity to directly communicate with a member of Congress, a nurses association's lobbyist could provide background on the member's political positions, information about what Congress is currently debating and what message would be most relevant, as well as talking points to help prepare for an interaction (see Chapter 10). This is the job of registered lobbyists: to prepare their members to be politically savvy through relationships or social capital. In relation to the big "P," political scientists have described these as grass tops.

Essentially, nursing needs to develop more grass tops. Grass tops are defined as citizens who have the "… greatest probability of influencing a legislator" (Goldstein, 1999, p. 61). The grass tops are constituents who have supported members of Congress either politically (worked on a campaign) or financially (provided an individual donation to a campaign), or who are leaders in their industry (Goldstein, 1999). Because a relationship with a member of Congress has been established, these constituents' voices will resonate loudly at the national and state levels. In fact, national organizations seek out their grass tops members to help drive an advocacy issue. Currently, two nurses hold high-ranking positions in the Obama administration and are leaders in their industry (grass tops): Marilyn Tavenner, MHA, RN, administrator of the Centers for Medicare and Medicaid Services (CMS) (the first nurse in history to head this agency), and Mary Wakefield, PhD, RN, FAAN, administrator of the Health Resources and Services Administration (HRSA). These nurses are excellent examples of grass top leaders who have significant social capital (not to mention intellectual and political capital).

Prior to her prestigious policy position at the national level, Ms. Tavenner was the Secretary of Health and Human Resources for the Commonwealth of Virginia and held numerous leadership positions for the Hospital Corporation of American (CMS, 2013). Administrator Tavenner built such strong political relationships that Representative Eric Cantor (R-VA) overwhelmingly supported her federal nomination by stating, "Marilyn Tavenner is eminently qualified to be the administrator of the CMS. She was an individual with a wealth of knowledge about the complexities of the health care system, and she came forward with solutions that actually made sense" (Congressman Cantor, 2013, p. 1). Representative Cantor was the Republican majority leader who supported a Democratic nominee for the CMS administrator, a shining example of the relationships Ms. Tavenner built with key policy makers across both sides of the aisle.

Dr. Wakefield came to HRSA from the University of North Dakota where she was associate dean for Rural Health at the School of Medicine and Health Sciences. Earlier in her career, she was the chief of staff for Senators Kent Conrad (D-ND) and Quentin Burdick (D-ND), was a member of President

Clinton's Advisory Commission on Consumer Protection and Quality in the Health Care Industry, and was a consultant to the World Health Organization's Global Programme on AIDS in Geneva, Switzerland (HRSA, 2013). Dr. Wakefield's expansive leadership career has been shaped by the relationships she developed (through trust, intelligence, and being politically savvy) that are necessary to rise to such respected positions. Dr. Wakefield often recounts a memorable story on how her political career first began. She was in search of an internship in Washington, DC, to help influence the policy process. Dr. Wakefield called Geraldine "Polly" Bednash, PhD, RN, FAAN (then director of Government Affairs for the AACN, former CEO of AACN) and asked if she had open internships. Dr. Bednash welcomed Dr. Wakefield to AACN. However, shortly after accepting the internship, Dr. Wakefield was informed that she had been offered an internship on Capitol Hill. Dr. Wakefield sought Dr. Bednash's guidance on which internship to take. Without hesitation, Dr. Bednash said Capitol Hill. There, Dr. Wakefield could build the necessary relationships and use her intellectual capital to inform policy makers on the nursing perspective from the inside (Wakefield, 2009).

Although Ms. Tavenner and Dr. Wakefield are excellent examples of grass top nurses, given their federal positions, they cannot lobby in the way discussed in this chapter. The reality is that the nursing profession does not have a strong grass tops network for federal advocacy (Begeny, 2009). Congressional staff and medical lobbyists note that grass tops play a significant role in securing support from members of Congress. One lobbyist helps illustrate the impact of grass tops by sharing this: "Grass tops are significant. The champions we had were the people who made the difference. It was a personal 'ask' to the member of Congress" (Begeny, 2009, p. 135).

To summarize, nursing can build its social capital by having individuals who are savvy (intellectual capital) and who have developed relationships with their elected representatives or staff, in other words, grass tops. The goal is to develop a meaningful relationship. That relationship will help the individual nurse be a valued and trusted resource to that member of Congress. At the core of social capital is developing a long-standing relationship.

Meaningful relationships can be nurtured through financial or personal volunteerism. If financially contributing to the campaign of a member of Congress is not feasible (discussed later), consider volunteering to work on the campaign. If your political views do not align with your current members of Congress, work on the campaign of their upcoming opponent. Also consider being an ever-present voice in your legislator's office, no matter his or her views or party affiliations. This activity can lead to and has led to nurses becoming a major resource and influence to a legislator, a governor, or staff member.

Offering time and expertise is a significant determinant in one's ability to have an effect on a member of Congress and his or her staff. These relationships do not form overnight. Do not give up even when you are told "no." Even when you have differing political leanings than the member of Congress, you can have the opportunity to educate the legislator or staff about issues that are important.

Relationship building takes tenacity, particularly when you are working with a congressional office that might not have the same viewpoint and may never support the issue at hand. This should never be a reason not to visit a member of Congress and his or her staff and pass on the opportunity to educate them about the issue and the importance to their constituency. "No" does not always mean never.

The Little "p"

Social capital can ensure policy change at the little "p" level in many of the same ways as the big "P." The goal is developing relationships with individuals making the policy decisions and with individuals who have intellectual and social capital themselves. It is critical to identify who those individuals are and how you can make the connection with them. Often at the big "P" level, the individuals with whom you want to develop relationships may be obvious, and at the little "p" level, it is sometimes less clear. At first, one may think of only the organizational hierarchy where you work as important in building social capital. Those relationships are vital. However, a good strategy is starting with your existing base of relationships and then broadening those relationships and networks. Consider all of your acquaintances as potential opportunities to extend your social capital. As your network grows, it extends to people who do not necessarily think like you or do the same job as you. You will become less insulated in your views, friendships, and networks.

As will be discussed in the next section on political capital, there is power in numbers. Building a network of colleagues (may be nurses or non-nurses) who agree with the premise of the policy change can better solidify the chances of its implementation. Demonstrating that more than one individual supports the policy change can influence the decision. Establishing this network can sometimes be done easily. Talking during a shift or during an after-hour socialization are some ways. Oprah Winfrey popularized the "book club" and thousands began discussing literature. Take a cue from this "en vogue" socialization to create a "policy club," "kitchen cabinet"—in other words, a network that can offer information and assistance.

Building social capital at the local level can be accomplished in a number of ways: attending continuing education programs provided by your employer, district nurses associations or other nursing groups, serving as a moderator for educational sessions, joining or participating in local organizations' social events or journal clubs, using break times to socialize with key leaders in your organization, or volunteering for your organization's community events. For example, one new graduate built social capital when she was asked by her nurse manager to volunteer for her hospital's community health fair 1 week before her employment start date, because of an unexpected emergency for one of the volunteers. The graduate had experience in organizing community events.

She fulfilled an important need in making the event a success while building important social capital.

A particularly effective way to learn about social capital is from a mentor. Mentors formally or informally can help you by advising you through stories and exemplars of how they were successful and not so successful in relationship building. Nurse leaders, like committee chairs, managers, or nurse executives, can serve as mentors. Successful nurse leaders embrace helping nurses with less experience as they will often tell you they owe their success to a mentor or mentors. They believe in paying it forward.

In summary, whether social capital is built at the state, national, or local level, the key is not necessarily quantity, but quality. As your network grows, it is important to monitor and continually scan for changes in opinions, relationships, and opportunities to advance your social capital. Just as in building any relationship, it takes time and commitment to establish a trusted long-term relationship. A visit or phone call once a year is not enough. Consistent, regular communication is necessary. At the big "P" level, consistently taking the time to send your legislators a new study or simply check in to offer assistance will establish that necessary connection. Moreover, creating opportunities to connect with your network at the little "p" level is also done through consistent purposeful communications. Simple measures to maintain a relationship yield great return on the social capital investment and can ultimately assist in creating policy changes.

POLITICAL CAPITAL

Political capital is influence. It can take multiple forms: financial, social, or intellectual. For the context of this section, political capital will be described as advocacy and "lobbying" efforts undertaken by nurses and the nursing profession.

The Big "P"

At the federal level, the Lobbying Disclosure Act (LDA) guidance defines lobbying contact as any oral, written, or electronic communication to a federal official as specified in the LDA (Office of the Clerk, U.S. House of Representatives, 2013, p. 15). Moreover, lobbying activities include "any efforts in support of such contacts, including preparation or planning activities, research, and other background work that is intended, at the time of its preparation, for use in [lobbying] contacts" (Office of the Clerk, U.S. House of Representatives, 2013, p. 14). Basically, any attempt to influence an official is considered lobbying. State laws also dictate what is considered lobbying in each state (see E-Resources for the National Conference of State Legislatures report). Lobbying is protected under the First Amendment as it allows for the right to "petition the government for redress of grievances" (Public Affairs Council, 2013).

Not all attempts by nurses to contact their representatives should be considered lobbying nor should these nurses be considered lobbyists. Since nurses are not paid to lobby, technically they are not considered registered lobbyists; however, they are advocates and can share their intellectual capital with legislators.

Lobbyists work for a cause or, often, an association or firm, and are paid to "lobby" members of Congress. These individuals must file lobbying disclosure forms to legally engage in this process and are deemed registered lobbyists. There is also variation on what a lobbyist can and cannot do under the LDA depending on where he or she works. For example, the ANA is a 501c(6) organization (trade association, defined under tax code) that can lobby, have a political action committee[4] (PAC), and endorse candidates (see E-Resources, Internal Revenue Service). Many other nursing associations are considered a 501c(3) organization (nonprofit); because of this status, they can only spend a certain portion of their annual revenue on lobbying and it cannot be a major component of the association's work, nor can they have a PAC, or endorse candidates.

The 2010 Supreme Court decision created controversy and confusion regarding the use of donated monies for political influence and the "Super-PAC" (Citizens United, 2010). Former chair of the ANA-PAC, Faith M. Jones, MSN, RN, NEA-BC, states, "A PAC is not a PAC is not a PAC." The ANA-PAC is not a Super-PAC; it is a trade association PAC. The ANA-PAC is composed of nurses who are ANA members. Through their contributions to the ANA-PAC, these nurses participate in the political process and support candidates at the federal level who support ANA's legislative agenda. The ANA-PAC is bipartisan and supports candidates based on the candidates' stand related to issues important to nurses, regardless of party affiliation. This PAC provides the avenue needed to stay abreast of issues, to be educated on a personal level, and to become an informed educator of patients and communities related to health care policy (F. M. Jones, personal communication, July 14, 2013). PACs may endorse candidates for office. The ANA-PAC engages in the endorsement process in order to enhance its political capital (see Policy on the Scene 7.2).

The ANA presidential endorsement process contributed to nursing's strong presence and influence in White House health care discussions. During Bill Clinton's presidency, this led to his appointments of nurses in key senior leadership positions. Beverly Malone, PhD, RN, FAAN (ANA president at the time), was appointed to serve as a deputy assistant secretary for health within the Department of Health and Human Services (DHHS), while Virginia Trotter Betts, MSN, JD, RN, FAAN (ANA past president), was appointed a member of President Clinton's Health Care Reform Task Force and senior advisor on nursing and policy to the secretary and assistant secretary in the DHHS. Clinton supported many of nursing's positions, including the creation of the President's Advisory Commission on Consumer Protection and Quality in the Health Care Industry, which today is known as the National Quality Forum (NQF). Endorsement of Barack Obama was timely with the most recent health care reform debate. The ANA president at the time, Rebecca M. Patton, MSN,

RN, CNOR, FAAN, was often invited to participate in the White House forums discussing health care. This in turn resulted in key provisions in the PPACA favorable to nurses and nursing.

Often when the term *lobbying* is heard, it carries a negative connotation until you understand that it is more than just slapping hands and giving money. Next, the concepts of grassroots, free riders, and coalitions will be introduced and clarified in relation to lobbying. The financial aspects of lobbying will be covered in the section "Financial Capital."

Grassroots

For the nursing profession, the single most powerful form of political capital is its grassroots. Utilizing grassroots is powerful no matter the issue at hand. In grassroots efforts, numbers matter; this is why the RN workforce size is so important. When comparing the number of employed RNs (using the most recent and similar year data, 2010), there were 2,737,400 RNs (Bureau of Labor Statistics [BLS], 2013a) as opposed to 691,000 physicians (BLS, 2013b). The RN workforce outnumbered the physician workforce by 396%.

POLICY ON THE SCENE 7.2: Enhancing Political Capital Through Endorsements
Lori Lioce, DNP, FNP-BC, NP-C, CHSE, FAANP, Clinical Assistant Professor and Simulation Coordinator, University of Alabama Huntsville, AL; Past Chair, ANA-PAC Board of Trustees

---

ANA's PAC (ANA-PAC) works to ensure that nursing's perspective is considered in policy decisions made on Capitol Hill through multiple strategies. The ANA-PAC trustees oversee political matters for the ANA, including the endorsement of candidates who can help accomplish work for the profession. As a PAC, the ANA-PAC is bipartisan in that it includes members of both major political parties. It works directly with political parties at the national level to recruit and support candidates. All federal candidates (Senate, House of Representatives, and the president) are considered for endorsement. Candidates who recognize and support nursing's role and efforts to educate, recruit, and retain nurses in the workforce are identified. During each election cycle, ANA-PAC endorses candidates who will best serve the interests of nurses and their patients. The process includes evaluating candidates' survey responses, assessing incumbents' legislative records on the ANA's priority issues, reviewing campaign polling and fund-raising information, and tracking races in newspapers. Each individual is judged using concrete endorsement criteria set forth by the ANA-PAC trustees. The final step in this process requires the SNA to approve candidate endorsement.

(continued)

For the presidential election, a special bipartisan Presidential Endorsement Task Force is appointed. The process, designed to be transparent, includes examining the voting records of viable candidates, drafting a questionnaire to gauge support for the ANA's core policy issues, conducting candidate interviews, polling SNAs, and polling the ANA members using a virtual voting booth. Detailed records are kept of all contacts and attempted contacts with candidates and/or their staff. Once all information is gathered, the Presidential Endorsement Task Force forwards its recommendation on to the ANA-PAC and the ANA Board for ratification. The presidential endorsement process is a strategy designed to enhance nursing's visibility and credibility as a significant player in health care policy discussions.

The ANA endorsement is considered highly valuable to the candidate even though not all endorsements include financial support. However, many include the maximum amount permitted by law. Each election cycle the ANA publishes the endorsements and encourages nurses to support candidates through their campaigns and in the voting booth.

Consider the impact nurses could make in their advocacy efforts compared to physicians. Political capital for nursing could be summarized in the long-standing adage: "power in numbers." The premise underlying this assertion suggests that numbers mean nothing if they are not maximized. In other words, the choice of the individual nurse plays a substantial role in building the profession's political capital. Engaging nurses as grassroots members can achieve this.

Grassroots involves "using interest group members (or the general public) to pressure congressional lawmakers to support a group's agenda" (Wilcox & Kim, 2005, p. 136). Grassroots can be in the form of letter-writing campaigns, coordinated calls to Capitol Hill, or face-to-face meetings with members of Congress or their staff (Wilcox & Kim, 2005). Grassroots can also include participating in a coordinated e-mail campaign, a lobby day, or protest (Kollman, 1998; Wilcox & Kim, 2005). One of the most effective forms of grassroots lobbying is a lobby day (Wilcox & Kim, 2005). Lobby days (also known as advocacy days) occur when professional associations coordinate their meetings for their members to meet with a legislator or his or her staff to advocate on behalf of a particular issue.

What Policy on the Scene 7.3 demonstrates is twofold: (a) the importance of expertise in developing relationships with members of Congress and (b) the need to adhere to the motto of "Come early, and often." Relationships do not occur overnight, and without the dedication to foster the connection, legislation to address the nurse faculty shortage may not have occurred. Additionally, this exemplar embodies the synergy between individual nurse experts and national nursing lobbyists. The nursing expert does not need expertise in all realms of the policy process to be successful. However, the savvy nurse does know when to utilize his or her network to help accomplish the desired outcome. In this case, the nursing lobbyist was able to act on the relationship that the members had created. This is another ringing endorsement for nurses to be engaged in nursing associations.

Research has shown that an organization with a large constituent base in a particular district or state can "gain the ear" of their member of Congress simply because their members are registered voters (Wright, 1996). As Goldstein (1999) suggests, "Grassroots communications demonstrate to legislators that traceability has been established" (p. 39). Traceability suggests that a large constituent voice has been registered with the member of Congress through calls,

---

POLICY ON THE SCENE 7.3: The Power of Grassroots: Come Early, and Often

Annually, the AACN hosts Advocacy Day for nursing school deans and directors to meet with members of Congress to share their expertise and discuss pressing issues facing the profession. Nursing school deans understand, first hand, that for over a decade, a major barrier impacting the number of students accepted into nursing school is lack of qualified nursing faculty. The faculty shortage in 2012, for example, has been identified as the leading reason that 79,659 qualified applications were turned away from both baccalaureate and graduate nursing programs (AACN, 2013).

One AACN member from Delaware was particularly adamant that the national nurse faculty shortage was inhibiting Delaware schools' ability to educate the nurses needed in the state. She met with her senator and shared examples, statistics, and research to support this issue. When she returned home, she remained in regular communication with the senator's office. Her persistence yielded significant results. The senator investigated the matter further while maintaining ongoing communication with the dean. Over the course of the year, legislation to address the nurse faculty shortage was drafted by the senator's office with the input of the Delaware dean and the AACN lobbyist.

Similarly, nursing deans and directors from Iowa presented their members of Congress with data about the negative impact of the nurse faculty shortage. One Iowa representative was convinced it was critical to address the issue and also worked with the AACN lobbyist to develop legislation to solve the problem. This particular provision was then included in the PPACA.

e-mails, or other methods such as visits, as seen in Figure 7.3. The effectiveness of grassroots is often measured by the quality and quantity of output by the constituents (Kollman, 1998; Thrall, 2006; Wilcox & Kim, 2005). This is where nursing can excel and demonstrate its power in numbers.

Congressional staff, medical lobbyists, and nursing lobbyists all believe grassroots to be a critical advocacy tool (Begeny, 2009). Yet nursing lobbyists have stated they had extreme difficulty mobilizing their grassroots networks. Simply stated, nurses did not respond to action alerts, which included requests like communicating with a member of Congress or participating in a lobby day event. It is clear that answering calls to action is an essential strategy that works—the challenge is to engage all nurses in joining the call to action. According to Begeny (2009, p. 123), "... nurses out in the field don't understand and don't appreciate the power of their voices and that lobbying is a part of being an advocate."

Goldstein (1999) suggests a number of methods to increase constituent engagement. First, Goldstein (p. 50) notes, "Citizens contact their legislators when someone asks them to and shows them how." In nursing, this is done by national groups, state nursing, or specialty organizations by e-mail communication. These action alerts, sent by organizations via e-mail, can take mere minutes to complete and the dividends are high.

If a member of Congress receives one letter on a particular issue, the constituent may receive a response back that was written by the health legislative aide thanking the writer for the message. The health legislative aide may never bring that issue to the legislator's attention because it represented only one voice from the district or state. However, if 50, 100, or 500 messages reach a congressional office, that is when the issue will be brought to the attention of the legislator. It is often questioned whether form e-mail messages to members of

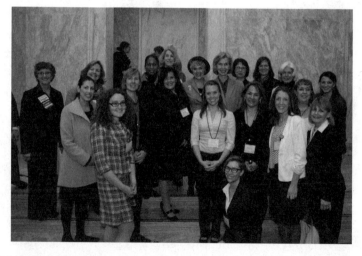

FIGURE 7.3 AACN deans, faculty, and students are featured with the co-chair of the House Nursing Caucus, Representative Lois Capps (D-CA).

Congress are actually effective and the answer is yes. As Goldstein (1999) points out, the quality and quantity must be high. How does one improve the quality of a form letter? That also takes mere minutes. The individual should consider personalizing action alerts by simply modifying the introductory paragraph to introduce himself or herself and indicate why the issue is important; this can increase the quality of the letter. See Chapter 10 for additional details on communicating with legislators. Again, nurses have the opportunity to grow their political capital by using strength in their numbers, but let us examine one of the barriers that is prevalent in nursing.

Free Rider Syndrome

With so much at risk, it is important to explore the reasons why nurses do not engage. Some may suggest time constraints, other competing priorities, or a lack of interest in policy work as factors. However, for nearly five decades, the political science community has described this as what Olson (1965) originally defined as the "free rider syndrome." Free riders are individuals who avoid bearing any of the costs or burdens associated with the actions required to get a benefit. This is common particularly in large groups.

With nearly 3 million practicing nurses, the free rider syndrome is not as easy to spot as in smaller groups. In small groups, it is easier to see when only a few individuals are doing the work and financially supporting the cause. As the group gets larger, members of the group will not notice if some are doing the work while others gain the benefits of that work. As an example, a nurses association sends an e-mail action alert to its 10,000 members requesting them to tell their member of Congress to increase funding for nursing education. Normally, 100 responses would be considered robust. However, there are 100 U.S. Senators and 435 members of the U.S. House of Representatives. With 100 letters, it is likely that some congressional offices did not receive a letter, some offices may have received only one or two, while other offices may have received 25. With 1% participating in this call to action, nursing education funds may not be increased as requested.

The free rider syndrome explanation for this lack of participation is that nurses are relying on the large group to do their work with excuses for their nonparticipation. Regardless of the explanation, lack of participation hurts the profession and ultimately hurts patients. For years, scholars have suggested the importance of an implied cost. Tversky and Kahneman (1981) propose that in order to elicit a more intense response, one must impress upon the individual constituent that he or she would suffer a personal cost. Additionally, some researchers suggest that in order to elicit greater grassroots intensity, interest groups have to raise the cost of not participating (Goldstein, 1999; Rosenstone & Hansen, 1993). A nurse, for example, may have finished all of the degrees that he or she set out to achieve. However, he or she may work in a setting that has a nursing shortage. That individual nurse may be experiencing the added stressors that come from working in a facility with a shortage of nurses: increased emotional distress and job dissatisfaction (Aiken, Clarke, Sloane, Sochalski, & Silber, 2002). So while the issue may not be directly relevant, there is the benefit to that particular nurse if he or she helps ensure there are more colleagues to join him or her in the care-delivery setting. That is why nurses associations often craft a message to show how their members could be personally affected.

To achieve the desired outcome, quantity is necessary for grassroots advocacy. Numbers matter and the only way to increase nursing's numbers are for the individual nurse to respond. The voice of each nurse does in fact make a difference; when nurses come together in coalitions, the impact intensifies.

The Power of Coalition Building

For decades, coalitions have been an effective strategy to build political capital. While the makeup, structure, and longevity of a coalition may vary, they demonstrate power in numbers. Coalitions are usually created to address an immediate issue (Nownes, 2001); for example, the passage of the PPACA. Most nursing associations at the national and state levels are involved with some coalitions to advance policy agendas. At the national level, for example, the Oncology Nurses Society (ONS) uses a number of partnerships to strengthen its influence. Two examples of ONS coalitions include Health Professions Nursing Education and the National Coalition for Cancer Research (Paul, 2008). These two examples from the many in which the ONS participates serve to show the diversity of coalitions. Another example is at the state level where nurse anesthetists represented by the Alabama Association of Nurse Anesthetists (2011) joined a national group by partnering with the Coalition for Patient's Rights.

A prominent example of a coalition is found in supporters of graduate nurse education. During the health care reform debates and after President Obama signed the PPACA into law, coalitions were formed to promote particular initiatives. The Center to Champion Nursing in America launched in December 2007 as a joint initiative of RWJF and AARP, "it was designed to strengthen the nursing workforce by raising awareness of nursing issues and building multistakeholder coalitions seeking solutions at the state and federal levels" (RWJF, 2012, p. 5). It was essential for the Center to network with national nursing associations to advance common goals. One of the priority goals focused on the opportunity to address the need to increase access to primary and acute care through the use of APRNs. This coalition proposed a plan to the national nursing associations representing APRNs and the organizations that represented higher education to secure Medicare dollars for the clinical training of APRNs. While a similar program had been attempted back in the 1990s during the Clinton administration by nursing leaders, the AACN, and the ANA, a second attempt was warranted, given the current legislative climate.

Over the course of many months, the national nursing associations and AARP negotiated a proposal that was then shared with congressional offices. Through established relationships with Senator Debbie Stabenow (D-MI) and Representative Lois Capps (D-RN), the nursing associations were able to demonstrate the demand for the program. By working together to achieve a common goal, this coalition successfully advocated the proposal's advancement. In this instance, it was the unique pairing of nursing and AARP, the largest consumer group, that spoke volumes. Through the work of this distinct coalition, nursing was able to successfully include provision for clinical training of APRNs in the PPACA.

Coalitions provide credibility for the needs of organized interests. Credibility can be developed in two ways. First, organizations with a similar membership can form a coalition. For example, a coalition of all nursing associations could advocate for federal nursing appropriations or a piece of legislation. This demonstrates credibility because nurses are speaking with a unified voice. The RWJF and Gallup study (2010) pointed out that health care opinion leaders felt that one of the ways for the profession to make its voice heard was to speak with a unified message. Often policy makers may become weary if only one organization is promoting an issue (Nownes, 2001). Additionally, a coalition of unlikely or unique partners could be developed. In the aforementioned instance, national nursing associations partnered with AARP, which is an example of a unique coalition.

Second, coalitions can reduce the level of conflict associated with an issue (Nownes, 2001). When conflict is minimal, an issue stands a better chance of being recognized and successfully moving through the policy process. As Price (1978) points out in his seminal work, an issue has a better chance of appearing on the congressional agenda if the degree of conflict among groups is low and public salience (or interest) is high.

Third, coalitions are extremely efficient, as they allow organizations to pool their resources (Nownes, 2001). Pooling of resources allows organizations to spend less if they were advocating for the issue on their own (Hula, 1995). This is critically important to the nursing profession. As will be discussed in the section on financial capital, nurses associations often do not have the same level of funding as other health professions associations. One of the advantages in creating coalitions is that they allow organizations to share resources in the forms of financial resources, lobbyists, expertise, and time.

While coalitions may be effective, it is important to know that they do not always work. Olson (1965), in his classic work, warns that the assumption that groups of individuals with common interests will usually work to further those interests is false and based on flawed logic. Just as in the case of grassroots, coalitions can also fall victim to the "free rider syndrome." As organizations convene to work on a particular issue and as that group grows, members of the coalition quickly decide if the benefits outweigh the necessary contributions. In a coalition of 50 organizations, there may only be 5 to 10 that actually do the work, while the others benefit. If incentives are not in place for the 5 to 10 organizations that actually do the work, they may not be willing to share their political capital. While Olson points out that altruism is sometimes the case, it is not the norm. Knowing that Congress places significant weight on coalitions and their ability to speak with one voice, many organizations are actively pursuing coalitions. Coalition work is an opportunity to network (build social capital) with others who share similar views on a particular issue. However, a coalition must be strong enough to have members that become engaged and find value in its work. See Figure 7.4 for key components in coalition building based on lessons learned by the author.

One example of a strong collaboration within nursing is the Nursing Community (Nursing Community, 2009). Started circa 2002, the Nursing Community was a group of national nurses associations that came together once a year to discuss the unified funding request for the Nursing Workforce Diversity programs (Title VIII of the Public Health Service Act). For over a decade, the Nursing Community has determined the funding request level for nursing

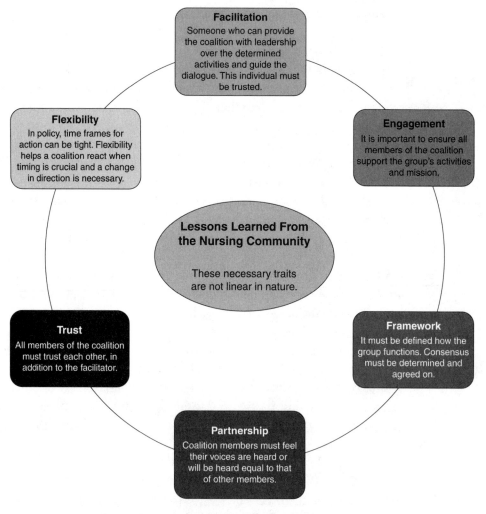

FIGURE 7.4 Keys to building an effective coalition.

education and advocated in a cohesive fashion to move this number forward. Over the years, this forum has strengthened its power from a loosely affiliated group that came together once a year to a coalition that drafts letters to congressional appropriations; hosts virtual lobby days, receptions and briefings on Capitol Hill; and visits with members of Congress who sit on the House and Senate Appropriations Committees.

Coalitions offer a prime opportunity to build political capital. However, not all coalitions are easily established or maintained. The common theme that has surfaced throughout this chapter is that all forms of capital are needed. When working in coalitions, trust (social capital) needs to be established and a common good must be identified. The ability of nurses to build coalitions as a form of political capital transcends across big "P" and little "p." To create a policy change at the unit, local, or state level, coalitions can be an effective tool. At the heart of coalitions is power in numbers.

The Little "p"

In many respects, building political capital starts at the local level. It is not uncommon for elected officials to work their way through a number of appointed or elected positions before reaching the state or national level. The processes of big "P" and little "p" can and, by necessity, often do overlap. Grassroots work by its very definition starts at the local level. In addition, free riders exist across all settings. They do not attend meetings, are often critical of discussions and decisions, and seldom offer solutions or get involved to resolve issues. Just as coalitions are important at the big "P" level, they are equally important at the little "p" level. An experienced nurse working to improve patient flow illustrates a little "p" example of political capital. This issue is problematic for many units, for example, emergency departments, ICUs, and postanesthesia care units. Each year, during the flu season, the need for timely discharges and transfers intensifies and becomes a major throughput issue. In anticipation of the flu season, a well-respected nurse convened a meeting with representatives from each unit. All agreed there was a need to recommend solutions to improve patient flow and formed a coalition, including staff from other departments. This group quickly assembled solutions that were implemented system-wide and in each department that improved patient flow and patient satisfaction.

To summarize, political capital is influence, which is essential to impact policy. Nursing must be strategic. Significant health care policy issues can benefit from the nursing perspective. When policy issues are identified, coalitions must be established, experts found, and resources pooled to achieve success.

FINANCIAL CAPITAL

Financial capital is often exemplified in the golden rule: "He who has the money, makes the rules" (Nownes, 2001). Nurses may be quick to point out that, compared to other industries and professions in health care, nurses do not have the "gold" that would allow the profession's voice to resonate loudest. In many cases, this is true. According to the BLS (2013a, 2013b), in 2010, physicians made approximately 2.5 times more money than RNs. This is clearly an important factor in the amount a nurse can contribute to a PAC[4] or donate as an individual contribution to candidates or causes. Nevertheless, financial resources are, without a doubt, a significant factor to organized advocacy and allow for a specific interest to be advanced.

The Big "P"

At the federal level, it is believed that money is the driving force in achieving space on the congressional agenda. As Berry (1999, p. 85) points out, "Space on the Congressional agenda is a precious commodity." Nursing's financial capital has not measured up to the capital of other health care professionals. Organizations' financial capital supports services such as professional registered lobbyists and provides resources to promote their agendas, such as studies to support an issue, expert analysis, and advocacy materials. Money also comes in the form of a PAC and individual contributions to members of Congress. Two forms of financial capital are lobbying and PACs.

Lobbying

As indicated earlier, lobbying serves to educate and influence members of Congress. Currently, there are 12,389 registered federal lobbyists in the United States working on issues from gun control to health care (Open Secrets, 2013c). This number has grown by 19% in 14 years. For the "health professions" category, there are 690 registered lobbyists (Open Secrets, 2013d). In 2012, the "health professions" organizations spent $78,605,157 on their lobbying efforts (Open Secrets, 2013d).

Comparing the top nursing (ANA) and physician (American Medical Association [AMA]) organizations, the ANA spent $1,678,797 on lobbying activities with five lobbyists in 2012, while the AMA spent $16,130,000 with 21 lobbyists in the same year (Open Secrets, 2013e, 2013f). The AMA spent 960% more on lobbying than the ANA and used 4.2 lobbyists for each ANA lobbyist (see Exhibit 7.4).

Top physician organizations outspent nursing's top organizations by 879% and had almost three lobbyists for every one nursing lobbyist. The impact can be seen with more lobbyists visiting members of Congress and their staff, more funding for studies to demonstrate the effectiveness of programs, more money to develop comprehensive lobbying materials, and resources to organize lobby days. Simply stated, physicians have more financial capital.

Political Action Committees

Some would argue that PACs hold much weight as a form of capital in helping to secure space on the congressional agenda. Exchange theories suggest that lobbyists and legislators engage in unspoken agreements or trades (Austen Smith,

EXHIBIT 7.4 LOBBYING DOLLARS SPENT IN 2012**: TOP FIVE NURSE AND PHYSICIAN ORGANIZATIONS

NURSE ORGANIZATIONS	LOBBYING DOLLARS SPENT	NUMBER OF LOBBYISTS*	BILLS LOBBIED	ISSUES LOBBIED
American Nurses Association	1,678,797	5	33	10
American Association of Nurse Anesthetists	1,060,000	10	30	4
American Association of Colleges of Nursing	145,000	6	7	6
Association of Rehabilitation Nurses	120,000	6	0	4
American College of Nurse Practitioners	93,800	1	91	3
Total	**3,097,597**	**28**	^	^
PHYSICIAN ORGANIZATIONS				
American Medical Association	16,130,000	26	54	14
American College of Radiology	3,559,650	15	6	4
American College of Emergency Physicians	2,912,171	10	89	16
American Academy of Family Physicians	2,597,215	13	16	20
American College of Cardiology	2,030,000	12	5	2
Total	**27,229,036**	**76**	^	^

*Includes lobbying firms but not state associations.
**Data compiled after every 2-year election cycle.
^Overlapping bills and issues lobbied.
Source: Open Secrets (2013d).

1996; Morton & Cameron, 1992). As the theory suggests, the trade between a member of Congress and a lobbyist is an implicit trade that mutually benefits both parties and is typically identified as a political campaign or PAC contributions to a member of Congress for their vote on a particular issue. Exchange theories have been described as "vote buying," while others viewed this as "buying" a member of Congress's time (Stratmann, 1998). This suggests that PAC contributions are made so lobbyists can discuss a specific issue with the hope of gaining their "vote." Some may question the level of effectiveness between PAC contributions and actions of congressional members, but there is evidence that PACs provide some level of access to legislators and their staff (Wright, 1990). As Berry (1999, p. 151) states, "Interest group leaders believe that PAC donations are well worth it because the money is converted into more face time with legislators and key aides, and they think that this interaction increases the chances that these congressional offices will do something on the group's behalf."

For the context of this discussion, the assumption is that PACs, to a certain level, influence and build financial capital. More importantly, it is a quantifiable data piece that clearly illustrates the gap in nursing's political expenditures. Nursing has PACs at both the national and state levels. In total, there are 128 PACs that are considered "health professions," and five of them are national nursing PACs. With the merger of the American Academy of Nurse Practitioners (AANP) and the American College of Nurse Practitioners (ACNP) (Open Secrets, 2013a), the number of national nursing PACs will be four. Compare this to the over 50 national physician PACs. Many state physician PACs and private companies lobby at the national level (Open Secrets, 2013b). Not only do physicians have more PACs, but they also significantly out spend the existing nurse PACs.

Nursing's largest PAC, which belongs to the American Association of Nurse Anesthetists (AANA), raised over $1.4 million in the 2012 PAC cycle (see Exhibit 7.5). AANA's physician counterpart, the American Society of Anesthesiologists (ASA), raised over $3.5 million in the same 2012 cycle (see Exhibit 7.5). The ASA raised 237% more than the AANA. The actual number of contributions per person was approximately 292% higher.

One could even compare the ANA, nursing's second largest PAC, which raised $767,212, to the AMA, which cleared $1,902,096 in the same 2012 PAC cycle (see Exhibit 7.5). The AMA outspent the ANA by 248% in donations to members of Congress during their election campaigns. This substantial difference is disappointing even though physicians generally make more money. Consider the potential impact of our financial capital if every nurse would contribute just one dollar in a PAC cycle.

PAC contributions for physician groups are quite robust. However, other health professions also see the direct benefit of PAC fund-raising. Some have greater PAC contributions despite having fewer members in their professions than nursing. The American Dental Association, the American Optometric Association, the American Physical Therapy Association, and the American Podiatric Association ranked 4th, 7th, 8th, and 10th, respectively, of the top ten 2012 PAC contributors (Open Secrets, 2013b). It is important to point out that AANA was ranked 11th in contributions.

The path for nursing to overcome the financial resources dilemma is clear. Organizations pay for lobbying activities through their membership dues and other sources of revenue generated by the support of their membership (i.e., conferences and publications). Numbers matter in achieving financial capital. Membership in national nurses associations is paramount. The individual nurse must determine where his or her money will be best spent, matching personal values and priorities.

It should also be noted that while the aforementioned information concerning PACs and lobbying relates to federal activity, trends are similar at the state level. At the state level, most nurse PACs and lobbying are done by SNAs.

EXHIBIT 7.5	NATIONAL NURSE AND PHYSICIAN ORGANIZATION 2012 ELECTION CYCLE PAC SUMMARY				
NURSE ORGANI-ZATIONS	RAISED	CONTRIBUTIONS TO FEDERAL CANDI-DATES	% TO DEMO-CRATS	% TO REPUB-LICANS	NUMBER OF DONORS*
American Association of Nurse Anesthetists	$1,483,434	$683,800	50	50	1,928
American Nurses Association	$767,212	$542,500	82	16	262
American College of Nurse Midwives	$173,407	$70,500	74	26	235
American Academy of Nurse Practitioners	$64,972	$63,050	65	35	17
American College of Nurse Practitioners	$24,965	$26,500	49	51	20
Totals	$2,513,990	$1,386,350			2,462
PHYSICIAN ORGANIZATIONS					
American Society of Anesthesiologists	$3,516,525	$1,404,650	36	64	5,644
American Medical Association	$1,902,096	$1,627,200	40	59	1,073
American College of Emergency Physicians	$1,880,101	$1,290,000	41	59	1,950
Ob-Gyn PAC	$1,021,599	$613,000	61	39	1,631
American Academy of Family Physicians	$891,041	$481,500	60	40	1,280
Total	$9,211,362	$5,416,350			11,578

*Gave over $200.
Source: Open Secrets (2013b).

Unions representing nurses may also lobby at the state level. Therefore, not only should nurses consider joining national organizations, but also state associations. This is important for APRNs where a unified voice at the state level is so critical to removing practice barriers. It is important for all nurses when unlicensed persons seek to represent themselves as "nurses" in states that do not protect the title "nurse" or "registered nurse." There are numerous issues addressed at the state level that require an ongoing and vigilant presence at the statehouse that benefit from the use of PACs and lobbying efforts. These same principles can be applied at the local level such as in the case of a school board, city council, or township board.

The Little "p"

Money speaks at all levels. While financial capital at the big "P" level receives a lot of attention, the financial impact at the little "p" level is often not fully realized. Contributions locally are just as important as at the national and state levels. Your personal contribution of time or money will be acknowledged and may lead to opportunities for influencing policy within your community. In particular, personal donations are strategic and can lead to future board appointments. Often there is the expectation for board members to support foundations and special events, causes, and programs. However, financial capital is not just about what you contribute. It is important to realize the opportunities that exist to fund and support your cause or policy. Foundations, hospital auxiliary boards, and alumni groups can be solicited for financial support.

To summarize, the first essential step a nurse can take to maximize the profession's political capital is joining the organizations that advance the voice of nursing at the national and state levels. Second, knowing the importance and significant gap in nurses' financial political capital, nurses should consider contributing to a PAC, to a member of Congress, or to both.

OPTION FOR POLICY CHALLENGE: Are Nurses at the Health Care Reform Table?

During the health care reform dialogue, national nursing associations individually and through multiple coalitions used their expertise (drawn from their membership) to advocate on behalf of the profession and America's patients. Contrary to rumors and speculation that nursing could not speak with a unified voice, nursing proved otherwise. The nurses associations' representatives involved in the process had significant capital in the form of intellectual, social, and political capital. It should be noted explicitly that each individual nursing association played its own unique role in shaping the provisions that were included in the final health care reform bill.

Because national nurses associations came together and stood united around a common set of recommendations, they were able to achieve many of the critical provisions in the PPACA [Pub. L. No. 111-148]. The effort was daunting, but yielded great dividends.

(continued)

Strategies for health care reform achieved results this time. Often recognized but inconsistently utilized, the nursing profession came together and remained focused on achieving meaningful results in health care reform. Whether working at the big "P" or little "p" level, these strategies, while complex and interrelated, can be used by nurses to achieve policy change. Selected strategies for health care reform are summarized here:

- Collaborating among stakeholders
- Presenting an unified nursing voice
- Establishing a common set of goals
- Determining a single set of priorities
- Developing framework for the group's actions
- Instituting a clear communication process

IMPLICATIONS FOR THE FUTURE

Nursing has remarkable potential to build and expand its capital. This is true of each individual nurse, as well as state nurses associations and national nurses associations. But the cornerstone of achieving this potential is the ability of the individual nurse to understand that his or her voice and resources (i.e., money, time, and expertise) are necessary for the greater good of the profession and patients, families, and communities. While many of the themes outlined in this chapter relate to capital focused on national advocacy, they translate to the work of each nurse. If one's goal is to change a standard in his or her hospital setting, how can relationships, coalitions, resources, and expertise be maximized?

Over the decades, nursing has made epic strides as a profession. Nurses are trusted and respected by the public, but as the RWJF (2010) opinion leader study pointed out, they must make their voices heard, and heard in unison. It was evident in the financial capital discussion that significant work is essential for nursing to be comparable with the lobbying efforts of other national health professions. This is within our reach by using our expertise and dedication to the patient.

KEY CONCEPTS

1. Nursing's capital must be grown and cultivated.
2. Nurses must value and appreciate the importance of the individual voice in building capital.
3. At the heart of the profession is patient advocacy. This innate trait should be used to improve the health of the nation at every level.
4. Nurses must not be intimidated or hesitant to offer their valued contribution to those in power. Nursing's expertise is a commanding form of capital.
5. Nurses must view political advocacy as a professional value, not something that is "dirty."

6. Whether social capital is built at the state, national, or local level, the key is not necessarily quantity, but quality.

7. For nursing, coalitions offer prime opportunities to build political capital. However, not all coalitions are easily established or maintained.

8. Nurses must invest in their nursing associations to ensure they have the resources to build the profession's capital.

9. Building capital is obtainable and necessary for every nurse as all politics are local.

10. Nurses must understand that policy change will continue to occur without the profession's insight if nurses do not build all forms of capital.

SUMMARY

If nursing wants a seat at the table when health care policy decisions are being debated and made, then it must invest in the efforts to obtain that seat. As the opening quote from Vice President Biden points out, "Don't tell me what you value; show me your budget." Nurses may say they value advocacy and policy work, but their budget often does not match up. Nurses and the nursing profession must get strategic and build capital through education and engagement of nurses. It cannot be left to a few to attempt the massive change that the profession wishes to achieve to truly impact health and wellness nationally and globally. Nursing can excel in this realm; however, nurses must first overcome any lingering stereotypes and historical sentiments that politics and policy are not appropriate for the profession. At the heart of the profession is patient advocacy, so why can this not be replicated at the local, state, and national levels? Nurses must establish a pathway that will create their own capital. In the end, it is power in numbers.

LEARNING ACTIVITIES

1. Identify your local, state, and federal legislators. Select one whom you want to visit. Identify the key points that you will discuss at the visit. Plan for a 10-minute visit and for a 20-minute visit. Consider how your visit will vary if you talk to a staffer or the legislator. Then make a visit to the office and report on the highlights of the visit.

2. Determine when Nurse Advocacy Day is held by your state nurses association and the process to register. Review resources that cover the material presented and the legislators who were encountered in last year's Nurse Advocacy Day. Register and attend.

3. In your work environment consider inviting a leader to coffee. Ask for recommendations and advice for becoming politically active. Specifically inquire about their pathways in policy and mentors.

4. Compare and contrast two advocacy tool kits. Compare one tool kit listed in Exhibit 7.1 and an additional one on the Internet. Explain why

you selected each and then compare and contrast the key features of each tool kit.

5. Develop a list of strategies to convince classmates of the importance of supporting a nurses association and its PACs at the state or national level.

6. Reread the sections on "free riders" and "grass tops." Consider whether you know people in either category. Develop talking points to challenge one "free rider" to join an advocacy effort with you.

NOTES

1. The Senate Finance Committee has jurisdiction over Medicare and Medicaid.
2. The House Ways and Means Committee has jurisdiction over Medicare and Medicaid.
3. At this time Representative Nancy Pelosi was the Speaker of the House of Representatives.
4. Political action committee is "An organization set up solely to collect and spend money on electoral campaigns. A type of organized interest" (Nownes, 2001, p. 231).

E-RESOURCES

Effective Coalitions

- Coalition for Patients' Rights. http://www.patientsrightscoalition.org
- The Nursing Community. http://www.thenursingcommunity.org
- RWJF and AARP's Future of Nursing Campaign for Action. http://campaignforaction.org

Lobbying Information

- Internal Revenue Service. http://www.irs.gov/Charities-&-Non-Profits/Lobbying
- National Conference of State Legislatures. http://www.ncsl.org/legislatures elections/ethicshome/50-state-chart-lobby-definitions.aspx
- Public Affairs Council. http://pac.org/ethics/Response-to-Abramoff-Scandal

PAC Information

- Open Secrets. http://www.opensecrets.org/pacs/pacfaq.php

REFERENCES

Aiken, L., Clarke, S., Sloane, D., Sochalski, J., & Silber, J. H. (2002). Hospital nurse staffing and patient mortality, nurse burnout, and job dissatisfaction. *Journal of the American Medical Association, 288*(16), 1987–1993.

Alabama Association of Nurse Anesthetists. (2011). Retrieved from http://www.alabamacrna.org/?p=729

American Association of Colleges of Nursing. (2013). *2012–2013 Enrollment and graduations in baccalaureate and graduate programs in nursing.* Washington, DC: Author.

Austen Smith, D. (1996). *Interest groups: Money, information and influence.* As cited in Mueller, D. C. (Ed.). (1997). *Perspectives on public choice.* Cambridge, UK: Cambridge University Press.

Begeny, S. M. (2009). *Lobbying strategies for federal appropriations: Nursing versus medical education.* Retrieved from http://hdl.handle.net/2027.42/64641

Berry, J. M. (1999). *The new liberalism: The rising power of citizen groups.* Washington, DC: Brookings Institute Press.

Bradbury-Jones, C., Sambrook, S., & Irvine, F. (2008). Power and empowerment in nursing: A fourth theoretical approach. *Journal of Advanced Nursing, 62*(2), 258–266.

Bureau of Labor Statistics. (2013a). *Occupational outlook handbook: Registered nurses.* Retrieved from http://www.bls.gov/ooh/healthcare/registered-nurses.htm

Bureau of Labor Statistics. (2013b). *Occupational outlook handbook: Physicians and surgeons.* Retrieved from http://www.bls.gov/ooh/healthcare/physicians-and-surgeons.htm

Centers for Medicare and Medicaid Innovation (CMMI). (2013). *Community-based care transitions program.* Retrieved from http://innovation.cms.gov/initiatives/CCTP

Centers for Medicare and Medicaid Services. (2013). *CMS leadership: Administrator: Marilyn Tavenner.* Retrieved from http://www.cms.gov/About-CMS/leadership

Citizens United v. Federal Election Commission, 558 US 310 (2010). Retrieved from http://en.wikipedia.org/wiki/Citizens_United_v._Federal_Election_Commission

Congressman Cantor. (2013). *Congressman Cantor statement on CMS nominee Marilyn Tavenner.* Retrieved from http://cantor.house.gov/press-releases/congressman-cantor-statement-cms-nominee-marilyn-tavenner

Des Jardin, K. (2001). Political involvement in nursing: Politics, ethics, and strategic action. *Association of Operating Room Nurses Journal, 74,* 614–628.

Gallup. (2009). *Honesty and ethics poll finds Congress' image tarnished.* Retrieved from http://www.gallup.com/poll/124625/honesty-ethics-poll-finds-congress-image-tarnished.aspx

Gallup. (2010). *In U.S., nurses at top of ethics list, lobbyists at bottom.* Retrieved from http://www.gallup.com/video/145199/Nurses-Top-Ethic-List-Lobbyists-Bottom.aspx

Gallup. (2011). Record 64% rate honesty, ethics of members of Congress low. Retrieved from http://www.gallup.com/poll/151460/record-rate-honesty-ethics-members-congress-low.aspx

Gallup. (2012). *Honesty and ethics in professions.* Retrieved from http://www.gallup.com/poll/1654/honesty-ethics-professions.aspx

Gallup. (2013). *Honesty/ethics in professions.* Retrieved from http://www.gallup.com/poll/1654/honesty-ethics-professions.aspx

Goldstein, K. M. (1999). *Interest groups, lobbying, and participation in American.* New York, NY: Cambridge University Press.

Health Resources and Services Administration. (2013). *Mary Wakefield, PhD, RN: Administrator, Health Resources and Services Administration, U.S. Department of Health and Human Services, Biography.* Retrieved from http://www.hrsa.gov/about/organization/biowakefield.html

Hinshaw, A., & Grady, P. (2011). *Shaping health policy through nursing research.* New York, NY: Springer.

Hula, K. W. (1995). Rounding up the usual suspects: Forging interest group coalitions in Washington. In A. J. Cigler & B. A. Loomis (Eds.), *Interest group politics* (4th ed., pp. 239–258). Washington, DC: CQ Press.

Kollman, K. (1998). *Outside lobbying.* Princeton, NJ: Princeton University Press.

Laschinger, H. K. S., & Havens, D. S. (1996). Staff nurse work empowerment and perceived control over nursing practice: Conditions for work effectiveness. *Journal of Nursing Administration, 26*(9), 27–35.

Manojlovich, M. (2007). Power and empowerment in nursing: Looking backward to inform the future. *OJIN: Online Journal of Issues in Nursing, 12*(1). Retrieved from http://www.nursingworld.org/MainMenuCategories/ANAMarketplace/ANAPeriodicals/OJIN/TableofContents/Volume122007/No1Jan07/LookingBackwardtoInformtheFuture.asp

Morton, R., & Cameron, C. (1992). Elections and the theory of campaign contributions: A survey and critical analysis. *Economics and Politics, 4,* 79–108.

Nownes, A. J. (2001). *Pressure and power: Organized interest in American politics.* Boston, MA: Houghton Mifflin Company.

Nursing Community. (2009). *Commitment to quality healthcare reform: A consensus statement from the Nursing Community.* Retrieved from http://www.thenursingcommunity.org/#/health-reform/4542347781

Office of the Clerk, U.S. House of Representatives. (2013). *Lobbying Disclosure Act Guidance.* Retrieved from http://lobbyingdisclosure.house.gov/amended_lda_guide.html

Olson, M. (1965). *The logic of collective action: Public goods and the theory of groups.* Cambridge, MA: Harvard University Press.

Open Secrets. (2013a). Nurses. Retrieved from http://www.opensecrets.org/industries/indus.php?ind=H1710

Open Secrets. (2013b). *PACs: Health professions.* Retrieved from http://www.opensecrets.org/pacs/industry.php?txt=H01&cycle=2012

Open Secrets. (2013c). *Lobbying.* Retrieved from http://www.opensecrets.org/lobby

Open Secrets. (2013d). *Lobbying: Health professions.* Retrieved from http://www.opensecrets.org/lobby/indusclient_lobs.php?id=H01&year=2012

Open Secrets. (2013e). *Lobbying: American Nurses ASSN.* Retrieved from http://www.opensecrets.org/lobby/clientlbs.php?id=D000000173&year=2012

Open Secrets. (2013f). *Lobbying: American Medical Assn.* Retrieved from http://www.opensecrets.org/lobby/clientlbs.php?id=D000000068&year=2012

Patient Protection and Affordable Care Act (PPACA) [Pub. L. No. 111-148], § 3026.

Paul, I. (2008). Coalition Participation Allows ONS to Influence Numerous Public Policy Issues. *ONS Connect, 23*(8), 21.

Price, D. E. (1978). Policy making in Congressional Committees: The impact of "environmental" factors. *The American Political Science Review, 72*(2), 548–574.

Public Affairs Council. (2013). *Explaining lobbying to external and internal audiences.* Retrieved from http://pac.org/ethics/Response-to-Abramoff-Scandal

Public Health Service Act [Pub. L. 78-410]. Title VII.

Rao, A. (2012). The contemporary construction of nurse empowerment. *Journal of Nursing Scholarship, 44*(4), 396–402.

Robert Wood Johnson Foundation. (2010). *Nursing leadership from bedside to boardroom: Opinion leaders' perceptions.* Retrieved from http://www.rwjf.org/en/about-rwjf/newsroom/newsroom-content/2010/01/nursing-leadership-from-bedside-to-boardroom-opinion-leaders-per.html

Robert Wood Johnson Foundation. (2012). *Center to Champion Nursing in America. A progress report.* Retrieved from http://www.rwjf.org/en/research-publications/find-rwjf-research/2012/08/center-to-champion-nursing-in-america.html

Rosenstone, S., & Hansen, M. (1993). *Mobilization, participation, and democracy in America.* New York, NY: Macmillan.

Stratmann, T. (1998). The market for congressional votes: Is timing of contributions everything? *Journal of Law and Economics, 41,* 85–113.

Thrall, A. T. (2006). The myth of outside strategy: Mass media news coverage of interest groups. *Political Communications, 23,* 407–420.

Tversky, A., & Kahneman, D. (1981). The framing decisions and the psychology of choice. *Science, 211,* 453–458.

Wakefield, M. (2009, October 25). *Acceptance Speech for AACN's Policy Luminary Award,* AACN Fall Semiannual Meeting, Washington, DC.

Wilcox, C., & Kim, D. (2005). *Continuity and change in the congressional connection.* As cited in P. S.Herrnson, R. G. Shaiko, & C. Wilcox, (2005), *The interest group connection: Electioneering, lobbying, and policymaking in Washington* (2nd ed.). Washington, DC: CQ Press.

Wright, J. R. (1990). Contributions, lobbying, and committee voting in the U.S. House of Representatives. *American Political Science Review, 84,* 417–438.

Wright, J. R. (1996). *Interest groups and Congress: Lobbying, contributions, and influence.* Boston, MA: Allyn & Bacon.

EIGHT

Changing Organizations, Institutions, and Government

Tim Porter-O'Grady
Kathy Malloch

> *The natural instinct is to think that innovation has to do with invention. That's the smallest part … the real essence of innovation is fresh thinking that connects with value creation. —Vijay Vaitheeswaran*

OBJECTIVES

1. Compare and contrast the differences between change and innovation and their relationship to policy advancement.
2. Explain the barriers and facilitators to policy development and implementation in the work of health care.
3. Examine the significance of team building and teamwork among health care stakeholders and the relationship to effective policy formulation.
4. Differentiate concepts necessary for translational policy formulation in both small- and large-scale change.
5. Evaluate lessons learned in the creation of health care policies.
6. Plan one's own future actions as a nursing leader in the continuing journey of effective health care policy participation, creation, and revision.

The work of change is inherent in making policy. While change is often challenging, there is no avoiding it. Understanding change is essential to health care policy, as many policies evolve from the ever-emergent nature of health care. Shifts in knowledge, relationships, economics, technology, and the environment are normative now and are projected to only increase in the future. Health care policies need to be current and appropriate to support safe and effective health care with the numerous changes that are ongoing. As nurses, the essence of our work is about change, innovation, and creating policies to support the expected work of patient care excellence. Nurses work with patients to change and improve their state of health on a continual basis. When, for example, a new technology or treatment is initiated, it is often the nurse in direct care who is the first to see the unforeseen impact to patients and nurses as they carry out new work and recognize the need for policy change. The numerous redesign of workflow that occurs when moving from paper to electronic documentation is one example of how policy with a little "p" is implemented.

The work of nursing is also about ensuring that established evidence and core beliefs for value-driven patient care are supported and drive the appropriate policy change and innovation in health care. The Institute of Medicine (IOM) *The Future of Nursing* report recommended that nurses should be prepared to lead change and advance health (IOM, 2011). Every nurse needs to be a partner in this work. In this chapter, theories of change, team building, translational policy formulation, barriers and facilitators to change, lessons learned from recent changes, the work of turning around failed attempts, and a brief discussion of unresolved issues and future opportunities are presented.

Changing policy requires careful thought, involvement of appropriate stakeholders, planning, and evaluation. The oversight of nurse licensure and regulation is complex. See the following Policy Challenge. The certified nurse midwife (CNM) is credentialed in both states, but questions are raised about where the practice occurs and whether the differences in regulatory requirements across states make sense for the recipients of our care. With the availability of the Internet, the exponential growth of telemedicine, and multistate case management, discussions have focused on the optimal process to assure safe and effective nursing practice. In addition to the Nurse Licensure Compact (NLC) in which 24 states are engaged, discussions have focused on both national nurse regulation and national nurse licensure. Each model has advantages and disadvantages. As you move through this chapter, consider what type of change or innovation might be needed for this work, the most appropriate processes to build effective team processes, the barriers and limitations to this work, and the desired outcomes from the perspective of all stakeholders.

POLICY CHALLENGE: Emergent Demand for Policy

A CNM provides well-woman and midwifery care for an obstetrical-gynecological practice in a small town near the border of another state. In her home state, where she delivers babies, she does not have complete prescriptive privileges. However, her practice has offices across the border where she sees patients in the office once a week. One day, the CNM's patient who regularly sees her across the border calls her office. Susan decides her patient needs a prescription for an antibiotic for a urinary tract infection.

This example raises a number of questions about interstate practice. Can the CNM phone the prescription into a pharmacy? Where is the CNM providing the service, at the CNM's location or at the patient's location? Must Susan see the patient for an emergency appointment in her home office? And while today we discuss policies for interstate practice, tomorrow we may want to apply those principles to practice across international borders. *See Option for Policy Challenge.*

THEORIES OF CHANGE

Every day, new evidence and new approaches in providing patient care are introduced with the expectation that these ideas are considered and implemented when appropriate. Nurses continually assess current work processes and explore new research and information to find and deliver the highest value patient care for the lowest cost—and this requires change as a basic competency for professional nursing practice. The implementation of new policies, adjustments to existing policies, or elimination of current policies must be necessarily grounded in evidence.

Nurse work requires that we become experts in advancing both change and innovation in the delivery of patient care services and the environment in which the care is delivered. Nurses must also be mindful that standing still, the opposite of change and innovation, is the beginning of the dying process, a process that is final and reflects the absence of life. In essence, standing still jeopardizes patient safety and quality. For example, many hospitals implemented 12-hour shifts as a means to retain nurses and provide more days off for their nurses. However, we now have research indicating that shifts longer than 12 hours are associated with worse job outcomes and lower quality and safety (Rogers, 2003), although some research does not indicate an impact on patient outcomes (Stone et al., 2007). Research indicates planned naps taken during night shifts are beneficial in improving alertness (Smith-Coggins et al., 2006). So, the question that is raised is whether employers of nurses will modify their policies and practices as they learn about the evidence regarding fatigue and its relationship to safety and patient outcomes. Standing still on evidence has the potential to jeopardize patient safety and quality. It raises the question about at what point the body of evidence is sufficient for implementing change within an organization and beyond through legislation and/or regulation.

Interestingly, in spite of the seemingly positive nature of change, much time and effort is spent in working to harness and minimize change given its often disruptive and uncertain nature. Learning to embrace both change and innovation is necessary to successfully navigate events and, ultimately, thrive in our ever-changing world. Successful advocates have mastered the competencies of embracing change and innovation.

There are numerous strategies, templates, and theories of both change and innovation available to assist nurses in understanding and advancing new ideas, specifically advancements in health care policy. Some theories are linear and devoid of the influences of the context, while others are more robust and include the multiple forces and interactions impacting the change or innovation process. Having an appreciation of the nature of theories of change and innovation provides a foundation for nurses to assume an active role in the policy process. What is also important to understand is that the multifaceted nature of change and innovation makes it nearly impossible to focus on all aspects of change simultaneously. Thus, our attempts to understand change and innovation are necessarily limited and incomplete—but necessary in the evolution of effective change and health care policy creation. To be sure, the change expert will integrate multiple facets of change to increase understanding of the concepts and processes involved in change and innovation.

An overview of the multiple descriptions and definitions specific to change and innovation is presented here to assist the reader in differentiating the concepts as well as to provide frameworks for readers to examine and consider their own change and innovation attributions when involved in this work. Descriptions of common terms related to change and innovation are presented in Exhibit 8.1 (Porter-O'Grady & Malloch, 2012). Change is more commonly referred to as a simple alteration of something, while innovation is considered a qualified type of change in which the alteration positively impacts future processes. A brief overview of selected traditional theories of change is presented in Exhibit 8.2; Exhibit 8.3 contains brief descriptions of selected theories of innovation and strategies to facilitate change and innovation. As indicated in Exhibit 8.2, innovation theories extend theories of change and add qualifiers to the type, space, and timing of change processes. Most of the traditional change theories tend to simplify the processes of change. The addition of theories of innovation (Exhibit 8.3) provides a more robust understanding of the complexities of change and innovation—and may, in fact, assist nurses in more eagerly embracing new ideas. Selected strategies for implementation are illustrated in Exhibit 8.4.

Regardless of the specific theory examined, there are common characteristics (Exhibit 8.5) across all of the theories that nurses will want to consider when planning and implementing policy change and innovation (Poole & Van de Ven, 2004). These include:

- *An alteration.* Both change and innovation involve an alteration of the present way of doing things. *Change* can be an event of moving an item from one position to another. *Innovation* adds qualifiers of the movement and includes benefits, irreversibility, and nuance.
- *Human agency.* Individuals or groups (*human agency*) range from one individual to groups to organizations.
- *Time parameters.* These include the rate of change, when change will occur, and the extent of the change. Change can be episodic or continuous depending on the drivers or mechanisms of change. Continuous change is

EXHIBIT 8.1   COMMON DESCRIPTIONS FOR CHANGE AND INNOVATION

- To make different; to undergo a transformation or modification (Merriam-Webster, 2014)
- The implementation of new or altered products, services, processes, systems, organizational structures, or business models as a means of improving one or more domains of health care quality (Agency for Healthcare Research and Quality [AHRQ] Health Care Innovations Exchange, 2013a)
- Anything that creates new resources, processes, or values or improves a company's existing resources, processes, or values (Christensen, Anthony, & Roth, 2004, p. 293)
- The power to redefine the industry; the effort to create purposeful focused change in an enterprise's economic or social potential (Drucker, 1985)
- A new patterning of our experiences of being together as new meaning emerges from ordinary, everyday work conversations (Fonseca, 2002)
- The first, practical, concrete implementation of an idea done in a way that brings broad-based, extrinsic recognition to an individual or organization (Plsek, 1997)
- A historic and irreversible change in the way of doing things; creative destruction (Schumpeter, 1943)
- Emergent continuity and transformation of patterns of human interactions understood as ongoing ordinary complex responsive processes of human relating in local situations in the living present (Stacey & Griffin, 2008)
- Fresh thinking that leads to value creation (Vaitheeswaran, 2007)
- Innovation is something new, or perceived new by the population experiencing the innovation, that has the potential to drive change, as well as redefine health care's economic and/or social potential (Weberg, 2009)

ongoing, evolving, and cumulative and episodic. Episodic change is infrequent, discontinuous, and intentional.

- *Level of change.* This refers to the size of the units of change and innovation and range from a unit of similar individuals to units of differing foci to organizations composed of multiple levels of groups.
- *Predictability of the change or innovation.* Some changes are planned, while other changes are unplanned. The range of planning includes the degree to which change can be choreographed, scripted, or controlled. Planned change is consciously conceived and implemented by knowledgeable individuals. There are attempts to improve a situation with targeted end points for the desired state. In contrast, unplanned change may or may not be driven by human choice or purposefully conceived, and it moves an organization in either a desirable or undesirable direction. Natural disasters, such as floods or hurricanes, can be the drivers of unplanned changes in resource allocations. Such events often force the reprioritization of resources and planned change processes. For example, changes may include funding priorities when federal funds designated for roads may be diverted to flood or hurricane relief. Or, as in the case with Hurricane Sandy in 2012, if a hospital with an obstetrical service closes, it impacts patients, nurses, physicians, and other staff. Patients may have to deliver their babies in a different facility. Displaced nurses need to be oriented

EXHIBIT 8.2 TRADITIONAL CHANGE THEORIES

Lewin (1947)—A common change theory using a force-field model where behaviors of driving and restraining forces push individuals in a particular direction. This model describes the change process as one of, first, unfreezing current behaviors; second, moving to a new position; and third, refreezing the new behaviors. For change to occur, there must be a shift in the balance between driving and restraining forces.

Lippitt, Watson, and Westley (1958)—Extends Lewin's model and emphasizes the role of the change agent, participation of those involved, communication, and problem solving.

Reddin (1970)—A seven-step technique with a participatory element that can be used by nurses to bring about change. The steps are diagnosis, mutual setting of goals, group emphasis, maximum information, discussion of implementation, use of ceremony and ritual, and resistance interpretation.

Havelock (1973)—Modifies Lewin's model and emphasizes the participative approach to effecting the desired change.

Spradley (1979)—Theory of change is based upon Lewin's theory; Spradley emphasizes constant monitoring of the change project.

Rogers (2003)—Extends Lewin's, Lippitt's, and Havelock's theories emphasizing the iterative nature of the decision-making process specific to change; change can be reversed or discontinued on the basis of interest and commitment to the new expectations.

to new facilities to provide for expanded capacity needs. Physicians may not have practice privileges at the facilities taking their patients. Finally, expectations and processes for implementing practice standards may differ when professionals from different facilities work together to meet patient needs. Both planned and unplanned changes can occur simultaneously at differing levels of an organization. Leadership teams can be strategically implementing a new electronic medical record using a project plan, while the larger community in which the organization exists can be experiencing unplanned economic, cultural, or nature-driven change from an unplanned perspective.

EXHIBIT 8.3 SELECTED THEORIES OF INNOVATION

- *Disruptive Innovation*: Helps create a new market and value network, and eventually disrupts an existing market and value network (over a few years or decades); displacing earlier technology; describes innovations that improve a product or service in ways that the market does not expect, typically first by designing for a different set of consumers in the new market and later by lowering prices in the existing market (Poole & Van de Ven, 2004)
- *Punctuated Equilibrium*: Depicts organizations as evolving through relatively long periods of stability-equilibrium or convergent periods—in their basic patterns of activity that are punctuated by relatively short periods of fundamental change—revolutionary periods (Tushman & Romanelli, 1985)

(continued)

EXHIBIT 8.3   SELECTED THEORIES OF INNOVATION (*CONTINUED*)

- *Organizational Logics*: Logic can be understood as the underlying cognition or mental model that configures a coherent thought, orders an argument, or arranges a system; dominant logic is defined as the way in which managers conceptualize the business and make critical resource allocation decisions—be it technologies, product development, distribution, advertising, or in human resource management (Drazin, Glynn, & Kazanjian, 2004)
- *Diffusion of Innovations*: Seeks to explain how, why, and at what rate new ideas and technology spread through cultures (Rogers, 2003)
- *Complex Adaptive Systems (CAS)*: Teleological in nature and portrays constructive change brought about by individual agents pursuing improvement in their individual fitness level, although fitness can also have global, aggregate components (Dooley, 2004)
- *Dynamics of Organizational Culture*: Built on Schein's theory, using artifacts, assumptions, and values, Hatch focused on the processes linking these elements, processes of stability and change, symbols, and the environment (Hatch, 2004)

- *Driver of the change or innovation.* Four drivers of change have been identified: life cycle, teleological, dialectical, and evolutionary. Life cycle change and innovation occur in sequenced stages much like the stages of life, from birth to death. The change has a clearly defined beginning and end. Teleological drivers emphasize social construction and the cycle of goal formation, implementation, and modification of actions of goals. Dialectical drivers involve a thesis and antithesis. This change process is iterative and emphasizes discussions and actions to confront conflict and determine the best option. The evolutionary change process is one of repetitive sequences of variation, selection, and finally retention. The emphasis is on competition for scarce resources (Poole & Van de Ven, 2004).

These essential characteristics of a change or innovation process—alteration type, agency type, time, level of impact, predictability, and driver—should

EXHIBIT 8.4   SELECTED STRATEGIES FOR CHANGE IMPLEMENTATION

- *The Deep Dive*: An area is selected for observation in multiple ways; workflows, photos, interviews, and observations are gathered by a team to analyze current processes and brainstorm new ways of doing the current work processes (Kelley, 2005)
- *Directed Creativity*: Situation is proposed to encourage and advance new ideas. For example, stakeholders are asked how to design a wound clinic if resources such as staff, space, and finances are unlimited (Plsek, 1997)
- *Mind Mapping*: Tool for collecting, organizing, and synthesizing large amounts of data in layers with complex relationships; useful for documenting connectivity, interdependencies, and emerging phenomena in health care
- *Scenario Planning*: Disciplined approach considering multiple conditions in various orders; a strategic planning method used to make flexible, long-term plans; allows inclusion of factors difficult to formalize, such as novel insights about the future, deep shifts in values, unprecedented regulations or inventions (Schoemaker, 1995)

(continued)

EXHIBIT 8.4   **SELECTED STRATEGIES FOR CHANGE IMPLEMENTATION** *(CONTINUED)*

- *Innovation Space*: Place or laboratory where inquiring minds collaborate to create a more livable and sustainable world focused on developing products that create market value while serving real societal needs; products that are progressive, possible, and profitable; the focus is often on biomimicry (Boradkar, 2010)
- *Prototyping*: Model built to test a concept or process or to act as a thing to be replicated or learned from; designed to test and trial a new design to enhance precision by system analysts and users; prototyping serves to provide specifications for a real, working system rather than a theoretical one (Endsley, 2010)
- *Brainstorming*: Process to generate ideas as a collective exercise; a good exercise generates 100 ideas; focuses on suspending judgment and criticism, freewheeling thinking, quantity of ideas, and building on the ideas of others (Endsley, 2010)

---

be determined for any anticipated policy change or innovation. The value of these processes is summarized in Exhibit 8.6.

Clarification of these characteristics provides critical insight into the anticipated trajectory of the process as well as potential barriers to the process. For example, if a dialectical or goal-driven change such as the funding for health care is framed as a life cycle change with a beginning and an end, significant frustration would occur each time a new iteration for funding is proposed—when in fact it is part of the change and innovation process.

Four exemplars using the drivers or motors of change and innovation are presented to enhance further understanding of these complex processes (Poole & Van de Ven, 2004).

The first exemplar is *life cycle* change and innovation. Consider the election or reelection of candidates to office. Using the five characteristics discussed previously, the change model would include:

> *Alteration*: An expectation for either new or sustained leadership as the current individual is reelected or the challenger is elected. Minimally, there would be a change in the elected official with potential for innovation of new policies.
> *Agency*: The focus is on the candidate or incumbent; a single entity or individual. There are also multiple groups involved in an election, including those very active in the campaign and election processes and those individuals able to vote for candidates.

EXHIBIT 8.5   **COMMON CHARACTERISTICS OF CHANGE AND INNOVATION**

- An alteration
- Human agency
- Time parameters
- Levels of change
- Predictability
- Driver

From Poole and Van de Ven (2004) and Porter-O'Grady and Malloch (2012).

EXHIBIT 8.6   THE VALUE OF CHANGE AND INNOVATION THEORIES
Moving ahead with a lot of good ideas without a framework to guide this complex work can be disastrous. Knowing whether there are multiple individuals and groups who could be supporters or obstacles is an important first step. Further, the extent of the change across units, organizations, or national groups further provides information about the length and complexity of the process. Knowing the time parameters and the drivers of the change provides important framework information that will facilitate change processes. Each of these concepts is derived from change and innovation theories that assist leaders to address complex policy change not as a simple linear change, but rather as a multidirectional and ambiguous process that needs all the guidance available.

Time parameters: Clearly defined by election guidelines and election dates. Some extended time might be required for vote counting in close elections. *Level of change*: Change is expected at multiple levels across the specific district or legislative area and will impact all of the parties involved in an election. *Predictability*: In general, elections are planned changes and occur at legislatively defined times. There are unplanned circumstances when an incumbent leaves office at a time outside of the established election times, thereby requiring the appointment of an individual to complete the elected person's responsibilities until the next election.

The second exemplar is based on a change or innovation known as the *teleological* driver. In this exemplar, the area of interest is the support for abortion. Goals are determined by selected groups to advance a particular position. Specific groups create initiatives and work to gain support for them.

Alteration: The intent is a change in acceptable behaviors and procedures. Innovation is most likely not considered.
Agency: The focus is a single entity or individual with an unwanted pregnancy. There are also multiple groups involved in supporting or opposing the proposed position.
Time parameters: These are determined by position advocates based on support and resources to advance the position. Start time could be when resources and support are available and stop time is when the goal is achieved or support and resources are exhausted.
Level of change: Change is expected at multiple levels at either the state or federal level.
Predictability: Typically, this is a planned change that evolves on the basis of support and resources for the initiative.

The third exemplar is *dialectical* change and innovation. This process is one of iterative discussions and actions to confront conflict and determine the best option. Development of health care policy specific to access, funding, and coverage is a dialectical change process.

Alteration: Both change and innovation may be included in this process, and new and creative ideas to support health care services emerge from debates and discussions.

Agency: Large-scale change involving national groups as well as state-based groups.

Time parameters: These are determined based on support and resources to advance the position. Start time could be when resources and support are available and stop time is when the goal is achieved or support and resources are exhausted.

Level of change: Change is expected at multiple levels across state and national groups, including groups representing providers, payers, and numerous other constituencies.

Predictability: Planned change is the backdrop for this initiative on the larger scale. At times, unplanned change may occur as smaller interest groups may emerge and facilitate or obstruct the progress in determining whether or not health care will be supported at a national level.

Dialectical change is illustrated by the process used to develop the Nursing Community's request for federal funding for nursing workforce programs under Title VIII (see Chapter 7, "Building Capital: Intellectual, Social, Political, and Financial"). For many years, nursing organizations would ask congressional leaders for different funding levels. Eventually, a process was put into place that resulted in a unified request that was championed by more than 50 nursing organizations, resulting in greater success in achieving the desired funding levels.

The fourth exemplar is an *evolutionary* change or innovation and can be identified in the processes to fund health care over time. Medicare was enacted into law in 1965 as amendments to the Social Security Act (U.S. Social Security Administration, 2012). In 1983, the Social Security Act was again amended to add Diagnosis-Related Groups, a prospective payment system, to control costs for Medicare patients (3M Health Information Systems, 2003). Most recently, a national payment system, the Patient Protection and Affordable Care Act (PPACA) of 2010, was implemented to cover all citizens from a value-driven perspective. An evolutionary driver is one in which a repetitive sequence of variation, selection, and finally retention occurs. This process is focused on the competition for scarce resources.

Alteration: Both change and innovation may be included in this process and new and creative ideas to support health care services or decrease costs emerge.

Agency: Large-scale change involving national groups as well as state-based groups.

Time parameters: These are determined based on the needs of the citizens and available support from the federal government.

Level of change: Change is expected at multiple levels across the specific district or legislative area and will impact all of the parties involved in an election. Also, providers, funder groups, and vendors will influence the process.

Predictability: This process is both planned and unplanned as needs change in the health status of citizens or changes in available resources.

These exemplars can greatly assist policy makers in determining the elements for consideration in a complex change or innovation process. The determination of the characteristics of the change or innovation provides essential information and strategies to advance the desired position with specific target actions and measures. While each driver or motor of change is presented as a discrete event, it is highly likely that more than one driver is involved in complex change. A change can begin as a life cycle change and quickly become a teleological or evolutionary change. In the next section, the critical components of teamwork in the policy process are presented.

SUCCESSFUL TEAM PROCESSES IN POLICY FORMULATION

In the era of recalibrating health reform policy and practices, building a foundation in collective wisdom is essential to both engaging stakeholders and assuring that concerted collective action operates in a way that demonstrates mutual understanding, commitment, and coordinated action (Nickerson, 2010). Often, development and initiation of new policies and collaborative action are waylaid from the outset simply because critical relational and communication requisites necessary to successful design and implementation of policy are not successfully addressed (Nohria & Khurana, 2010). Here, the details of good team dynamics are critical to the collective ability to establish effective principles, set good direction, and implement concerted action (Finkelman, 2012).

A number of components of policy team dynamics are essential to effective formulation, translation, and implementation of good policy (Matheson, 2009). From initial formative stages of group development to the definitive phases of policy implementation, each of the elements necessary to good group process must be effectively addressed if related processes are to bear fruit. Each stage of the policy team process is dependent on the previous phase in a way that exemplifies the cascade of related elements in the building of a successful trajectory toward effective policy application and implementation (Bodenheimer & Gumbach, 2012). See Exhibit 8.7, which highlights the critical cascade of stages essential to establishing a good policy process.

Determining the Foundational Need

Policy should not be lightly undertaken or superficially addressed. Policy has serious implications with regard to organizational constructs, political variables, social trajectory, and individual life. Since much legal, regulatory, and administrative direction and discipline is grounded in the fulfillment of particular policy, the use of policy for making change at any level must be carefully considered and well developed. Whether the policy covers a broad range of society or a narrower population or group, it has the potential to impact action

EXHIBIT 8.7   ESSENTIAL PHASES OF POLICY TEAMWORK

- Determining the foundational need
- Setting the table with the right stakeholders
- Defining clear expectations
- Enumerating context, timeline, powers, and deliverables
- Effectively delineating methods and terms of engagement
- Ensuring a good fit between team tools and dynamics
- Agreeing collectively about the product of teamwork
- Determining when the team's work is done
- Establishing good mechanisms for handoff and bringing closure to the work

and behavior in a disciplined and definitive manner with the hope of creating an effective and consistent response to an overarching need.

Policy assumes that some aggregated good will be advanced and the action based on the policy will lead to more appropriate or effective patterns, conditions, or behaviors. In the absence of these essential improvements or enhancements, the development of policy as a mechanism for codifying action should be avoided. It is preferable that a protocol for administration of a particular drug be authorized by the involved clinicians rather than having a universal policy that would require more prescribed processes and/or a time requirement. For example, some facilities require that pain medication orders specify different dosages for mild, moderate, and severe pain intensity ratings in the absence of any empirical evidence that a specific dose is effective for pain levels within a certain range. This removes the expectation for nurses to use professional judgment in assessing pain and is potentially unsafe. The ability to shift a protocol when evidence demands is easier and more focused than making a policy change, which has broader implications for both time and resources. There is a whole range of other approaches to establishing consistency and patterns of practice through use of protocols, standards, quality metrics, or evidentiary dynamics (Hayes, 2006). The lack of careful consideration with regard to the use of policy, its general overuse, and its inappropriate use ultimately creates diminishing value, adherence, and ownership. The larger the number of policies that are created, the less value each policy represents.

While policy can certainly be viewed as foundational, it should also be seen as critical. Policy should not be easily or superficially conceived and applied. Good policy reflects sound principles and establishes a floor for systematic and universal applications and actions in a given set of circumstances. The point to establishing policy is to generate a firm set of principles upon which process and action scaffolding can be constructed in a way that ensures a consistent response to principle-related issues, yet provides sufficient individual flexibility to render critical judgment that adapts action to inherent circumstantial vagaries (see Policy on the Scene 8.1). Policy should not be rote, inflexible, pedantic, or unchanging. Policy works best when it represents a principle or a set of principles that inform human judgment and that uses the policy that flows from it to guide effective related human action (Bardach, 2011).

Policy formation should be rare and policies should be few in number. Policy sets general rules for action within which standards, protocols, and processes can be more clearly and specifically designed to guide human action. A policy statement such as "the American Nurses Association Code of Ethics for Nurses forms the foundation for all ethical decision making made within the nursing ethics committee of this organization" provides an example of the simplicity, clarity, and directness of a good policy statement. Policies need to be briefly stated, succinct, specific, and clear. The rationale for a policy should be generally understandable, be acceptable, and reflect a rational basis for subsequent action. The reason for the policy should be evident, clear, and logical in a way that could be found generally acceptable to most persons. The need for it should be obvious and understandable to all those to whom the policy relates. The need for a policy should be reasonably obvious and reflect a generally understandable premise upon which it is built.

Setting the Table With the Right Stakeholders

No policy should be formed that reflects or impacts the processes or actions of individuals without their representation or participation in its formation. Good policy assumes a measure of ownership, engagement, and investment. If any said policy is to have significant impact on the action of individuals or groups and they do not share a role in its consideration and formulation, no commitment or buy-in is the price paid. It is at this point that many leaders and organizations pay a significant price in nonadherence or noncompliance with appropriate and well-thought-out policy that lacked only the engagement and investment of those upon whom it had an impact (Schuman, 2006).

Setting the policy table involves a goodness of fit between policy and policy makers. The leader setting the table must know how deliberation and formation need to be informed and what varieties of capacity will be necessary in order to adequately serve the process (Exhibit 8.8).

Those with knowledge related to the policy arena and others with understanding regarding the structural, organizational, and contextual impact considerations influencing effective policy design must be carefully incorporated into the process. While there may be a core group of team members at the policy table who need to be consistently present by virtue of their stake, there are other members at the policy table who may be either situationally or influentially present depending on the breadth or significance of contribution the policy formation requires. The policy leader must also be aware of the design process, knowing just when particular representation or interface needs to occur in the decisional flow and who best needs to play a decisive role at a particular point in the process that helps facilitate the policy dialogue and decision making. Group membership is

POLICY ON THE SCENE 8.1: ThedaCare, Appleton, WI

Recognizing the need to transition health care delivery in a values-driven equation challenged ThedaCare, a community health care system, to recognize that essential health reform policy changes would ultimately require institutional, structural, and practice changes in its health system in Appleton, Wisconsin. Policy foundations at the center of this change responded to three drivers: (a) delivery of care that is designed around the patient; (b) payments based on values and outcomes; and (c) transparency of treatment quality and cost. This policy foundation provided a framework for the convergence of strategic organizational and delivery efforts to transform the service model into a collaborative care system. The collaborative care partnership resulting from this new policy and strategic focus consisted of a team of nurses, physicians, pharmacists, and a case manager who together would meet with patients in a 90-minute admission process developing an integrated coordinated plan of care. The team-approach intent was to advance patient-centered communication and clinical interaction, and to eliminate duplication and silo-based approaches to care delivery. The central effect was to make the patient the coordinator of his or her care and build partnerships around a patient-coordinated plan. This policy and team practice shift resulted in a decrease of 10% to 15% in the average length of stay and cost per case reductions from 15% to 28%. The structure of the environment was redesigned, rooms were reconfigured, and clinical processes were restructured to reduce waste and improve efficiency and quality.

The impact of ThedaCare's policy shift in the local setting represents the following key elements:

1. Policy must reflect environmental shifts, which recalibrate and reconfigure demand for a shift within the system. Systems policy response should tightly reflect environmental demands and translate them into action and performance in the organization.
2. Changing policy must affect the life of the organization at all levels: (a) strategic decisions that drive systems changes; (b) operational decisions that address structure, process, finance, resource management, and leadership; and (c) practice decisions that affect clinical protocols, care partnership, care practices, evaluation of impact, and changes that advance patient care.
3. Policy informs practice when it changes patterns of interaction, role expectations, personal behavior, interprofessional interaction and relationship, and the role of the patient in day-to-day decision making.

> ## EXHIBIT 8.8 GETTING STARTED WITH STAKEHOLDERS
>
> Critical elements for the core team selection process include:
> - Senior-level representatives who have strategic authority
> - Policy issue experts who reflect content competence
> - Stakeholders who have a personal/impact investment in the policy decision
> - Innovators who see a unique way of delineating, translating, and applying policy
> - Representatives upon whom the policy has an impact and/or will be responsible for its implementation

a fluid and dynamic circumstance requiring good group management and continual recalibration of the players in the process in a way that best fits the circumstances and needs of the process at any given moment in time. Recognizing this strong need for fit between process and player alerts the group leader to the need for constant assessment of dialogue, decisions, and the goodness of fit with participants and contributors to the group dynamic (Taylor, 2011). This is illustrated by the Agency for Healthcare Research and Quality (AHRQ) On-Time Quality Improvement Program for Long-Term Care involving the use of design teams composed of core members to provide expertise and ad hoc members who provide expertise related to specific aspects of care processes. This model has been used successfully to reduce falls, prevent pressure ulcers, promote pressure ulcer healing, and avoid hospital transfers (AHRQ, 2013b).

Enumerating Context, Timeline, Powers, and Deliverables

Important to policy group dynamics and team behavior is the establishment of clarity with regard to the premises and purposes driving the work of the team. While this is common to all group processes, what is especially important to policy groups is a deep and clear understanding of the drivers, circumstances, and conditions necessitating the establishment of principle and the formation of policy. Understanding contextual issues and policy drivers provides the umbrella that serves to frame dialogue and deliberation and to formulate a backdrop for intent, which serves to provide a rational basis for the formation of policy. The conditions and circumstances that create the need for principle and consistency and underpin policy formation help the participants clarify both whether and how use of policy will result in desirable outcomes. If, on the one hand, the dialogue demonstrates that a less directive or interventional set of choices could better address the issues of concern, the need for policy is abrogated and less intensive methods can be applied. If, on the other hand, the contextual realities point to a specific need for policy formation, providing the backdrop helps more strongly elucidate the appropriateness of this choice.

Ensuring clarity of purpose and laying the foundations for deliberation rest in the hands of planning leaders. Much of this activity is initially generated prior to the formation of the policy team. Much of this work establishes the basis for the initial dialogue team members around further refinement and clarification of purpose and direction following their initial group activities. Some of the early elements and issues that need to be addressed and that establish the foundations for dialogue and deliberation are:

- General summary of the issues and concerns, which provide both reason and purpose for undertaking a policy initiative
- Level of specificity with regard to the mandate, charge, and powers for setting policy and direction established within the group's purview
- Brief but clear indication of organizational leadership support for the work, deliberation, decisions, and actions of the policy group as a part of the clear charge to the group
- Some primary establishment of the parameters within which the policy team operates that provides the contextual framework within which policy teamwork expectations are located
- Clear and precise delineation of the time parameters within which the policy team works with some clear delineation of the termination date for its work
- General indication of the performance expectations and products anticipated from the work of the policy team that narrowly articulates the expectations for change and the anticipated positive impact or consequence of the policy work

Rather than narrowly constricting the ability of the policy team to undertake as wide a range of actions as necessary to inform and guide policy, an original charge from leadership establishes the floor upon which team construction, membership, and initial discourse are based. Establishing as much specificity and clarity as possible at the outset of the purpose and work of the policy team ensures that the team is clear about the thinking of current leadership and the depth of their reflection and intention in response to the need underpinning the formation of the policy team (Cheung, Mirzaei, & Leeder, 2010). It should be understood that, while this floor is established, it is not a fixed position as subsequent discussion by the policy team, further informing its deliberation and introducing new realities impacting policy formation, will ultimately alter the way issues and concerns are perceived and addressed by the team.

Effectively Delineating Methods and Terms of Engagement

Once the issues and drivers are clarified, stakeholders are identified and members selected, and the table set for policy deliberation, it becomes important to focus on methodology and process rules. In many cases, team dynamics around policy formation are liberally sprinkled with strong feelings, bias, preexisting positions, and definitive points of view. The goal of all teamwork is to find points of reference that lead to opportunities for consensus and agreement in a way that moves the team through the course of its work (Dunin-Keplicz & Verbrugge, 2010). Successfully doing so is neither accidental, serendipitous, nor simply emergent. Rather, the products of innovation and creativity in thought, dialogue, and serious deliberation emerge from well-thought-out methodology and processes that provide discipline for the dialogue and accelerate the opportunity for the emergence of the seeds of innovation (see Exhibit 8.9).

Team leaders must be as deliberate about methods and approaches as they are about the selection and inclusion of participants. Balancing the team with those who have much to contribute to its work requires that there be participants with widely variable styles of reflection and communication. Team leaders must be aware of the personality characteristics and vagaries of the participants they have pulled together and adapt methods and approaches that maximize the contribution of each, yet facilitate the synergy of ideas through use of the disciplines and methods of good discourse and distributive decision making. At the same time, policy team leaders must also use techniques that help the team work through deliberative conflicts, contrasting ideas, group confabulation, heading off course, process "dead space," and relational crisis.

While there is much contemporary discussion concerning emergent leadership and team innovation and creativity, much of the current evidence suggests that formal team leadership is best determined in advance of team process (Gratton & Erickson, 2007). Who these individuals should be must be balanced against organizational concerns, strategic imperatives, role locus of control, team facilitation competence, and team trust. Much of the work of team leadership occurs before and beyond team interaction and involves intensive processes of facilitating teamwork, assessing/evaluating effective team processes, anticipating and planning team dynamics and processes, and developing useful and productive team methodologies. Certainly, there must be a goodness of fit between the policy team methodologies, work efforts, process, and progress. As to whether those dynamics interface well and produce a satisfactory product is often dependent on the effectiveness of these leadership activities.

EXHIBIT 8.9   THE DISCIPLINED TEAM

All members of the team need to take ownership and accountability for the team's performance and functioning. Some considerations for the policy team to ensure good structure and effective process include:
- Is everyone clear on the purpose and the charge to the team?
- Are the terms of interaction specific and clear?
- Are members clear of their obligations for participation?
- Are the time parameters for the team process clearly outlined?
- Are methods and processes for the team's work understood and useful?
- Are the mechanisms for measuring progress specific and effective?

Ensuring a Good Fit Between Team Tools and Dynamics

Managing highly creative and strongly motivated team members provides a set of challenges that requires rigorous group process skills. The effectiveness of teamwork can be significantly diminished or extended if those designated to facilitate such processes do not have the requisite skills to move the group successfully through the vagaries of group dynamics. Good process relates to not only facilitating the progress of the group's work but also helping to create synthesis of effort, strong and creative bonds of reflection and deliberation, useful methodologies and techniques for problem solving, crisis management, and solution seeking. Policy groups are especially challenging because of the high degree of personal interest issues, political bias, and individual values investment. In the policy-setting process, leaders will often confront issues and concerns that make sense to particular individuals, yet, at the same time, serve to alienate or challenge other group members. Values differences often create the most intractable positions and require sensitive and delicate maneuvering to keep participants fully invested and on track toward problem resolution (Deleuran, 2011).

Policy team leaders cannot expect that they will be universally skilled in all of the arenas of group process and problem solving. Some flexibility must be applied with regard to the inclusion of content and process experts from outside the core group periodically providing unique skills that help move the team past potential logjams and critical barriers to effective deliberation. Additionally, access and adaptation of a wide variety of communication and deliberative techniques, as well as process tools and innovations, help keep the group dynamic focused yet sufficiently innovative to avail themselves of the most useful supports that consistently move the team toward achieving the positive products of its work. Policy development reflects a continuum of stages before full implementation can be achieved. For example, the PPACA (2010) was originally seen as a single-payer approach. Through political process, the Act is instead a compromise that expands access and establishes a foundation (a "policy door") that subsequent policy and legislative deliberation will refine and adapt.

Collective Agreement Regarding Teamwork Product

While the purpose, mission, and drivers of the formation of the policy team are often determined prior to the formation of that team, the team does have an obligation both at the outset and during the process of deliberation to ensure that the goals and anticipated results of the work are legitimate, are viable, and fulfill the purpose for which they were formed (Fitz-enz, 2009). Often, the purpose for which a policy team is formed appears clear at the outset and provides a definitive foundation upon which that work will build. At the same time, the work and processes of the team's deliberation, interaction, knowledge generation, work processes, and development yield new facts, insights, and clarity that alter original notions and substantially affect the original purpose for which they were formed. In the interests of transparency and truth, policy teams often determine that initial insights used to establish their work may not accurately reflect the theory of the case or adequately represent the full range of issues, which will differently influence appropriate decision making and subsequent solutions. The policy imperative originally perceived may no longer be accurately reflected subsequent to deeper and more intensive assessment, subsequently changing both the premises and the terms of engagement. Should this occur, policy team leadership may need to "time out" the team's work process in order to provide an opportunity for interaction and recalibration with senior leadership who initially charged the team with its work.

Process always shifts the initial design. Whatever the originating charge for a team's work, its progress ultimately adjusts the initial design for it and creates opportunities to rethink the relationship between original design and implementation. Flexibility and fluidity between purpose and deliberation do not mean the loss of purpose. Progress may actually help reinform purpose in a way that both refines and adjusts it to better reflect emergent reality. This ability to "trust the process" means that leaders must develop a foundational understanding that the risk of implementing a policy change using team dynamics can often be best represented by conclusions not originally conceived by those driving the policy change. The result may either be a recognition that there is no justifiable need for the policy itself or an entire shift in the character and content of the policy resulting from the policy team's work.

Within the team itself is the continual obligation to periodically but regularly review its progress against its charge. Here again, the team's deliberation and progress may alter key elements of the policy process and determine significant enough factors to shift original expectations, creating the demand for new insights and the high possibility of a shift in strategy and approach.

Determine When the Team's Work Is Done

Policy decisions and developments unfold along a continuum. It is incumbent upon policy team leadership to clearly monitor the team's progress and help the team delineate along the way what progress has been made and at what stage they are in achieving their policy goals. All policy team activities must be moderated and measured against the team's initial charge. Whether the policy is local, institutional, or broad based, the same parameters of measuring progress and satisfying intent operate for team leaders.

An often-seen detriment or deficit in policy development is the continuing and sometimes endless wrangling over whether policy goals have been met. Often driving such conflicting views is the uncertainty around whether the points of policy decision making have fulfilled the policy intent and hopes of those who initiated the process. One of the characteristics of negotiation and compromise in deliberation and decision making relates to the personal acknowledgment of the difference between the ending point of policy discussion and decision making from those perceptions present at the initial charge for policy formation. As the policy process becomes increasingly informed by the team's deliberation, data gathering, and new knowledge generation, original insights, notions, and directives become differently informed and call the policy team to recalibrate its charge, inform leadership, and, ultimately, make the most correct policy decision (Tunis, 2007).

Harnessing the policy team around final decision making is the role of team leadership. It is the obligation of the policy team's leader to direct and manage its work and to help it discern when that work has reached a critical juncture. The leader must determine whether its original charge has been substantially addressed. The leader asks whether deliberations have led to a point of demarcation where further work would lead the team away from the contextual framework for the policy or where their work has obtained substantial value or impact as a reflection of the issue that it was intended to address. The team leader must always work to keep dialogue and decision making clearly within the parameters of the policy charge and validate that concluding decisions and impact demonstrate a fulfillment of the original purpose and intent. As with all such directed and time-limited work, the policy team terminates its function at the conclusion of this final decision making and with its report to the systems leadership who gave it its charge.

Establishing Good Mechanisms for Handoff and Bringing Closure to the Work

The importance of clinical handoffs is well described in the literature (Bennett, Probst, Vyavaharkar, & Glover, 2012; Clarke et al., 2012; Maxson, Derby, Wrobleski, & Foss, 2012; Staggers & Blaz, 2012). In policy teamwork, the linkage to handoff is just as critical. Good policy affects values, actions, and outcomes and therefore should never be lightly addressed.

Policy also represents the principal foundation upon which it is grounded and challenges organizations and people to be continuously aware of the principles, which guide thought and action and inform correct choices. At the same time, policy is not fixed. If it is, it is as much an impediment to growth, development, and transformation as any other structural and behavioral element in an organization. For example, some state nursing boards have regulations that specify the number of clinical hours in nursing programs. The introduction of high-fidelity simulation has changed the nature of laboratory instruction in nursing. Having great specificity in laboratory requirements may be a hindrance to programs seeking to substitute some of their clinical hours with simulation. Policy should never be looked at as finite or rigid, or even unchanging. These insights alone create pushback and reaction from those who see policy as inflexible, finite, and fixed. When policy is used as a weapon rather than a tool, it becomes an impediment to engagement, advancement, and appropriate meaningful change (Cooperrider, Whitney, & Stavros, 2008). This is illustrated by policies related to medication error reporting in the past that focused on individual blame and efforts to shift to a more reasoned approach that examines the nature of the error in the context of the system and the riskiness of the behavior that may have led to the error (Vogelsmeier, Scott-Cawiezell, Miller, & Griffith, 2010). Similarly, zero-tolerance and punitive policies result in an atmosphere where nurses with substance abuse problems are reluctant to ask for help (Monroe & Kenaga, 2011).

Handoffs in the case of policy development relate specifically to follow-up occurring after the work of the policy team and subsequent to the decisions they've made regarding specific policy. There is no value in establishing policy if it does not directly influence decisions and behaviors. The intent of policy formation is ultimately to establish principled foundations that drive particular decisions and actions. Policy team leadership and executive leadership should undertake the following steps to ensure good linkage between the decisions of the policy team and the actions of organizational leadership:

1. A clear presentation and delineation of the policy team's work and decisions collectively shared with involved organizational leadership in a way that best articulates the considerations, value, and meaning of both deliberation and decision making on the policy team.
2. A specific delineation of "next steps" of the organizational leadership and the subsequent decisions and actions related to their role, which follow up or advance the policy team's work and decisions.
3. Development of a follow-up and/or implementation process that translates policy decisions or directives into an organizational initiative that establishes the foundations, principles, and drivers that make the policy a part of the organization's operating milieu.
4. Identify and outline metrics that serve as the frame for measuring performance and compliance with policy and principle in all the places to which the policy is directed. Measures should reflect real-time progress associated with inculcating the policy in the practices and behaviors of the organization and people to which it is directed.
5. Establish a long-term mechanism for measuring the value and effectiveness of the policy and determining both the need and time for alteration and change; note that both the organizational dynamics and practice shifts create a demand for policy change.

Whether talking about national policy or local work unit policy, the processes associated with its planning and implementation are consistent. The implications of policy represent the same set of characteristics regardless of how broadly their impact is experienced. It is simply a matter of degree, not of process. Those establishing national health policy are driven by the same rules of engagement as those attempting to lay the foundations for a practice policy. Reflection on the need for policy and the implementation of policy must always be carefully considered. Policy should not be developed as a vehicle for codifying, controlling, and circumscribing every single element of human behavior.

In guiding and governing the work of professions, precedence must always be given to the role of critical thinking and judgment moderated by the circumstances and conditions driving particular response. Policy should always be more strongly related to the establishment and/or codification of principle rather than to the formation of directives. In the contemporary age, policy has all too often been used as a vehicle for establishing behavioral strictures and as a reaction to personal or process error that would be better addressed by enhancing critical thinking skills and good judgment than by constructing rigid policy boundaries that eliminate the capacity to think, adjust, and adapt. Policy has often been used in place of accountability and effective discipline; in doing so, it has acted as a poor substitute for managing human behavior. The work of the policy team should reflect this understanding, validate the principal foundation of policy, and limit the use of policy as a unilateral mechanism for control and discipline (Stone, 2011). For example, some facilities restrict the use of smartphones and the Internet while nurses are on duty, resulting in nurses being unable to access current information for clinical treatments and medications to provide safe care. Keep in mind that policy gives direction to action; it is not the action itself. As indicated in this chapter, action refers to the processes and mechanics of translating policy into protocols, practices, and processes. Examples of simple policy statements are illustrated in Exhibit 8.10.

Note that each policy statement is declarative, simple, and directive. Not included in the policy statement itself are the rationales, procedures/methodologies, definitions, responsible persons, and so forth. Each of these elements is a subset to the policy and serves to provide an expanded explanatory and

---

EXHIBIT 8.10 EXAMPLES OF SIMPLE POLICY STATEMENTS

A member's eligibility and benefits must be verified each time he or she receives hospital services. The hospital's Voice Response Unit (VRU) is always available 24 hours a day, 7 days a week.

The community health service requires that all services performed on behalf of its members be provided in a culturally sensitive manner, including to those with limited English proficiency or reading skills, diverse cultural and ethnic backgrounds, and physical or mental impairment.

All decisions about practice standards, policies, and protocols related to orthopedic nursing care are made by the orthopedic unit practice council.

All members of the professional nursing staff must be credentialed annually through the Credentials Committee of the Nursing Quality Council.

All nursing clinical policies, protocols, and practices must be based on the appropriate specialty nursing standards of practice and specifically enumerated and/or referenced in the body of the text.

The Patient Protection and Affordable Care Act (PPACA) requires that the value case be made for all episodes of care and includes the contribution made to desirable outcomes by all members of the health care team.

methodological foundation for acting upon and implementing the policy; they are not themselves the policy.

TRANSLATING POLICY INTO ACTION AND IMPACT

Much effort and resources are utilized to plan, change, and initiate policy. Federal legislation such as the 2010 PPACA demonstrates both the significance and the breadth of social impact of significant policy efforts. The time and resources associated with harnessing social, political, and economic forces and converging them around particular policy initiatives are not only considerable but also personally demanding at every level of society (Hartley, 2012). The economic and social capital invested in such efforts concentrate change forces and marshal societal responses that represent considerable expenditure of intellectual, emotional, and political "noise." Intellectual noise is characterized by conflicting ideologies regarding a particular policy; emotional noise relates to how people "feel" about a position or a policy; political noise relates to the variety of power positions people take to influence the content and exercise of a policy.

Health care change at every level of consideration is a "hot button" issue. Because of both the personal and social issues implicated in health care services, all people have a vested interest in the translation and application of health to their own personal experience. Everyone has a viewpoint on some element or consideration of health care. Complicating this particular view are individuals' social and political perspectives, which inform their personal expectations related to the health system in general and health service at the more personal level. Even if people judge a health policy change as appropriate or even essential, their capacity to understand or embrace the change may be moderated by their view of its personal demand or impact. The social good is always viewed through the lens of personal value. Therefore, translation and implementation of shifts in policy at every level of consideration must incorporate a deep and abiding understanding of the vagaries of health policy as it is translated into personal experience. See Policy on the Scene 8.2.

This is just as true for a point-of-service practice change as it is for a transformative federal health policy change. While each represents a different level of social intensity, both demonstrate the same human characteristics in response to the requisites for a modification or adjustment in existing patterns of behavior.

For the change agent at any level of policy change, there are some basic considerations that should almost always be incorporated into the processes and dynamics of any policy shift:

1. No matter the breadth, depth, or complexity of a policy change, the policy maker must always be prepared to translate it into the simplest elements of description that will satisfy the most basic level of understanding of those

upon whom it will impact. If the owner of response to any policy change cannot describe it in personal terms, he or she cannot engage its implementation.

2. Clarity is a fundamental companion to understanding. If the policy can be presented in component parts or as a cascade of action and impact, understanding can be more easily obtained. Here again, clarity is best informed through how it is succinctly described in terms of personal impact.

3. Understanding and acceptance of a policy change is best obtained when individuals can judge that it has value and meaning at the personal level. The more effectively the policy can be applied to a net aggregated improvement in the personal experience and in a language that articulates positive personal impact, the easier it is to embrace it.

4. Ultimately, all policy is local, regardless of where it originates or its breadth. Suggesting how good a policy is for the country is not nearly as effective as demonstrating how valuable the policy is for the individual. All policy is seen through the lens of each individual and is thus modified to the perception that best reflects personal values and perspective.

5. In addition to suggesting what a policy means, it is vital to define what a policy does. Clearly, policy change will alter experience and behavior in a specific and defined manner. This alteration is of concern to the individuals and groups around whom these actions and responses must coalesce. The individual needs to know what he or she must do and how he or she must change in order to act congruently with the requisites of the policy.

6. Individuals and groups need to sense a generalized awareness that they will be better as a result of the policy change. Suggesting that "things" will be better represents a generalized amorphism, which will keep people disengaged and suspicious of the "real" value of the suggested change. Any policy change that requires personal energy but does not attain some level of personal benefit or threatens the "safe" status quo will have a short tenure.

POLICY ON THE SCENE 8.2: Beth Israel Medical Center Parish Partnership, Newark, NJ

One of the nation's major policy and health issues relates to obesity, especially in urban and minority communities. Costs associated with health issues related to obesity continue to grow at an accelerating and alarming rate. Beth Israel Medical Center recognized the significance of this problem for its community. Using their partnership position as a leader of health in the community, they saw their engagement as a policy imperative to fully participate in advancing their community's health and reducing obesity's impact. The administrative and clinical leadership knew that establishing a partnership with community leaders and especially church leadership was important. Therefore, they initiated a program reflecting their commitment to affect obesity by responding with their "Beth Challenge" approach. Beth Israel runs a garden market that grows healthy foods and makes them available to inner-city residents in the surrounding Beth Israel community. They are also constructing a greenhouse to make their farm produce available year-round and to use it as a laboratory for educating schools and children about nutrition and obesity prevention. Engaging with the national policy to improve population health and specifically to reduce obesity, Beth Israel translated that policy into institutional and community policy priorities in a way that exemplified the hospital's accountability for advancing health. The hospital also serves to transform its operating and clinical environment from emphasizing treatment and illness care to one focusing on advancing the health of the community that Beth Israel serves.

Policy implications for the community initiative include:

1. Governmental and social policy addressing population health forms the frame within which health service providers operate that requires policy translation within the culture and characteristics of the community of service. Systems and institutions must translate social policy in a way that has specific meaning and value for the communities for which they are accountable.
2. Health systems, representing their community membership, demonstrate application of health policy through active models and programs, which best represent their convergence with the particular and unique community health needs. This process makes them available as the centerpiece of community direction and action in bringing policy to life and advancing its potential for positive impact.
3. Health systems provide an opportunity for the translation of policy that demonstrates new models, programs, and innovations that refocus delivery structures, as well as services that create models with the potential for replication and adaptation in other settings and communities across the country. This translation and application of policy results in innovation hubs that aggregate community to community and ultimately have an impact on shifting national health practices.

7. All individuals associated with any policy change express and need to play some part in the design and initiation of policy that directly impacts their lives. Good policy formation is generative, engaging, and invests stakeholders in the processes associated with its formation. Suggesting to stakeholders impacted by a policy that they can only be involved in its implementation creates "late-stage engagement" and delays their capacity

to incorporate it as part of their personal values and behavior. The closer a policy can be formulated to where it will have impact, the more likely it will be both embraced and successfully initiated.

This growing understanding of the essential "locality" of policy formation and implementation over this past decade has challenged historic notions of centralized approaches to policy management (Winowiecki et al., 2011). Much of the devolution to regions and states of policy decision making with regard to national health reform and Medicaid reform is an example of the shift. In addition, the Centers for Medicare and Medicaid Services (CMS) Center for Innovation best demonstrates this point-of-service approach to model building and policy formation through the generation of innovation initiatives in a wide variety of local settings. Models such as accountable care organizations, medical home delivery systems, community care delivery models, and nurse navigator continuum-of-care approaches all demonstrate point-of-service approaches. In addition, the CMS is attempting through the Patient-Centered Outcomes Research Institute (PCORI) to fund the building of a framework for comparative effectiveness in order to compare and contrast clinical approaches based on research and clinical evidence that can validate preferred approaches and best practices (PCORI, n.d.). All of these models demonstrate an approach that serves to permit the aggregation of local efforts to be evaluated in a way that helps define common elements and characteristics. This effort better defines those policies and practices that converge to inform appropriate policy formation and more effectively suggest those policies and practices that can be best replicated across a larger number of settings. Organizational efforts have suggested this less "top-down" and more "center-out" approach yields better engagement and ownership suggested by crucial policy change.

FACILITATORS AND BARRIERS TO CHANGE AND INNOVATION

In addition to the barriers and facilitators noted in the effective teamwork section of this chapter, there are both subtle and overt barriers and facilitators that can render the policy process either effective and impactful or dismantling. Gaining an appreciation of the significance of both facilitators and barriers to change and innovation further supports the advancement of new ideas.

Facilitation of change results from multiple factors including knowledge and understanding of the intended change, personal or professional investment in the intended change, and active involvement in creating the intended change. Facilitation of change results when goals and values are mutually supported and the personal impact of the change or innovation is acceptable to the individual. To be sure, there is nothing more frustrating than learning about an intended change that will impact your work after the change has been formulated and proposed. When key stakeholders are involved in creating the rationale, processes, and expected outcomes of new or revised policies, support for the proposed change is more likely to be facilitated and supported. An exemplar is the work done by nursing associations in supporting legislative agendas. Consider the work and processes in the clarification of the role and advancement of certified registered nurse anesthetists (CRNAs). In clarifying the scope of practice of CRNAs across the country, involvement of key stakeholders is essential. For example, collaboration with physicians and pharmacists in the discussion of changes as well as with drafting of the language of the bill is an essential step in facilitating the change process. It is also important to note that this type of scope of practice documentation in the legislative process typically requires more time than anticipated.

Consider the length of the actual times in which legislative bodies are in session and the available time frames for which changes can be submitted. Fitting change processes into legislative schedules requires significant collaboration and teamwork prior to the start of the session; being strategic and timely in this work are essential. Ensuring that key stakeholders are knowledgeable and able to support the proposed change cannot be accelerated without some anticipation of loss of support.

A second factor that generates support for change is one in which personal or professional practice is supported or enhanced. To be sure, change and innovation often arouse emotions and passionate pleading for one choice or another. When one's choice is sustaining the current reality, barriers to considering and adopting new ways are quickly raised. Fear of what the change might result in as well as avoidance of risk taking contributes to resistance. These barriers to change and innovation are most often related to personal comfort with the current situation. Our personal baggage includes everything from once-valid beliefs and practices that have outlived their usefulness, to misinformation and misconceptions that we've accepted (even embraced) without much examination or thought or evidence.

Consider the implementation of regulations specific to the need for a collaborative relationship with nurse practitioners. Each state varies in its requirements for nurse practitioner collaboration. Some states do not recognize clinical nurse specialists in their nurse practice acts or regulations. Similar to the work in clarifying the role of CRNAs, developing practical and safe practices from the policy perspective requires collaboration of physicians, nurses, payers, and insurers. To achieve the goal of decreasing the level of supervision, support and facilitation from multiple stakeholders is needed. Consideration specific to individuals as practitioners, groups of practitioners, organizations using the services, and payers reimbursing for the services all needed to be included.

In spite of the best preparation and planning, resistance to change and innovation occurs. As noted in Exhibit 8.11, resistance to change occurs in many formats from the outspoken, verbal reactions to the subtle, nonverbal, indirect avoidance of the issue. In general, individuals resist change when there is a perceived threat to their safety and security or position. The culture of an organization or the leadership style can also impede change and innovation

---

EXHIBIT 8.11 RESISTANCE TO CHANGE: UNCOVERING COMPETING COMMITMENTS

Individuals often state they are supportive and want to participate in change or changing; however, the change does not happen. Consider the following underlying assumptions that get in the way of individuals moving forward with change.

- Stated commitment: I want to be a team player, but I am struggling with making this happen as I know I don't collaborate enough. I make unilateral decisions too often and I really don't take people's ideas and input into account.
- Competing commitment: I am committed to being the one who gets the credit and to avoiding the frustration or conflict that comes with collaboration.
- Big underlying assumption: I assume that no one will appreciate me if I am not seen as the source of success. I assume nothing good will come of me being frustrated or in conflict.

Using your understanding of change and innovation, the process and dynamics, the strategies to manage resistance, and the tools of innovation, how would you and your team address these types of resistance and, more importantly, how could the team be proactive in minimizing this resistance in the planning phase for a new policy?

(Schein, 2004). Some barriers or resistors to change and innovation are covert and difficult to uncover. Resistance to change and innovation can result from subtle competing commitments (Kagan & Lahey, 2001). Consider the situation in which an individual indicates that he or she is a team player; however, feedback from others indicates that the individual dismisses the ideas and input of others and seldom asks for assistance. According to Kagan and Lahey (2001), the competing commitment for the individual is that he or she is internally committed to getting the credit for work and avoiding the frustration or conflict that comes with working with others. What is even more important is the assumption that the individual believes no one will appreciate him or her unless he or she is seen as the source of success; nothing good will come of being frustrated or in conflict. Consider the potential competing values involved in supporting pro life or pro choice. Professionally, a nurse might support pro choice; however, from a personal faith perspective, alignment of values is with pro life, thus creating a very challenging situation for the nurse. As a person, the nurse may have been raised in a religion strongly supportive of life, while as a professional nurse, the challenges of teenage pregnancy and casual sex have garnered her support. These competing values often make it difficult to understand which side of the policy debate an individual will eventually choose.

Finally, resistance can emerge as a result of outdated systems or information that obstructs one from considering a different alternative. If electronic communication is believed unreliable and a violation of privacy, individuals will resist until secure electronic line information is fully disseminated. Sometimes the most challenging aspect is determining the source of the resistance. The resistance could emanate from personal knowledge to levels of trust to skills in managing conflict and negotiation. Being able to differentiate personal knowledge or professional resistance provides information to move from jaded nostalgia about the past or knowledge deficits to increasing engagement in the change and innovation processes. Exploring resistance is a critical part of the change and innovation process. Interestingly, the resistance to change and innovation often occurs when there is little stakeholder engagement, sharing of knowledge and ideas, and team building. Strategies to decrease resistance include sound principles of team building, working to understand the rationale, and competing commitment that results in resistance and allowing adequate time for discussion and collaboration.

LESSONS LEARNED

Given the complexity of policy change, it is not surprising that creating and sustaining policy changes specific to nursing practice are not always successful on the first attempt. Numerous lessons can be learned from both successful and unsuccessful changes. What is important is that we learn and share lessons from each and every policy change process at the local, state, and national levels. The importance of collaboration, allowance of chaos and noise during the dialogue to allow voices to be heard, negotiation, compromise, and overall comfort with the evolutionary process of change cannot be overstated. Equally important is the recognition that new information emerges during the process and this new information needs to be considered in the continuation of the process in order to achieve the desired goals.

The implementation of the NLC provides many policy process lessons (National Council of State Boards of Nursing [NCSBN], n.d.). In this section, the characteristics and processes of the NLC innovation process are outlined as the basis to determine where the gaps in support occurred, guides for celebration of successes, and lessons learned that facilitate course correction in the future.

The characteristics of this planned, teleological change are described as an innovation to be completed by large groups at the state and national levels. At the outset of this initiative, key leaders at the NCSBN described the purpose of the NLC and sought to involve and educate others as to the anticipated outcomes. This early collaborative process was critical in gaining support for the state-based model. The time frame was open ended depending on the levels of acceptance of the innovation and legislative schedules. Using the Nine Essential Phases of Policy Team Work guidelines, the NLC process proceeded in the following manner:

1. Determining the foundational need
   The NLC group determined that the three drivers were supporting this licensure approach; telehealth, multiple shared borders among states, and maintenance of multiple licenses were burdensome (Dorsey & Schowalter, 2008). The increasing mobility of the population further supports

national licensure. The intent of the NLC is to provide a nationally recognized licensure system in which licensure is state based and state enforced (NCSBN, 2012).

2. Setting the table

Representatives from NCSBN member boards met with the then president of the American Nurses Association (ANA), representatives of the American Nurses Credentialing Center, and numerous other nursing organizations.

3. Defining expectations

The expectations of the NLC were identified as simplification of governmental processes, removing regulatory barriers, and increasing access to safe nursing care. States expected to be able to share complaint and investigative information and impact patient safety in a more timely manner. Standardizing state regulations is believed to further support mobility, telehealth, and timely resolution of complaints to positively impact patient safety.

4. Context, timeline, powers, and deliverables

The education of state boards, professional associations, and citizens groups along with individual nurses occurred over time. The timeline for full implementation was deemed dependent on state boards of nursing gaining the appropriate support for the NLC and legislative support to enact the appropriated statutes. Powers rested with each board of nursing in determining whether or not to move forward with the NLC. The deliverables or outcome was the successful implementation of legislation for the NLC and successful creation of administrative policies to support the processes of multistate licensure.

5. Methods and terms of engagement

Each board of nursing determined the appropriate time for advancement of the NLC.

6. Team tools and dynamics fit

Strategies and dynamics included information documents, local and national presentations with open dialogue to understand the issues surrounding the process.

7. Agreement of outcome

The outcome of NLC is participation of all of the boards of nursing to achieve the identified goals. This outcome was identified by the originating NCSBN committee.

8. Completion of work

Work would be completed when legislation was enacted in all 50 states and implemented at each board of nursing.

9. Handoff mechanisms for closure

Once legislation is enacted, the oversight is handed off to the NLC administration for oversight of the compact processes.

Since 2000, 24 states have joined the NLC. While nearly half of the states have adopted and enacted the NLC, others have not. The lessons learned are both positive and negative. Successful enactments resulted from collaborative work among constituencies, sensitivity to legislative timelines, and the work of champions for the NLC. Many legislators saw the NLC as a means to mediate the nursing shortage and advance the health care of their constituents. In contrast, many lessons were learned and are still being learned. Step 2 of the process addresses the importance of key stakeholders. Resistance was quickly evident from labor organizations representing nurses in many states. States with high union membership believe that increasing the mobility of nurses was not necessarily a positive outcome, but rather this new mobility would facilitate strike breaking. However, when there have been strikes in states not within the NLC, employers have been able to bring in fully licensed nurses who live in other states to work in their facilities. Another lesson is related to the context and intent of the NLC. Some states' attorneys general believed that the implementation of the NLC would be abandonment of a state's rights; therefore, in so joining the compact, an illegal action was committed. Another interesting area of resistance from state boards of nursing is that the loss of revenue from nurses being licensed in multiple states would negatively impact the state boards' budgets and decrease their ability to effectively discipline nurses.

These lessons and sources of resistance provide valuable input into the continuing process to enact this complex legislation. To be sure, the competing commitments for union membership, preservation of state funds, and states' rights issues will need to be examined and mediated in order for more states to enact this legislation.

CONFRONTING FAILED POLICY AND REENERGIZING ENGAGEMENT

Each of us can enumerate the sometimes devastating and lingering effects of a truly failed policy. Most policy failures represent an inadequate application of the processes, terms of engagement, and the cautions briefly pointed out in this chapter. Policy most often fails because some process associated with its formation was in some way flawed (Latin, 2012). While the challenges of policy implementation can be daunting, adherence to good process from the outset can facilitate implementation and reduce both the intensity and vagaries associated with making policy work (see Exhibit 8.12).

Policies fail for specific reasons. Often a policy is doomed for failure at the outset, driven by the primary process failure in the establishment of *inappropriate objectives* (Richtermeyer, 2010). In health care, the focus of a policy is often on service provision directed to specific populations rather than to clearly defined and well-articulated health outcomes, expectations, or impact. Establishing strong helmet laws to reduce accidental head injury is not nearly

EXHIBIT 8.12 ESSENTIAL ELEMENTS IN THE POLICY PROCESS

Policy teams can enhance the success of their proposed policy through use of a brief checklist, which focuses on policy progress. Some important items on the checklist include:
- Specificity and clarity of the policy
- General understanding of the policy and its implications
- Appropriateness of the policy to the issue it is attempting to address
- Significance of the policy and its impact
- Strategic and systemic commitment to the policy
- Perceived fairness and value of the policy
- Evaluation of effectiveness of the policy
- Flexibility of the policy to change, when necessitated

as specific a policy objective as is the establishment of such laws in an effort to reduce crippling and costly brain damage. In addition, health laws that focus predominantly on particular elements of cause or prevention are more strongly and effectively defined than those emphasizing treatment. For example, a policy stating that, because of the potential for devastating head injury, helmets are always required for manual or motorized cycles is a stronger and more deterministic policy than one that simply relates to treatment availability for head injuries in general. There must be a clear cause-and-effect relationship in policy formation (no helmet leads to inevitable head injury) that goes beyond the root cause (e.g., there is always a risk of head injury with manual or motorized cycles), and also identifies double-loop learning (the thinking and perceptions that lie beneath determination of cause). Double-loop learning, in this case, would suggest that a policy reflects an abiding understanding of the perennial risk in riding manual or motorized cycles, indicating a clear need for a concerted and specific response to this risk. The best policy is that which addresses both the risk and causative factors. In a specific way, policy efforts are not wasted as when they are directed to issues of effect (correction, accommodation, reaction, and recidivism).

A second leading failure for policy initiatives is the provision of *asymmetrical information* to those who are impacted by the policy. The classic example in the United States is the duplicity shown by drug companies when recommending use of their drugs to the general population. While this information may be objectively correct, its accuracy and veracity are particularly limited when viewed through the lens of individual patient conditions, circumstances, and drug interactions. The fact is that one of the most prescribed powerful psychotropics is prescribed by family physicians and internists because of patient demand rather than carefully delineated clinical need. Or in the case of a notable erectile dysfunction drug, it is generally prescribed for those who want it but who present little evidence of actual erectile dysfunction; advertising a side effect of prolonged action led to a boon in demand. Both are examples of this information asymmetry resulting in behaviors that have little relationship to purpose or intent.

A third threat to the integrity of policy formation is the issue of *moral hazard*. There are a large number of cases in the United States where Food and Drug Administration (FDA)-approved drugs have been used for "off-label" purposes or where the data supporting the use of drugs for specific purposes have been inadequate or inaccurate. Often the interests in generating a large volume of sales or the exciting potential effects of one of these drugs overwhelms careful judgment with regard to appropriateness, safety, and efficacy. Problems lie both in policy, which governs the approval process, and in issues with the effectiveness related to countering opportunity enthusiasm, elements of groupthink, or inadequacies in review or process leading to a negative impact or outcome.

Often driving policy failure are issues of *adverse selection* with regard to who, how, and where policy is managed and executed. Often the formation of policy portends a legitimate response to a public need. On the other hand, however, that good intention is lost in the dynamics of politics, competition, lowest bidder vendor selection, hidden agendas, and so on. Implementation and application of policy can be disciplined through clear management, budgetary parameters, and precise metrics, which validate the relationship between intent, impact, and outcome expectations. Careful selection of partners and stakeholders (especially users of potential products who can bring to the table insights regarding implications for application and predict complications and vagaries prior to their widespread adoption) in the translation and implementation of particular policies can go far in avoiding many of the vagaries associated with the selection of process and players resulting in the demonstration of effective policy implementation and the related achievement of successful outcomes (see Exhibit 8.13). Examples can relate to whole hosts of scenarios, which could include selection of safety needles and/or safe sharps, lay use of catheters or other insertable devices, wound care treatment products and supplies, colostomy and fistula products, and therapeutic dietary regimens, among others.

An important challenge to policy effectiveness lies in the intensity of the relationship between *efficacy (power to produce an effect)* and *effectiveness (the desired result)*. Costs and service requirements of particular policies often demonstrate that there is only a tangential relationship between the significance of resource demands and the resulting value of the policy. Often there is little relationship between the costs associated with implementing the policy and the resultant positive effects of the policy. This set of circumstances is not infrequent. Once such resource-intensive policies are generated and patterns of behavior are subsequently developed, it becomes even more cost-intensive to accommodate, adjust, or correct such policies. Cost–benefit relationships must be clearly delineated at the policy formation stage as a way of ensuring a net positive relationship between the human and resource costs of a policy and the value of its impact. A classic example of the conflict between policy and resources is that which relates to the wide variety of nursing staffing mechanisms and approaches. Frequently, policies related to staff-to-patient ratios do not include valid measures of

---

EXHIBIT 8.13	SUGGESTIONS FOR AVOIDING POLICY FAILURE

- Make sure the use of policy to address the behavior is necessary
- Define objectives in a way that clearly relates to policy outcomes
- Make sure there is a tightly related interaction between cause and effect in policy formation
- Define a clear relationship between cost–benefit and outcome efficacy and effectiveness
- Invest and engage stakeholders in policy design and construction
- Ensure that there is an effective communication model that affirms a strong relationship between intent and implementation
- Establish a continuous and ongoing mechanism for monitoring policy effectiveness and relevance

---

preparation, competence, intensity, and demand, resulting in generalized staff-to-patient ratios that may not best fit the clinical conditions or requirements of particular patients or populations. As a result, wide variation exists in the appropriate use of resources and goodness of fit with patient needs.

One of the most challenging circumstances to the successful implementation of policy is that related to failure *to effectively communicate*. When good policies are introduced, the relationship between design and implementation becomes critical. Often the breakdown in effective handoffs and the thorough and complete generation of relevant information related to the character, content, and intent of the policy gets lost or altered in the process. In effect, frequently the policy being implemented is not the policy designed and either the structure of implementation leads to a perversion of the policy or the processes of application implement a policy format that looks little like its origination. The disciplines of communication must be as well addressed as any other factor of implementation and demands as intensive a focus as any component of the policy development and implementation process if this error is to be avoided.

Finally, one of the most critical areas of concern for successful policy implementation is the one that relates to the *failure to monitor policy performance effectiveness*. As policies moved into the rituals and routines of organizational systems and human practices, they often devolve into patterns of behavior and action that little resemble the purpose, intent, or origination that drove policy formation. There is often a policy driving the ritual related to a particular nursing practice; for example, frequency of blood pressure or cardiac rhythm monitoring for a particular patient population may be reduced or increased based on new evidence or science that better informs that protocol, yet nurses may fail to adjust their practices because of established rituals or a lack of availability of the evidence that would change those practices, or just long-standing habits that are ingrained into workflow patterns. Therefore, monitoring policy application is as critical an element to the long-term viability of policy formation as is the detail and veracity associated with initial policy design and implementation. The long-term vagaries associated with policy translation, practices, scenario changes, and adjustment in circumstances affecting the policy are critical variables that affect both the legitimacy and sustainability of policy.

A structured, regular, consistent review of individual policy (and policy sets) is an essential corollary to effectively managing policy that can serve to determine the continuing value and relevance of policy as it is applied. There is nothing more destructive to value and meaning of policy in human action than the continuation of behaviors and actions subsequent to policy requirements that are no longer relevant or viable. This complication is often seen in the duplication of effort between electronic medical record documentation and paper records. Often nurses are duplicating similar data in both record systems. Sometimes, this duplication of documentation operates for the convenience of particular providers, which ultimately keeps them from integrating the documentation system and advancing the utility and engagement of digital documentation. Similarly, some institutions may bar nurses from using cellphones while on duty. Yet, nurses are now using their personal smartphones to access online information about medications, diseases, and laboratory tests as well as applications to help patients manage their illness. Limiting access to such resources could have a negative impact on the quality of care received by patients. Policy is as dynamic as the circumstances it addresses; when those circumstances change and policy fails to change along with them, people become cynical, lax, and non-compliant, and their action becomes increasingly situational (Scott, 2004).

OPTION FOR POLICY CHALLENGE: Interstate Practice Policy Needs

As you have read and reflected on the policy challenge at the beginning of the chapter and the contents of this chapter, there are now many options for consideration in evaluating nursing licensure policy models. Begin the process by using strategic team processes to define the type of change or innovation that is needed for advanced practice nurses to work seamlessly across state borders. Most likely, this work would be driven by teleological or goal formation and dialectical forces. In this early formation process, recognizing if this work is an expectation or if it is still open for both rejection and acceptance is an important step given the strong feelings of current supporters and opponents. In this case, either a change or an innovation could be possible. Change would be appropriate if the current licensure model is merely translated to a national model; an innovation model would be appropriate if the model for licensure was reinvented in a new, different way. In examining the case of the CNM in the beginning of the chapter, think about the nature of the change if both states signed on to the NLC. Think about how the change process would be different if we moved to a model of national licensure, not only for

(continued)

registered nurses and advanced practice nurses, but also for all health care professionals. The nature of this complex change requires time parameters in a planned process, the levels of participation from local, to state, and to national collaboration. And, if national licensure were implemented, could such a model provide the foundation for global credentialing?

As the infrastructure and teams are formed and the processes are selected, the translation of policy formulation is a critical step in gaining maximum engagement of stakeholders. The stakeholder process is illustrated by the Future of Nursing Campaign to ensure that all nurses are practicing to the full extent of their education and training (Initiative on the Future of Nursing, 2011) and differences in opinion about the location of one's practice (ANA, 2013). To be sure, key stakeholders would want to be aware of the lessons learned in the current processes engaged by 24 states in forming the NLC. Barriers and facilitators would also be identified and recognized by stakeholders in this complex work. These are just the beginning steps of a complex process!

IMPLICATIONS FOR THE FUTURE

Policy formation and policy changes are rarely the result of linear approaches or even sequential dynamics where the stages of policy are logically determined. While it is true policy formation is a discipline, the generation of policy and the machinations influencing its formation are often surreptitious and tangential. Looking through the "windows" of social dynamics, it is often easy to see the emergent character of demand for policy as a result of changes in conditions, circumstances, scenarios, or interactions (see Option for Policy Challenge). Leaders must be available during such occurrences and recognize when the forces they represent aggregate sufficiently to challenge current policy and practice.

The changing digital landscape will play an important role in the future of policy formation and change. Nothing could be more clearly indicative of a changing social milieu and technological context for policy formation than social media and the innovative and dynamic opportunities for connection it represents. Throughout the globe, overwhelming political, social, and economic circumstances have been both challenged and reacted to through predominantly online media mechanisms. The emergence of digital reality has created a whole new set of challenges and opportunities for democratic action, decision making, discourse, cooperation convergence, and social revolution. The breadth of connections and interaction that a universal media such as the Internet provides creates an entirely different social construct, diminishing the two-dimensional value of borders, boundaries, limited access, and human communities. The universality of the human condition and human interaction has emerged as the critical centerpiece of these digital tools whose most widely used purposes are connection, communication, linkage, networking, convergence, and relationship.

Dialogue and discussion related to existing policy circumstances and conditions, policy efficacy, legality, appropriateness, and legitimacy now have a broad constituency with mutual access to information and resources in a way that more broadly informs policy discussion and decision making. At every level of communion from international to regional to local, policy implications can be explored over a large constituency of stakeholders, providing a medium for enhanced engagement with a more vigorous interaction and collective convergence achieving a higher level of veracity of fact and truth. Not only does the digital reality create increasing opportunities, but it also ultimately creates an accelerating demand for connection, participation, and stakeholder engagement.

Because of the access and opportunity for interaction, the mechanisms of policy formation can now be more functionally refined as policy makers become more aware of the multifocal "streams" of interacting forces that serve to inform, discipline, and direct the processes of policy formation. Advocacy for particular approaches and views becomes more transparent as information is more available to all the stakeholders. As data provide increasing clarity around implications and choices, solutions become more emergent and visible across stakeholder groups, creating a greater potential for agreement and ratification.

At every level of policy deliberation and formation, the use of the digital infrastructure and tools provides a more dependable and sustainable format for the establishment of principles and for more strongly universalizing policy, protocols, and best practices. Whether it is an international conflict over the management of immigration or citizen flow across national boundaries or a very local decision around a particular patient care practice, policy can now be more "universalized" and the evidence and rationale for supporting and sustaining it can be more generally promulgated and accepted. Furthermore, when evidence suggests the need for refinement or change in a policy, the digital environment makes it possible to make such adjustments "just in time" so they can be immediately reconfigured and applied (Tucker, 2010).

KEY CONCEPTS

1. Change is an alteration of something, whereas innovation is a type of qualified change that impacts future processes and includes benefits and nuances.
2. Important features to identify in the change process include knowing supporters and obstacles, the extent of the change, time parameters, drivers, levels of change, and its predictability.
3. Types of drivers of change include life cycle change and innovation (e.g., election cycle), teleological change (e.g., advancing a position), dialectical change

(e.g., iterative development), and evolutionary change (e.g., repetition of variation, selection, and retention).

4. Successful team processes in policy formulation include determining the foundational need; setting the table with the right stakeholders; enumerating context, timelines, power, and deliverables; effectively delineating methods and terms of engagement; ensuring a good fit between team tools and dynamics; collective agreement regarding teamwork products; determining when the work is done; and bringing closure to the work.

5. Translating policy into action and impact requires simplicity, clarity, illustrating how the policy impacts individuals, illustrating the policy's value for individuals, describing exactly what will happen as a result, indicating that the policy will make things better, and involving stakeholders at the outset.

6. Change is facilitated by understanding the intended change, personal and professional investment, and active involvement.

7. Resistance to change takes many forms, may be difficult to uncover, and may result from competing commitments.

8. There is value in sharing lessons learned from policy implementation at the local, state, and national levels.

9. Policy failures most commonly result from an inadequate application of processes, inappropriate objectives, asymmetrical information, poor communication, poor implementation, or failure to monitor policy effectiveness.

10. The changing digital landscape will impact how policy is formulated and implemented in the future.

SUMMARY

Health care policy is an essential societal component and requires stakeholders knowledgeable in the basic processes of change and innovation. Nurses, in particular, are critical stakeholders in facilitating effective team building to ensure that the best interests of all community members are served. To be sure, effective teams are best able to translate policy formulation while understanding the barriers, facilitators, and historical lessons learned from policy processes. As the nation moves to a reformed model of health care, the future is filled with opportunities for nurses to create the essential health care policies and avoid the creation of non-value-added policies.

LEARNING ACTIVITIES

1. Select an issue of personal importance to you that can be addressed with a change in policy. Describe the intellectual, emotional, and political noise associated with the implementation of a policy change related to the issue.

2. Describe a potential policy change for the selected issue: (a) the actual change or alteration, (b) human agencies (individual or organizational), (c) time parameters, (d) level of change, (e) predictability, and (f) drivers of change (life cycle, dialectical, teleological, or evolutionary).

3. With the selected issue, identify all the potential stakeholders or stakeholder groups who have an interest in the outcome of a policy change related to the issue, describe their position on the issue, and explain the rationale for their position. For each stakeholder, determine whether the issue is a serious one, as well as if the stakeholder is for, against, or neutral with regard to the policy change.

E-RESOURCES

- Aid on the Edge of Chaos: Exploring Complexity and Evolutionary Sciences in Foreign Aid. http://aidontheedge.info/2011/04/20/six-theories-of-policy-change
- Helena Temkin-Greener on Teams and Teamwork in Health Care: Using Evidence to Inform Policy. University of California Irvine Open Courseware. http://www.youtube.com/watch?v=FhMWh2qU7WY
- Institute of Developmental Studies: Theory of Change and Outcome Mapping. http://www.slideshare.net/ikmediaries/theory-of-change-and-outcome-mapping-for-intermediary-work
- Team Effectiveness Assessment: How Good Is Your Team? http://www.mindtools.com/pages/article/newTMM_84.htm

REFERENCES

3M Health Information Systems. (2003). *All patient refined diagnosis related groups (APR-DRGs): Methodology overview.* Retrieved from http://www.hcup-us.ahrq.gov/db/nation/nis/APR-DRGsV20MethodologyOverviewandBibliography.pdf

Agency for Healthcare Research and Quality. (2013a). *AHRQ innovation exchange: Inclusion criteria for health care policy innovations.* Retrieved from http://innovations.ahrq.gov/inclusion/policy.aspx

Agency for Healthcare Research and Quality. (2013b). *On-time quality improvement program.* Retrieved from http://www.ahrq.gov/professionals/systems/long-term-care/resources/ontime/index.html

American Nurses Association. (2013, April). *Nurse Licensure Compact (NLC).* Retrieved from http://nursingworld.org/MainMenuCategories/Policy-Advocacy/State/Legislative-Agenda-Reports/LicensureCompact/INLC-TalkingPoints.pdf

Bardach, E. (2011). *A practical guide to policy analysis: The eightfold path to more effective problem-solving.* Washington, DC: CQ Press College.

Bennett K. J., Probst J. C., Vyavaharkar, M., & Glover, S. (2012). Missing the handoff: post-hospitalization follow-up care among rural Medicare beneficiaries with diabetes. *Rural and Remote Health, 12*: 2097. (Online). Retrieved from: http://www.rrh.org.au

Bodenheimer, T., & Gumbach, K. (2012). *Understanding health policy* (6th ed.). New York, NY: McGraw-Hill.

Boradkar, P. (2010). Transdisciplinary design and innovation in the classroom. In T. Porter-O'Grady & K. Malloch (Eds.), *Innovation leadership: Creating the landscape of health care* (pp. 109–134). Sudbury, MA: Jones and Bartlett.

Cheung, K. M., Mirzaei, M., & Leeder, S. (2010). Health policy analysis: A tool to evaluate in policy documents the alignment between policy statements and intended outcomes. *Australian Health Review, 34*(4), 405–413.

Christensen, C. M., Anthony, S. D., & Roth, E. A. (2004). *Seeing what's next: Using the theories of innovation to predict industry change* (p. 293). Boston, MA: Harvard Business School Press.

Clarke, D., Werestiuk, K., Schoffner, A., Gerard, J., Swan, K. Jackson, B., ... Probizanski, S. (2012). Achieving the "perfect handoff" in patient transfers: Building teamwork and trust. *Journal of Nursing Management, 20*(5), 592–598.

Cooperrider, D. L., Whitney, D. K., & Stavros, J. M. (2008). *The appreciative inquiry handbook: For leaders of change* (2nd ed.). San Francisco, CA: Barrett-Koehler.

Deleuran, P. (Ed.). (2011). *Conflict management in the family field and in other close relationships: Mediation as a way forward*. Portland, OR: International Specialized Book Services.

Dooley, K. J. (2004). Complexity science models of organizational change and innovation. In M. S. Poole & A. H. Van de Ven (Eds.), *Handbook of organizational change and innovation* (pp. 354–373). New York, NY: Oxford University Press.

Dorsey, C. F., & Schowalter, J. M. (2008). *The first 25 years: 1978–2003*. Retrieved from https://www.ncsbn.org/25Years_13.pdf

Drazin, R., Glynn, M. A., & Kazanjian, R. K. (2004). Dynamics of structural change. In M. S. Poole & A. H. Van de Van (Eds.), *Handbook of organizational change and innovation* (pp. 161–189). New York, NY: Oxford University Press.

Drucker, P. (1985). The discipline of innovation. *Harvard Business Review, 63*(5), 67–72.

Dunin-Keplicz, B., & Verbrugge, R. (2010). *Teamwork in multi-agent systems: A formal approach*. Hoboken, NJ: John Wiley & Sons.

Endsley, S. (2010). Innovation in action: A practical system for results. In T. Porter-O'Grady & K. Malloch (Eds.), *Innovation leadership: Creating the landscape of health care* (pp. 59–86). Sudbury, MA: Jones and Bartlett.

Finkelman, A. W. (2012). *Leadership and management for nurses: Core competencies for quality care*. Boston, MA: Pearson.

Fitz-enz, J. (2009). *The ROI of human capital: Measuring the economic value of employee performance*. New York, NY: AMACOM.

Fonseca, J. (2002). *Complexity and innovation in organizations*. London: Routledge.

Gratton, L., & Erickson, T. (2007). Eight ways to build collaborative teams. *Harvard Business Review, 85*(11), 100–111.

Hartley, D. (2012). *Social policy*. London: Polity Press.

Hatch, J. J. (2004). Dynamics in organizational culture. In M. S. Poole & A. H. Van de Van (Eds.), *Handbook of organizational change and innovation* (pp. 190–211). New York, NY: Oxford University Press.

Havelock, R. G. (1973). *The change agent's guide to innovation in education*. Englewood Cliffs, NJ: Educational Technology Publications.

Hayes, M. T. (2006). *Incrementalism and public policy*. Lanham, MD: University Press of America.

Initiative on the Future of Nursing. (2011). *IOM recommendations*. Retrieved from http://thefutureofnursing.org/recommendations

Institute of Medicine (IOM). (2011). *The future of nursing: Leading change, advancing health.* Washington, DC: The National Academies Press.

Kagan, R., & Lahey, L. L. (2001). The real reason people won't change. *Harvard Business Review, 78*(10), 85–92.

Kelley, T. (2005). *The ten faces of innovation.* New York, NY: Doubleday.

Latin, H. (2012). *Climate change policy failures: Why conventional mitigation approaches cannot succeed.* Hackensack, NJ: World Scientific.

Lewin, K. (1947). Frontiers in group dynamics: Concept, method, and reality in social science, social equilibria and social change. *Human Relations, 1(1)*, 5–41.

Lippitt, R., Watson, J., & Westley, B. (1958). *The dynamics of planned change.* New York, NY: Harcourt Brace.

Matheson, C. (2009). Understanding the policy process: The work of Henry Mintzberg. *Public Administration Review, 69*(6), 1148–1161.

Maxson, P. M., Derby, K. M., Wrobleski, D. M., & Foss, D. M. (2012). Bedside nurse-to-nurse handoff promotes patient safety. *Medsurg Nursing, 21*(3), 140–144, quiz 145.

Merriman-Webster. (2014). Dictionary: Change. Retrieved from http://www.merriam-webster.com/dictionary/change

Monroe, T., & Kenaga, H. (2011). Don't ask don't tell: Substance abuse and addition among nurses. *Journal of Clinical Nursing, 20*(3–4), 504–509.

National Council of State Boards of Nursing (NCSBN). (n.d.). *Nurse licensure compact.* Retrieved from https://www.ncsbn.org/nlc.htm

National Council of State Boards of Nursing (NCSBN). (2012). *Nurse Licensure Compact (NLC) fact sheet for legislators.* Retrieved from https://www.ncsbn.org/2012_NLCA_factsheet_legislators.pdf

Nickerson, J. A. (2010). *Leading change in a Web 2.1 world: How ChangeCasting builds trust, creates understanding, and accelerates organizational change.* Washington, DC: Brookings Institution Press.

Nohria, N., & Khurana, R. (Eds.). (2010). *Handbook of leadership theory and practice: An HBS centennial colloquium on advancing leadership.* Boston, MA: Harvard Business Press.

Patient-Centered Outcomes Research Institute (PCORI). (n.d.). *National priorities and research agenda.* Retrieved from http://www.pcori.org/research-we-support/priorities-agenda

Plsek, P. E. (1997). *Creativity, innovation and quality.* Milwaukee, WI: ASQC Quality Press.

Poole, M. S., & Van de Ven, A. H. (Eds.). (2004) *Handbook of organizational change and innovation.* New York, NY: Oxford University Press.

Porter-O'Grady, T., & Malloch, K. (2012). *Leadership in nursing practice: Changing the landscape of healthcare.* Sudbury, MA: Jones and Bartlett.

Reddin, W. J. (1970). *Managerial effectiveness.* New York, NY: McGraw-Hill.

Richtermeyer, S. B. (2010, February 8). Top 5 reasons why strategic initiatives fail. *Industry Week, 1,* 1.

Rogers, E. M. (2003). *Diffusion of innovation* (5th ed.). New York, NY: The Free Press.

Schein, E. (2004). *Organizational culture and leadership.* San Francisco, CA: Jossey-Bass.

Schoemaker, P. J. H. (1995). Scenario planning: A tool for strategic thinking. *Sloan Management Review, 36*(2), 25–40.

Schuman, S. (2006). *Creating a culture of collaboration: The International Association of Facilitators handbook.* San Francisco, CA, Jossey-Bass.

Schumpeter, J. A. (1943). *Capitalism, socialism, and democracy* (6th ed.). London: Routledge.

Scott, G. (2004). Public policy failure in health care. *Journal of the American Academy of Business, 5*(1/2), 88–94.

Smith-Coggins, R., Howard, S. K., Mac, D. T., Wang, C., Kwan, S., Rosekind, M. R., … Gaba, D. M. (2006). Improving alertness and performance in emergency department physicians and nurses: The use of planned naps. *Annals of Emergency Medicine, 48*(5), 596–604.

Spradley, J. P. (1979). Spradley's theory of change. In L. A. Roussel & R. C. Swansburg (Eds.), *Management and leadership for nursing administrators* (5th ed.). Sudbury, MA: Jones and Bartlett.

Stacey, R., & Griffin, D. (Eds.). (2008). *Complexity and the experience of values, conflict and compromise in organizations.* New York, NY: Routledge.

Staggers, N., & Blaz, J. W. (2012). Research on nursing handoffs for medical and surgical settings: An integrative review. *Journal of Advanced Nursing, 69*(2), 246–262.

Stone, D. (2011). *Policy paradox: The art of political decision-making.* New York, NY: W.W. Norton & Company.

Stone, P. W., Mooney-Kane, C., Larson, E. L., Horan, T., Glance, L. G., Zwanziger, J., & Dick, A. (2007). Nurse working conditions and patient safety outcomes. *Medical Care, 45*(6); 571–578

Taylor, J. (2011). *Decision management systems.* Philadelphia, PA: IBM Press.

Tucker, P. (2010). Remaking education for a new century. *The Futurist, 44*(1), 22–25.

Tunis, S. (2007). Reflections on science, judgment, and value in evidence-based decision making: A conversation with David Eddy. *Health Affairs, 26*(4), 500–515.

Tushman, M. L., & Romanelli, E. (1985). Organizational evolution: A metamorphosis model of convergence and reorientation. In L. L. Cummings & B. M. Staw (Eds.), *Research in organizational behavior* (Vol. 7, pp. 171–222). Greenwich, CT: JAI Press.

U.S. Social Security Administration. (2012). *The history of Medicare.* Retrieved from http://www.ssa.gov/history/corning.html

Vaitheeswaran, V. (2007). An interview with Vijay Vaitheeswaran. *The Economist.* Retrieved from http://www.economist.com/ node/9934754

Vogelsmeier, A., Scott-Cawiezell, J., Miller, B., & Griffith, S. (2010). Influencing leadership perceptions of patient safety through just culture training. *Journal of Nursing Care Quality, 25*(4), 288–294.

Weberg, D. (2009). Innovation in healthcare: A concept analysis. *Nursing Administration Quarterly, 33*(3), 227–237.

Winowiecki, L., Smulder, S., Shirley, K., & Remans, R. (2011). Tools for enhancing interdisciplinary communication. *Sustainability: Science, Practice & Policy, 7*(1), 74–83.

NINE

Activating the Advocacy Plan

Jeanette Ives Erickson
Deborah Colton
Marianne Ditomassi

*There are those who look at things the way they are, and ask why ... I dream of things
that never were, and ask why not?—Robert Kennedy*

OBJECTIVES

1. Appraise different scenarios for activating an advocacy plan in clinical practice and the public policy arena.
2. Analyze collaborative strategies for effective advocacy in activating a plan.
3. Evaluate opportunities to develop and use influence when activating a policy plan.
4. Create opportunities for clinicians to share expertise with health policy leaders.
5. Develop steps of an action plan to impact policy processes and outcomes.

Activating a plan is a pivotal step in the policy process. Having a plan and giving careful thought to the phases of the plan, as well as the key stakeholders at each phase of the way, are integral to the success of the plan. The plan and the details, of necessity, will depend on the particular policy issue and the environment for bringing that policy issue forward in either the big "P" or little "p" arena. This chapter is designed to help you develop the knowledge and competencies necessary to successfully activate an advocacy plan. This chapter particularly builds upon the lessons learned about setting the agenda (see Chapter 6, "Setting the Agenda") and implementing the change process (see Chapter 8, "Changing Organizations, Institutions, and Government"). Activating a plan is an iterative process that often requires constant monitoring, shifting, and balancing in order to be responsive to changes that can derail or stall a plan. Involving others along the policy journey and detailed preparation are essential to maximizing success.

The phases of activating the advocacy plan both within organizations and within the public arena are natural extensions of nursing knowledge and skills. Be it in the development of new models of care delivery, influencing within an organization for resources, speaking to the media on an important issue to nurses, or testifying before an important committee, nurses have the skills and firsthand knowledge acquired from day-to-day practice to make a difference. The practical work and the need for activating an advocacy plan are illustrated by the challenges of running an emergency department (ED) in today's complex health care environment (see the following Policy Challenge).

POLICY CHALLENGE: Improving Patient Flow in the Emergency Department
Nancy Bonalumi, MSN, RN, CEN, FAEN, President, NMB Global Leadership, LLC, Past President, Emergency Nurses Association

We have all seen headlines like these about ED care:

"Crowded emergency department leads to deadly delay for patient."
"Overcrowding in the emergency department leads to long waits, increased costs."
"Patients admitted to the hospital on days when there is emergency department crowding are more likely to die."

ED overcrowding has a negative impact on patient outcomes, including but not limited to suffering due to inadequate pain management (Pines & Hollander, 2008), delay in administration of thrombolytics (Diercks et al., 2007), delay in antibiotic administration for patients with community-acquired pneumonia (Sikka, Mehta, Kaucky, & Kulstad, 2010), and increased mortality (Jo et al., 2014). ED crowding disproportionately affects racial and ethnic minority populations as indicated by more ambulance diversions in hospitals that serve large minority populations (Hsia et al., 2012).

Patients in the ED reflect a microcosm of the issues encountered in our health care system. Delays and untimely treatment not only influence patient satisfaction, but can also have profound influences on the quality of care and lead to a cascade of events that impedes the ability of the ED to move patients out of the ED either to a hospital unit or toward discharge. Bottlenecks created by systems stretched to the limits and poor communication between units contributes to problems in the delivery of care. Financial consequences include canceled or delayed procedures, patients leaving without being seen (LWBS), patient boarding, and patients needing more emergent care due to the delays. Consultations may be difficult to complete in a timely fashion because of interruptions to physicians' regular schedules. Admission processes are unnecessarily complex and duplicative. Despite designing policies to address these issues, if there is not adequate plan activation, old habits will persist and work-arounds will replace the new policies. Patients and family members will be dissatisfied, and staff members will continue to be disgruntled. Ultimately, these forces have a negative impact on the quality of care (Bernstein et al., 2009).

Since the 2006 publication of the Institute of Medicine's (IOM) 3-volume report, *The Future of Emergency Care in the United States Health System* (IOM, 2008), stakeholders in emergency care have been keeping patient flow in and out of the ED a high-profile concern for health care leaders. While few national- or state-level strategies have been implemented, health care systems have increased efforts to improve the movement of patients through the ED. Nursing has an important role to play in decreasing the adverse consequences of ED crowding and attention to improvements in care processes, backed by strong policies. Activating an advocacy plan is essential for achieving success in addressing the complexities of a problem such as ED overcrowding.

See Option for Policy Challenge.

We offer a practical approach for developing and implementing an advocacy plan for initiating policy changes. We examine environmental considerations, resource assessment, successful strategies for activation of the plan, rolling out the plan, unexpected turn of events, and how to sustain the plan.

ENVIRONMENT FOR ACTIVATING THE PLAN

The environment where your plan is activated can include the work environment of an organization like a hospital, an office, or a health department; external organizations or groups such as a professional association or consumer group; or a new environment, when a new structure or group is created. Each of these environments has unique features that can be harnessed in the implementation of the advocacy plan. These varying environments can be a critical driver for the success of such efforts and tailoring the plan to capitalize on the strengths of the environment is critical to success in influencing a particular course of action or policy. The role of the organizational structure for leadership and empowerment, and the environment outside of the structure of the organization, as well as a new structure that might be created are important factors in the success of an advocacy plan.

Organizational Environment

Leadership and empowerment are two key facilitators of the advocacy process (Richardson & Storr, 2010). Leadership is defined as the ability to influence others (Whitehead, Weiss, & Tappen, 2010) and engage them as partners in the development and achievement of shared visions (Redfern, 2008). Leadership plays a fundamental role in creating conditions to promote work engagement (Spence Laschinger & Leiter, 2006).

Empowerment is an interpersonal process whereby the correct information, support, resources, and environment exist, enabling the formulation of increased personal ability and effectiveness to set and achieve organizational goals (Hawks, 1992). In the context of patient care, this is translated as the extent to which nurses possess the power to influence those around them to deliver safe, effective care.

In many health care organizations, a collaborative governance structure is the umbrella for the decision-making process. "Collaborative governance is the decision-making process that places the authority, responsibility and accountability for patient care with the practicing clinician," and the goal of collaborative governance is to "facilitate communication and optimize staff participation in decision-making across disciplines" (Ives Erickson, Hamilton, Jones, & Ditomassi, 2003).

The impact of a collaborative governance structure on staff empowerment has been explored (Barden, Grifiin, Donahue, & Fitzpatrick, 2011; Bina et al., 2014; Brody, Barnes, Ruble, & Sakowski, 2012). In our study of staff across disciplines, participation in a collaborative governance committee resulted in significantly higher empowerment and fostered self-growth and organizational development (Ives Erickson et al., 2003). By engaging nurses in the work of the organizations, they further develop problem-solving skills to address patient care issues and implement important policy changes. Research examining Magnet hospital outcomes has demonstrated the value of creating empowering social structures that enhance nurses' abilities to take ownership and leadership for enhanced practice. The empirical evidence indicates that strong nursing leadership at all levels in the organization strengthens practice behaviors (Manojlovich, 2007).

Policy on the Scene 9.1 is an example of collaborative governance in action as staff nurses identified an opportunity to address a practice need. This staff nurse initiative illustrated the invaluable impact nurses can have on practice through advocacy. In this situation, nurses used research to close the gap between evidence and practice by raising awareness of the importance of sleep and rest and changing unit policies and practices in the process. The positive feedback from patients and their families gave the nurses a sense of satisfaction as well as affirmation that their interventions were meaningful. The success of a little "p" initiative engaged the staff in the policy process and provided them with the confidence that they could influence other practices through the policy process.

Outside the Organization: Professional Associations

Participation in professional and specialty associations is another way to use the resources in the environment to activate an advocacy plan. Professional

POLICY ON THE SCENE 9.1: Quiet Time for Mothers and Their Newborns, Massachusetts General Hospital
Boston, MA

Nurses on our clinical units recognized the need for quiet time on the clinical unit. We knew that the results of our patient satisfaction surveys indicated that noise and lack of rest were an issue.

The chief of sleep medicine at Massachusetts General Hospital (MGH) had published a study in the *Annals of Internal Medicine* finding that electronic sounds were the most likely sounds to disrupt sleep in healthy volunteers. Our staff nurses on our newborn-family unit championed efforts to create a quiet time on their unit. Quiet time is when staff members make a concerted effort to provide dedicated time and space on the unit for quiet along with minimizing interruptions. Quiet time is an hour or perhaps 2 hours when the lights are dimmed, doors are closed, and interruptions by nurses, doctors, and other staff members are minimized. Quiet time creates a calming effect on patients and respects the patients' need for rest and healing. We also installed a device that provides the staff with information about noise levels on our units. The "Yacker Tracker" flashes green, yellow, and red lights based on the decibel level. The staff placed signs on the unit and the patient room doors, "Quiet Time: Resting Is Healing." This practice change initiative has led to the development of policies about noise and use of quiet time on other units. A beautiful painting was created by their artist-in-residence with the phrase, *quiet, the children are healing*. In addition, MGH received positive publicity, in local and national media, for our efforts, boosting the nurses' confidence about initiating practice changes.

associations enable nurses to articulate values, integrity, practice recommendations and standards, and social policy, and to demonstrate advocacy and self-regulation (Matthews, 2012). The American Nurses Association (ANA) is the organization in the United States that gathers and coordinates ideas, convenes meetings from individuals and from the nursing specialties and associations, deliberates regarding these ideas, and develops the ideas. Because the ANA uses a deliberative and democratic process to develop its positions, nurses have the opportunity to provide input into the development of the profession's foundational policy documents, the *Code of Ethics for Nurses* (ANA, 2001), *Nursing's Social Policy Statement* (ANA, 2010b), and *Nursing: Scope and Standards of Practice* (ANA, 2010a) (see Chapter 2, "Advocating for Nurses and for Health") as well as position statements on issues of key importance to the profession. Not only does this organization provide a wealth of information to their members, the nursing community, and the public, but it also provides resources when activating a plan and opportunities to work together to activate a plan.

Some professional associations have limited resources for advocacy initiatives, but provide member services such as specialty-specific standards and education and/or an annual conference and membership meeting. Other associations dedicate resources to formulate position statements, develop formal policy agendas, engage their members in advocacy, and provide specific resources to enable its members to take action on specific issues. Larger associations may have staff members in various roles related to lobbying or government relations. These associations provide members with tool kits with actionable items to enable members to easily participate in the implementation of an advocacy plan. Examples of tool kits and resources for advocacy related to specific issues are listed in Exhibit 9.1. These tool kits include resources such as newsletters, sample letters to legislators, guidance in establishing teams to implement a particular advocacy strategy, and recommendations for policy implementation.

EXHIBIT 9.1 SPECIFIC-ISSUE ADVOCACY TOOL KITS

ORGANIZATION	SPECIFIC ISSUE	LINK
American Association of Critical-Care Nurses	Alarm Fatigue	http://www.aacn .org/dm/practice/ actionpakdetail .aspx?itemid= 28337&learn=true
American Nurses Association (ANA)	Advanced Practice Registered Nurse (APRN) Consensus Model	http://www.nursingworld .org/consensusmodel
Association of periOperative Nurses (AORN)	Patient Handoffs	http://www.aorn .org/Clinical_ Practice/ToolKits/ Safe_Patient_Handling/ Safe_Patient_Handling_ Tool_Kit.aspx
National Association of School Nurses (NASN)	Childhood Obesity	http://www.nasn .org/Continuing Education/Live ContinuingEducation Programs/SchoolNurse ChildhoodObesityToolkit
National Council of State Boards of Nursing (NCSBN)	APRN Consensus Model	https://www.ncsbn .org/4213.htm
Office for Victims of Crime, Office of Justice Programs, U.S. Department of Justice	Sexual Assault Response Team (SART) Tool Kit: Resources for Sexual Assault Response Teams	http://ovc.ncjrs.gov/ sartkit/about.html

(continued)

EXHIBIT 9.1 SPECIFIC-ISSUE ADVOCACY TOOL KITS (CONTINUED)		
ORGANIZATION	**SPECIFIC ISSUE**	**LINK**
United States Breastfeeding Committee	Exclusive Breast Milk Feeding	http://www.usbreastfeeding. org/HealthCare/ HospitalMaternityCenter Practices/ToolkitImplementing TJCCoreMeasure/ tabid/184/Default.aspx

Professional nurses associations unite individuals to create power and influence in the political arena. The Organization of Nurse Leaders (ONL) in Massachusetts includes over 700 nursing leaders who collectively employ, manage, and influence over 40,000 nurses and health care workers; their voice is powerful and has been heard. The ONL Government Affairs Committee has led numerous efforts to initiate policy agendas and to influence the passage of legislative bills while advocating on behalf of nurses and patients. Most recently, the ONL and the Massachusetts Department of Higher Education led an effort that resulted in awarding Massachusetts a $300,000 national grant from the Robert Wood Johnson Foundation (RWJF) to help current and future nurses seeking to advance their academic preparation within the nursing profession. While this is a small amount, it is a step toward garnering wider support for this initiative and the growing effort to move policy forward regarding baccalaureate preparation for 80% of the registered nurse workforce by 2020.

At the local level, health care organizations benefit from supporting nurse manager and staff nurse involvement in professional organizations. Nurses can develop leadership competencies, which in turn can be very productive for the organization. Involvement in organizations, boards, and other key groups is also a strategy to influence their direction and participate in activating numerous advocacy plans to address issues pertinent to the mission (see Chapter 6). A nurse's advocacy journey through involvement in professional organizations is illustrated in Policy on the Scene 9.2.

Creating New Environmental Structures

New structures, like coalitions, may be created for an advocacy plan when there is a specialized need to bring representatives from diverse constituencies. While we generally think of coalitions as groups of organizations, coalitions may also consist of representatives of diverse organizations, but the organizations themselves might not be a formal member of the coalition (see coalitions in Chapter 6).

An example of a new environmental structure is the development of coalitions across the states as illustrated by the Center to Champion Nursing in America (CCNA), an initiative that is supported by AARP, the AARP Foundation, and the RWJF. The goal is to ensure all Americans have access to

POLICY ON THE SCENE 9.2: An Advocacy Journey
Gino Chisari, DNP, RN, Director, Norman Knight Center for Clinical and Professional Development, Massachusetts General Hospital, Boston, MA

I began working at my current organization almost three decades ago. My goal was to complete the licensed practical nurse program. Little could I have imagined that all these years later, I would be a DNP graduate of the school affiliated with our hospital. I often think to myself, "what a journey this has been!"

None of us achieves this success alone. If we are lucky, we have many people who encourage, support, champion, mentor, guide, and coach us along the way. This began for me with a wonderful faculty member who became a role model for all of the things I aspired to be as a nurse. I was supported by my organization to earn an associate's degree in nursing, to enroll in a baccalaureate nursing program, and to obtain a master's degree. Upon completion of my master's degree, I soon became aware of the value of membership in professional organizations. It was suddenly in my DNA! My first membership, as a new faculty member, was with the Massachusetts/Rhode Island League for Nursing. I was encouraged to "stretch myself" by actively participating.

My roles also evolved over time as well, including those of clinical nurse specialist and clinical educator. I was appointed to the Board of Registration in Nursing (BORN). I now appreciate how important the voice of a nurse is when deciding on policy matters affecting both patients and nurses. I left my hospital position to become the BORN nursing practice coordinator. My chief nurse appreciated the unique experience this role would provide by counseling, "If you don't go, you won't know when it's time to come back."

When my BORN tenure ended, I had the opportunity to return to my current health care organization. It remained important to me both personally and professionally to continue promoting a loud, strong voice for nurses across the state and to remain involved with professional activities focused on moving nursing's agenda forward in the state. With support and mentorship, I joined the ONL–Massachusetts/Rhode Island and began serving on a committee. I am currently the cochair of the Nurse of the Future Nursing Core Competencies Committee, a role that places me in a wonderful position to champion nursing in Massachusetts.

I am also a member of the Massachusetts Association of Registered Nurses (MARN), and its Health Policy Committee. My work with MARN, ONL, and BORN resulted in my election as MARN president. This role provided me with a seat on the statewide steering committee for the Massachusetts Action Coalition. When I think of my humble beginnings in nursing 29 years earlier, I appreciate the support, mentorship, and guidance that resulted in my successful nursing career today.

high-quality care, with nurses contributing to the full extent of their capabilities. Another goal is to ensure that 80% of registered nurses (RNs) have a bachelor's degree by 2020.

While the structure is formalized on the national level, the futures of nursing initiatives are being implemented through state and local coalitions. Each of these groups has a different internal structure and operating principles. Some state coalitions have made significant progress and others are just beginning their work. The CCNA website provides details about state activities as well as resources for coalition members. The Nebraska State Coalition has made significant progress publishing guidance on the use of models to guide the development of partnerships and coalition building as well as a framework for data collection and analysis to identify challenges and opportunities (Cramer, Lazure, Morris, Valerio, & Morris, 2013). In addition, CCNA provides resources and tools for members of state and regional action coalitions.

The Massachusetts Action Coalition is focused on the goal of ensuring that 80% of registered nurses achieve a baccalaureate degree by 2020. The strategy for achieving this goal includes evaluating academic curricula in order to identify programs and resources and develop scholarships for all nurses to advance their education.

Nurses, other health care professionals, and consumer groups may form temporary or informal coalitions or groups to advance an issue. A council or ad hoc task force might be formed, which bands together to address a specialized issue. An example might be a parent–teacher–nurse group to support healthy food choices in a school cafeteria. Another example is the Environmental Health Committee of the Pennsylvania State Nurses Association, which was formed to advocate for healthy environments for patients and their families.

ASSESSING RESOURCES

The degree of sophistication that can be achieved with an advocacy plan will depend on the resources and support available for implementation. Regardless of the environment for the implementation of an advocacy action plan, whether it be a health care association, a professional association, or an informal group, it is necessary to assess resources and identify those resources that are available or could be available as well as those resources that will need to be acquired in order to implement the plan. The assessment of resources includes people or manpower, data, finances, and communication capabilities.

People and Manpower

The assessment of people resources and the sheer manpower to implement the advocacy plan includes examining the expertise of volunteers, staff members of organizations, and individuals who could potentially contribute to the cause.

Volunteer expertise includes determining who is interested in the issue and potential sources of volunteers. For example, a state may have several nurse practitioner groups, based either on region or on specialization, as well as a state-wide organization. When an issue involves prescriptive privileges, individuals from all of these groups, as well as members of the state nurses association, may wish to take part in an initiative. Other advanced practice nurses may wish to join because advancing a cause for one advanced practice group will help all advanced practice groups in terms of political capital (see Chapter 7, "Building Capital: Intellectual, Social, Political, and Financial"). The ANA has the Nurses Strategic Action Team (N-STAT), which notifies nurse activists of pending issues and votes so that they can contact their legislators in a timely and strategic manner.

Included in assessing volunteer expertise is ensuring individuals understand the dynamics of the policy issue being advanced for the action plan. For example, if an association or professional group wants to take on the responsibility of being more systematic in evaluating proposed legislation to determine whether the group supports, opposes, or has no position on it, then the members need to have training and guidelines for making a decision or making a recommendation for a board that ultimately makes the decision. To facilitate the process, the group might create talking points or a background document for the issue. A group or association might organize regional town halls to raise awareness of an issue, or someone may need to research previous positions of the group in order to provide a historical perspective of the group's position on the issue and how changes in the issue and policy proposals have evolved over time. The strategies that are used to assess volunteer expertise depend on the information that is available to an organization, which might include a member database or speaker's bureau or some other systematic way of gathering information. Larger organizations will have the capacity to conduct member surveys or obtain systematic feedback on an issue. Smaller groups, of necessity, will use more informal means such as networking, e-mail, or media outlets such as Facebook or Twitter to obtain information. It is important that the volunteer activities are a match with the organization's mission as well as the volunteer's interests.

Manpower resources also include staff members of health care organizations or associations. Staff members may include nurses who have direct experience with the issue or ancillary staff such as secretaries or administrative assistants who can be released to devote time to an issue. If a health care organization wants to have staff nurses with direct patient care responsibilities involved in an issue, then consideration needs to be given to protected time for such activities. For example, advancing a policy issue might be a component of a clinical nurse specialist's regular job duties, but obtaining staff input, particularly on a substantive level, requires provision of time for the activities. Things to consider in using staff members are determining the kind of work that is needed, the tasks that could be accomplished by different staff members, whether the need is ongoing or on a temporary basis, and whether any tasks could be grouped together (New York City, n.d.).

Consideration should be given to marshaling the forces of additional volunteers who are willing or have capacity to support the activation of a plan. This might include family members who have connections to media outlets, students, family members of volunteers with computer or webpage skills, or people who might be willing to provide short-term service for the plan. Individuals who teach at universities and colleges may be able to provide introductions to faculty members who place students in internships or externships in fields such as communications, computer science, business, or media. Universities and colleges may have volunteer offices that serve as a clearinghouse for students desirous of being involved in community service.

Data Resources

Data are important in any policy endeavor. Data may take the form of findings from research, evidence-based projects, or quality improvement processes in providing the foundation for a policy position (see Chapter 5, "Harnessing Evidence in the Policy Process") or details or background information that can support the plan. Data sources can include research on priorities, demographic characteristics, and other details in support of an issue. For example, the National Sample Survey of Registered Nurses (NSSRN) provided demographic data for RNs every 4 years from 1980 to 2008. This was supplemented in many states with the establishment of nursing or health care workforce centers. Some states are working with state agencies charged with licensure renewals to incorporate key questions that will assist with obtaining workforce data; this data is useful in evaluating the effectiveness of strategies to implement *The Future of Nursing* recommendations (IOM, 2011). Nurses will need to examine other sources of key national data for workforce planning (Auerbach, Staiger, Muench, & Buerhaus, 2012).

Data may not only include characteristics about nurses, but also information about the impact of an issue, or the number of people affected. Ensuring that one has the right data and the latest data can facilitate the development of information and other support materials in activating the advocacy plan. For example, a hospital may examine its own pressure ulcer rate in comparison with national benchmark data from the National Database of Nursing's Quality Indicators® (NDNQI), or its own workers compensation cases for nurses with back injuries to make the case for purchasing ceiling lift equipment. See also environmental scanning in Chapter 4, "Identifying a Policy Issue."

Economic Resources

Economic resources require a realistic appraisal of what will be needed to implement the advocacy plan. This will include supplies, materials, and personnel time, both paid and unpaid. Organizations typically budget financial resources to implement advocacy programming and, at times when additional resources are needed, will divert resources from other priorities or seek external funds. Health care organizations may have resources to finance a policy initiative. Some organizations, such as a professional association or a nonprofit organization, may not have significant financial assets. However, they may be able to obtain financial assistance through community organizations designed to assist nonprofits with their business processes or join a coalition that will have greater combined resources. While large foundations such as the RWJF or the Kellogg Foundation may fund major initiatives, smaller foundations may be a resource for policy initiatives or pilot projects that have policy implications in their own communities. Local affiliates of national organizations (e.g., March of Dimes, Susan G. Komen for the Cure, and American Heart Association) and hospital foundation or auxiliaries are some resources to consider.

A relatively new strategy for obtaining resources is crowd-sourcing. Crowd-sourcing is derived from "outsourcing to the crowd" whereby solicitations are taken to a larger group outside a formal structure:

> ... A type of participative online activity in which an individual, an institution, a nonprofit organization, or company proposes to a group of individuals of varying knowledge, heterogeneity, and number, via flexible open call, the voluntary undertaking of a task. (Estellés-Arolas & González-Ladrón-de-Guevara, 2012)

While crowd-sourcing involves asking people for ideas and help in solving problems, it can include soliciting for donations (Brabham, 2008). Crowd-funding or crowd-sourced fundraising refers specifically to soliciting for donations for a specific project. Examples include Give Forward, GoFundMe, Indiegogo, Kickstarter, and Weeve. Kickstarter funds creative projects. For example, the Air Quality Egg, funded through Kickstarter, involves the use of a sensing network that allows anyone to collect air-quality data related to urban air pollution (Kickstarter, n.d.). This has the potential to create a network of advocates interested in addressing the problems associated with air pollution in communities around the world. The Global Partners in Care, an organization for funding global hospice and palliative care partnerships uses crowd-funding to fund pain relief efforts. (Global Partners in Care, n.d.) While crowd-funding is a relatively new phenomenon, its potential for financial support of advocacy for health policy is largely untapped.

Communication Resources

Communication is essential throughout plan activation. The goal is to mobilize staff, members of organizations, and the public in order to implement all phases of the activation step. Communications include the management of internal and external relationships, as well as messaging. In addition, free or inexpensive resources can be investigated such as community bulletin boards, radio or television talk shows, mail list servers, and public service announcements (see Chapter 10, "Working With the Media: Shaping the Health Policy Process").

A town hall or well-publicized event can also be used to communicate important messages about a policy issue. Town halls are open forums that are an opportunity to provide information about an issue to the community while allowing for dialogue with key stakeholders.

The degree of formality of a town hall will depend on the overall goal and how the town hall is being used to advance a particular policy. Often, the forum is a panel discussion followed by questions from the audience. With advertising savvy, a town hall or workplace forum draws additional supporters who are interested in and supportive of your positions or proposed policy.

Readiness Assessment

The assessment of readiness for activating the plan includes a number of components that will help to determine the capacity of the group to take action. Understanding the organization or group's knowledge, skills, and resources is essential for activating the plan, whether it is a little "p" bedside policy change or a big "P" policy that involves proposing legislation. The Alliance for Justice has developed resources for advocacy, including an Advocacy Capacity Tool (Bolder Advocacy, n.d.). The organization focuses on using its expertise on equity in the federal judiciary, but provides resources for advocacy capacity assessment as well as understanding the laws and regulations impacting the advocacy work of nonprofit organizations at the local community, national, and international levels. The assessment of readiness includes ongoing activities to ensure that you have the latest intelligence on the issue and to create a mechanism for ongoing environmental scanning.

Understanding the available resources, the needed resources, and assessing readiness can be used to empower and support individuals involved in activating the advocacy plan.

STRATEGIES FOR ACTIVATING THE PLAN

An advocacy plan can take many forms, depending on the desired goals, whether it is a public policy goal or the achievement of a policy change within an organization. However, common to all plans are goal refinement, applying influence, strategic issue framing, and audience targeting of your message for an audience. In each of these endeavors, it is important that nurses are strategic in activating the plan. Nurses advocating for a policy are going to need to make decisions related to who, what, when, and where in order to make the best use of strategy to move an issue forward. Exhibit 9.2 compares and contrasts strategic and nonstrategic methods to advancing an issue.

Goal Refinement

Goal refinement is an ongoing process. It involves specifying the "what" as illustrated in Exhibit 9.2. While the initial problem identification and

EXHIBIT 9.2 COMPARISON OF APPROACHES FOR ADVANCING AN ISSUE

	STRATEGIC	NONSTRATEGIC
Who	Taking it to a shared governance nursing council, or nurse manager	Complaining to the chief surgeon or chief of medicine
What	Targeted issue focused on a doable solution or discrete problem	Huge laundry list of all the ills associated with the problem
When	When related reports indicate the issue is a problem that when solved could improve outcomes or when a precipitating event occurs	Same time as when a major change initiative such as an electronic medical record is introduced, or 3 months after national publicity on a topic
Where	Privately, or in a small group	In front of other staff members, or the person's supervisor

agenda setting might be a more laborious and intense process, it is essential to continue to modify and refine advocacy goals. You need to determine what it is you want to change and the extent of the change that is possible within the context of the environment for the particular policy goal. For example, during the White House discussions that took place in 2009 regarding health care reform, it was apparent that both the expansion opportunities for advanced practice nurses, such as demonstration projects with the nurse-managed health centers and school-based health centers, and addressing inequities in reimbursement for nurse practitioners could not be accomplished in a single piece of legislation (R. M. Patton, personal communication, September 8, 2013). Hence, efforts were focused on expanding opportunities for advance practice nurses' recognition and role in a reformed health care delivery system.

While there may be uncertainty with regard to the effectiveness of a plan, at some point you will need to make the decision to move forward. You will need to refine the plan as you move along as new information becomes available and the circumstances change. Regardless, activating the plan should be based upon the best available evidence, and consideration needs to be given to the fact that you may need to change course and revise strategies and/or goals. Barkhorn, Huttner, and Blau (2013) developed a framework for the assessment of an advocacy plan that includes conditions for a successful policy campaign. Exhibit 9.3 illustrates how this framework can be used in the assessment of the conditions for an advocacy plan for the implementation of a safe patient handling and mobility campaign.

The assessment of the safe patient handling and mobility campaign indicates that there are a number of conditions that are favorable for the activation of the advocacy campaign that can be used to marshal the forces to move the initiative forward.

EXHIBIT 9.3   ADVOCACY ASSESSMENT FRAMEWORK FOR A SUCCESSFUL POLICY CAMPAIGN

FRAMEWORK CONDITIONS	APPLICATION TO SAFE PATIENT HANDLING AND MOBILITY
1. Functioning venue(s) for adoption: The relevant legislative, legal, and regulatory institutions are functioning sufficiently for advocacy to be effective	Stimulated by American Nurses Association's (ANA) work, Handle With Care Campaign in 2003 (ANA, 2013a), 11 states have passed some form of laws or developed rules/regulations in the years between 2003 and 2011. See http://www.nursingworld.org/ MainMenuCategories/Policy-Advocacy/ State/LegislativeAgenda-Reports/State SafePatientHandling
2. Open policy window: External events or trends spur demand for the solution	Years of research indicates nurses are at high risk for injury due to handling patients and the trend over decades has not changed. A 2011 survey of RNs indicates that 80% report working despite experiencing frequent musculoskeletal pain (ANA, 2013b)
3. Feasible solution: A feasible solution has been developed and shown to produce the intended benefits	12th Annual Safe Patient Handling East Coast Conference in Orlando in 2012 determined the need of a framework for universal standards
4. Dynamic master plan: A pragmatic and flexible advocacy strategy and communications plan is ready for execution	A work group was convened in June 2012 hosted by the ANA Department for Health, Safety and Wellness. Subsequently, drafts of standards, definitions, and language were developed. Resulted in a publication titled *Safe Patient Handling and Mobility: Interprofessional National Standards* (http://nursingworld. org/DocumentVault/Occupational Environment/SPHM-Standards-Resources/ Sample-of-the-SPHM-book.pdf)
5. Strong campaign leader(s): Central advocates can assemble and lead the resources to execute the strategy and communications plan	Members of the work group included care providers and administrators; professional association members and staff; experts in the field (consultants); and representatives from several major U.S. federal agencies (e.g., U.S. Department of Veterans Affairs)
6. Influential support coalition: Allies can sway needed decision makers and help the campaign leader to pursue the solution	A coalition was formed at the national level: the Coalition for Healthcare Worker and Patient Safety (CHAPS). An example of a statewide coalition is the Oregon Coalition for HealthCare Ergonomics (OCHE)

(continued)

EXHIBIT 9.3	ADVOCACY ASSESSMENT FRAMEWORK FOR A SUCCESSFUL POLICY CAMPAIGN *(CONTINUED)*	
7. Mobilized public: Relevant public audiences actively support the solution and its underlying social principles		The ANA has taken the lead in activating the advocacy plan including press releases and public vetting of the final draft of the proposed safe patient handling and mobility standards
8. Powerful inside champions: Decision makers who can overcome the opposition support the solution and its underlying principles		Key champions include the ANA, International Organization for Standardization, The Joint Commission, National Institute of Occupational Safety and Health, Occupational Safety and Health Administration, Department of Defense, Department of Veterans Affairs, Association of Occupational Health Professionals
9. Clear implementation path: The implementing institution has the commitment and the ability to execute the solution		Federal legislation was introduced; the *Nurse and Health Care Worker Protection Act* of 2013 (HR 2480)

Adapted from Barkhorn et al. (2013).

Applying Influence

The nursing profession has outstanding leaders (see the ANA American Hall of Fame). This distinguished tradition continues today with many individuals taking on a leadership role in their work setting, in the larger community, and in society (see Chapter 12, "Serving the Public Through Policy and Leadership"). Nurses who have become active policy advocates and who have significant accomplishments in improving health care have learned to recognize that they can effectively influence policy development and implementation.

Being a leader involves using influence in order to achieve goals. Influence is the ability of an individual to sway or affect another person or group (Adams & Ives Erickson, 2011). The development of advocacy skills can be enhanced with the development of leadership and an understanding of the process of influence. The Adams Influence Model (AIM) provides a framework for understanding how various factors, attributes, and processes support nurses to influence and impact individuals and/or groups (Adams, 2009). The AIM serves not only as a guide for nursing practice, education, policy, research, and theory, but is also a framework that can be used for the development of a focused organizational effort for activating the plan. By applying the factors and attributes of the AIM, nurses can develop and influence strategies and become health care advocates in the political arena.

The AIM highlights the relationship between two parties. The first party is the influence agent, for example, the nurse with knowledge and skill of health care that seeks to influence a decision. The second party is the influence target: likely the policy maker (including legislators, staff, or other political leaders or groups) who is the focus of the effort and has a role in setting the ultimate policy. The AIM, in Figure 9.1, illustrates the relationship between the nurse (influence agent) and the policy maker(s) (target of influence). The influence process begins at the center with the influence agent who knows or perceives to know the target and chooses influence tactics based on the issue, the situation, and his or her perceptions of the target; the influence target has perceptions of the influence agent informed in part by the tactics chosen and then provides feedback. Either influence is achieved or the influence agent can choose to begin the process again. The three outer rings demonstrate the importance of personal (ability to influence personal knowledge of policy), interpersonal

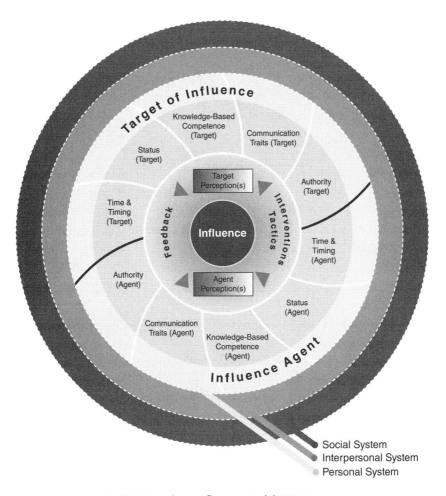

FIGURE 9.1 Adams Influence Model (AIM).
Reprinted with permission from Adams (2009).

EXHIBIT 9.4 AIM INFLUENCE FACTORS AND ATTRIBUTES

FACTOR	ASSOCIATED INFLUENCE ATTRIBUTES	ALIGNED NURSE ATTRIBUTES FOR INFLUENCING POLICY
Authority	Access to resources Accountability Responsibility	Extended education Understanding of patient experience Accountability for care delivery
Communication Traits	Confidence Emotional involvement Message articulation Persistence Physical appeal environment Physical appeal self Presence	Experience in communication in challenging situations involving patients and their families
Knowledge-Based Competence	Aesthetic knowledge Empirical knowledge Ethical knowledge Personal knowledge Sociopolitical knowledge	Empirical knowledge (science, nursing) Personal experience Capacity to envision needed improvements Commitment to ethical and moral judgment Understand role of socioeconomic status in access to health care
Status	Hierarchical position Informal position Key supportive relationships Reputation	Highly respected and trusted Expertise in relationship building
Time and Timing	Amount of time to sell an issue Timing to deliver the issue	Experience in selecting actions based upon competing priorities

(prior interactions between influencer and target), and social (organizational culture) systems.

Both the agent and the target possess the same influence factors and attributes although these may be titrated in different amounts for the agent and target depending on the issue. As Exhibit 9.4 illustrates, five factors are in play in any effort to influence policy: (a) authority, (b) communication traits, (c) knowledge-based competence, (d) status, and (e) use of time and timing. By considering these elements, nurses can develop a well-organized plan for working in and activating a plan to implement a policy. It amounts to finding the right spokesperson with the appropriate knowledge and authority, who communicates clearly, consistently, and effectively at the right moment(s) in time. Very often nurses don't believe that they have the power to use influence. However, Exhibit 9.4 illustrates how nurses' attributes are aligned with attributes for using influence. Because of this alignment, nurses are in an ideal position to use influence in policy development and to be quite successful at it. Ultimately, it is the entire social system and the organizational culture that needs to be considered in developing strategies to influence policy direction.

Activating the plan involves preparing nurses to use influence and engage in the policy process. We posit that nurses can use the same skills of developing leadership and influence to master the political world of their workplace and adapt them for context in mastering the political world in communities, states, and even at the national and international levels. See Policy on the Scene 9.3 for a staff nurse's description of how becoming involved in issues related to pain management at work was transferred to influencing the political world in her area of specialization. Developing the competencies to activate the policy plan will facilitate the development of personal efficacy. Careful planning can increase the likelihood for success in assuming the advocacy role and help nurses contribute to the delivery reforms that will take place in our lifetimes. Health care organizations and professional associations play important roles in facilitating the leadership development to influence the policy process.

Strategic Framing of the Issue

Success in implementing health policy is contingent upon the development and activation of a plan that is specifically targeted using proven strategies tailored for the particular action needed. Some of these strategies may be the culmination of years of efforts to achieve the desired change. For example, efforts to reduce tobacco use include (a) policies and funds to promote education about the hazards of smoking in schools, (b) workplace smoking cessation programs, and (c) smoke-free environments. Each of these requires the support of different constituencies and different strategies tailored to achieve the policy action. However, commonalities among strategies can be used in short- and long-term efforts to achieve policy goals. Framing the issue is an important step that takes advantage of the needs and desires of various stakeholders and/or constituencies impacted by the advocacy plan.

Once you have identified goals, the ideal path to solutions, and the potential opposition, it is time to frame your issue in a way that provides the greatest likelihood of advancing your targeted policy agenda and attaining your goals. As indicated with the AIM, knowledge of the issue, situation, and perceptions of the target determines the strategies that are used in framing the issue. The policy issue should be framed within the context of existing policy agendas whenever possible. Framing the issue is not just for legislative audiences. Regulators, executive agency staff, judges, potential jurors, executives, and the public are not only listening to the problems and solutions on policy makers' agendas, many may have their own policy agendas, or they might be more receptive to the agendas of others, depending on how they understand the problems as described.

POLICY ON THE SCENE 9.3: Influencing Policy Development
Gayle Peterson, RN-BC, Staff Nurse
Massachusetts General Hospital, Boston, MA

As a staff nurse on a hematology/oncology unit, I have a personal and professional interest in patients' rights, pain management, and ethics in health care. It is necessary to advocate for people who may not have a voice, especially in the area of adequate pain medication. Because of this, I serve as a human rights commissioner for my city and have participated in work regarding the Clean Air Act in my state.

Twelve years ago, this interest led me to become a member of the American Society for Pain Management Nursing. I became active in the organization and eventually became president of the Massachusetts chapter. When the American Nurses Credentialing Center offered certification as a pain management nurse, I became certified. I joined the Massachusetts Pain Initiative, was a member of their legislative committee, and eventually became a board member. I was very interested in a bill requiring physicians and other primary care providers to receive pain management education. I also spoke directly with senators about a legislative proposal to ban the use of oxycodone, an effective pain medication for cancer patients that does not cause drowsiness. My clinical interest emerged into something much bigger. Competent in pain management, I was concerned about trends, not only in the local practice environment, but also in the broader community. This knowledge and concern led to my participation in advocacy groups. My direct knowledge of care delivery and the impact on patients' well-being were core to our success.

Later I learned that my professional nursing organization, ANA Massachusetts, the ANA state affiliate, had a Health Policy Committee and I joined those organizations as well. My nursing director was instrumental in my participation in these organizations, encouraging my work and allowing me scheduled time off and/or paid time off to attend meetings and to go to the State House when important legislative activities occurred. I was also supported to attend the Nurse in Washington Internship (NIWI). The internship made me more aware of the policy issues of concern to nursing.

Over the past few years, I have become active in the ANA. I was elected to the House of Delegates for three terms and became a member of the Congress on Nursing Practice. More recently, I was a Policy Institute fellow and member of the work group that revised the ANA *Principles for Delegation*. Going forward, I have been named to the task force that will revise the *Code of Ethics for Nurses* and serve on the ANA board. In these roles, I have personally grown and have contributed. The investment of time has positively influenced who I am and has enhanced my clinical practice.

How we construe the problem is "linked to the existing social, political and ideological structures at the time" (Birkland, 2011, p. 71). Not only must advocates remain mindful of the prominent and broader issues already on the "agenda," such as the White House's attention in 2012 to the economy, health care, education, energy, and the environment, but advocates must frame their issue to maximize the likelihood that the issue will be important to stakeholders and within the context of their values in order to motivate people to action. For example, Americans have generally and historically valued individualism, freedom, and free enterprise over socialism and, some would say, even community.

Nurses seeking to define an issue that requires public attention should not only highlight how their solution advances patient safety, improves access to care, and/or achieves cost efficiencies in delivering health care, but might also take heed of how the traditional American values may or may not be consistent with your group's proposed solution. For example, given recent political changes in traditionally strong labor states such as Wisconsin, Michigan, and Ohio, a proposal for staffing legislation might resonate with legislators and the public if it is framed from a patient safety perspective rather than as a labor issue. Influencing which committee receives a bill or a policy proposal might be important in determining whether it ever gets out of committee or sees a vote.

Framing an issue is an ongoing process. While consistency in messaging is needed, one needs to be mindful of the changing context for a particular issue. A recent study determined that the environmental consequences of climate change may not have as much of an impact as a message about the public health consequences of climate change; that message is more likely to result in an emotional reaction that is supportive to mitigating the effects of climate change (Myers, Nisbet, Maibach, & Leiserowitz, 2012). So, while we use research to make the case for a particular policy action, we can use research to help inform the strategies that are important to key policy makers. Framing an issue involves focusing on a specific aspect of an issue to emphasize a particular dimension. For example, *The Future of Nursing* report (IOM, 2011) recommends that nurses should practice at the full extent of their education and training. This message is designed to specifically counteract opposition to removing barriers for advanced practice registered nurses (APRNs) and fears that they are unprepared for their responsibilities. While traditional efforts have focused on the legislative arena, nurse practitioners are expanding their efforts to lobby the administration to require the inclusion of nurse practitioners in health insurance exchanges (Appleby, 2013). See Exhibit 9.5 for examples of how an issue can be framed.

Defining policy solutions and framing within an existing issue agenda strengthens the priority given to an issue within a given political context. Given the political climate in anticipation of implementation of the Patient Protection and Affordable Care Act's (PPACA) provisions, policy solutions designed to improve patient safety, access to care, and cost-effectiveness are likely to be better received than initiatives that do not address any of these goals. Legislators

EXHIBIT 9.5 FRAMING AN ISSUE

BROAD TOPIC	IMPACT ON HEALTH	STRATEGIC FRAMING
Climate change	Health consequences of global warming	Weather-related disasters, emerging infectious diseases
APRN scope of practice and full practice authority	Access to care	Uninsured in a local community, antitrust issues impacting APRNs; removal of collaborative agreements, provider neutral language
Nurse shortage	Reduced musculoskeletal injuries	Cost of workmen's compensation
School nurse–pupil ratios	Healthy children, reduced teen pregnancies	Higher educational attainment of school children
"Nurse" title protection	Preventing the public's confusion about the qualifications of nurses	Protecting the public from unsafe practitioners
Certified registered nurse anesthetists (CRNAs) as sole providers	Access to obstetrical, surgical, interventional diagnostic, trauma stabilization, and pain services	Closure of rural hospitals

and executive branch officials are wary of historical "turf war" bills advanced by various professional groups.

While framing is designed to have issues resonate with key policy makers, it is necessary to ensure that members of the team advancing a policy agenda are prepared with key facts. This is frequently accomplished with the creation of talking points to provide easily remembered and succinct information about the proposed policy change. Talking points may be done on an informal basis when preparing for a meeting or they may be more formal as when preparing nurses to visit legislators on Capitol Hill. Organizations and associations may prepare talking points that are for general distribution to the public and legislators, with more detailed backgrounders so that the individual nurses speaking to the issue can quickly learn the salient facts and answer potential questions (see Chapter 10).

Targeting an Audience

Identifying the best audience for a policy issue goes hand in hand with framing an issue and is the "who" of being strategic. While framing an issue is designed to make the policy goal resonate with the audience, targeting the audience is a careful and strategic analysis of the key decision makers and those who are in a position to influence the key decision makers. Thus, targeting the audience involves strategizing to frame an issue for a particular constituency in a way that motivates decision makers to take action. In a hospital setting, it might be a chairperson of a committee, a particular department head, or a board member. In the regulatory arena, it might be an administrator of an agency. In Congress, a state legislature, or city council, it might be the chairperson of a committee for a bill. In the community, the target audience might be members of key agencies or community boards.

Framing an issue for a group of legislators may be different from framing an issue for school board members. Legislators collectively may have different demographic characteristics than their constituents. In a study of state legislators' priorities, the top-rated factor in determining health issues of importance was constituents' needs followed by evidence of scientific effectiveness (Dodson et al., 2013). In this particular sample, 63% of the state legislators were aged 55 years and older, and 76% were male. Thus, activating a policy plan should include considerations for targeting decision makers, the nurse community, and the general public for support for the desired policy.

Nurses seeking policy changes locally or within their health care organizations also need to be mindful of the ideologies and biases of the decision makers. Kingdon's (2011) research indicates that policy solutions must be "acceptable in the light of the values held by members of the policy community" (p. 143). When selling the need for a new policy designed to improve patient safety to the chief financial officer of a health care facility, nurse leaders will need to speak to the financial bottom line that can be realized from the new policy (e.g., reduced readmissions [which are not paid for by Medicare] and fewer costly medication errors). When seeking adoption of the policy by staff, nurse leaders will need to frame the policy as advantageous to the staff (as well as the patients). For example, a new hand-washing policy needs to include support from leadership, facility-wide campaign, staff traffic patterns, availability of sinks for hand washing, education for multidisciplinary teams, and patients so it will more likely be implemented by members of the team.

Targeting an audience involves learning about its characteristics as well as being strategic about the location and timing for a presentation. This information can be obtained through direct interaction such as when making visits to a legislator's office, and consultation with colleagues and policy makers. Examination of websites and other publicly available information about the decision maker provides information about positions and values. For example, a legislator's website can provide information about legislative committee memberships and expertise. Other sites can provide information on specific votes cast for certain bills. Very often, legislators will have had contact with health professionals and nurses through their own illnesses or experiences with family members. This information can be used to develop messages that take advantage of these important details. The when and where of targeting an audience will depend on the current milieu for the issue and other issues on policy makers' agendas. For example, something seemingly simple might be the placement of an issue on an agenda for a meeting, whether it is part of another agenda item, or it stands alone. Location factors might include whether members of an audience are on their home turf, or whether a meeting is public or private.

ROLLING OUT THE PLAN

Once the details of the plan have been developed, it is time to roll out the plan, take the story on the road, and publicize the issue in the appropriate venue. These actions include using activities that might be very commonplace and seemingly simple such as creating narratives, providing leadership through chairing meetings, and building relationships with key decision makers. With each step, a number of anticipated or unanticipated barriers need to be overcome.

Creating Narratives

Any advocacy plan includes enhancing the visibility of an issue. Nurses can bring their real-world experiences to bear in the discussions through the creation of narratives. While media strategies are critically important (see Chapter 10), nurses need to be adept at developing narratives that make issues real and understandable across a spectrum of audiences. Encouraging nurses to share their stories about their clinical practice and their impact are an effective means of empowering nurses to become advocates for their patients and for the profession.

A clinical narrative is a first-person story that describes a specific situation and includes the "thoughts, intentions, interpretation of events, chronology and outcomes" (Benner, 1984). Narratives help us understand practice through reflection, by making it visible, by uncovering hidden aspects of the practice, and by sharing with the larger community clinical knowledge, caring practices, and the complex environment in which we practice. In health care organizations, narratives can be used to strengthen nurses' abilities to voice their concerns and to speak up about extraordinary situations. They are used to make the case for a policy initiative by serving to inform and influence colleagues, members of other disciplines, management, board members, and the public. As it happens, the way in which a nurse communicates through a narrative is also an extremely effective way to communicate in the policy arena—by telling an important first-person story, in a clear and concise way that the uninitiated can easily understand. Narratives can be used external to a health organization, as when talking with a reporter, visiting a legislator, or framing testimony for a legislative hearing. We are increasingly seeing the use of narratives in books about clinical practice in nursing, medicine, and other health care disciplines. The prestigious health policy journal, *Health Affairs*, has a long-running column, "Narrative Matters," designed to capture the stories of patients, families, and their caregivers (Iglehart, 1999). Nurses have shared their narratives in this column (Swan, 2012). Characteristics of situations that make good clinical narratives that may be included in advocacy plans are listed in Exhibit 9.6. These characteristics, derived from the work of Benner and her colleagues (2011) in selecting narratives, can be used to select compelling narratives for policy makers.

As you write the narrative, provide background for the reader; this can include time of day, the setting where it took place, and what was occurring. Focus on what you were thinking, using "I" rather than "we." The narrative gives the reader insight into the practice and it also provides the opportunity to *reflect* on practice—what the nurse did and why. The story that is told is the right one for that person at that time (see Theresa Brown's suggestions for blogging in Chapter 10).

For many nurses, the idea of writing a narrative is paralyzing. They worry that their story is not enough: It is not extraordinary enough, it is not long enough, and it is not perfect. Nurse leaders can create an environment that is nonjudgmental, that values and respects practice at all levels, and that offers encouragement and support as nurses share their narrative. As one chief nurse officer (CNO) writes in the Policy on the Scene 9.4, encouragement and support for the voice of nurses is critical.

Telling one's story is not without its caveats. Suzanne Gordon and Bernice Buresh, both journalists who have written extensively about issues in nursing, indicate that nurses need to be more vocal and visible by telling their stories in a way that represents nurses as knowledgeable and competent. In their classic book, *From Silence to Voice*, Buresh and Gordon (2013) take nurses through a step-by-step process of developing and refining narratives to more effectively capture the realities of nurses' work.

Building Momentum

Building momentum pushes an issue into the policy limelight, much like the tipping point described by Gladwell (2000). For example, needlestick prevention passed in a critical number of states before it was possible to achieve passage at the federal level. On the other hand, North Dakota had baccalaureate entry for nursing practice from 1986 through 2003 (Smith, 2009). Nurses in Oregon, Montana, and Maine initiated efforts for baccalaureate entry, but were unsuccessful. The failure to create an action plan to accompany the ANA 1965 position statement on baccalaureate entry (Elliott, June 2010) and the lack of momentum with other states adopting baccalaureate entry contributed to failure in these implementation efforts and the ultimate demise of baccalaureate entry in North Dakota. Several ways to build momentum include marshaling forces, visiting legislators, seeking out organizational leaders, and policy maker events.

EXHIBIT 9.6   ELEMENTS OF GOOD NARRATIVES

- Portrayed excellence in nursing
- Described practice breakdowns, errors, or moral dilemmas
- Raised issues and problems
- Illustrated differences made by nurses
- Provided opportunities for learning new perspectives
- Etched into memory

From Benner, Hooper-Kyriakidis, and Stannard (2011).

Marshaling Forces to Advance a Policy Position

We need to take the time to strategically identify where to focus efforts and choose issues that are important to the profession and for which a nurse would be a respected, knowledgeable advocate. Dig deeper, learn more, and understand what needs to be changed and why, as well as who has the authority to actually make the change. Consider who potential allies are, ask why the policy you advocate for (or would like to prevent) has not been adopted, and decide whether you have the interest and stamina to see the issue through to its conclusion. Integral to any plan are opportunities to have direct interaction with lawmakers, policy makers, and key decision makers. Key strategies are visiting legislators, having legislators visit your facility, and participating in legislators' or policy makers' activities.

POLICY ON THE SCENE 9.4: Nurses Telling Their Stories
**Karen Haller, PhD, RN, FAAN, Vice President for Nursing and
Patient Care Services, The Johns Hopkins Hospital, Baltimore, MD**

Institutional leaders all work closely with local media—television, news, and magazine journalists—and will find it relatively easy to set some standards. For example, no photos leave the institution for publication without full identification of those in the picture. Gone are the days of identifying two people in a photo as "Dr. Jones and a nurse."

I have learned over time, however, that some ownership of nursing's absence in the media rests with us. When Hopkins has a media-worthy story about new and innovative patient care, physicians step forward readily, although just as often the nurses demure. Medical practice consists of many instances of individual heroism in the service of patients or science, but nursing practice is collective and collaborative. The media loves heroes.

(continued)

When nurses do step forward and are recognized for their role in a patient's care or tell their stories, they often convey to me their "embarrassment" in front of colleagues who did just as much as they did. The 24/7 teamwork of nursing practice works against identifying an individual hero, or any one nurse willing to accept that label that the media so loves.

I continue to encourage articulate nurses to step forward and represent us all. Some are more comfortable with the lights, cameras, and microphones. We need them to step forward and accept the accolades that all Hopkins nurses—and the profession—have earned. Along the way, they educate the public with a more accurate and balanced view of nurses' value to society.

Recently, I thanked nurses who appeared on National Public Radio's local affiliate and were cited in the Southwest Airlines magazine, *Spirit*. I thanked a nurse who allowed a photojournalist to follow her at work, to school, and at home. They represent us all, and are heroes because of it.

Visiting Legislators

The experience of state of Massachusetts with nurse staffing ratios illustrates this point. Beginning in the late 1990s, a Massachusetts nursing union started urging state legislators to mandate nurse-staffing ratios in state law rather than leave the authority for this decision in the hands of hospitals and the nurses caring for patients. In 2003, the first legislative committee approved this proposal. Clinical nurses at MGH were concerned that legislation would limit their autonomy. To an organization with a nearly 200-year tradition of patient-centered nursing excellence and a strong collaborative decision-making philosophy and culture, the concept of government intervention into nurse staffing decisions seemed directed at removing the autonomy and accountability for practice from the patient's nurse. The CNO led the effort to learn more, involving staff nurses throughout the organization—all of whom would be affected by any potential policy change. The nursing leadership made it a priority to include briefings on the topic at regular staff meetings, always leaving time for questions and discussion. Staff nurses were encouraged to be active in local nursing leadership groups and to share the importance of nurses having control over their practice, including having a voice in resource allocation. Nurses also needed to be knowledgeable about how nurse-staffing decisions were being made at the MGH to help them determine whether to be active advocates for retaining nursing authority over staffing and opposing mandated ratios. While it was recognized that, for some nurses, staffing ratios might appear to be the only viable solution given their practice environment, it was just not the case for MGH.

With the initial homework done, it was important to begin educating existing nursing groups—nursing leadership, staff nurse advisory committees, collaborative governance groups, and others—about the issues and what was at stake. Clinical nurses are the core role group to address clinical nursing practice challenges and opportunities. Involving clinical nurses sends an important message about the value of collaborative decision making and that nurses are well qualified to speak to the media and to policy makers.

The ability to deliver a clear and consistent message is important in all settings and circumstances and is especially important for a nurse who is also a public policy advocate. Presentation skills can be learned. Training helps participants understand how to organize clear messages and practice their delivery skills (see Chapter 10). A leadership coach helped MGH staff nurses prepare for nurse-staffing testimony before the Massachusetts legislature, stressing the importance of understanding the audience, clear communication, and using voice and body language. As the coach noted, they were not to "put things on," but to bring more of what they know. This encourages speakers to bring to the table what already exists in them—to be more of their real and vital selves, to understand and inhabit each circumstance with clarity, presence, and the power that actors have to touch hearts and minds, to interact effectively with others, and to command the attention of audiences.

Influence is the essence of leadership and nurses need the ability to communicate and influence in order to participate in policy making and achieve their political and policy goals. The visibility of nurses committed to MGH's approach to staffing was key in influencing lawmakers. This was challenging, because legislators had difficulty in understanding that nurses are not unified on a particular position. Obviously, unity among nurse groups would be highly desirable. However, when that is not the case, and it does not look like it will be achieved for a particular issue, it is important to be prepared with facts that are presented in a professional and compelling manner and that the people who are affected by the proposed policy or legislation are integrally involved in activating the plan.

Visiting legislators and providing testimony was one component of MGH's strategy. Since building new relationships takes time, capitalizing on existing relationships is key, just as it is in delivering patient care. As part of this process, it is important to identify any existing personal connections with important opinion leaders and public policy decision makers—a nurse who is active in her town government, or went to school with a legislator's child has an entré and built-in credibility. Getting to know the decision makers, educating about issues, solving the inevitable constituent patient care and employment questions that arise, and alerting them to breaking news—good and bad—at your institution are excellent ways to foster these relationships.

Seeking Out Organizational Leaders

Invitations to visit and see your institution can also be extremely effective. Often, extending these invitations is a routine responsibility of the chief executive officer (CEO). Finding ways to expand these so that other role groups play a central role is very useful. Examples include invitations to shadow a nurse on an inpatient unit, explain how patient acuity is calculated for staffing, observe surgical procedures, or tour services that are unique to your organization (an inter-professional approach to a particular disease, a specialized cancer treatment, or cutting-edge technology). During the Massachusetts debate on nurse-staffing ratios, it became clear that legislators didn't know much about how hospitals actually determine nurse staffing. Several key legislative leaders—including the chairs of two important health care committees—were invited to visit the hospital. One such visit focused exclusively on the question of how the nursing department determines staffing levels for a hospital unit and included a hands-on demonstration of the computer-based patient acuity measurement system that is used to decide staffing on each unit. During another visit, a legislator met with a small group of staff nurses who came well prepared to explain why they did not believe a one-size-fits-all approach to staffing ratios was good for their patients.

These two meetings were extremely effective: the first, because it gave the legislator valuable information about how staffing decisions are made that could be shared with colleagues and, in the process, reassure them that the decision was not arbitrary and, the second, because it made clear to the legislator that opposition to ratios extended to nurses practicing at the bedside who were worried about what it would mean for their patients. The proposed legislation on staffing ratios is an unfinished story in nursing not only in Massachusetts, but also across the country. This is typical in activating a plan. While some plans may end in legislation, the passage of a law is only the beginning of the regulatory process and evaluation of the law's outcomes. Other plans, like MGH's, which was focused on staffing autonomy, illustrate the ongoing process of policy development. More than 10 years later, no other state besides California has passed staffing ratio legislation. However, many states have introduced legislation on both safe staffing (nurses contributing to staffing decisions) and staffing ratios, supported by representatives of different nurses' groups.

Policy Maker Events

U.S. Senator Edward Kennedy (D-MA) was particularly adept at using another approach to building relationships and educating leaders. He regularly sponsored "teach-ins," in which hospital leaders from important states came to Washington, DC. Kennedy would convene their senators for a common briefing on an important issue of the day. The obvious advantages of these events are efficiency; it's an opportunity to highlight your organization in your legislator's turf; policy makers get a consistent message; and the common experience creates some accountability among the leaders who attend. Publicity about any visits, in your newsletters, will be appreciated and can be shared with the political leader as well.

DEALING WITH THE UNEXPECTED

In any advocacy plan, there may be an unexpected turn of events or unintended consequences. For hospitals, these may be sentinel events; for advanced practice nurses, it may be a report of less than desired outcomes; for anesthesia providers, it may be a lapse in infection control practices leading to potential widespread outbreak of disease; or for nurse educators, it may be a loss of accreditation status. These events require an immediate response and transparency. The public wants and needs to be assured that something is being done about the situation and that your organization's staff will provide safe care. Transparency provides information and helps to restore trust. See Policy on the Scene 9.5 for an example of how an unfortunate event was used to activate a plan to address alarm fatigue.

The organization's commitment to transparency and continuous improvement led to numerous policy changes within the MGH. In addition, openly sharing this unfortunate story—by contributing to the literature and speaking in public forums—has helped other institutions address system gaps as well as inform technology changes and national agendas that can lead to improved care. Influencing immediate action while being transparent to system challenges is highly reflective of the time and timing factor of the AIM (see Figure 9.1). The time to address the issue and the timing at which to do so was immediate and pertinent. This situation initially required immediate action. The emphasis on clear message articulation and key supportive relationships of the senior leadership team provided status and optimized communications. While inherently it is a challenge to have specific knowledge-based competence around an unforeseen issue like the monitor alarms, the knowledge-based competence around systems action, transparency, and leadership is an imperative in influencing success when dealing with unexpected serious events (Ives Erickson, 2010). While this issue was addressed within the MGH organization at the little "p" level, alarm hazards are a problem faced by many organizations. The Emergency Care Research Institute (ECRI), a patient-safety organization, lists alarm hazards as the top health technology hazard for 2013 (ECRI, 2012). The American Association of Critical-Care Nurses has a tool kit on alarm fatigue (see Exhibit 9.1), and the National Association of Clinical Nurse Specialists established an Alarm Fatigue Task Force. Alarm hazards as an issue of this magnitude can be ideally addressed with an interdisciplinary team of stakeholders from many organizations moving it into the big "P" of the policy arena.

SUSTAINING THE ADVOCACY PLAN

With many issues and efforts to move forward, it usually takes years of effort and success to achieve policy goals. The path may be circuitous or not very direct, but persistence is important. A single policy achievement is only one step of the process. Incrementalism is a credible strategy for achieving sustainable results.

POLICY ON THE SCENE 9.5: Transparency as a Means of Activating a Policy Plan

MGH is a 971-bed academic medical center that is consistently ranked in the top five of *U.S. News & World Report*'s rating of hospitals (2014) for providing high-quality care; in addition, it has been designated as a Magnet institution since 2003. In 2010, an unfortunate incident occurred. A nurse discovered a patient to be unresponsive and without a pulse (Ives Erickson, 2012). Emergency efforts were immediately undertaken but, despite these best efforts, the patient died. Questions arose after the event about why the nurses did not hear the monitor alarm, which should have alerted them to deterioration in the patient's condition. To the dismay of all involved, the initial investigation found that the alarm had inadvertently been turned off. Because clinical nurses were free to bring system issues forward, they raised their voice to identify an organization-wide problem. The CNO, with members of the clinical community, conducted a thorough investigation and defined and implemented preliminary action steps. Within hours, the alarm off-switch on 1,100 monitors was disabled to prevent this unfortunate event from ever happening again, not only at the MGH but, ideally, anywhere. To achieve this, a multifaceted interdisciplinary workgroup structure was created to identify recommendations to improve physiologic monitoring systems and responses to ensure a safe, evidence-based, and reliable monitoring program for patients. This new committee of stakeholders was asked to (a) critically review practice standards, evidence-based practice, and research on physiologic monitoring and alarm management; (b) make recommendations regarding criteria for, and management of, physiologic monitoring; and (c) review recommendations for patient placement standards/criteria.

At times, achieving only small steps is possible. Today we are witnessing independent practice for advanced practice nurses knowing this was not a possibility when these roles were first conceived years ago. When implementing a plan, there is constant consideration of the pros and cons for possible solutions or compromises. Often, the implementation of a policy provides the first opportunity to learn if the policy will be effective in the manner it was conceived and desired. Throughout this process, the leaders responsible for activating a plan need to give careful thought to how to sustain interest and effort in the plan and what adjustments are needed in order to achieve the desired goals.

Sustaining interest involves creating an interest among key legislators, stakeholders, and decision makers. Strategies to sustain interest include maintaining contacts with key leaders, sending newsletters or updates, and developing press releases on the topic (see Chapters 7 and 10). In general, work on expanding your influence by meeting new people and building coalitions. Networking never ends.

Sustaining interest involves keeping the supporters of your plan engaged in continuing the work. Transparency in sharing information and providing your team members with progress updates is essential. As with any issue, some individuals who were once leaders will drop out and new leaders will emerge. It is important that your plan includes consideration to succession planning and ongoing leadership development to ensure the policy agenda will continue.

Knowing the challenges to achieve success in changing policy, the likelihood becomes more difficult. In those instances, it is useful to propose a pilot project with the suggested policy change. This would allow you to collect data. More realistically, a pilot would provide you with preliminary information about the policy as well as challenges, foreseen and unforeseen, in implementing a policy. This information may lead to a revision in the policy or the strategy for getting it implemented.

Finally, any advocacy plan needs periodic revision and regrouping through an evaluation process. This may be accomplished formally, with an evaluation tool, or informally, depending on the nature of the plan. This will provide you with the necessary information about your stakeholders, your organization, the external environment, and the impact of your plan. Having new information and the latest information will empower you and your team members as your plan is refined and implemented. While it is important to deliver a consistent message and preferably a unified message, the plan may need revision depending on new circumstances. Being strategic at the big "P" or little "p" level is a constant shifting, gauging, being aware of the environment, being aware of the concerns of your patients and colleagues, as well as being aware of the concerns and challenges faced by key policy decision makers. It is an iterative process and most successful when the people who are most affected by the issue are involved.

OPTION FOR POLICY CHALLENGE: Improving Patient Flow in the Emergency Department
Nancy Bonalumi

The policy plan needs to be activated to improve patient flow. Activities must include analyzing the current problem, developing a problem statement, and establishing appropriate goals. A sample problem statement is "ED crowding increases length of stay (LOS) beyond national benchmarks. It extends waiting time for patients to see a provider, creates dissatisfaction for patients and significant others, costs the health care system revenue and increases liability risk if patients leave without being seen." The next step is to identify project goals such as national ED throughput benchmarks or internal targets to establish

(continued)

specific metrics such as arrival to provider, provider to disposition decision, admission decision to in-patient bed, and patient satisfaction scores.

The improvement agenda requires key ED internal and external stakeholder involvement. The agenda should first focus on streamlining activities and services to reduce LOS. Examples include use of care protocols; decreasing turnaround time for testing; and reporting, evaluating, and designating a distinct ED area for patients with mild or low acuity illness and injury.

An ED in central Florida was experiencing many of these efficiency challenges. By using work teams composed of process stakeholders and facilitated by consultants, the organization gained large-scale support for implementation of a hospital-wide improvement agenda. Throughput accountabilities and processes were redesigned. As a result, ED arrival to provider time improved by 29%, overall ED LOS improved by 23%, and patient satisfaction scores improved by more than 200%. Additionally, bed-requested to bed-assigned times improved by 62% and hospital discharges before 3:00 p.m. increased from 34% to 59%. A culture of accountability emerged at all organizational levels for individual roles in efficient patient flow. Staff nurse involvement in developing work flow solutions provided buy-in and support for new processes that demanded behavior changes.

ED patient experience has a direct financial impact on a health system's bottom line. The patient's perception of care is a component of the Centers for Medicare and Medicaid Services (CMS) Hospital Consumer Assessment of Healthcare Providers and Systems (HCAHPS) scorecard. This measurement is currently derived from patients admitted to the hospital; their overall impression of care begins in the ED. There is significant financial risk if satisfaction scores do not meet the HCAHPS target. In 2015, ED-specific data (Consumer Assessment of Healthcare Providers and Systems [CAHPS]) will begin for all patients who are cared for in the ED, placing even greater pressure on hospitals to meet these CMS standards to avoid penalties. The pace of improvement for ED patient flow will continue to quicken to stay ahead of these requirements.

IMPLICATIONS FOR THE FUTURE

Nurses have unique professional skills to activate an advocacy plan. Therefore, greater involvement by nurses at the grassroots level is needed. Resources are increasingly limited and plans need to be creative, strategic, and well thought out, anticipating desired and unintended consequences. In some instances, establishing or joining coalitions will certainly add resources, support, and credibility, particularly coalitions that include other health care professional and consumer groups. State nurses associations will have greater visibility with efforts to advance *The Future of Nursing* recommendations (IOM, 2011) because their established networks and partnerships provide an ideal infrastructure to support these initiatives. State-based affiliates of specialty nurses associations will also have greater opportunities for visibility through partnerships and coalitions.

Greater emphasis will be placed upon mentoring recent graduates, involving them in policy through (a) shared governance at their place of employment, (b) professional associations, and (c) community organizations to lead advocacy plan efforts. Many recent graduates have been involved in service learning. This means that they are accustomed to providing service. However, nurses who have had service learning experiences may not have necessarily thought about service as a means to influence policy. In addition, many recent graduates of undergraduate, graduate, and doctoral programs have been involved in projects related to policy change, but upon graduation, this enthusiasm has not been marshaled for further engagement in the policy process. These graduates are an ideal resource as organizations seek to vitalize their advocacy efforts.

Advocacy plans in an increasingly wired society will involve greater use of technology and social media. However, attention will need to be paid to how to include individuals living in remote areas and those who do not have Internet access. Data analytics will increasingly become part of advocacy plans. Therefore, strategies need to be designed for seamless data collection when plans are developed, initiated, and evaluated.

The implementation of many policies important for nursing and health policy will be implemented at the state level. Often, laws and regulations must be enacted in a critical number of states before they capture the attention of policy makers at the national level. As organizations make improvements in certain policies, it may take time for the value of these improvements to achieve widespread recognition and then be adopted, as we saw with the Magnet Recognition Program®. Likewise, when new programs, laws, or regulations are established, it may take years for related policies and procedures to be implemented. For example, the implementation of many policies related to the PPACA will be at the state level. Nurses are a crucial link in helping the public to understand how the PPACA is applied, promoting the shift in emphasis to preventive care and advocating for policies to achieve the goals of a transformed health system. According to the AAN (2010), the national goals of a transformed health system that improves access, improves quality, and controls costs "cannot be achieved without maximizing the contributions of nurses." It is not only the contributions of nurses that need to be maximized, but also their roles in activating and sustaining advocacy plans to enhance nursing practice and promote the health of the public.

KEY CONCEPTS

1. Activating a plan is a pivotal step in the policy process.

2. The environment for activating a plan can be a health care organization, a professional association, or an entirely new structure developed for the specific policy issue; each has unique features to be considered in plan activation.

3. Shared governance provides opportunities to address policies as well as serving as a vehicle for implementation of a plan.

4. Participation in a professional association enables nurses to activate plans in an organized and systematic manner, providing resources, tool kits, and an infrastructure for activities.

5. New structures and/or coalitions may be created in order to energize support for an advocacy plan.

6. Resources that need to be assessed for an advocacy plan include people and manpower, data, economic resources, and communication abilities, as well as the overall readiness or capacity for action.

7. Activating the advocacy plan involves the use of multiple strategies including goal refinement, applying influence, framing an issue, and targeting an audience.

8. The AIM involves the assessment and understanding of the interplay of authority, communication traits, knowledge-based competencies, status, and timing to effectively advance an advocacy plan.

9. Rolling out the plan includes creating narratives and building momentum.

10. Strategies to build momentum include marshaling forces to advance a policy position, visiting legislators or key policy makers, seeking out organizational leaders, attending policy maker events, and bringing policy makers to your organization.

11. Dealing with the unexpected such as unanticipated adverse events or an unintended consequence requires superb communication, an immediate response, and transparency to restore trust.

12. Sustaining an advocacy plan may take years with numerous refinements and reiterations of the advocacy plan as the implementation of the policy or related policies unfold.

13. Incrementalism may be a strategic choice that allows a plan to move forward and slowly build momentum.

13. The use of technology and new media for communication will help nurses to garner support from a wider audience in implementing the advocacy plan.

14. Future initiatives will require greater involvement by nurses at the grassroots level, including new graduates who have unique experiences and competencies to offer that can be harnessed to enhance the success of an advocacy plan.

SUMMARY

Nurses, long champions for their patients, must now become champions and indeed experts in implementing plans for advocacy. Consistently involving nurses and widening the circle of involved nurses are key to implementing an advocacy plan. Each environment—be it workplace, professional associations, or within the larger community at the state, national, or international level—has its own unique circumstances and challenges in implementing an advocacy plan. The establishment of a new policy, law, or regulation may only represent the initial phases of a plan that addresses a critical issue.

Consistently articulating the importance of advocacy from within the profession and equipping nurses with practical tools will facilitate the activation of an advocacy plan. The AIM provides a useful framework for understanding, articulating, and using influence to help nurses gain the knowledge needed to advance health care policy issues and successfully persuade key decision makers. Involvement in professional organizations and advocacy groups provides nurses with the additional competencies and confidence to advance policy goals.

Understanding the environment, assessing resources, and being strategic and systematic in the rollout are all critical to an advocacy plan's success. Activation of a plan is not a single activity, but an ongoing process that needs to be sustained through constant refinement, involving those directly impacted by a policy, and engaging decision makers. It involves ongoing work, an ability to respond to the unexpected, and a tolerance for ambiguity as policies are moved forward.

LEARNING ACTIVITIES

1. Write a personal narrative to use to support a policy at your work, locally in your community, or for a state or federal legislative action. Include it in your portfolio.
2. Identify an issue you support at the big "P" level, identify the target audience, and then examine websites and other publicly available information about the decision maker in order to determine information about the decision maker's positions and values.
3. Examine one of the tool kits listed in Exhibit 9.1, identify personal talking points that you can speak to, and review them with a colleague where you work.
4. Locate a recent news story that highlights the growing issues surrounding injuries among nurses and other health care workers related to safe patient handling and mobility. Then click and read about *Safe Patient Handling Under Hot Issues* (www.rnaction.org/site/PageNavigator/NSTAT/nstat_homepage?ct=1&ct=1). After reading both the story and the suggested activities, pick one, do it, and share what you learned with classmates.

5. Select an issue at the big "P" level and identify groups that would be good strategic partners or members of coalitions that would advance a policy position and why these groups should be involved.

6. Select an issue at the little "p" level and then determine how the members of the task force to oversee the issue should be selected. Identify the people who should be on the task force and what roles need to be represented, and provide the rationale for your selections.

7. Describe the strategies you would use for activating a plan to implement a policy change for the issues selected in 5 and 6. Include who, what, when, and where (see Exhibit 9.2).

E-RESOURCES

- American Heart Association. *How to schedule and conduct a successful meeting with your elected officials.* http://www.youtube.com/watch?v=Q320LHS847w
- American Nurses Association. *Policy and advocacy.* http://www.nursingworld.org/MainMenuCategories/Policy-Advocacy
- Bolder Advocacy. http://www.bolderadvocacy.org
- Frameworks Institute. http://www.frameworksinstitute.org
- Future of Nursing Campaign for Action. http://campaignforaction.org
- Illinois Education Association. *Tips for talking to legislators.* http://www.youtube.com/watch?v=8TtAe-_rs5U
- Initiative on the Future of Nursing. *Action coalitions.* http://www.thefutureofnursing.org/content/action-coalitions
- National Association of Clinical Nurse Specialists (NACNS). *Coalitions.* http://www.nacns.org/html/coalitions.php
- NSTAT. http://www.rnaction.org
- Prevention Institute. *Prevention and equity at the center of community well-being.* http://www.preventioninstitute.org
- Rising Voices. *Featured guide: Social advocacy tool kit for activists and non-profits.* http://rising.globalvoicesonline.org/blog/2012/05/28/featured-guide-social-advocacy-toolkit-for-activists-and-non-profits
- Robert Wood Johnson Foundation, Nurses & Nursing. http://www.rwjf.org/en/topics/rwjf-topic-areas/nursing.html
- UNICEF. (2010). *Advocacy tool kit: A guide to influencing decisions that improves children's lives.* http://www.unicef.org/evaluation/files/Advocacy_Toolkit.pdf
- Video for Change Tool Kit. http://toolkit.witness.org

REFERENCES

Adams, J. M. (2009). *The Adams Influence Model (AIM): Understanding the factors attributes and process of achieving influence.* Saarbrüken, Germany: VDM Verlag.

Adams. J. M., & Ives Erickson, J. (2011). Understanding influence: An exemplar applying the Adams Influence Model (AIM) in nurse executive practice. *Journal of Nursing Administration, 41*(4), 186–192.

American Academy of Nursing. (2010). Implementing health care reform: Issues for nursing. Washington, DC: Author. Retrieved from http://www.aannet.org/assets/docs/implementinghealthcarereform.pdf

American Nurses Association. (2001). *Code of ethics for nurses.* Silver Spring, MD: Author.

American Nurses Association. (2010a). *Nursing: Scope and standards of practice* (2nd ed). Silver Spring, MD: Author.

American Nurses Association. (2010b). *Nursing's social policy statement: The essence of the profession.* Silver Spring, MD: Author.

American Nurses Association. (2013a). Safe patient handling and mobility. Silver Spring, MD: Author. Retrieved from http://www.nursingworld.org/Mainmenucategories/workplacesafety/Healthy-work-environment/SafePatient/SPHM-Trifold-Brochure.pdf

American Nurses Association. (2013b). *Safe patient handling and mobility: Interprofessional national standards across the care continuum.* Silver Spring, MD: Author.

Appleby, J. (2013, September 8). Nurse practitioners try new tack to expand foothold in primary care. *Kaiser Health News.* Retrieved from http://www.kaiserhealthnews.org/Stories/2013/September/09/nurse-primary-care-slowed-by-insurer-credentialing.aspx

Auerbach, D. I., Staiger, D. O., Muench, U., & Buerhaus, P. I. (2012). The nursing workforce: A comparison of three national surveys. *Nursing Economics, 30*(5), 253–260; quiz 261.

Barden, A. M., Griffin, M. G., Donahue, M., & Fitzpatrick, J. J. (2011). Shared governance and empowerment in registered nurses working in a hospital setting. *Nursing Administration Quarterly, 35*(3), 212–218.

Barkhorn, I., Huttner, N., & Blau, J. (2013, Spring). Assessing advocacy. *Stanford Social Innovation Review.* Retrieved from http://www.redstonestrategy.com/wp-content/uploads/2013/02/Spring_2013_Assessing_Advocacy_No_Links.pdf

Benner, P. (1984). *Novice to expert: Excellence and power in clinical nursing practice.* Upper Saddle River, NJ: Prentice Hall.

Benner, P., Hooper-Kyriakidis, P., & Stannard, D. (2011). *Clinical wisdom and interventions in acute and critical care: A thinking-action approach* (2nd ed.). New York, NY: Springer.

Bernstein, S. L., Aronsky, D., Duseja, R., Epstein, S., Handel, D., Hwang, U., & Society for Academic Emergency Medicine, Emergency Department Crowding Task Force. (2009). The effect of emergency department crowding on clinically oriented outcomes. *Academic Emergency Medicine, 16*(1), 1–10.

Bina, J. S., Schomburg, M. K., Tippetts, L. A., Scherb, C. A., Specht, J. K., & Schwichtenberg, T. (2014). Decisional involvement: actual and preferred involvement in decision-making among registered nurses. *Western Journal of Nursing Research 36*(4), 440–455.

Birkland, T. A. (2011). *An introduction to the policy process: Theories, concepts, and models of public policy making* (3rd ed.). Armonk, NY: ME Sharpe.

Bolder Advocacy. (n.d.). *Tools for effective advocacy.* Retrieved from http://bolderadvocacy.org/tools-for-effective-advocacy

Brabham, D. (2008). Crowdsourcing as a model for problem solving: An introduction and cases. *Convergence: The International Journal of Research Into New Media Technologies, 14*(1), 75–90.

Brody, A. A., Barnes, K., Ruble, C., & Sakowski, J. (2012). Evidence-based practice councils: Potential path to staff nurse empowerment. *Journal of Nursing Administration, 42*(1), 28–33.

Buresh, B., & Gordon, S. (2013). *From silence to voice: What nurses know and must communicate to the public* (3rd ed.). Ithaca, NY: ILR Press.

Cramer, M. E., Lazure, L., Morris, K. J., Valerio, M., & Morris, R. (2013). Conceptual models to guide best practices in organization and development of State Action Coalitions. *Nursing Outlook, 61*(2), 70–77.

Diercks, D. B., Roe, M. T., Chen, A. Y., Peacock, W. F., Kirk, J. D., Pollack, C. V., Jr., & Peterson, E. D. (2007). Prolonged emergency department stays of non-ST-segment-elevation myocardial infarction patients are associated with worse adherence to the American College of Cardiology/American Heart Association guidelines for management and increased adverse events. *Annals of Emergency Medicine, 50*(5), 489–496.

Dodson, E. A., Stamatakis, K. A., Chalifour, S., Haire-Joshu, D., McBride, T., & Brownson, R. C. (2013). State legislators' work on public health-related issues: What influences priorities? *Journal of Public Health Management and Practice, 19*(1), 25–29.

Elliott, J. E. (2010, June). *ANA Past Presidents Panel Discussion.* American Nurses Association House of Delegates. Washington, DC: American Nurses Association.

Emergency Care Research Institute. (2012). Top 10 health technology hazards for 2013. *Health Devices, 41*(11), 1–23.

Estellés-Arolas, E., & González-Ladrón-de-Guevara, F. (2012). Towards an integrated crowdsourcing definition. *Journal of Information Science, 38*(2), 189–200.

Gladwell, M. (2000). *The tipping point.* Boston, MA: Little Brown.

Global Partners in Care. (n.d.). *Funding hospice and palliative care partnerships globally.* Retrieved from http://crowdfunding.globalpartnersincare.org

Hawks, H. J. (1992). Empowerment in nursing education: Concept analysis and application to philosophy, learning and instruction. *Journal of Advanced Nursing, 17*(5), 609–618.

Hsia, R. Y., Asch, S. M., Weiss, R. E., Zingmond, D., Liang, L. J., Han, W., … Sun, B. C. (2012). California hospitals serving large minority populations were more likely than others to employ ambulance diversion. *Health Affairs, 31*(8), 1767–1776.

Iglehart, J. (1999). "Narrative matters": Binding health policy and personal experience. *Health Affairs, 18*(4), 6.

Institute of Medicine (IOM). (2008). The future of emergency care in the United States health system. *Academic Medicine, 13*(10), 1081–1085. doi: 10.1197/j.aem.2006.07.011

Institute of Medicine (IOM). (2011). *The future of nursing: Leading change, advancing health.* Washington, DC: The National Academies Press.

Ives Erickson, J. (2010). A nurse leader's perspective on disaster preparedness and response: Experiences from Haiti. *AONE Voice,* May.

Ives Erickson, J. (2012). Leading a highly visible hospital through a serious reportable event. *Journal of Nursing Administration, 42*(3), 131–133.

Ives Erickson, J., Hamilton, G., Jones, D., & Ditomassi, M. (2003). The value of collaborative governance/staff empowerment. *Journal of Nursing Administration, 33*(4), 251–252.

Jo, S., Jin, Y. H., Lee, J. B., Jeong, T., Yoon, J., & Park, B. (2014). Emergency department occupancy ratio is associated with increased early mortality. *The Journal of Emergency Medicine 46*(2), 231–249.

Kickstarter. (n.d.). *Air quality egg.* Retrieved from http://www.kickstarter.com/projects/edborden/air-quality-egg

Kingdon, J. W. (2011). *Agendas, alternatives, and public policies* (Update 2nd ed.). Glenview, IL: Pearson Education.

Manojlovich, M. (2007, January 31). Power and empowerment in nursing leadership; looking backward to inform the future. *OJIN The Online Journal of Issues in Nursing, 12*(1), Manuscript 1. Retrieved from http://www.nursingworld.org/MainMenuCategories/ANAMarketplace/ANAPeriodicals/OJIN/TableofContents/Volume122007/No1Jan07/LookingBackwardtoInformtheFuture.asp

Matthews, J. H. (2012, January 31). Role of professional organizations in advocating for the nursing profession. *OJIN: The Online Journal of Issues in Nursing, 17*(1), Manuscript 3. Retrieved from http://nursingworld.org/MainMenuCategories/ANAMarketplace/ANAPeriodicals/OJIN/TableofContents/Vol-17-2012/No1-Jan-2012/Professional-Organizations-and-Advocating.html

Myers, T. A., Nisbet, M. C., Maibach, E. W., & Leiserowitz, A. A. (2012). A public health frame arouses hopeful emotions about climate change [Letter]. *Climatic Change, 113*(3–4), 1105–1112.

New York City. (n.d.). *Building capacity for using volunteers.* Retrieved from http://www.nyc.gov/html/mocs/downloads/pdf/nonprofit_help/16_NYCSERVICE%20Cap%20Bldg%20Document%2002%2001%2011.pdf

Pines, J. M., & Hollander, J. E. (2008). Emergency department crowding is associated with poor care for patients with severe pain. *Annals of Emergency Medicine, 51*(1), 6-7.

Redfern, L. (2008). Symposium in tribute to a nursing leader. *Nursing Research, 57*, S1–S3.

Richardson, A., & Storr, J. (2010). Patient safety: A literature review on the impact of nursing empowerment, leadership and collaboration. *International Nursing Review, 57*, 12–21.

Sikka, R., Mehta, S., Kaucky, C., & Kulstad, E. B. (2010). ED crowding is associated with an increased time to pneumonia treatment. *American Journal of Emergency Medicine, 28*(7), 809–812.

Smith, T. G. (2009, October 5). A policy perspective on the entry to practice issue. *OJIN: The Online Journal of Issues in Nursing, 15*(1). Retrieved from http://www.nursingworld.org/MainMenuCategories/ANAMarketplace/ANAPeriodicals/OJIN/TableofContents/Vol152010/No1Jan2010/Articles-Previous-Topic/Policy-and-Entry-into-Practice.html

Spence Laschinger, H. K., & Leiter, M. P. (2006). The impact of nursing work environments on patient safety outcomes. *Journal of Nursing Administration, 36*(5), 259–267.

Swan, B. A. (2012). A nurse learns firsthand that you may fend for yourself after a hospital stay. *Health Affairs, 31*(11), 2579–2582.

U.S. News & World Report. (2014). US News Best Hospitals 2014–2015. Retrieved from http://health.usnews.com/best-hospitals/rankings

Whitehead, D. K., Weiss, S. A., & Tappen, R. M. (2010). *Essentials of nursing leadership and management* (5th ed.). Philadelphia, PA: F. A. Davis.

Working With the Media: Shaping the Health Policy Process

Pamela F. Cipriano

If you don't exist in the media, for all practical purposes, you don't exist. —Daniel Schorr, commentator, National Public Radio

OBJECTIVES

1. Design a media strategy to advance a current policy issue.
2. Develop effective written communication (letters, press releases, op-eds, policy briefs, etc.) to convey a message to the public and policy makers.
3. Examine methods to develop successful relationships with radio, television, and print media.
4. Prepare a story with resources for the media and the public using the Internet.
5. Appraise the evolving impact of social media's impact on shaping the policy process.

The media, love them or hate them. This commonly heard phrase aptly describes the reaction to the strong influence the media exerts in shaping public opinion. The media can rapidly build support or swiftly derail well-intentioned ideas. Society relies on traditional media to inform us by exposing the truth and reporting news and events. Social media and other types of user-generated content, however, are instruments of influence with a broad reach to a vast audience. Social media is unbridled by traditional reporting ethics as well as the rigor and formalities of publishing and scripting. With instantaneous dissemination channels, social media can trigger a tsunami of interest in a subject, which in turn can compel traditional media to cover an issue. Converged media, or a merging of traditional and newer social media, blends the two platforms to garner the attention of the public by being provocative and quick to respond to controversial activities.

This chapter explains how to work with the media and, in particular, how to develop the tools to communicate effectively to various audiences, along with pointers to ensure that actions will lead to the intended results. Using proven techniques to work with the media helps nurses in all settings think critically and strategically about establishing and maintaining relationships with the media. It is important to look for as well as create opportunities to broadcast messages important to the public welfare and advancement of the profession. Nurses can take advantage of digital communication and social media platforms to reach a broad audience and establish a greater presence never before possible. The process for establishing presence is illustrated in the Policy Challenge.

POLICY CHALLENGE: *The Future of Nursing*

On October 5, 2010, Dr. Harvey Fineberg, president of the Institute of Medicine (IOM), and Dr. Risa Lavizzo-Mourey, president of the Robert Wood Johnson Foundation (RWJF), unveiled the report *The Future of Nursing: Leading Change, Advancing Health* (IOM, 2010d) at the National Press Club in Washington, DC. The 1-hour 7-minute live briefing was also webcast, telecast, recorded, and later archived for Internet access. Coverage, however, was not limited only to this briefing. Also appearing that day along with the initial prepublication full report (IOM, 2011) were other media releases including (a) a press release (IOM, 2010e), (b) recommendations (IOM, 2010d), (c) a chart on barriers to nurse practitioner practice (IOM, 2010c), and (d) two report briefs (IOM, 2010a, 2010b). The report was the culmination of a 2-year study of the need to transform the nursing profession so that nurses could, in turn, help transform health care. Expected to be controversial, the report did not disappoint. It set off a firestorm of opposition from some physician groups while being hailed by nurses and many others who believed the time had come for nurses to take a greater leadership role in addressing the changes needed to create a more sustainable and effective health care system (American Academy of Family Physicians [AAFP], 2010; American Association of Colleges of Nursing [AACN], 2010; American Medical Association, 2010; Chen, 2010; Tri-Council for Nursing, 2010). Physician groups opposing some of the recommendations did not attack the report directly and in some cases suggested agreement with the report's direction.

Strategic planning with individuals influential with the media was used to draw positive attention to this issue. A prominent physician member of the Steering Committee, John (Jack) Rowe, MD, professor of Health

Policy and Management at the Mailman School of Public Health, Columbia University, and former chairman and chief executive officer (CEO) of Aetna, Inc., in strong support of the report in its entirety, proclaimed that the report "is not about doctors, is not about nurses, but is about the patients" (Watman, 2010). He promoted the timely and important role nurses should assume to meet the needs of a growing population of patients who will be insured and in need of primary care. By supporting the removal of scope of practice barriers so that nurses can practice to the full scope of their education and training, he made an offensive move to fend off criticism and resistance from physician groups who oppose any expansion of registered nurse practice that is not directly under physician supervision.

Esteemed chairperson of the initiative, Donna Shalala, PhD, president of the University of Miami, and former U.S. Secretary of Health and Human Services, reinforced a similar view that advancing nursing care is good for the health of the nation. She did not mince words proclaiming, "While the report says nursing, it's really about health care. ... It's all about the patient and no one knows this more than nursing." Known as a fierce and powerful leader, Shalala underscored the imperative that nurses help lead the transformation of health care.

While nurses could have spread the message of *The Future of Nursing* report and stress the significance of the far-reaching recommendations, commentary and support from credible allies helped promote the legitimacy of the message and decrease any notion of self-serving actions. Anticipating areas of denunciation by other groups made it essential for nurses to have strong voices aligned and ready to acclaim the recommendations and refute the criticism that was sure to come.

The success of these media strategies is illustrated by the high demand for the report at the time of its release, making history by temporarily shutting down the IOM servers. This was nursing's moment, the media were hooked, and the country was watching. The challenge now is mobilizing for action.

See Option for Policy Challenge.

THE MEDIA AND HEALTH POLICY

Nurses have always embraced advocating for patients (see Chapter 2, "Advocating for Nurses and for Health"). The time has come to advocate for health care policy with the same vigor and tenacity to realize the vision for an improved health care system where nurses are leading change. Nurses need to be knowledgeable about the media and how to use it to advocate for their issues. Strategies for using the media include a variety of written as well as digital approaches such as news releases, letters to the editor, opinion editorials, editorial board meetings, interviews, and holding a media event.

The Media and Nursing

Why is it essential for nurses to engage the media? Starting with grassroots efforts to initiate changes in our communities, nurses can exert influence to achieve little "p" and big "P" changes alike by utilizing the media to spread their messages, thereby influencing as many people as possible. We want to shape the continuing development of nursing and health policy. We have a responsibility to convey our current thinking and opinions and stimulate action to effect better health policy to serve our communities and the nation. Public policy advocacy means speaking up. An essential focus throughout this book is creating or changing laws and policies to advance nursing and promote health.

One of nursing's greatest role models, Florence Nightingale, was viewed as an astute political actor (McDonald, 2006). She was credible, determined, well connected, deliberate, and did not shy away from controversy. She was able to influence social changes not only in health care delivery, but also in working conditions. Her approach included obtaining information from reliable sources, discussing the content with experts, then writing her views and recommendations. From her prolific letter writing, to issuing meticulous reports she had vetted with colleagues, using statistics, and developing innovative visual representations of data, she was able to influence opinion leaders and politicians despite her lack of formal degrees and her station as a woman. She knew the importance of garnering support and tapped her extensive network of friends and colleagues to accomplish her agenda for change. In Nightingale's time, it was the power of the pen. Today, it is the power of the Internet. We can use her strategies along with our modern methods of communication to achieve our goals.

Media Advocacy

Working with the media to have your message heard, advance opinions about issues, and influence policy decision makers is considered "media advocacy." When we promote a nursing or health care issue, we seek to educate the public, influence policy makers, and steer public viewpoints. Media advocacy combines mass communication with community advocacy. By using a range of media with purposeful strategies, groups can evolve episodic news stories into reframed public health issues. When children were dying from drunk-driving accidents, a far-reaching media advocacy campaign shined a spotlight on the dreadful effects of drunk driving, eventually resulting in stiff laws and long prison sentences for offenders. Effective media advocacy addresses gaps in power and resources to effect changes that will improve health and health care (Winett & Wallack, 1996). Media advocacy requires building skills for using the media as a tool to pursue social change and shift power within a community.

Planning your approach to media advocacy involves a number of steps and strategies to get the desired outcome. One approach is to follow the steps of "Got Me," including the goal, objectives, target audience, message, and evaluation as outlined in Exhibit 10.1 (Wallack & Dorfman, 1996). These steps are complementary and aim to inform the media in a clear and concise manner so your message is understood and amplified.

Spreading information about issues no longer relies on only one-way mass communication via the traditional media of radio, television, film, books, and newspapers. Instead, consumer-generated messages flood the Internet. Individual content experts are able to use new digital distribution channels to court public opinion. A multitude of opportunities exists to use print, audio, and video in traditional presentations along with various newer technologies such as webpages, pod casts, online conferencing, blogs, smartphone applications, and postings on social networking sites.

The media is a powerful messenger to policy makers, as well as the public. Mainstream news media heralds issues to policy makers and non-news entertainment media, particularly through television and newspapers. Coverage of issues creates awareness and exerts major influence over public sentiment. Politicians are attentive to the media as well because they know their constituent voters pay attention and are influenced by what they see and hear (Ensign, 2011). Media outlets, many of which align exclusively with liberal or conservative ideologies, choose to cover issues and related opinions as a means of shaping the public policy agenda. Fictional television dramas can provide public health as well as health policy information. Controversial or sensitive issues

EXHIBIT 10.1   "GOT ME" APPROACH TO MEDIA ADVOCACY

Goal	Establish common ground among the group that describes what you plan to accomplish
Objective	Define the set of actions that will achieve the goal
Target audience	Tailor the message to the audience: • Those with power to change policy • Influential interest groups • General public
Message	Help the media get an accurate message: • Clearly state the concern • Identify impact or threat and frame as the value to the community • Propose the policy solution(s)
Evaluation	Assess the success of your media advocacy approach to advancing your message

Adapted from Wallack and Dorfman (1996).

such as death, drug abuse, rare diseases, and any major tragedy may evoke an emotional response, drawing in viewers.

Unfortunately, these shows also portray nurses in various roles that may or may not depict the image nurses find attractive or accurate. When researchers analyzed television and other media coverage of nurse roles (2000 to 2009), only in a few instances did the media portray nurses accurately (Truth About Nursing, 2009). Only a few television shows depicted strong role models who advocate for patients. Infrequent coverage of powerful nurse leaders in health care is dwarfed by distorted portrayals of nurses as sex symbols. Such stereotypes increase the challenge of nursing practice understood and policy messages taken seriously. Media campaigns are used to spread a message quickly to a large audience. Campaign messages may include providing public health information and advisories, announcing event promotions, asserting viewpoints, or declaring pro or con positions to current issues. Social media may also be used to create a rapid short-term gathering both physically and virtually in support of a cause, policy, or to raise issue awareness.

Simple techniques such as having a letter or editorial published can capture media attention. The more coverage secured in the media, the more potential influence is gained. Targeting multiple means of exposure for media coverage garners the attention of policy makers from local to national elected officials. For local or state issues, media can help publicize opinions, information, or events. Maintaining contact with local reporters as well as radio and television personalities helps familiarize them with your expertise and content and can lead to coverage of your issues on a regular basis.

Media advocacy involves not only planned activities to initiate a policy change, but also activities that arise as a result of current events. A multipronged approach can garner widespread publicity and support. Media advocacy can be used for different types of situations or health policy initiatives. Media advocacy combines mass communication with community advocacy. An example of media advocacy is illustrated by the case of two nurse whistle-blowers from Texas in Policy on the Scene 10.1.

GUIDELINES FOR WORKING WITH THE MEDIA

Whether you want to contact the media as an individual or as a representative of a group, first become familiar with the type of media you believe will help convey your message. For local issues, knowing the interest and track record of the print and broadcast media coverage of public health issues is important. Become acquainted with the reporters and, if possible, cultivate relationships that can lead to more longitudinal coverage of an issue. If your reach is to Congress, contacting papers and media outlets that cover politics and reach a broader audience will be necessary.

Organizations should maintain an updated current media contact list. If you hold events, maintain a sign-in list and follow up with media representatives

POLICY ON THE SCENE 10.1: Media Advocacy: Triumph of Nurse Whistle-Blowers

The case of registered nurses Anne Mitchell and Vicki Galle, working in Winkler County, Texas, captured the attention of local nurses, community leaders, law enforcement officials, and public policy officials, as well as the national media as this story unfolded. The Texas Nurses Association (TNA) initiated a legal defense fund for these two nurses. TNA was joined by the American Nurses Association (ANA) in expanding the nurses' defense strategies and utilizing national media. Both nurses were fired by their employer. Local government officials retaliated by indicting both nurses on criminal charges, and then prosecuting Anne Mitchell for misuse of information. The video, *Fighting for Nurses Who Speak Up for Patients* (ANA, 2011a), chronicles the events and media coverage that revealed the injustice levied on these nurses and their remarkable victory overcoming their unlawful firing and prosecution. The ultimate victory was passage of legislation in Texas that protects nurses who engage in patient advocacy from retaliation by any person. This triumph of the two nurses who were indicted for blowing the whistle on what they believed, and was later proven to be, substandard care by a physician demonstrates the broad reach and power of the media.

to thank them for attending. National directories are also available for a fee to locate media outlets. Examples are listed in Exhibit 10.2. Media directories are also available by state, which can be easily found by typing media directory and the state into a search engine.

It is also important to seek resources in your community and establish relationships before a pressing issue becomes news. Traditional (newspapers, radio, television, and Internet) and nontraditional (electronic bulletin boards, blogs, corporate and community organization newsletters, etc.) media reach different audiences and help replicate your message. Get to know your local newspaper editorial staff, talk radio personalities, and television broadcasters. Health care organization public relations (PR) and marketing staffs may be less familiar with how to promote nursing stories, so it is important for you to familiarize them with issues important to nurses as well as nursing interest stories. For example, invite your organization's PR staff to attend events such as nursing research presentations, awards ceremonies, advancement celebrations, and community service days. Request that a consistent person be assigned to cover nursing events to avoid a repetitive learning curve. PR staff members make excellent partners and are familiar with writing guidelines and have usually already established relationships with local media representatives. Since it is their job to make an

EXHIBIT 10.2	MEDIA DIRECTORIES AND RESOURCES	
DIRECTORY	**WEBSITE**	**DESCRIPTION**
Burrelles*Luce*	http://www.burrellesluce.com	Media outreach, monitoring, and reporting
Cision (formerly provided Bacon's Media Directories)	http://www.cision.com/us/	Sources provide information about more than 1 million media outlets
Gale Cengage Learning	http://www.gale.cengage.com	Directory of Publications and Broadcast Media, 2013, Edition 149
Gebbie Press	http://www.gebbieinc.com	Media directories for print and broadcast; media tips
Hudson's Washington News Media Contacts Directory	http://www.greyhouse.com/hudsons.htm	Washington, DC, directory plus issue-specific directories for numerous health care topics
New Media Yellow Book	http://www.leadershipdirectories.com	Directories for online, print, and list feeds for media contacts
Vocus	http://www.vocus.com	Software increases visibility and reach of media coverage and distribution

organization look good in the public eye, you can help make their job easier by being a resource and alerting them to newsworthy stories.

As you work with the media, it is helpful to make yourself available in a timely manner to reporters seeking information, interviews, or quotes; this helps journalists respond to tight deadlines. These stories do not always have much lead time. Remember, you are responding "on the record" so your comments can be used and quoted. Being prepared when a hot issue breaks allows for immediate coverage and premier positioning of nursing's response. If you initiate the media contact, your message must be clear and concise. Using personal experiences makes examples more compelling and easily understood. Avoid health care jargon to enhance clarity.

MESSAGE DEVELOPMENT

Your message is a value proposition so you must explain why an issue is important, what is at risk, and why one should care, as well as why someone should act. The more closely you can align the message with others who share your values and concerns, the more support you will engender. Being prepared with a plan is the starting point for advocating an issue.

Professional associations provide a wealth of background information for their members such as fact sheets, issue briefs, policy analysis, and talking points. These may be combined into a comprehensive resource allowing one to be prepared when making a plan, outlining goals and objectives, and crafting an effective message. Knowing the overall goal of the actions you are taking on an issue allows you to identify appropriate audiences and the most effective types of media to reach them. Your goal may be to introduce a new issue and ask others to join in action. Or you may want to express a position or opinion about a current issue in your community or on a state or national agenda. Your plan to develop a clear and simple message will include the steps in Exhibit 10.3.

Developing a Case Statement: Tell Your Story

A simple compelling story often captures attention. Telling your story starts with the facts and builds on what your audience knows and believes. Case statements are often used in fundraising circles, but involve a simple compelling story that captures the essence of your values and what you are trying to address with policy. Try to establish a personal connection, one that inspires an emotional attachment on the part of the audience. Often issues are depicted as having a threat, a victim, good guys and bad guys, and a real or potential solution. Drawing the lines and explaining your side helps define what's at stake. Define the actions you want to take that will solve a problem. Linking solutions to problems, and explaining how the audience can help, advances an action agenda.

Talking Points

As the emotional debate rages, talking points are a useful tool to focus the message on facts, which will in turn educate media sources, internal and external

---

EXHIBIT 10.3   STEPS TO DELIVERING A SUCCESSFUL MESSAGE

1. State your goal clearly
2. Identify your audiences
3. Define your issue—the issue must draw attention and be considered "newsworthy"
4. Include only one main message with no more than three underlying themes of support
5. Confine your message to 30 seconds or less so that it is memorable
6. Frame your statements so your message connects to the greater public's interest
7. Be strategic when proposing a solution
8. State the support sought
9. Compel the audience to be concerned about your issue
10. Use humanizing examples and/or analogies
11. Match your message and language to the audience
12. Repeat your message frequently and consistently in all communications
13. Evaluate your message effectiveness

stakeholders, and the public. Talking points are a short list of arguments that succinctly summarize your arguments for or against an issue. Advocating for advanced practice nurses to pursue unencumbered roles in primary care is an example of a contentious issue that garners media attention as states debate changes in state practice act legislation. Fueled in part by the clear recommendation in *The Future of Nursing* (IOM, 2011a) to remove barriers to practice, but rooted in the belief that these nurses do not require direct supervision by physicians, nurses have embraced media advocacy as a key component of their success strategy to achieve changes needed for more independent practice. The American Association of Nurse Practitioners, in collaboration with four other national nurse practitioner associations, issued a discussion paper and talking points in response to a report issued by the AAFP in 2012 titled *Primary Care for the 21st Century*, which perpetuates a physician supervision model of care and ignores evidence of quality outcomes of care delivered by nurse practitioners (see Exhibit 10.4).

Messages should not be about "spin"; however, it is common to use rhetoric that gets a key message across. When the Florida Nurse Practitioner Network (2012) endorsed a candidate for a state House seat, they used their press conference as an opportunity to transmit key messages. They repeated consistent language used in *The Future of Nursing* report recommendations that underscored the need to remove barriers to advanced practice. Points made at their press conference bear close similarities to the talking points issued by the American Association of Nurse Practitioners.

The "Pitch": Getting Your Story Heard

Getting your story heard can be achieved with a succinct, powerful, 25- to 35-word description of your subject and position, answering what your issue is about, who is the target of your issue, why anyone should care, why your position is different, and what your qualifications are for making the pitch. Otherwise known as an elevator speech, it is an ideal way to pitch newsworthy information (see Chapter 2). These terms describe the concise wording one would use in a theoretical encounter with a captive audience when you have less than a minute to make a lasting impression (Pagana, 2013). Brevity is key to getting your message across.

The pitch can be made in writing, in person, or via telephone. When pitching your story, follow these five rules: (a) introduce yourself, your credentials, and your affiliations; (b) inform them of your story idea; (c) ask if it is a good time to talk; (d) offer your brief description of what, who, and why; and (e) confirm follow-up plans.

Written pitches by letter or e-mail should be no more than one page. Present the issue in a concise manner and establish relevance and timeliness to the audience. Include a simple description of your story and provide names of contacts, resources, and appropriate contact information. Other preparations include compiling supporting documents, developing talking

---

EXHIBIT 10.4   **TALKING POINTS: NURSE PRACTITIONERS AND THE FUTURE OF PRIMARY CARE**

Recently, the AAFP released a document suggesting that nurse practitioners need to participate in patient care as members of teams under the supervision of physicians. It implied that nurse practitioners functioning autonomously and at the top for their license would lead to a two-tiered health care system that would expose patients to inferior care.

Listed below are recommended talking points for nurse practitioners to use when confronted with questions regarding the opinions expressed by the AAFP:

- Nurse practitioners are highly qualified health care providers who undergo rigorous educational preparation that enables them to diagnose and treat acute and chronic illness as well as provide preventive care to their patients. A significant magnitude of studies has demonstrated the high quality of nurse practitioner care.
- The patient is the focus and center of *all* nurse practitioner practice.
- Nurse practitioners support and participate in team approaches to patient care based on the following concepts:
  - Health care teams consist of patients and their health care providers
  - The health care team does not belong to a single provider
  - Health care teams are dynamic, with the needs of the patient directing who best can lead the team at any given point of time
  - Flexible frameworks are required for innovation and creation of emerging models to provide high-quality care
- Current research on innovative nurse practitioner-led models of care demonstrates the success of nurse practitioners as team leaders for primary care.
- Studies have demonstrated that nurse practitioners are adequately educated/prepared to provide safe, high-quality primary care to their patients. All nurse practitioner educational programs are at the graduate level (master's, postmaster's, or doctoral degree). Programs of study are based on strong scientific foundations including evidence-based practice and the management of complex health systems. These programs of study clinically build upon the bachelor's program in nursing. Population focus is determined at the time of entry into the graduate program (e.g., family, adult/gerontology, pediatrics, and women's health).
- Care coordination is a hallmark of nurse practitioner care. Coordinated care delivery comes in many forms: nurse practitioner-led teams are one of the available and successful delivery models for team-based care.
- Nurse practitioner practices meet the criteria for the primary care medical home: patient-centered, comprehensive, coordinated, accessible high-quality, and safe care.
- Nurse practitioners can make significant contributions to reducing the primary care shortage if they are able to practice to the full extent of their educational preparation.

Reprinted with permission from the American Association of Nurse Practitioners (2012).

---

points, and determining who is available to be interviewed. However, when working with television stations, plan on no more than 15 to 30 seconds of coverage and prepare recommendations for video coverage that support your story.

You must be clear about identifying who you are, your credentials, and in what capacity you are speaking. Identify whether you are acting as an individual, as a concerned citizen, or as an official spokesperson of an organization or group. It may be useful to have personal calling cards prepared for use when business cards with your employer's name are inappropriate.

Reporter Calls

When a local issue breaks, or if your organization is on the critical path of a story line, being prepared for reporter calls puts you in a prime position to respond. Reporters are looking for access and information, not an adversarial relationship. Some due diligence is essential to preparing your ideas and being sure you will be able to anticipate the request of the reporter as well as the timeline for responding. Understanding the reporter's interest and familiarity with the subject as well as the priority for the story will provide clues about the amount of information you will need to provide. Information to gather from the reporter is reviewed in Exhibit 10.5. Ask clarifying questions before providing answers. Never argue, but stick to your message. If it is a negative story, additional preparation may be necessary, but in general, take some time to prepare thoughtful responses. Indicate you will get back to the reporter within the designated time frame. Do not repeat a negative statement or question because it may inadvertently get associated with you or your organization.

Sound Bites

A short 10- to 20-second statement comprises a sound bite that you may develop, or that the media may distill from longer stories. Sound bites should support your proposition. You can promulgate them as short quotes and use them repeatedly in conversations or interviews. Anticipating what might be used in a negative perspective is helpful as well; try to avoid providing ammunition for your opposition.

Press Releases and Advisories

Press or news releases are intended to convince reporters to cover a story. Reporters scan news releases to gauge interest in potential stories. Bloggers, policy experts, and the public also pay attention to press releases for basic information on issues. This section includes techniques for writing releases and provides examples where press releases can provide new information as well as correct misinformation.

EXHIBIT 10.5   THINGS TO KNOW BEFORE RESPONDING TO A REPORTER

- Topic of interest
- Type of information you are being asked to provide
- What information the reporter has already gathered
- Importance of the story
- Who has the expertise and experience to give the best interview
- What background information is available and can be shared publicly
- Deadline for the story

The Inverted Pyramid

Widely used for more than a century, many news writers use the inverted pyramid guide as depicted in Figure 10.1 in response to readers' desire for fast-paced delivery of information that holds their interest. In this style, the most important information is provided up front. The content covers the five W's and H: who, what, where, when, why, and how. The amount of content diminishes as do the sizes of the three areas of the pyramid. Alternatively, presenting a story that is idea-driven or reported in chronological order may be appropriate for more human interest stories rather than breaking news.

Writing a Press Release

The standard format for a press release provides quick access to all the information a reporter needs and indicates how to get in touch with the author. To grab a reporter's attention, start with one or two strong leading sentences that will convince the reporter the issue has news value. Address who and what in the first sentence. Throughout the story, address when, where, why, and how. Follow the introductory paragraph with one that begins to communicate feeling; using a quote helps personalize the message. The concluding paragraph typically includes a quote. Above all, the information must be credible and defensible. Once the entire release is written, devise an eye-catching headline. It can have up to 10 words, and subheadlines are acceptable as well. Purposeful inclusion of positive or negative words can shape the reader's opinion of the story. A sample list of positive and negative words in Exhibit 10.6 illustrates the power of adjectives; the same impact applies to oral presentations.

Important items to consider when issuing a press release are displayed in Exhibit 10.7. When faculty and doctoral students from the University of California, Los Angeles (UCLA), School of Nursing presented research findings and symposia at the distinguished Western Institute of Nursing annual conference in 2013, the institution issued a press release highlighting the work of UCLA scholars who are redefining the state of the science in women's and cardiovascular diseases as well as other topics affecting vulnerable populations (Perry, 2013). Advanced practice nurses can help prepare this type of press release as

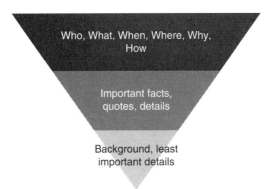

FIGURE 10.1 Journalism inverted pyramid.

content experts and authors of work being shared at conferences and research symposia. Also, as volunteers for professional organizations, nurses are well positioned to author press releases about news events, advisory or advocacy statements for pending legislation, or interpretation of health information of interest to the public. When sending a press release to a media outlet, additional materials such as a background paper or tip sheet may be used to convey facts on a subject and can provide more information than a brief press release.

Nursing organizations actively disseminate press releases on a variety of topics throughout the year to address issues from responses to tragic events; to notable events and funding awards; to congratulatory accolades; to expressing positions on issues of major import at the local, state, or national level depending on the scope and reach of the organization; and for recognition of major legislative victories. The ANA in the first half of 2013 had already issued over 35 press releases covering topics such as the U.S. Supreme Court ruling on marriage equity, release of the collaborative National Standards for Safe Patient Handling and Mobility, and applauding the confirmation of Centers for Medicare and Medicaid Services (CMS) administrator Marilyn Tavenner, to name a few. These can be viewed on NursingWorld (www.nursingworld. org/FunctionalMenuCategories/MediaResources/PressReleases), a site that is updated regularly. Other national nursing organizations routinely issue press releases to address major issues facing nursing, health care, and the well-being of the American public. A press release can also be used to "set the record straight" as was done by the AACN in January 2013 in response to an article published by Cable News Network (CNN) Money, offering an overly pessimistic view on new nursing graduate employment. AACN's press release (www.aacn.nche.edu/news/articles/2013/cnn-article) addressed factual errors and informed readers of more accurate sources of information. As a result, CNN amended the original article in less than 10 days and supplied new data from credible sources believed to be more accurate reflections of new graduates' job-seeking experiences.

EXHIBIT 10.6   POSITIVE AND NEGATIVE OPINION WORDS

POSITIVE WORDS	NEGATIVE WORDS
Acclaimed	Abysmal
Appealing	Angry
Beneficial	Callous
Courageous	Despicable
Distinguished	Difficult
Effective	Disastrous
Flourishing	Dishonest
Generous	Expensive
Impressive	Ill-conceived
Knowledgeable	Terrible
Quality	Tired
Respected	Unhappy
Successful	Unpleasant
Transformative	Weak

> **EXHIBIT 10.7   SAMPLE PRESS RELEASE CONTENTS**
>
> - Organization's name
> - Use letterhead if possible
> - Contact information
>   - Contact person
>   - Company name
>   - Phone and fax numbers
>   - E-mail address
>   - Website address
> - Headline—catchy
> - Release date
> - City, state, followed by lead sentence
> - Body of message
>   - Powerful introductory paragraph
>   - Quotes
>   - Organization "tag" (standard paragraph describing organization or goals highlighted in the release; may be in italics)
>   - Symbols indicating end of the release at bottom center of page
>   - For more than one page, use "—more—" at the bottom of the page and abbreviate headline at the top of the second page; repeat contact information at the end
>   - At the conclusion use "END" or "###" to indicate end of content

Press Advisories

Press advisories alert the media to a pending event. For example, an organization may want to invite the press to cover an upcoming convention. The International Council of Nurses (2013) issued a press invitation to secure coverage of the 2013 Quadrennial Congress in Australia and followed up with a press release announcing the meeting highlights 1 month in advance. A hospital or nursing school may want to alert the press to a release of research findings or innovations important to improving care. The announcement should be brief but arouse interest without exposing the whole story. Be sure to include the sponsor (who), subject (what), time (when), place (where), and relevance (why), as well as contact information. A press advisory may also ask media representatives to respond if they are planning to cover the event. If you have provided more than a week's advance notice, plan to send a follow-up message 1 to 2 days before your event. E-mail transmission is common for both press releases and advisories.

When sending information to media audiences via e-mail, limit the text to 500 words or about five paragraphs. Expert audiences will accept longer releases of one to two pages. Avoid sending the key information only in an attachment. Place a short headline in the subject line of the e-mail using the most important attention-grabbing words. Include URL links to additional information sources. Mirror the format of a press release. Both the advisory and the e-mail should begin with contact information followed by the headline and then body of the release. Do a test of your e-mail because formats may change with transmission.

When sending to multiple media representatives, place the names as blind copies so addresses are not shared without permission. Releases and advisories sent at slower business times will receiver greater attention. Aim for late morning.

Nurses rarely have difficulty establishing credibility. Despite the portrayal of inaccurate stereotypes on TV and other entertainment, the mainstream media recognizes and respects nurses' expertise. Academic degrees, certifications, and job titles convey a certain status and should be used when contacting the media. When representing an organization, pick an appropriate leader or spokesperson.

MESSAGE DELIVERY

Effective message delivery includes knowing your audience and their interest in your story, as well as how to deliver a message using a specific medium. Each of these media—written, voice, or visual—requires specific strategies to enhance policy impact.

Knowing Your Audience and When Your Story Is of Interest

Knowing the right medium for reaching the target audience guides media strategies. If you are taking your message to a broad audience, it may need to be tailored in several different ways to reach different groups. Questions to bear in mind for any audience include: What is important about this issue that someone should make others care? Of what interest is this to the targeted audience? What will capture the attention of this audience? Is it a friendly audience or one that bears convincing? What actions can I expect or request the audience to pursue? Is the timing right?

The reporter's or your target's response to a conversation with you can reveal if or when you have piqued their interest. According to Fitch and Holt (2012), immediate silence is not a good sign but an initial response of "Really?" means the reporter wants to hear more, and a "Wow" is promising for a print story and is your cue to get ready to respond with an interview or additional materials; a "Holy shit" is a top-drawer response that is almost a guarantee of a print coverage.

Policy Makers

Reaching local policy makers may require tracking down someone at a home or work address as they often fulfill public duties as a part-time responsibility. Reaching state and national policy makers may mean initially getting to their staff as the preferred communication route. Response times may vary. Federal officials have a chief of communication and dedicated communications staff, as well as issue-specific staff. Many have someone assigned to cover health care issues. The more potent your message, the greater likelihood policy makers will take note and listen. Successfully getting on the public's agenda will also almost ensure getting on a policy maker's agenda. The messages are synergistic for focusing attention on health issues and concerns that affect large constituencies. The typical vehicles for delivering your message to policy makers include letters, e-mails, opinion editorials, background papers, blogs, press releases, and published articles, all of which can be made available to the individual and their staff.

General Public

The use of broadcast media (both television—news and non-news—and radio), newsletters, newspapers, bulletin boards, and social media can reach the general public. Offering nursing's response to time-sensitive issues, or weighing in to a larger debate, can bring attention to nursing's interest in and viewpoints about public health issues and the welfare of the general public as well as nurses. While most consumers will have interest in nursing's message, it may be only situational and, thus, calls for aiming the message for broad appeal. Nurses should also weigh in on current events that relate to the public health and well-being in order to solidify nursing's role of advocacy in the eyes of the public. Issues like smoking cessation, gun violence, and legalization of marijuana have struck a chord and nurses, as opinion leaders, can provide a viewpoint that shapes local sentiment and brings the perspective of a trusted professional. Following the shootings in Newtown, Connecticut, in December 2012, the American Academy of Nursing (AAN) issued a statement expressing shared grief in the loss of innocent lives and provided practical guidance (www.aannet.org/pr-12-18-12-child-stress) for decreasing stress and anxiety for parents and children.

Public service announcements, or PSAs, are an effective way to spread your message at no cost to your organization. The announcement must benefit the community; most often, it is used to announce a nonprofit community event or service. The announcement can be in written form or presented in audio or visual format. If transmitted electronically, radio or television coverage is typically a short spot less than 1 minute in length. Similar to press releases, the PSA includes the typical who, what, where, when, and why.

Journalists

Most of the exposure we seek for delivering our message is through journalists. Press releases, letters to the editor, opinion editorials, e-mail communications, interviews, and media events target the health and general interest media with the intent to have our story published or broadcast. Multiple channels increase the odds of successfully disseminating your issue and opinions. Journalists are also relying more on social media as a source of information.

Delivering Your Message—Put It in Writing!

As previously discussed, written communication about an issue in your words or expressing the position of an organization is a simple tool that can deliver a powerful message. Written formats provide asynchronous contact and can be sent to multiple media sources at the same time to maximize coverage.

Letters to the Editor

Newspapers and journals accept letters that offer commentary on other published articles or issues of current interest. Letters are also used to respond to criticism, offer a different view on a recently covered topic, correct inaccuracies, or add interesting content to a recent story. A letter to the editor is simple and focuses on one key point. Plan on a short letter of about 150 words that succinctly describes your ideas; check the editorial specifications as the limit may vary. If referencing a previous article, include a brief explanation so readers will connect your letter with the original source. Send letters quickly and in close proximity to the event or article you are addressing. Include your name, address, telephone contact numbers, and e-mail for follow-up information.

See the letter to the editor of the *Courant* newspaper in Exhibit 10.8 written by a nurse practitioner asking for support for advance practice nurses.

Opinion Editorials

Op-eds appear *opposite* the editorial page in a paper and aim to evoke an emotional response from the reader. The targeted opinion piece opens with a strong statement or argument and offers a clear point of view. They can be used to persuade public sentiment or to defend a particular policy position. Op-eds are more successful when they are written about current issues that appeal to readers with an urgency for understanding and action. Tips for a successful op-ed are displayed in Exhibit 10.9.

Be sure to check the policies and submission guidelines for your chosen publication. Making contact with the editor to introduce yourself and your topic in advance may increase the likelihood of publication. For local publication, a strong association with a local angle will increase your editorial appeal. See the sample opinion article in Chapter 1, "Leading the Way in Policy."

Organizational Policy-Oriented Newsletters

Many different types of nursing groups use newsletters as an effective vehicle to reach a specific target audience. The content must match the target audience's interests and include items that are newsworthy. Newsletter contents should also follow the inverted pyramid style of an effective headline followed by the five W's and H, then the supporting information in descending order from most to least important. Newsletter design should focus on a primary issue and fulfill a need for information. A persuasive argument or point of view creates interest. Ensure the accuracy of the content to earn the trust of your audience. Hardcopy newsletters are becoming less common, giving way to electronic ones that arrive quickly and at a lower cost. Newsletters, in general, can be read asynchronously at someone's leisure, making them more effective than media such as radio, television, and social media where content is updated and older coverage may be available for only a few days.

Electronic newsletters require some additional preparation, including addressing visual display differences for electronic in-box formats, offering

---

EXHIBIT 10.8   LETTER TO THE EDITOR OF *THE COURANT,* HARTFORD, CT, MAY 24, 2013

LETTER: State Must Untie Advanced Practice Nurses' Hands

With 400,000 new patients expected to enroll in health insurance plans in Connecticut under the Affordable Care Act, it's imperative for the legislature to pass a measure to untie the hands of advanced practice registered nurses (APRNs) to allow them to keep the practices they currently have and provide an opportunity for other APRNs to start practices. APRNs are diagnosticians and prescribers in both psychiatric and primary care practices and other areas of medicine. In Connecticut since 1999, they have been able to establish practices and be responsible for their own patient care. But practices have actually closed, others are at risk, and still others are prevented from opening. The reason is old language in the APRN practice act that requires a written collaborative agreement with a physician for all APRNs except certified registered nurse anesthetists. This agreement does not require consultation, although collaboration is ongoing with specialists and physicians and other providers. In recent years, many APRNs have been unable to find physicians willing to sign such an agreement, and APRN practices cannot open or remain established without one.

The IOM, the National Governors' Association, and the Federal Trade Commission have all published reports recognizing such barriers and have urged states to change their laws so independent APRN practitioners are available to patients. To date, 18 other states have acted. It is time for Connecticut to do the same.

Lynn Rapsilber, Torrington (2013)

The writer is chairwoman of the Connecticut Coalition of
Advanced Practice Nurses.

Reprinted with permission from the *Hartford Courant.*

EXHIBIT 10.9   KEY POINTS FOR GETTING AN OP-ED PUBLISHED

- Provide author's credentials and expertise
- Develop a catchy title
- Incorporate data/statistics, expert testimony, or other resources
- Describe a personal story or analogy
- Create an engaging flow of ideas
- Close with a strong final sentence culminating the argument/position
- Limit reading time to under 5 minutes; 700 to 800 words

other versions such as HTML, and an opt-in process to receive the newsletter. Sending frequent electronic editions can increase your reputation as a top-of-mind source of information. The same format can be used to send special messages highlighting a release of distinct urgent information. Many professional organizations have electronic newsletters.

The ANA *SmartBrief* is an excellent example of an opt-in electronic newsletter for members addressing current newsworthy items with URL links to retrieve in-depth information. It offers an optimized mobile version of the newsletter as well as an in-box e-mail version. ANA members can sign up at www.nursingworld.org/Smart-Brief.aspx to receive this daily collection of handpicked news sources for current trends and issues; it is also offered to non-nurses at a small annual subscription fee.

Policy Briefs, Backgrounders, and Tip Sheets

A policy brief succinctly states a position. The target audience is policy makers who seek facts and arguments about an issue from trusted sources. A brief, as its name implies, is concise, and quickly conveys the important policy facts and implications, poses questions for policy makers to consider, and proposes arguments substantiating one's position on the issue. An effective policy brief is persuasive and well organized. The contents of a policy brief are addressed in Exhibit 10.10.

Issuing a policy brief on an emerging issue positions your organization as an opinion leader on a subject. For example, the AAN issued a brief to capture the attention of policy makers as well as influential stakeholders such as leaders at the CMS about the need for clear definitions of care coordination and transitional care. They also emphasized that reimbursement should be available for contemporary, evidence-based team–based models of care coordination that utilize the most appropriate caregiver as the leader based on a patient or family's needs; nurses can and are leading such models today. The brief, *The Imperative for Patient, Family, and Population Centered Interprofessional Approaches to Care Coordination and Transitional Care* (AAN, 2012), was shared widely throughout the nursing and health policy communities.

A media backgrounder addresses one topic and is written without bias. It usually includes a fact sheet with statistics, timeline of related events, contact information, and description of sources. Backgrounders should be no more than three to four pages, with facts appearing in an easily identifiable format such as bulleted notes so a reporter can easily identify salient points. Longer papers such as white papers, reports, or analyses are not expected to generate a rapid response. Tip sheets or fact sheets that provide either facts at a glance or

---

EXHIBIT 10.10 CONTENTS OF A POLICY BRIEF

- Introduction
  - Overview
  - Statement of the problem or objective
  - Argument or thesis
  - Clear statement of position
- Recommendations (placed at the beginning)
- History and relevant background
- Analysis
  - Critique of arguments, alternate viewpoints, and quality of evidence
  - Cite evidence that supports your thesis and recommendations
- Conclusion
  - Argument
  - Call for action
  - Summary statement

an exhibit that expands upon the contents of a policy brief are helpful materials that add depth to other formal statements.

The ANA provided a media backgrounder, toolkits, and multiple other resources about its campaign to protect nurses through improved needlestick safety and prevention. The materials for the press served a dual purpose of also educating nurses, other health care workers, employers, and policy makers as part of a well-orchestrated campaign to alleviate unnecessary and sometimes life-threatening sharps and needlestick injuries.

Consistent updating of tip sheets and fact sheets advances an ongoing agenda by having information at the ready when there are new developments around a current issue, or when an organization wants to refresh coverage of their position. Several organizations calling attention to the nursing workforce and other messages embodied in the recommendations of *The Future of Nursing* report provide information in the form of fact sheets easily accessible from websites. One example is Quick Sheet (http://campaignforaction.org/evidence/quick-facts), which is found at the Center to Champion Nursing in America (CCNA) website.

Letters, E-Mails, and Announcements

Letters and e-mails to public officials and other influential leaders also accomplish the goals of informing them of issues and opinions. Letters should be targeted, simple, and direct. It is best to use official letterhead for correspondence or construct professional-looking stationery for print or electronic transmission. Aim to impress your target audience by opening with a declarative statement that conveys your issue clearly. Bullet points and other punctuation that draw attention to your points, such as headings, underlines, and italics, are acceptable. Personalizing your message will be most effective. As with other forms of communication, be specific about the action you are requesting; create the opportunity for a response.

Delivering Your Message—Voice and Visuals

Live presentations provide the opportunity for powerful message delivery. With videography the message can be rebroadcast and quickly made available to remote audiences.

Images

Visual images can also help transmit a message that words alone cannot convey. Availability of portable high-quality still and video cameras has made the use of visual images an integral part of messaging today. Photographs are commonly used in newsletters, on websites, and in social media, as well as supplied to print media outlets. In the absence of live footage, television stations may also use still photos.

Obtaining permission with a signed photography/videography release form is essential for using pictures of individuals not associated with your organization. A professional photographer owns the copyright to photos and must grant permission for you or your organization to place the image on a website or reuse a photo. In addition to any required fees, the site or publication gives attribution to the photographer.

Speeches

Speeches at scheduled meetings may get the attention of a reporter with advance promotion of a well-known or important presenter or the announcement of breaking news. Reporting of controversial expert knowledge or revealing important findings also helps guarantee coverage. As with press conferences, advance materials will enable the reporter to judge the importance of covering your meeting. Typically nursing media representatives will cover a limited number of national meetings, but regional, state, and local meetings will draw fewer reporters in the absence of a high-profile speaker or topic.

Arranging time after a presentation for an invited speaker to grant interviews to the press can provide a personal angle and more in-depth content for a reporter. Seasoned speakers may or may not have honed their interview skills, so you would want to work with the interviewer to limit the subject matter to what was presented at the meeting and a specific area of expertise. Having your own spokesperson in attendance also allows for an additional perspective to represent your organization in the event there is a discrepancy with the speaker's comments and it is important to provide the distinction.

Organizations want to have experts at the ready for interviews of all types—live or taped, radio or television, and for print coverage. When a hot topic emerges, have your most articulate spokesperson available and prepared for impromptu or scheduled interviews. Many organizations maintain a speaker contact list or advertise a speaker's bureau. Consider signing up with your availability dates and times. Remember to keep your expertise and contact information up to date.

Interviews

The fastest way to circulate your information is on the radio. Not surprising, the best times are listening hours during morning and evening commutes (6 a.m.–10 a.m. and 4 p.m.–7 p.m.). The morning audience tends to be almost 3 times larger than afternoon. Radio interviews are usually short, less than 5 minutes; questions are direct and predictable—you can help shape them by talking with the radio show host in advance or sending in questions that address the topic you will discuss. Radio interviews can also be done over the phone. Television and the use of video add emotional intensity. Television, in particular, is part show as well as part content. Like radio, interviews can be live or taped. If live, being prepared to respond to an emerging issue is critical. If taped, there is typically more time to prepare and stage the interaction. Timely topics include connections to a current news story, or new development in health care or your organization.

Maintaining readiness and being available are critical to getting radio or television coverage as new topics and changes emerge. Scheduling appearances on live talk shows can reach a broad audience. Always remember to research your host so you can know the style of questioning and the audience. Different media offer different approaches to transmit your message. The most rapid form of traditional media dissemination is radio, followed by television and print. The Internet allows for combining the speed of broad transmission with inclusion of visual as well as print messages. The impact and attributes of each form are reviewed in Exhibit 10.11.

Preparing for an Interview

Securing a coveted interview carries the responsibility of keen preparation. Do your homework. Determine the reporter's questions in advance and understand his or her key areas of interest. Know what type of work your reporter has recently covered. For radio and television, know the name of the host, show, station, and any other guests who may be appearing with you. Listen in advance to anticipate the style of the interviewer, pace, format of the show, audience or call-in questions, and length of the segment.

Before the interview, review previous statements on your topic and be clear on positions. Select the best person to do the interview, someone who can speak with authority on the subject; that individual may have name recognition or a specific position identified with your organization. Work with the reporter or host to prepare the person who will do the interview. Write talking points and rehearse your messages, including sound bites. Write down and rehearse personal stories, anecdotes, and the answers to anticipated questions. Ideally, media personnel will try to be balanced; therefore, identifying the counterarguments to your issues and potential responses will enhance the interview. Remember, anything you say can be repeated on television, radio, or the newspaper, so you want to be well prepared. Offer a fact sheet with your sound bites and have additional background information prepared.

When working with a reporter, know the deadline. Offer a list of questions to the reporter you would like to have covered, and ask if the reporter will also provide you with a set of anticipated questions. It may be beneficial to establish

EXHIBIT 10.11   COMPARISON OF MEDIA TYPES

MEDIUM	ATTRIBUTES
Radio	Fast, local access to large audience; brief coverage of issue
Television	Impact visual adds to emotional force
Print	Longevity, depth, and ability to be archived
Internet	Convergence of all types of media on demand

the setting and time frame that works best for your spokesperson to be prepared and relaxed, taking into consideration any deadlines or schedule constraints.

During the interview, keep your responses short, clear, crisp, and remain calm. Never get defensive or angry. When responding to questions, state your main message as succinctly as possible followed by supporting points. Be enthusiastic. Use simple, easily understood language—no jargon or acronyms. Be comfortable with slight pauses between questions and resist the urge to fill in the silence as it may lead to regrettable statements made in haste. If you detect any inaccuracies on the part of a reporter or interviewer, you should politely make the correction. Don't be afraid to say, "I don't know" when it applies. If questions are negative, redirect the focus of the question saying something like, "The real question is …," and return to your main message on the issue.

Appearing on Camera

Television adds the dynamic of managing your appearance, voice, and overall impression with your audience. A successful on-camera interview appearance requires attention to appearance and actions. Standard rules of dress include keeping clothing simple and professional. Clinical attire such as scrub suits and laboratory coats are worn only in settings reflecting patient contact or in settings that are in immediate proximity to the event you are covering such as a disaster response or inhospital press event. For example, nurses caring for victims in the aftermath of the Boston Marathon bombings were interviewed at a local receiving hospital in scrub suits, laboratory coats, and with stethoscopes around their necks (ABC Action News, 2013). The video image conveyed a temporal proximity to the events as well as a sense of high-technology care brought to bear in this unthinkable emergency.

When appearing on television, show energy and enthusiasm, make purposeful eye contact, maintain good posture, use gestures appropriately, and speak clearly. More detailed guidelines are specified in Exhibit 10.12. Practice your interviewing skills by getting a colleague to videotape you or use your own smartphone or camera. As you watch your practice performance, look for positive motions, animation, comfortable posture, and good eye contact. Be sure you are not speaking too quickly and listen for clear enunciation of each word.

Press Conferences and Briefings

Press conferences, also called news conferences, are planned for the release of a significant story or development. When the RWJF and IOM PR staff planned the press conference to announce the report from *The Future of Nursing*, they planned for a complex set of leader presentations, printed media kits, live coverage on site plus streamed video, availability of web materials, and a high-profile location, the National Press Club. The long-awaited report in itself would have drawn media attention, but headlining the event with the prestigious leaders of the commission and sponsoring organizations guaranteed immediate widespread coverage.

EXHIBIT 10.12   GUIDELINES FOR APPEARING ON CAMERA

- Appearance
  - Dress simply and look professional
  - Wear solid blue shirts rather than white, gray, or brown
  - Avoid solid white, black, and large prints
  - Avoid flashy jewelry that would reflect in lights
  - Consider makeup usage
  - Scrubs, uniforms, or laboratory coats should be worn only if filming in a care setting

- Energy
  - Show energy and enthusiasm
  - Raise the volume of your voice up 15%

- Eye contact
  - Maintain direct eye contact as much as possible
  - Look at the interviewer, not into the camera (unless it is a camera-only interview)
  - Eyes should not be excessively blinking, darting, or staring

- Posture
  - Sit straight and lean slightly forward; never swivel in chair
  - Keep feet planted or cross legs at the ankles even though many views are of only the upper body
  - Position one foot slightly ahead of the other when standing to keep from rocking or swaying
  - Be aware of arms and hand positioning to avoid a defensive posture
  - Keep arms open when seated to convey energy

- Gestures
  - Control body language including facial expressions that could be misinterpreted
  - Avoid nervous gestures or mannerisms
  - Use arm and hand gestures strategically in live interviews
  - Smile but do not overdo with a forced expression
  - Don't clasp hands, which may convey closed attitude and nervousness

- Voice
  - Practice diaphragmatic breathing to deliver a fuller voice
  - Use careful diction to be understood
  - Speak at a pace that can be understood
  - Change inflection appropriately

- Interview responses
  - Deliver, then reinforce the key messages
  - Maintain truthfulness
  - Be respectful
  - Avoid being defensive

Press conferences are not always complex, but all require a compelling story and careful planning. In addition to respected speakers, audiovisuals can be used not only to help tell the story but also to seize the attention and emotions of the audience. Both positive and negative visuals can evoke a response. The palm-sized preterm infant, the injured accident patient saved from the clutches of death, and the handcuffed perpetrator of a crime are powerful symbols of the human condition. Whenever possible, include other participants in the press conference who will draw in your audience such as children, heroes, or favorite personalities.

Select a venue that supports the space for video cameras and reporters. Consider the need for adequate sound and lighting, depending on whether the medium is radio or television. Also, examine access to electrical outlets and allow for open space at the rear of the room for cameras. A podium and front table to accommodate all of the speakers sets the stage for the conference. Be careful the venue is not too large so that chairs remain empty—empty chairs send an inaccurate message of lack of interest. Popular venues include press clubs, hotels, public buildings, and settings that will highlight or complement the topic such as a clinic, hospital, neighborhood, or other location within easy access of media offices.

Schedule the event so it avoids any major holidays or conflicting popular local or regional events. The same schedule restraints affecting reports apply to press conferences. Best times are late morning (10 a.m.–12:00 p.m.) with Tuesdays, Wednesdays, and Thursdays being less busy.

E-mail or fax a media advisory several days prior to your event to secure greater participation. Be sure to have extra printed materials available. Preparing your presenters is fundamental to any public speaking. Maximize coverage of your own events by quickly posting video or audio and pictures on your website and reuse materials in other publications.

Specially planned briefings give journalists background information on an issue you want them to cover. The briefing will establish your role as a trusted source of information on an issue that captures the public's attention. The content can be used to identify an emerging issue, update any key developments on a current issue, or present organizational policies and positions. Briefings are usually informal and offer the chance to build relationships and rapport with media representatives.

Both briefings and press conferences imply that there is important information forthcoming. Keeping a briefing small allows reporters to ask questions meaningful to their particular media outlet. Press conferences by nature include a larger number of participants other than the press such as key stakeholders. Nurse practitioners in Florida, who held a press conference in 2012 to announce their endorsement for candidate Kim Kendall while she was running for election in House District 17, articulated key issues related to removing practice barriers such as broadening prescriptive authority that their candidate would support (Florida Nurse Practitioner Network, 2012). The conference served a dual purpose of educating other voters plus solidifying their voice of support for their chosen candidate.

Press conferences and briefings require careful planning, execution, and follow-up. Whether you are a seasoned PR professional or volunteer, following the tips in Exhibit 10.13 will help ensure a successful event.

EXHIBIT 10.13   TIPS FOR A SUCCESSFUL PRESS CONFERENCE

Initial planning
- Identify target media outlets/individuals
- Choose a strategic date and time
- Write the press advisory
- Select an accessible, familiar location
- Identify and secure speakers
- Schedule speaker lineup

Groundwork
- Pitch the event; send press advisory 1 to 2 weeks in advance
- Contact media outlets to determine attendance
- Prepare media kit materials
  - Press release
  - Background information
  - Speaker biographies
- Prepare on-site visuals (charts, photos, and slides) and precheck all equipment
- Confirm event venue setup

Hold the event
- Record the list of press in attendance
- Collect information from press representatives for post-event needs
- Distribute press release and/or full media kits on arrival

Same-day follow-up
- Post press release and related material on website
- Post video and provide links
- Follow up with response to reporters' additional needs
- Summarize coverage for future reference
- Appropriate written and verbal acknowledgments

Tracking
- Collect inventory of all media coverage
- Prepare final summary for archives

Adapted from Fitch and Holt (2012).

Disaster Recovery—When Bad News Happens

Tragedy, macabre events, and wrongdoing all capture media attention. It is disheartening when the story implicates one of our own. The darker side of nursing, when a nurse strays from his or her contract with society and intentionally inflicts harm, or when negligence or human error results in a sentinel event or near miss, becomes newsworthy. All too often reporters use the generic term *nurse* without more accurate identification of the qualifications of a person believed to have done harm or acted in a way unbecoming to a law-abiding professional. In years past, gut-wrenching stories have shocked the public and health care community, such as the case of serial killer and nurse Charles Cullen (Associated Press, 2006).

In November 2007, news of a 1,000 times overdose of heparin given to three babies at the renowned Cedars Sinai Hospital in Los Angeles hit the airwaves. Two of the babies were twin newborns of actor Dennis Quaid. Celebrity websites and national news picked up the story immediately. Fortunately, there was no long-term consequence of the heparin dose, but in response to the situation, Quaid became a champion for safety in health care. News of his children's medication error and his quest for improving health care safety followed him for months, dredging up the incident over and over. Appearances on *The Oprah Winfrey Show* and the cover of *AARP Magazine* also kept the story in the spotlight for 3 years. A year and a half after the event, Vice President and Chief Nursing Officer Linda Burnes Bolton met with Quaid to share the implementation of a barcode medication administration Cedars had installed (Nurse.com, 2009). Burnes Bolton accepted the event as a "wake-up call" and was able to demonstrate turning what could have been a devastating error into a learning event, which was the catalyst for implementing technology to make care safer.

When bad news happens, organizations must tell the truth, admit to mistakes, and express remorse (see Chapter 9, "Activating the Advocacy Plan"). Aim for full disclosure. The public and the organization want to get the facts straight and move on to repair and healing. Most negative stories are 1-day events. If prolonged, the multiday event, or one that spans months and years, can be trying for any organization and requires effective PR management. Handling negative stories is part of the skill set held by PR professionals. It is unpleasant and embarrassing to have to deal with patient abuse or harm, safety violations, or illegal behavior. If surprised by a negative issue raised by a reporter, remain calm and suggest you need time to check out the facts and respond. As you gather facts, be planning your strategy, which may include a brief written statement or an interview. Sometimes an independent third party is effective as a spokesperson who can defend the organization. If your group is truly in crisis management mode, a communication plan is essential and will vary based on the magnitude of the blunder.

When your organization experiences a crisis, leaders must inform their internal constituents as well as keep an open channel to the media. It is important to generate a response quickly and be prepared to define the event, say what you are doing to address the situation, and let others know if you need their help. Top leaders must be visible. In addition, identify a team of individuals capable of interacting with the media. Anticipate questions and prepare talking points. Integrate social media into your plan to keep a variety of constituents informed with frequent updates. Remember, your organization's values and ethics will be judged by your response.

INTERNET AND SOCIAL MEDIA

Electronic media have changed how we communicate with each other. Media provide numerous channels of communication and connectedness with our family, friends, peers, and communities. Each format has unique advantages and disadvantages. Each can be key in the policy process.

Internet and Websites

The Internet provides rapid access to an endless source of information. The Internet is the core structure that supports the World Wide Web (WWW or W3), the window to millions of sites across the globe. The WWW is an application supported by the Internet. WEB 2.0 describes the current version of the interactive WWW with access to a myriad of remote software. Also referred to as a social web, people are interacting through sites such as blogs, social networks, social news, and wikis. These social media tools are evolving and new ones are constantly being developed. They enable human interaction and are a place to tell your story, often on your own terms.

Your website address on the Internet serves as the anchor for information about you and your organization. Maintaining current information in various formats including stories, news updates, videos, photographs, and links to other resources secures your position as a source of information. Reporters, policy makers, other colleagues, rival organizations, and the public use the Internet to gather insights and critique what your organization represents and has to offer in terms of expertise and influential opinions. Kalisch, Begeny, and Neumann (2007) reviewed over 150 websites focused on nursing in 2004, comparing them to coverage in 2001, and found over 70% acknowledge nurses as intelligent and possessing specialized knowledge and skills. Sixty percent were positive with descriptions of nurses as trustworthy, competent, and accountable.

Many organizations have online communities that provide not only information, but also interaction through message boards, surveys, blogs, and links to other resources. ANA's NurseSpace (American Nurses Association, 2012) is an example of a community with both open and members-only content.

Social Media Tools

The Internet has made possible rapid communication, collaboration, and connections with others on a real-time basis. The digital communication platform of Web 2.0 offers tools to participate in active dialogue through user-generated content and sharing of personal as well as professional information. More and more organizations are finding the engagement in social media an important adjunct to the more static website-based information for the distribution of professional content. Given the diverse preferences for communication among generations, social media helps reach segments of audiences that may not follow traditional sources such as print materials.

The use of social media tools by health care organizations has been growing rapidly. Just 10 hospitals were using social media in 2006 compared with 762 in 2010 (Ressler & Glazer, 2010). Hospitals, associations, consumer groups, and many health care businesses have started using popular social media accounts such as Facebook and Twitter, placing icons on their web pages to link readers to their sites. Businesses may also use LinkedIn, a professional networking site, to provide news and updates about their work as well as encourage ongoing connections. For many of these sites, push e-mails direct readers or followers to visit the sites often to stay informed.

A media convergence revolution is in motion. More and more multiple platforms will be used together. Current and emerging tools will make information and interactive communication available from single sites where video, live streaming, the ability to toggle to social media links, chats, messaging, and static more traditional information will reside together on a single site. Already social media sites have formed partnerships to provide live streaming from traditional television sites, impacting immediate access to news that reaches a mobile multigenerational audience. Rapidly evolving technology makes information portable and its device agnostic, allowing the public to choose how and when they receive information whether from their smartphones while on the go or from the comfort of watching television in their homes.

The possibilities for policy applications are endless. Nurses can employ these converged techniques when reaching coworkers, student groups, public gatherings, or association members. When planning strategies to promote a policy, nurses are challenged to consider new methods that increase your reach to target audiences locally, nationally, and even globally. Nurses planning for the future will consider technology changes an essential component. Facebook, Twitter, blogs, Really Simple Syndication or Rich Site Summary (RSS) feeds, and (QR) codes are some of the current popular free tools that have revolutionized real-time information sharing with the public.

Facebook

Started in 2004, Facebook connects people with other individuals or businesses (Facebook for Business). Boasting more than 1 billion users, businesses are sharing news, photos, and promotions with their followers. The primary use of Facebook in health care is for casual connection and information sharing, as it makes posting of messages, photos, and videos easy. However, an example of using Facebook to change policy is the Obesity Action Coalition's (OAC, n.d.) efforts to remove the restriction on Boy Scouts who are obese from participating in the 2013 National Jamboree. As previously noted, it is also useful to advertise events. However, many hospitals have Facebook pages as well as nursing organizations.

Twitter

Twitter, considered a micro-blogging service, is a vehicle to connect with other people and share timely news, opinions, and updates. The focus of Twitter is on the message. It may be personal opinion posted as blast communication that can contain as many as 140 characters, or photos and links can be sent via this medium, also. Regular media sources use Twitter as an additional means of drawing attention to stories, people, and connecting with audiences on the go. When you sign up to access a Twitter account, you become a "follower." Twitter posts are sourced in major search engines allowing access to real-time information. Just as is true with other blogs, one must consider the value of the source. Some popular nursing Twitter feeds include the ANA Government Affairs and *NursingWorld* Twitter feeds (twitter.com/nursingworld) and *American Nurse Today* (twitter.com/AmerNurse2day).

Twitter has many uses such as updating followers on an ongoing event or issue. Rapidly sharing information on critical issues (e.g., drug safety alerts, potential epidemic developments, or emerging disasters) is another benefit. Health care providers can also tweet to their patients and other followers about new developments in care or reminders about self-care. The use of Twitter for health policy is burgeoning.

Blogs

Blogs may have a broad or narrow topic focus or be issue specific. Blogs mirror the historic model of one voice, one view on an issue. You can either pitch a blogger to cover your content or offer your own blog. The author/writer, or blogger, can do a deeper dive on issues and needs to be ready as the content expert to answer tough questions. While most bloggers usually have expertise on a subject, nothing requires a blogger to be an expert; the follower will need to differentiate the credible expert from an individual who proliferates a dialogue with opinion only and not verified facts.

The number of blogs is growing exponentially. Bloggers want to attract interest to their topics and opinions on a regular basis, bringing loyal followers to a website. They can repurpose content as well, adding their own perspectives. Frequent updating is expected in order to attract new visitors and maintain repeat visitors to a blog website. Bloggers must heed the caution not to rant or face loss of credibility and interest among readers. With reliable facts, blogs can be a trusted source of information about nursing and health care (see Policy on the Scene 10.2).

RSS Feeds

RSS feeds began in 2000. News aggregators collect and download information to your e-mail inbox. As a receiver of information, you subscribe to selected feeds by using a RSS reader on your computer that allows downloading and display of the feeds. Typically you would want the latest headlines or pertinent information about subjects you routinely follow such as health policy, nursing practice, health care reform, or a specialty area. RSS feeds specifically allow you to get information effortlessly and read it at your leisure. As a generator of information, you can maximize traffic to your website by supplying your headlines to aggregator sites, which in turn send information to all their subscribers. You can also use programs to create an RSS feed for your website. Constructing the feed to place your website content into RSS syndication starts with preparing a list of content articles, including headlines, the URL, and brief description. This information is put into a simple XML file, the language used for RSS format. Submit the file to a service that makes content available to other users. Once approved, commit to regular updates of your content and know how often the service refreshes its feeds.

RSS feeds are a quick and easy source that alleviates the need to manually search sites for all the latest news and information on popular topics. Symbols indicating that an RSS feed is available are depicted in an orange box and may be either the sound wave graphic, XML depicting the language, or letters RSS.

QR Codes

A "QR" code is a type of two-dimensional barcode read with a special application on smartphones and some tablets. Originally developed for marketing, QR codes have become a tool used for social media that can be used to connect people in ways that have not been fully explored. The code can provide access to prewritten text, connect to a website, send an e-mail or a text message, and receive a telephone number or make a call. The codes have a characteristic square pattern arrangement of modules. Codes can appear anywhere a user might want to seek more information such as magazines, signs, giveaways at meetings, flyers, and any print materials.

Providing QR codes on your organization's materials that link to information important to policy makers is one way to take advantage of this technology. As you prepare briefs, backgrounders, and policy briefs, organizations can create their own QR code to link back to more issue-specific information on their websites. *The American Nurse, Clinical Psychiatry News*, and other publications now include QR codes. Another easy way to provide a link for policy makers to information about you and your organization is to provide a QR code on the back of your business card.

The ubiquitous nature of smartphones makes it essential that organizations think about using this technology for quick linkages and recovery of information. QR code readers are available as free smartphone applications, as is a QR code generator to create your own code. Free programs for both readers and generators are easily found using a web search.

The College of Health and Human Development at Penn State designed QR codes for patients and families to contact hospital officials in the moment regarding their experiences both positive and negative. The "Real-Time Care Experience Feedback" project helps patients express concerns as well as to receive immediate answers and follow-up from hospital staff (Penn State, 2012). Improving the patient experience is expected to help hospitals when patients rate them on satisfaction surveys that contribute information evaluated as part of CMS's value-based purchasing program. Another potential use is placing QR codes on equipment that links to related policies and procedures.

POLICY ON THE SCENE 10.2: Story of a Nurse Blogger
Theresa Brown, PhD, RN, Blogger

I started writing regularly for the *New York Times* blog called "Well" in 2009. My writing experiences for the *Times* provide useful lessons for any nurse wanting to write/blog for a larger audience. Nurses writing their stories and opinions matter because our profession needs more national visibility to affect health care policy. Blogging about "working short" or an injury from lifting a heavy patient gives face and voice to policy initiatives such as guaranteed staffing and safe patient handling laws. For the public to care about nurses' concerns, we need to make them real. Writing can do that.

When I began writing about nursing I felt I had a mission: to educate the public about what nurses really do. I might say then that the first rule of writing about your work as a nurse is to have a goal. You could aim to educate people, give voice to patient struggles, make sense of our chaotic health care system, or all three at once, but know why you want to write. Having a purpose beyond the merely personal will keep you motivated.

The second rule of writing about your work as a nurse is, tell the truth about your experience without breaking the law. We all know what the Health Insurance Portability and Accountability Act (HIPAA) is. Never include protected health information (PHI) in a blog post. You can disguise a patient's body type, age, diagnosis, and even gender, depending on what information is central to your story.

The third rule of nurse blogging is, don't worry about the size of your audience. Nursing is historically underrepresented in mass media and often inaccurately represented in popular media, so any writing about nursing that is well intended and true makes real nursing more visible to the public. If you maintain a blog and the only three people who read it are your mom, your first-grade teacher, and your best friend, those three people will know a lot more about nursing than they used to, thanks to your writing.

Motivated by policy concerns, I recently made the switch to writing for the Opinionator blog at the *Times*. In my Opinion columns I've considered the dangers of physician bullies ("Physician Heel Thyself," May 7, 2011), how misguided it is to use patient satisfaction scores as indicators of quality ("Hospitals Aren't Hotels," May 14, 2012), and whether there really is a July effect (July 14, 2012).

Special Uses of Social Media

Social media (e.g., Facebook, Twitter, RSS feeds, and QR codes) can be used to announce and publicize an event such as inviting participation in a flash mob. While the term *flash mob* usually connotes inclusion of impromptu music and dance, a simple Twitter mob can be formed to spread a message and come together for public awareness. Flash mobs have been used to support fund-raising events, recognize cancer survivors, raise awareness of a cause, and assemble demonstrations such as protesting the closure of a Long Island Hospital in New York (News 12 Brooklyn, 2013).

Challenges for Using Social Media in the Workplace

Many organizations have adopted policies to direct appropriate use of social media to protect the patients, staff, and institution. Protecting patient confidentiality, adhering to laws governing privacy, and maintaining appropriate patient–professional boundaries are typical areas addressed in policy. Numerous organizations around the world have issued guidelines about the use of social media, stressing how to avoid problems (ANA, 2011b; Barry & Hardiker, 2012; National Council of State Boards of Nursing, 2011).

Organizations have invoked policies to protect patients, staff, and their reputations. As with any new medium, a few individuals have abused it and some have used social media without understanding its implications. As a result, some policies have been overly restrictive and have not allowed people to explore the potential positive uses of social media. Following accepted guidelines and etiquette for proper communication, as well as being tech savvy, will lead to effective use of social media such as Facebook and Twitter.

OPTION FOR POLICY CHALLENGE: Implementing *The Future of Nursing* Report Recommendations

Following release of *The Future of Nursing* report in 2010, RWJF engaged the CCNA to shoulder the implementation of a national campaign to create momentum for policy change and solidify the long-term impact of enacting the recommendations of the report with creation of the Campaign for Action (2013). The campaign boasts 51 state action coalitions comprising state and local stakeholders. Together with numerous partners, the coalitions are aggressively promoting diversity, strengthening workforce data, removing practice barriers, promoting interprofessional collaboration, and enhancing academic progression in nursing. The campaign is generating a steady stream of success stories across the country.

Through a well-orchestrated multimedia strategy, the campaign is spreading news of the implementation of *The Future of Nursing*'s recommendations on a regular basis. Coalition members, supporting organizations and partners, together with RWJF and the AARP, maintain a robust website with dashboards, essential information, links to news coverage and events, fact sheets, resource directories, and an online community. A vital toolkit for communications includes resources for strategic planning and communication, as well as guides for working with social media, developing effective media materials, letters to the editor, opinion editorials, and general media outreach strategies. These guides are referenced in the E-Resources section of the chapter.

Almost 3 years after its release, *The Future of Nursing* report continues to hold the record for the most downloads from the IOM site. Implementation of the report recommendations is having a profound effect on nursing and health care. To implement these recommendations, individual nurses must take action. Nurses can have spin-off conversations in blogs, letters to the editor, and use social media among other strategies to catapult action and reaction back into the limelight with each new feat whether it is a skirmish or success story.

IMPLICATIONS FOR THE FUTURE

Without question, the use of media has changed people's behavior. What is critical for the future is taking advantage of media advocacy to influence not only individual behaviors, but also public policy that creates social change. Studies about social media have primarily focused on increased use and not effect. Nurses and others can study the implications of using media to influence public opinion, health policy, and legislation. Further work is needed by nurses as new media is developed to envision ways that it can be used to promote policy and advance nurses' roles in advocacy.

In perusing the Internet for illustrations of nurses in the media, there is a noticeable presence of union activity, feel-good congratulatory stories, and notices of new educational programs. Nurses also have a responsibility to proliferate stories, photos, videos, and electronic links to content describing the expertise and efforts of nurses to advance health policy issues. Every letter, background paper, policy brief, and presentation that addresses a current issue should be converted into media that is shared, archived, and repurposed. Taking advantage of the media means greater exposure of nursing's views and builds support for nursing's role in advancing health care policy.

KEY CONCEPTS

1. Nurses can use the media to reach a broader audience and establish a presence in the community.

2. Nurses have a responsibility to convey their vision, current thinking, and opinions to stimulate actions to effect better policies that serve our communities and nation.

3. Media advocacy combines mass communication with community advocacy.

4. Media advocacy includes working with the media to have your message heard, advance opinions about issues, and influence policy decision makers.

5. Working with the media includes cultivating long-term relationships with their representatives.

6. The "Got Me" approach—goal, objective, target, audience, message, and evaluation— can be used to guide media advocacy.

7. Message content needs to be short, concise, provide key details, and define the main issue using no more than three themes of underlying support.

8. Effective messages may include case statements, talking points, the "pitch," and a sound bite.

9. Responding to media representatives includes preparation on the who, what, when, where, why, and how of the story and preparing important facts and background using a format known as the journalism inverted pyramid.

10. Standardized formats for press releases and press advisories help in getting attention for a policy issue.

11. Messages should be specifically crafted for a target audience, which may include policy makers, the general public, and journalists.

12. Letters to the editors, opinion editorials, organizational policy-oriented newsletters, policy briefs, backgrounders, tip sheets, letters to policy makers, and announcements can all be used to garner support for an issue.

13. Careful orchestration of events such as press conferences can maximize their impact.

14. An effective disaster recovery plan can help mitigate the impact of a negative event.

15. Effective use of social media has the potential to maximize influence on policy makers.

16. Use of multiple media modalities can maximize the impact of media advocacy efforts, which has the potential to change the power differential in communities.

17. Nurses' use of media advocacy has the potential to change the power differential in communities.

SUMMARY

Media advocacy is a vital tool that can change the power differential for nursing and health in our communities and across the national landscape. Nurses, more than ever before, are recognizing the importance of working with the media to advance their messages and positions and are stepping up efforts to use traditional as well as nontraditional forms of media. A comprehensive plan is critical for bringing an issue to the public's attention, and then shepherding the crusade for desired policy outcomes through systematic efforts using all types of media communications.

Nurse leaders, together with their employers, professional associations, academic partners, and community organizations, can advance their views and positions through organized efforts to reach out to the media on a consistent basis. It is important to cultivate relationships with media representatives, make periodic contact to raise issues, provide background information, stand ready to address emerging issues, and give advance notice of developments important to the community related to nursing and health care. The same strategies for cultivating relationships with media representatives can be used to develop relationships with PR staff within one's organization.

Nurse leaders have a responsibility to learn the skill set needed for working with the media. Combining knowledge of media advocacy, ability to express ideas in writing and oral presentations, as well as use of current and emerging Internet and other social networking resources can have a profound impact on influencing local policies as well as more comprehensive national policy and politics.

LEARNING ACTIVITIES

1. Retrieve a set of talking points from a nursing organization. Assess the ways the media has covered the topic since the release of the talking points. Critique the impact of the talking points on the current state of the issue. Consider whether multiple nursing organizations have issued similar talking points.
2. Analyze positive and negative words used in coverage of a current health issue in a local, state, or national newspaper (print or electronic). Rewrite two to three paragraphs using your own selection of words.
3. Retrieve an electronic health policy–oriented newsletter. Critique the contents to assess: Is the story newsworthy? Do the authors use the inverted pyramid or other writing style?
4. Using Exhibit 10.10, critique a recent policy brief. What are its strengths? How could it have been improved?
5. Select a previously published issue or current health care concern and submit a letter to the editor of a newspaper of your choice. Indicate the rationale for your selected paper.

6. Write an elevator speech about why you believe nurses should be leaders in transforming health care. Share it in small groups, electronically or in person; offer critique.
7. Write a press release for an organization that is holding a conference to release evidence-based practice recommendations that will improve care.
8. Identify at least five media outlets (either local, state, or national) and the contact person for each.

E-RESOURCES

- American Nurse Today. http://www.americannursetoday.com/blogs
- American Nurses Association NurseSpace. http://www.ananursespace. org/ANANURSESPACE/BlogsMain/Blogs
- American Nurses Association Social Networking Principles Toolkit. http://www.nursingworld.org/FunctionalMenuCategories/AboutANA/ Social-Media/Social-Networking-Principles-Toolkit.aspx
- Berkeley Media Studies Group Resources: Media Advocacy 101. http:// www.bmsg.org/resources/media-advocacy-101
- Disruptive Women in Health Care. http://www.disruptivewomen.net
- E-Advocacy Summit. http://www.eadvocacy.org/aboutus.html
- Future of Nursing Campaign for Action. Communications Tools. http:// campaignforaction.org/resource/communications-tools
- HealthWorks Collective. http://healthworkscollective.com
- Institute of Medicine. *The Future of Nursing Leading Change, Advancing Health* [Press release]. http://www.iom.edu/Reports/2010/ The-Future-of-Nursing-Leading-Change-Advancing-Health/ Report-Release.aspx
- Kaiser Family Foundation Health Policy Communications. http:// www.kaiseredu.org/Tutorials-and-Presentations/Health-Policy-and- Communications.aspx
- Nurse.com. http://blog.nurse.com
- On the Spot Media Training and Coaching. http://www.onthespot mediatraining.com
- Theresa Brown, Opinionator, *The New York Times*. http://opinionator. blogs.nytimes.com/author/theresa-brown
- Theresa Brown, RN. http://www.theresabrownrn.com

REFERENCES

ABC Action News. (2013, April 7). *Local nurse treated Boston bomb victims* [YouTube video]. Retrieved from http://www.youtube.com/watch?v=5HukObcWGjk

American Academy of Family Physicians. (2010, October 5). *Talking points for responding to the IOM's report on the future of nursing*. Retrieved from http://azafp.org/wp-content/ uploads/2010/10/talkingpointsiomnp.pdf

American Academy of Nursing. (2012). *The imperative for patient, family, and population centered interprofessional approaches to care coordination and transitional care*. Retrieved from

http://www.aannet.org/assets/docs/PolicyResources/aan_care%20coordination_3.7.12_
email.pdf

American Association of Colleges of Nursing. (2010, October 5). *AACN applauds the new
IOM repo*rt [Web press release]. Retrieved from http://www.businesswire.com/news/
home/20101005006711/en/AACN-Applauds-Institute-Medicine-Report-Calling-
Transformational

American Association of Colleges of Nursing. (2013, January). *AACN responds to CNN
article on the employment of new nurses.* Retrieved from http://www.aacn.nche.edu/
news/articles/2013/cnn-article

American Association of Nurse Practitioners. (2012). *Nurse practitioners and the future
of primary care, and nurse practitioners and the future of primary care: Talking points.*
Retrieved from http://www.aanp.org/component/content/article/82-legislation-regulation/
policy-toolbox/np-policy-essentials/445-aanp-and-the-np-roundtable-joint-statements

American Medical Association. (2010, October 5). *AMA responds to IOM report on future
of nursing* [Web news]. Retrieved from http://www.ama-assn.org/ama/pub/news/news/
nursing-future-workforce.page

American Nurses Association. (2011a). *Fighting for nurses who speak up for patients* [Video].
Retrieved from http://www.nursingworld.org/FunctionalMenuCategories/AboutANA/
Nursing-Video-Gallery/Fighting-for-Nurses-Who-Speak-Up-for.html

American Nurses Association. (2011b). *Principles for social networking and the
nurse.* Retrieved from http://www.nursingworld.org/MainMenuCategories/
ThePracticeofProfessionalNursing/NursingStandards/ANAPrinciples.aspx

American Nurses Association. (2012). *ANANURSESPACE* [Online community]. Retrieved
from http://www.ananursespace.org/Home/?ssopc=1

Associated Press. (2006, 2 March). *Nurse who killed 29 sentenced to 11 life terms* [NBCnews.
com]. Retrieved from http://www.nbcnews.com/id/11636992/ns/us_news-crime_and_
courts/t/nurse-who-killed-sentenced-life-terms

Barry, J., & Hardiker, N. (2012, September 30). Advancing nursing practice through social
media: A global perspective. *OJIN: The Online Journal of Issues in Nursing, 17*(3),
Manuscript 5. doi:10.3912/OJIN.Vol17No03Man05. Retrieved from http://www.
nursingworld.org/MainMenuCategories/ANAMarketplace/ANAPeriodicals/OJIN/
TableofContents/Vol-17-2012/No3-Sept-2012/Advancing-Nursing-Through-Social-
Media.html

Campaign for Action. (2013). *Future of Nursing™ Campaign for Action at the Center to
Champion Nursing in America.* Retrieved from www.campaignforaction.org

Chen, P. (2010, November 18). *Nurses' role in the future of health care* [Web health views].
Retrieved from http://www.nytimes.com/2010/11/18/health/views/18chen.html?_r=0

Ensign, J. (2011, July 10). *Nurses and advocacy: Working with the med*ia [Web blog post].
Retrieved from http://josephineensign.wordpress.com/2011/07/10/nurses-and-advocacy-
working-with-the-media

Facebook. (2014). Homepage. Retrieved from https://www.facebook.com

Fitch, B., & Holt, C. J. (Eds.). (2012). *Media relations handbook for government, associations,
nonprofits and elected officials* (2nd ed.). Alexandria, VA: TheCapitol.Net.

Florida Nurse Practitioner Network. (2012, July 29). *St. Johns County press conference* [You-
Tube video]. Retrieved from http://www.youtube.com/watch?v=xx4A6ln30yo

Institute of Medicine. (2010a). *The future of nursing: Focus on nursing education* [Report
Brief]. Retrieved from http://www.iom.edu/Reports/2010/The-Future-of-Nursing-
Leading-Change-Advancing-Health/Report-Brief-Education.aspx

Institute of Medicine. (2010b). *The future of nursing: Focus on scope of practice* [Report Brief]. Retrieved from http://iom.edu/Reports/2010/The-Future-of-Nursing-Leading-Change-Advancing-Health/Report-Brief-Scope-of-Practice.aspx

Institute of Medicine. (2010c). *The future of nursing, leading change, advancing health* [Report Brief]. Retrieved from http://iom.edu/Reports/2010/The-Future-of-Nursing-Leading-Change-Advancing-Health/Report-Brief.aspx

Institute of Medicine. (2010d). *The future of nursing, leading change, advancing health. Report recommendations* [HTML document]. Retrieved from http://iom.edu/Reports/2010/The-Future-of-Nursing-Leading-Change-Advancing-Health/Recommendations.aspx

Institute of Medicine. (2010e) *Health care reform and increased patient needs require transformation of nursing practice* [Press release]. Retrieved from http://www.nationalacademies.org/onpinews/newsitem.aspx?RecordID=12956

Institute of Medicine. (2011). *The future of nursing. Leading change, advancing health.* Washington, DC: National Academies Press. Retrieved from http://www.nap.edu/catalog.php?record_id=12956

International Council of Nurses. (2013, April 18). *Thousands of nurses to gather in Melbourne to increase equity and access to healthcare* [Press Release]. Retrieved from http://www.icn.ch/images/stories/documents/news/press_releases/2013_PR_03_Congress_opens.pdf

Kalisch, B. J., Begeny, S., & Neumann, S. (2007). Image of the nurse on the Internet. *Nursing Outlook, 55*(4), 182–188.

McDonald, L. (2006). *Florence Nightingale and public health policy: Theory, activism and public administration.* Retrieved from http://www.uoguelph.ca/~cwfn/nursing/theory.htm

National Council of State Boards of Nursing. (2011). *White paper: A nurse's guide to the use of social media.* Retrieved from https://www.ncsbn.org/2930.htm

News 12 Brooklyn. (2013, 21 June). *Long Island College hospital doctors, nurses form flash mob to demand hospital stay open* [Video news]. Retrieved from http://brooklyn.news12.com/news/long-island-college-hospital-doctors-nurses-from-flash-mob-to-demand-hospital-stay-open-1.5543828

Nurse.com. (2009, March 23). *Cedars-Sinai CNO addresses medical errors on* The Oprah Winfrey Show. Retrieved from http://news.nurse.com/apps/pbcs.dll/article?AID=2009303230023

Obesity Action Coalition. (n.d.). Obesity Action Coalition is on Facebook. Retrieved from https://www.facebook.com/ObesityActionCoalition

Pagana, K. D. (2013). Ride to the top with a good elevator speech. *American Nurse Today, 8*(3). Retrieved from http://www.americannursetoday.com/article.aspx?id=10086&fid=10018

Pennsylvania State University, College of Health and Human Development. (2012). Penn State team's QR code wins REACH Challenge. [Press Release]. Retrieved from http://www.hhdev.psu.edu/news/2012/MHA-REACH-Challenge.html

Perry, L. (2013). *UCLA nursing research on women and heart disease among key topics at nursing conference.* Retrieved from http://newsroom.ucla.edu/portal/ucla/gender-science-in-heart-disease-244990.aspx

Rapsilber, L. (2013, May 24). Letter: State must untie advanced practice nurses hands. *Hartford Courant.* Retrieved from http://articles.courant.com/2013-05-24/news/hcrs-15026hc--20130520_1_aprns-practices-affordable-care-act

Ressler, P., & Glazer, G. (2010, October 22). Legislative: Nursing's engagement in health policy and healthcare through social media. *OJIN: The Online Journal of Issues in Nursing, 16*(1). doi:10.3912/OJIN.Vol16No01LegCol01. Retrieved from http://www.nursingworld.org/MainMenuCategories/ANAMarketplace/ANAPeriodicals/OJIN/

TableofContents/Vol-16-2011/No1-Jan-2011/Health-Policy-and-Healthcare-Through-Social-Media.html

Tri-Council for Nursing. (2010, October 14). *Tri-Council for nursing calls for collaborative action in support of the IOM's future of nursing report* [Press release]. Retrieved from http://www.prweb.com/releases/2010/10/prweb4655424.htm

The Truth About Nursing. (2009). October, November, and December 2009. *News on nursing in the media.* Retrieved from http://www.truthaboutnursing.org/archives/2009/oct_nov_dec.html

Wallack, L., & Dorfman, L. (1996). Media advocacy: A strategy for advancing policy and promoting health. *Health Education Quarterly, 23*(3), 293–317.

Watman, J. (2010, December 7). *The future of nursing/the future of the IOM report* [Health Agenda]. Retrieved from http://www.jhartfound.org/blog/the-future-of-nursingthe-future-of-the-iom-report

Winett, L., & Wallack, L. (1996). Advancing public health goals through the mass media. *Journal of Health Communication, 1,* 173–196.

ELEVEN

Applying a Nursing Lens to Shape Policy

Joanne Disch
Mathew Keller
Eileen Weber

There are thousands of opportunities for nurses to be connected to policy-making groups where they can make a difference for patients at a committee or board level. If they don't do it, someone else will.—Susan Hassmiller

OBJECTIVES

1. Examine how the intersection between policy, politics, and nursing impacts practice.
2. Analyze the essential features of a nursing lens as applied to policy.
3. Identify ways a nursing perspective can aid policy development and implementation.
4. Describe skills essential for formal and informal policy involvement.

Policy is "the deliberate course of action chosen by an individual or group to deal with a problem" (Anderson, 2006). Policies exist at unit (microsystem), organizational, and societal levels. They are developed through processes that are individually driven or collectively based. They can address social issues, organizational effectiveness, or health. Up to this point, the role of nurses in policy development and implementation at all three of these levels has been inconsistent. Donna Shalala (2012, p. 3) notes, "Health reform will only be achieved if nurses are unrelenting in pursuing their rightful place in policy leadership in partnership with others who are also committed to accessible, safe, effective, and equitable health care."

In early days, nurse leaders advocated for better health care for the public and established policies for the effective running of health care systems, whether they were field hospitals or community centers. Florence Nightingale created change through "behind-the-scenes management of the committees and doctors" and skillful persuasion through her correspondence with influential people. Nursing leaders who followed, such as Katharine Densford (1890–1978),

359

advised presidents on expanding nursing capacity (the Cadet Nurse Corps), creating innovative programs of education for nurses in universities, and working to advance professional nursing through her presidency of the American Nurses Association (ANA) as it voted to support collective bargaining and to integrate Black nurses into its membership. There is growing evidence of nursing influence on public policy, as reflected by nurses leading national organizations and advancing public policy in state and national legislatures. Additionally, nurses are increasingly assuming positions as senior leaders within their own organizations. Yet there are many more opportunities for nurses to be more actively involved, and their absence not only diminishes nursing's impact but also results in suboptimal policy outcomes.

The purpose of this chapter is to examine the intersection among policy, politics, and nursing, and to identify ways in which the particular contributions of a nursing perspective can aid policy development and implementation. The concept of "the nursing lens" will be used as a framework throughout the chapter, and numerous examples of the impact of this lens will be provided. The following Policy Challenge illustrates how a nurse in a non-nursing position uses her nursing lens to work with others at the national level to deal with a high-profile health issue.

POLICY CHALLENGE: Nursing Lens Helping People Understand and Support Complex Federal Legislation

In 2003, President Bush signed into law the Medicare Prescription Drug, Improvement, and Modernization Act (also called the Medicare Modernization Act or MMA), the largest overhaul of Medicare in the public health program's 38-year history. It passed by a close margin, was bipartisan, and yet was bitterly divisive for its proponents and opponents. The national board of AARP, formerly known as the American Association for Retired Persons, voted to support this bill after intense dialogue, substantial briefings, and numerous educational sessions. At the time, I (JD) was a member of the board. In fact, AARP aggressively promoted its passage, which angered many of its members. Approximately 50,000 AARP members resigned their membership, numerous members publicly ripped up their membership cards, and many others wrote scathing, sometimes threatening, e-mails and letters to the board and staff.

However, the vote to support the legislation was just the beginning of the board's work.

It was incumbent upon us to go out and meet with the public in town hall meetings, listen, hear their anger and concerns, and explain why the board had supported this controversial legislation. Several of these meetings were held with largely antagonistic audiences who felt that they were losing something. In actuality, much was being gained by the public, but it was difficult to understand. Facing audiences who are antagonistic, hostile, frustrated, and angry is something that many nurse leaders have had to do within their own organizations or professional associations. Several key points have to be remembered.

1. In situations such as this, the reaction is rarely personal but arises more out of fear, ignorance, misunderstanding, or other political reasons.
2. Listening carefully to what people are saying is crucial. Refrain from responding quickly with an answer or retort.
3. Periodically sum up what you are hearing to let the audience know that you understand the issue(s) from their point of view.
4. As best you can, prepare ahead of time for what issues you will hear and what might be possible compromises or solutions.
5. Speak simply in terms and words that the audience can understand.
6. Be honest in terms of what the change can accomplish. Acknowledge where there may be unresolved issues or work still to be done.
   See Option for Policy Challenge.

POWER TO INFLUENCE: POLITICS

United and armed with solid data and a common goal, this story shows how a nurse can use sizable influence to educate and shape opinions on major health policies in our country. The AARP board had power and they used it proactively to help get support for making major changes to Medicare for the first time in 38 years. Power is essential to influencing those around nurses, including patients and colleagues.

"Powerless nurses are ineffective nurses ..." (Manojlovich, 2007). Studies have shown that powerlessness is associated with several poor outcomes for nurses and patients alike. Power is essential for politics. Indeed, in its broadest and most informal definition politics "is the practice and theory of influencing other people on a civic or individual level."

Politics is a word derived from the Greek word *politikos* ("of, for, or relating to citizens") (Politics, n.d.). This term began to be used in English in the mid-15th century. Politics is not a dirty word: It is a misunderstood word. It is often the butt of jokes of comedians and late-night talk show hosts and often conjures up images of bipartisanship, finger pointing, and distortion of facts. More narrowly and formally defined, politics refers to the skills and techniques used to run government. Both definitions of politics are applicable to nursing. In this chapter, understanding the nurse's role both informally and formally is highlighted.

Every day nurses work to influence individuals. Talking with patients who have a poor prognosis, with students who are struggling in class, or with employees who are receiving negative feedback are just a few examples of the complex conversations where nurses exert influence. The skill sets to intervene in these work situations are learned and honed throughout our nursing careers.

The work of "influence" is a necessary political skill that can be cultivated and honed much like the skills used in working with patients, students, and employees. Yet these latter skills are often perceived as easier than putting oneself in a position that is uncomfortable or unfamiliar such as giving an elevator speech or sitting down to dinner with an executive. Less recognized by many nurses is the potential of political power where nurses work and live. Informal politics are carried out when we encourage colleagues to support a policy change at work, give an elevator speech to the chief executive officer (CEO) about an initiative we are undertaking, or sit with a board member at a luncheon. There are numerous opportunities to carry out informal politics (see Exhibit 11.1).

EXHIBIT 11.1 21 TIPS TO EXPAND YOUR INFLUENCE

Create one-on-one opportunities to meet people; get to know someone better

1. Attend a nursing forum or staff meeting at work and talk with someone you don't know.
2. Invite a colleague to coffee to gain his or her perspective on a key organizational issue.
3. Invite an adversary to lunch as Disch (2014) suggests. While you might not agree on issues, you learn about the person's point of view.
4. Invite a local faculty member or dean to accompany you for coffee.
5. Take a new employee to a coffee break during the first week of work.
6. Make an appointment with a senior administrator to better understand a controversial decision, and offer your perspective.
7. Sit down with the clinical preceptor in your area and ask to better understand the curriculum and how nursing student experiences can be improved.
8. Ask a physician colleague about his or her ideas for improving care on the unit.

Demonstrate your support

9. Join a professional nursing organization outside your work setting.
10. Volunteer to help with a recruitment event or nursing program.
11. Invite a co-worker to join you in helping at a community project.
12. Write a thank-you note to a nurse colleague who effectively handled a difficult patient situation.
13. Write a note complementing a supervisor on handling a difficult personnel issue.
14. Offer to cover for a nurse colleague, while he or she attends a nursing meeting.
15. Volunteer to be a nursing student preceptor.
16. Tell someone that he or she has done a good job.
17. Offer to help someone who is struggling.

Expand your knowledge

18. Attend nursing or organizational information sessions.
19. Familiarize yourself with the organization's mission, vision, values, and strategic plan.
20. Invite a colleague who is in a nursing education program to share with you what is being learned.
21. Subscribe to two professional nursing journals and read each issue.

Being skillful in engaging in the formal political process often starts with, and is strengthened by, engaging in acts of informal politics. In her book, *Becoming Influential*, Eleanor Sullivan, PhD, RN, FAAN (2012, p. 94), describes the power of small talk, which she points out is "neither small or unimportant." Rather, it is an opportunity for equal sharing between two people, for exchanging ideas and making connections, and for possibly laying the groundwork for future, more important conversations. To get started, simple questions of interest can be used such as, "How long have you been in nursing?" or "What intrigued you about becoming a physician?" At a conference with relative strangers, you could ask, "Is this the first time you're attending this meeting?" Follow-up comments or questions can be used to elicit more information and allow the conversation to evolve on its own. Small talk is about finding mutual connections and not indicating how important one is, or how much one knows. Before attending a key meeting or event, it is a good idea to anticipate who might be there and generate a few comments to make or questions to ask.

Nurses also must be involved formally in politics as well as informally. In the current era of health care reform, there is no better time for nurses to pursue politics. "The fact is, nurses who pursue politics offer something that candidates without their experience simply cannot: a firsthand and accurate accounting of what happens on site in medical institutions, in private practice, and in home health care environments" (Lyttle, 2011, p. 19). In spite of the importance and the stories in this book that highlight nurses who hold elected or appointed positions, the fact remains that not enough nurses are involved in politics. Adding to the complexity of the issue is that men are underrepresented in nursing and women traditionally are underrepresented in politics. In the United States, only 1% of congressional members (out of 535) are nurses and no nurses are senators (see Exhibit 11.2).

The need for nurses to be active in politics is a unifying theme globally. In the Nordic countries, females represent 40.8% of elected officials; rates in the remainder of Europe, sub-Saharan Africa, Asia, and the Arab states are, respectively, 17.45%, 16.6%, 16.4%, and 8.8% (International Council of Nurses [ICN], 2010). To the end of helping nurses in this capacity, the ICN Nurse Politicians Network (NPN) was developed as a forum for nurse politicians worldwide (see www.icn.ch/networks/overview).

All nurses need to understand politics, work locally to influence their practice, and participate in formal politics at least at the level of being informed of local (community and work), state, and national issues and voting at all levels. Then they can seek progressive roles as time and expertise dictate. These roles can range from volunteering for political campaigns, to seeking appointments, to running for office. Advanced practice registered nurses (APRNs) are uniquely positioned not only to be proactive in politics because of the constant challenges faced in being able to practice using the full extent of their education and training, but also to mentor, teach, and role model the value of the nursing perspective to nurses, administrators, and the public across the spectrum of settings.

EXHIBIT 11.2 NURSES IN CONGRESS

Karen Bass serves California's 37th district in Congress. She is a member of the Democratic Party. She was sworn in as a member of the 112th Congress in January 2011. She is the former speaker of the California Assembly and was the first African American woman to lead the California Assembly. Congresswoman Bass became a nurse and ultimately a physician's assistant. Current committees can be viewed at http://bass.house.gov/about-me/committees-and-caucuses

Diane Black serves Tennessee's 6th district in Congress. She is a member of the Republican Party. She was sworn in as a member of the 112th Congress in January 2011. She is a former member of the Tennessee State House and State Senate. Since 1971, Congresswoman Black worked as a nurse, including time in the emergency department, until 1998 when she was elected to Tennessee's Legislature. Current committees can be viewed at http://black.house.gov/about-me/committees

Lois Capps serves California's 24th congressional district. She is a member of the Democratic Party. She was sworn in as a member of the 105th Congress in March 1998. She founded the Congressional Nursing Caucus in 2003 and continued to serve as a caucus co-chair. A registered nurse (RN) since 1959, Congresswoman Capps worked as a school nurse in the Santa Barbara public schools; nursing instructor in Portland, Oregon; and head nurse at Yale New Haven Hospital while attending graduate school. Current committees can be viewed at http://capps.house.gov/about-me/committees-and-caucuses

Renee Ellmers serves North Carolina's 2nd district in Congress. She is a member of the Republican Party. She was sworn in as a member of the 112th Congress in January 2011. Since 1990, Congresswoman Ellmers worked as an RN, as surgical intensive care nurse, and then as clinical director of the Trinity Wound Care Center. Current committees can be viewed at http://ellmers.house.gov/committee-assignments

Eddie Bernice Johnson serves Texas's 30th congressional district. She is a member of the Democratic Party. She was sworn in as a member of the 103rd Congress in January 1993. She is the first RN elected to the U.S. Congress. As of 2013, she is the 17th chairperson of the Congressional Black Caucus. An RN since 1956, Congresswoman Johnson worked as Chief Psychiatric Nurse at the Dallas Veterans Administration Hospital (the first African American to hold that position). After 16 years, she entered public life. Current committees can be viewed at http://en.wikipedia.org/wiki/Eddie_Bernice_Johnson

Carolyn McCarthy serves New York's 4th congressional district. She is a member of the Democratic Party. She was sworn in as a member of the 105th Congress in January 1997. Since 1964, Congresswoman McCarthy worked as a licensed practical nurse in an intensive care unit (ICU). Current committees can be viewed at http://www.carolynmccarthy.house.gov/carolyns-committees1

THE NURSING LENS

What differentiates nurses from others when engaging in the political process are the insights and experiences about health, illness, resiliency, and the human condition gained through their nursing careers. Disch (2012, p. 170) calls this the *nursing lens*, or a "viewpoint from which someone sees things holistically, considering the person, population or community in the larger context." With this perspective, nurses seek personalized solutions that are pragmatic and realistic. Nurses can readily size up situations and people, as well. The nursing lens also enables nurses to be particularly effective in establishing effective interpersonal relationships that help people achieve their goals and do their very best work. With this lens, nurses understand the human condition with all of its intricacies and complexities. Finally, nurses can devise solutions or access resources where none seem to exist.

Examples of nurses using their nursing lens abound. Over the past few years, a growing number of leaders with a nursing background have stepped forward to make significant contributions in highly visible senior leadership roles, taking a big "P" role in national organizations beyond nursing, in government, and in industries outside of health care (see Exhibit 11.3). Each of these leaders would affirm that one of the strengths of his or her success is rooted in the foundation of the nursing profession, the way nurses view the world, and the skills and attitudes he or she has developed over the years based on that perspective (see Chapter 12, "Serving the Public Through Policy and Leadership").

Two nurses who demonstrate the power of the nursing lens are Mary Sumpmann, MSN, RN, and Mary Jo Kreitzer, PhD, RN, FAAN. When Mary Sumpmann became the administrator of a National Cancer Institute Comprehensive Cancer Center she was the only director who had a background as a nurse. She is adamant that her success is largely due to her nursing background and her ability to establish systems for coordinating the work of numerous researchers and creating personalized processes for patients moving through the complexities of cancer therapies. Examples of her ability to identify what patients and families need, and then successfully create, include her development of the role of care coordinator 20 years ago, her creation of a one-stop triage phone line for

---

EXHIBIT 11.3 NURSE LEADERS IN PROMINENT POSITIONS

Maureen Bisognano, MS, RN, President and CEO of the Institute for Healthcare Improvement

Carol Z. Garrison, PhD, RN, Past President of the University of Alabama in Birmingham

Jennie Chin Hansen, MSN, RN, FAAN, CEO of the American Geriatrics Society and Past President of AARP

LTG Patricia Horoho, MSN, MS, RN, FAAN, the Surgeon General and Commanding General of the United States Army Medical Command

Judy Murphy, RN, FACMI, FHIMSS, FAAN, Deputy National Coordinator for Programs & Policy at the Office of the National Coordinator for Health IT, Department of Health and Human Services

Jeannine Rivet, MPH, RN, FAAN, Executive Vice President of UnitedHealth Group

Marilyn Tavenner, MPH, BSN, Administrator for the Centers for Medicare and Medicaid Services

Mary Wakefield, PhD, RN, FAAN, Administrator of the Health Resources and Services Administration

answering questions and providing triage, and her installation of the first Patient/ Family Learning Center in the country that provides training to help families care for the complex needs of cancer patients in the home.

Mary Jo Kreitzer is director of the Center for Spirituality and Healing (CSH) at the University of Minnesota. This interprofessional center coordinates integrative health and medicine programs and initiatives in the Medical School, School of Nursing, College of Pharmacy, and other units within the Academic Health Center and throughout the university. The CSH is a founding member of the Consortium of Academic Health Centers for Integrative Medicine. Of the 57 centers that are now members of the Consortium, the University of Minnesota Center is the only center led by a nurse. The CSH is distinct from other centers in several ways. From the time that the Center began in 1995, it has been engaged in interprofessional education, research, and care model innovation. While the initial focus of the Center was on transforming the health care system through the integration of complementary therapies, culture, and spirituality, the focus has broadened over time to stimulating change and innovation not only within the health care system, but also within organizations and communities. Dr. Kreitzer's nursing lens brings a whole-person/whole-system perspective that informs the current work of advancing well-being within people, organizations, communities, and systems. As Dr. Kreitzer and her colleagues apply whole systems leadership concepts and principles into practice, they are as likely to be active at the bedside, in the boardroom, in the research laboratory, as they are interacting with media to advance bold and innovative ways of thinking, practicing, and leading. They also model the belief that nursing leaders employing their nursing lens pursue their goals through an interprofessional approach, welcoming colleagues from all disciplines and departments while affirming that nursing is an equal partner in any endeavor.

In addition to the nursing lens being a way to characterize nursing's unique contributions, it also describes the invaluable input that nurses bring to policy work. "Because of the way that nurses think, view situations holistically, engage diverse stakeholders, craft pragmatic yet innovative solutions and understand the human condition, our input and this perspective is vitally needed in boardrooms, at policy tables and in senior leadership positions" (Disch, 2012, p. 170). Claire Fagin provides a thoughtful reflection on the nursing lens and the unique perspective that women and nurses bring to leadership situations. In Policy on the Scene 11.1, she responds to a question posed to her after completing her term as interim president of the University of Pennsylvania, the first woman— and nurse—to hold this position. In fact, she was the first woman and nurse to be president of *any* Ivy League university.

Nurses have a unique lens because of their interface with patients, knowledge of equipment, and the central role they play in the day-to-day and often minute-to-minute safety of not one but literally millions of people every day worldwide. These experiences and our holistic approach to care facilitate and influence our perception and understanding of problems and help us determine and evaluate solutions. It is not simply a sum of nursing's expert knowledge. Compare this with intellectual capital in Chapter 7 "Building Capital: Intellectual, Social, Political, and Financial." The nursing lens when applied to each phase of the policy-making process results in a unique perspective in recognizing and identifying a problem, formulating policy, implementing the policy, and monitoring and evaluating the results (see Chapter 1, "Leading the Way in Policy"). A nurse in practice today, Carrie Gavriloff, MSN, RN, Ed, administrative director of the NeuroDevelopmental Science Center at the Akron Children's Hospital, states, "Nurses have the ability to influence healthcare policy, but to do so, we must speak up. As we advocate for patients while they are in our direct care,

---

POLICY ON THE SCENE 11.1: On Nurses, Women, and Leadership
Claire Fagin, PhD, RN, FAAN, Dean Emeritus, University of Pennsylvania School of Nursing, Philadelphia, PA

Some aspects of the woman as administrator and leader were similar to my experiences as a successful nurse. All too often after nurses have performed lifesaving, or life improving, functions during a patient's hospitalization, the comment made by patient and family is, "the nurses were so nice." Well, the nurse's niceness was lucky for everyone, but it was not niceness that facilitated what appeared to be their effortless acts. What mattered most in the person's hospitalization was that these nice nurses were using knowledge, skill, experience and smarts in a graceful and smooth way that often prevented their being noticed for what they were. … What seems to be misunderstood or not understood is how we use our personality attributes within the context of carefully designed strategies for accomplishing goals. The strategies in my case had to do with opening communication internally and externally, building responsibility and accountability, establishing relationships with Penn's wide public, healing the "open" wounds that were apparent, and identifying and dealing with more covert problems. Humanity, warmth, empathy, and other expressionistic characteristics undoubtedly helped and in some cases were essential to the strategies I chose. However these qualities alone do not do the job. Strategic planning … included setting goals, steps and timetables for their accomplishment, and sharing information about their achievement. … Nothing was left to chance or hope.

Reprinted with permission from Fagin (2000).

we must remember too that we have the ability to bring positive outcomes even outside of our care." Nurse Gavriloff did speak up. She used a nursing lens that led her to a letter, strategically cosigned by the pharmacy director and medical services vice president, to be sent to the Food and Drug Administration (FDA) and the Association for the Advancement of Medical Instrumentation (AAMI) that positively impacted safety and brought a nursing lens to an untapped international health care venue (see Policy on the Scene 11.2). These efforts to change policy about tube connections, specifically the color and shape of connectors, for feeding tubes resulted in Gavriloff and the inpatient pharmacy manager being invited to an international meeting of 40 representatives from the FDA and companies like

---

POLICY ON THE SCENE 11.2: Unique Lens of Clinical Care

November 16, 2009

Hillary Woehrle
Association for the Advancement of Medical Instrumentation
1110 North Glebe Road, Suite 220
Arlington, VA 22201-4795

Dear Ms. Woehrle,

Akron Children's Hospital recommends that the AAMI reconsider its decision to adopt the color purple as the standard color for enteral feeding supplies, to prevent tubing and catheter misconnections.

We instead recommend that orange be the standard color for enteral tube feeding sets and that luer-lock connection is removed from the sets. A mechanism that prevents enteral sets from being connected to intravenous (IV) set luer-lock connections must be developed.

The patient safety issue of tubing and catheter misconnection errors first reached clinical areas through the Joint Commission's Sentinel Event Alert System. The root cause attributed to these errors is the ability of IV luer-lock tubing to connect with non-IV tubing (i.e., enteral feeding sets) along with health care provider fatigue and lack of practitioner knowledge of the tubing misconnection errors (Simmons & Graves, 2008).

Although one recommended prevention measure has been to not color code medical tubing, health care staff have become familiar with industry color coding to distinguish different types of medical tubing. For example, Akron Children's Hospital purchases yellow epidural tubing, purple power peripherally inserted central catheter (PICC) line tubing, and orange enteral (oral) tubing.

Covidian's marketing of the color purple for enteral tubing to match the United Kingdom standard for enteral tubing color has led to confusion and increased risk for a tubing connection error. There have been documented errors of purple enteral tube feeding sets being confused with power-injectable PICC line tubing (purple).

The Institute for Safe Medication Practices (ISMP) has stated that "purple is not an official standard for either enteral feeding equipment or PICC lines." Further, the American Society for Parenteral and Enteral Nutrition (ASPEN) recognizes that "color-coding enteral connectors (for which there is no current authorized standard color) simply alerts the clinician that this is not an IV connector, but does not prevent the misconnection." To truly prevent tubing misconnections, it must be impossible to connect enteral feed tubing to IV tubing. We recommend that the enteral connectors be made square or triangular in shape. By having a dissimilar shape, providers will be unable to take a triangle or a square and place it into the circle of the luer connection.

Thank you for your consideration of these recommendations. We look forward to your response as we work together to improve patient safety.

Sincerely,

Michael W. Bird, MD, MPH, Vice President for Medical Services
Carrie Gavriloff, MSN, RN, Ed Education Coordinator, Nursing Products
John Lepto, RPh, Director, Pharmacy Services

Nestle and Dannon. Gavriloff was the only nurse at the meeting and she used her nursing lens to advocate for safety measures not only for patients within hospital settings, but also when patients went home with tube feedings. A summary of the story appears in the *Akron Beacon Journal* (Powell, 2010). The publicity the story received also demonstrated to the public the role of nursing and the unique perspective of the nursing lens.

BEYOND ELECTED POSITIONS

There are many roads to advocacy and politics. However, many visualize one road when they think of politics and they assume that road is a straight path that means running for and getting elected to a public office. In reality, elected positions reflect only a small number of political opportunities. Many political roles are less visible, but are vital to nursing and to health care policy development. Nurses do, and many more can, hold appointed positions or volunteer

---

EXHIBIT 11.4 **READINESS TIPS WHEN SEEKING APPOINTMENTS OR NOMINATIONS**

1. Learn the particular process that the organization uses to select its members
   a. Identify specific eligibility requirements (e.g., education, experience, or political affiliation)
   b. Review disqualifiers and conflicts of interest
   c. Have others review any written responses
   d. Consider professional consultation for advice when applying for prominent positions

2. Increase visibility of your expertise or experience that relates to the organization's mission and goals
   a. Attend organization's functions
   b. Participate in meetings and other processes
   c. Introduce yourself to organizational leaders

3. Know the organization and review relevant documents
   a. Website and printed materials
   b. Current structure and organization chart
   c. Mission and goals
   d. Current and sensitive issues under consideration

4. Demonstrate your interest by attending and supporting events, programs, and fundraisers

5. Network with individuals who have influence on or knowledge of the selection process: current board members, organization leaders, and community or legislative leaders

6. Review other considerations for selection like money or time donations

---

for positions. One can be appointed to an office or a committee, but in many situations, especially at the little "p" level, one can volunteer for membership on boards, committees, and task forces.

Whether contemplating or seeking an appointment or a staff position, or volunteering for an advocacy position, there are steps nurses can take to develop their skill set and position themselves to be ready to move forward as they become aware of opportunities (see Exhibit 11.4). When invited for an interview, the nurse should be thoroughly prepared. This preparation includes learning about the organization's history, priorities, and culture; writing several drafts of the application; having the application critiqued; participating in a mock interview; preparing answers to anticipated interview questions; and developing several questions for the interview team (Disch, 2007).

Political Appointments

Many of the nurse leaders listed earlier in Exhibit 11.2 have held or hold appointed positions, for example, Judy Murphy and Marilyn Tavenner. There are numerous federal, state, and local appointments that would benefit from the nursing lens and there are some positions that can only be filled by a registered nurse (RN). State boards of nursing, for example, are primarily filled by gubernatorial appointment. Each state will have regulations that specify the number of RNs and APRNs necessary for the full board complement. See Chapter 3, "Navigating the Political System," for additional details about boards of nursing.

States will differ slightly in the process of appointments and the rules may vary for how APRNs are appointed, if at all, to the state board. Wyoming, for example, has no regulations about APRNs holding positions on the Wyoming State Board of Nursing, but does have an Advanced Practice Advisory Board to provide advice on APRN matters. It is composed of a representative from each of the four APRN groups with appointments made after application to the Board of Nursing (National Association of Clinical Nurse Specialists [NACNS], n.d.).

Volunteer and Staff

The work of nurses associations has been instrumental in the policy strides made in nursing and health care. Essential to association successes are the countless staff members and volunteers committed to the mission and goals. There is strong conviction in what the association stands for and accomplishes. Associations provide numerous opportunities for political activism and visibility. Without the time, resources, and money of associations, the collective work on policy and advocacy could not be accomplished. It is the values of the members that propel ideas into actions to achieve policy goals. Therefore, engagement as an association member is an effective means of developing your nursing lens. While much of our discussion has focused on nurses presenting a nursing lens to a wider circle beyond nursing, there is considerable policy work to be done in influencing the public's understanding of a nursing lens through the policies and positions of nursing organizations.

As one volunteer example, the ANA uses Professional Issues Panels to inform the decisions on practice and policy issues made by its board of directors. Each panel is led by a steering committee that is informed by a larger advisory committee. This facilitates widespread input as well as a rigorous process to ensure quality of the recommended positions or actions.

Numerous similar opportunities exist within specialty nurses associations to shape policy agendas. Many associations have legislative committees in which volunteers play a critical role. While the legislative and practice committees are directly aligned with policy issues, other association activities provide opportunities to influence policy. For example, nominations to select leadership, bylaws to describe essential operations and functions, conference planning to showcase new ideas, and selecting liaisons to legislators and policy tables all provide opportunities to use the nursing lens.

Some committees have long-standing histories whereas others are more recent. In 2012, for example, the Nurses' Organization for Veterans Affairs (NOVA) initiated a legislative committee to provide a voice for legislation related to veterans and to the nurses who are employed in the system. At the state or regional level, many nurses associations have a parallel legislative structure that relies on nurses to focus on local issues and candidates. Each of the APRN groups has within their respective associations plentiful positions

EXHIBIT 11.5	SELECTED ASSOCIATIONS REPRESENTING APRN LEADERSHIP AND ADVOCACY LINKS	
ASSOCIATION	**LEADERSHIP/STRUCTURE**	**ADVOCACY LINK**
American Association of Nurse Anesthetists (AANA)	https://www.aana.com/aboutus/Pages/Board-of-Directors.aspx	https://www.aana.com/advocacy
American Association of Nurse Practitioners (AANP)	http://www.aanp.org/about-aanp/board-of-directors	http://www.aanp.org/legislation-regulation
American College of Nurse-Midwives (ACNM)	http://www.midwife.org/ACNM-National-Structure	http://www.midwife.org/Advocacy
American Nurses Association (ANA)	http://www.nursingworld.org/FunctionalMenu-Categories/AboutANA/Leadership-Governance	http://www.nursingworld.org/MainMenuCategories/Policy-Advocacy
National Association of Clinical Nurse Specialists (NACNS)	http://www.nacns.org/html/leadership.php	http://www.nacns.org/html/advocacy-policy.php
National Association of Pediatric Nurse Practitioners (NAPNAP)	http://www.napnap.org/volunteer-Leaders	http://www.napnap.org/advocacy

that often have too few volunteers, but provide numerous advocacy opportunities (see Exhibit 11.5).

Staff members within associations are often equally committed to the purposes and mission of the association. They serve in multiple capacities and are essential to the operation and continuity of the association. Staff can be an invaluable resource. Those staff members who are RNs bring added value by incorporating their nursing lens to their role.

Work and Community

Often the best place to start down the path toward the roles just described is local committee work in the work setting and the community. Many of the nurses who tell their stories in Chapter 12 relate how they began their involvement early in their career by serving on committees. Whether the career path is in practice, education, administration, research, or a combination, the pathway to leadership is often found in committee work. Committee work not only provides opportunities to build political skills but also often helps develop necessary networking skills and provides opportunities for mentoring and mentorship. Committees are often looking for members and chairs to lead committees both in the work environment and within their local communities. Committees can also be an effective way to help identify needs related to policy. Policy on the Scene 11.3 highlights the value of a nursing lens in a committee focused on solving a patient safety problem.

POLICY ON THE SCENE 11.3: The Color of Safety
Franchesca Charney, MSHA, RN, CPHRM, CPHQ, CPSO, CPPS, DFASHRM, Director of Educational Programs, Pennsylvania Patient Safety Authority, Harrisburg, PA, Color of Safety Task Force, Pennsylvania

A simple process, applying a color-coded wristband, led to a potentially dangerous event. A patient at a Pennsylvania hospital had a yellow wristband applied signifying a "do not resuscitate" order. The nurse who placed the wristband also worked at another hospital where yellow indicated that the extremity was not to be used for blood draws or IV access (Pennsylvania Patient Safety Authority, 2005). The patient had an event and was almost not resuscitated. In another instance, a color-coded wristband indicated a patient had clearance for surgery when the consent was not signed. Fortunately, a "time-out" corrected the mistake. These near-misses exposed an opportunity to make processes safer. It was logical to involve stakeholders at facilities who transfer patients among them to standardize color-coded wristband use.

The Color of Safety Task Force began with representatives of eight facilities. Members were either nurses or quality improvement/patient safety officers; many served in both roles. Even though the facilities were in competition with one another, this issue could only be addressed by working together. It was our commitment to our patients' safety that inspired us to act.

We first identified only two sources of potential problems: patients who are routinely transferred between facilities to receive a different service or level of care and clinicians who may not work at just one facility. We soon learned about multiple inconsistencies in meanings, colors, and use of color-coded wristbands.

We surveyed Pennsylvania hospitals and ambulatory surgical centers, learning that 78% used color-coded wristbands to convey critical clinical information such as allergies and falls risk (Pennsylvania Patient Safety Authority, 2005). Some wristbands had written information, while others

(continued)

did not; some had incomplete information. Color-coded wristbands were also worn to support charitable causes. Our team brought a real-world nursing lens to the table in addressing this problem with potentially harmful consequences.

Recognizing safety risks associated with lack of standardization, we "banded" together and expanded to include 13 hospitals. We were systematic, using available resources including the Pennsylvania Patient Safety Authority, their safety reports, lessons learned, the wristband survey results, and evidence-based risk reduction strategies.

Our efforts focused on risk reduction strategies: standardizing policies related to colors, admission and pre-registration emergency department wristbands, community and charitable cause bands, patient refusals, and handoffs; using consistent procedures; and educating patients, staff, and families. Our education efforts needed to reach national health professions associations, local charitable organizations, and community newspapers, as well as the many health care agencies in our region. We created a tool kit, including (a) an administrative manual, (b) community education materials and letters, (c) patient education protocols, (d) staff competencies, (e) documentation forms, and (f) equipment procurement guidelines (Color of Safety, 2009). We realized that our regional borders were fluid. So, we worked with the American Hospital Association (AHA) and the American Society of Healthcare Risk Management. Our work received a Pennsylvania Patient Safety Authority Board of Directors commendation. What started as a "small" regional project resulted in policies implemented across the country. The Department of Defense adopted our Color of Safety policies in military hospitals. The United Kingdom and Australia are also using our color-coded wristband system.

Often committee work can seem daunting; finding a mentor and getting familiar with fulfilling expectations is critical. Without guidance, committee members can lose sight of the work of the committee or valuable time can be lost while members try to gather a sense of the committee. Both veterans and new members can benefit from formalizing the committee orientation process. Each committee should be clear on what role it has in policy making and review in relation to its purpose and functions.

Providing an orientation that is tailored to the responsibilities of the committee will help members make solid ongoing contributions. The responsibility of orienting new members may most easily be led by the chair, but in some cases, such as an orientation to a governing board, the orientation may initially be as extensive as a half- or whole-day orientation by key members of the committee or staff that support its work. Some of the key elements to include in an orientation are (a) purposes, functions, and relationships to organizational structures;

(b) ongoing and special projects; (c) attendance requirements, meeting schedules, and use of alternates; (d) time commitments; (e) process for establishing agenda items; (f) parliamentary procedures; (g) process for minutes, recording, access, and approval; (h) access to key documents; (i) any training requirements (e.g., human subjects training); and (j) confidentiality and conflicts of interest.

To be effective, committee work often requires work outside of meetings, including reading, discussing ideas with people outside the committee, reporting to other committees, and sometimes ongoing education. Helping new members balance their time between committee work required by their work role and committee work that falls outside of work is a delicate balance that is easily overlooked when orientation is provided.

Stepping into one committee position can open many doors whether you volunteer to work for a community organization like the United Way or a woman's shelter or volunteer for the policy committee or research committee at work. Many organizations also have foundation or directors' boards, thus providing the introductory skills necessary for increasing the number of nurses on prominent health care boards.

The Road Less Traveled

Nontraditional, entrepreneurial, and executive roles such as presidents, health sciences deans, and business owners are just a few of the titles that reflect the diversity of roles that nurses hold that often are overlooked when advocacy and politics are discussed. These roles are often overlooked because individuals mistakenly think that nurses in these roles have left the nursing lens behind. Nurses in these positions often hear from nurses in more traditional roles who state they could not consider such atypical roles as it would mean "giving up nursing" and the opportunities to advance nursing. Yet leaders (like those listed in Exhibits 11.2 and 11.3) find they do have many opportunities to have a positive impact on patients and nurses in their roles, even though they may be seen as less traditional. Entrepreneurs are owner-managers of companies that provide nursing services. These services may include direct care clinical services or educational, research, or other consultative services. With their nursing lens and their span of authority and responsibility, they have found advocacy opportunities beyond what they imagined early in their careers. In Policy on Scene 11.4, Kathy Player describes how she followed a nontraditional path.

BOARDS

In the report, *The Future of Nursing: Leading Change, Advancing Health*, the need for nurses in leadership positions is outlined as a key strategy for advancing health care (Institute of Medicine [IOM], 2011). One leadership position that has been specifically targeted and is getting much attention is the need for nurses to serve on boards. This is not a new issue; in fact, the Robert Wood Johnson Foundation (RWJF) created a program, Pipeline to Placement: Nurse Leaders in the Boardroom, as a national effort to increase the number of nurses prepared to serve on influential boards (RWJF, 2007).

POLICY ON THE SCENE 11.4: Walking a Nontraditional Path in Nursing

Kathy Player, EdD, MSN, MBA, MS-C, RN, Vice-President and Chief Academic Officer of Health Sciences, Midwestern University, Phoenix, AZ

The first decade of my nursing career started off on a traditional path as I went to work in a hospital setting, but within a few years I realized that furthering my education would be essential. I completed both my master's and doctoral degrees and found I had three job offers. I accepted the most unlikely position; I moved from being a director of psychiatric services to working as a director of a start-up RN-BSN program, an important shift in the scheme of my career path.

I held dual reporting lines to the deans of nursing and professional studies. Within 2 years, a reorganization left me with a choice to continue in the position heading the RN-BSN program or take a promotion to a chair position in professional studies within the business college. It was an agonizing decision to shift from the nursing college to the business college, but an offer I couldn't refuse, as I was again drawn to the idea of new challenges and responsibilities.

However, in this case, the challenges were on a grand scale. The university was on the brink of bankruptcy. The 50-year-old institution was quickly sold (within 2 months) to a group of investors who had to turn around a $25 million debt. This resulted in several 180-degree changes that included moving from nonprofit to for-profit status and from a traditional academic environment to an entrepreneurial one. Times were chaotic, but I recall knowing that if the university made it through the other side successfully, the leadership lessons learned would be remarkable. In times of change, opportunities abound, and within 6 months of the purchase I was promoted to dean of business. Over the years, I also held roles as associate provost, provost, and president.

While going up the career ladder I stepped up to run for president of the Arizona Nurses Association (AZA), which later led to running for a board position on the ANA. These state and national boards gave me experience in running a campaign, lobbying in Washington, DC, and navigating the politics of nursing's agenda within a bureaucratic system, while also providing the venues that strengthened my public speaking skills. While president of the AZA, a mentor encouraged me to apply to the Robert Wood Johnson Foundation (RWJF) Executive Nurse Fellows Program. The boards and fellowship seemed intimidating when first suggested but I embraced the risk and, in time, these became huge stepping-stones in my professional development.

I certainly did not envision myself becoming president of a publicly traded university, or a coauthor and author of several books, nursing textbook chapters, and articles, let alone having a career that would allow me international travel to promote the nursing profession. Neither holding board seats nor the fellowship brought salary, so these professional opportunities all occurred while advancing on the executive ladder. The rewards of being a change agent and part of something larger such as proactively moving nursing bills through the House and Senate made the hours all worthwhile.

One of the most powerful observations was the lack of young nurses "at the table," pushing nursing's agenda forward into the future. I sat next to nurses who would have liked to retire and pass the torch, but few were coming up behind to accept it. To an energetic nurse wanting to make a difference, I found an environment that welcomed and embraced my energy, passion, and enthusiasm. The field is wide open for those interested in advancing the profession. This is where strategy and leveraging opportunity overlap.

As an executive in higher education, I am around nursing students who frequently ask for career advice. More specifically, they will ask the questions: "How did you do it?" "Do you miss working in nursing?" I share my story here and relate how there are many paths one can take in carving out a career. My path focused on keeping all options open with an understanding of my strengths and passions. In hindsight, the journey has been strategically serendipitous, if there is such a thing, and doors opened that I never would have imagined. I tactically leveraged the opportunities that came as a result of great mentoring from those far wiser than me.

Getting on Boards

The two major ways through which nurses become invited to serve on boards are the same mechanisms for which other leaders are invited: relationships or a valued perspective/expertise that they bring. Relationships operate from either a personal connection with the person(s) populating the slate of nominees or a referral from an intermediate party. The valued perspective or expertise can reflect something very specific such as an accounting background or something broad such as being a member of a particular community. As it relates to this chapter, the nursing lens is a perspective that is holistic, relationship-based, insightful, understands both the human condition and how systems (particularly in health care) do or do not work, and is innovative in thinking of creative options or solutions. Thinking back on my own career, these are the two factors that were involved in my invitation to serve on the boards of which I've been privileged to serve (JD).

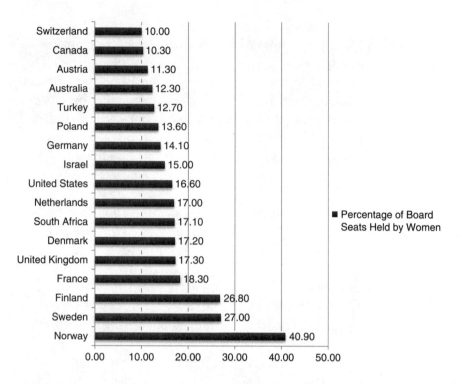

FIGURE 11.1 Corporate board seats held by women, by country.

Reprinted with permission from Catalyst (2013, May 31).

Having said this, however, a concurrent reality is that nurses are not always in proximity to decision makers who are inviting nominees to serve. This may be due to class differences, occupational silos, or other factors. There are also biases as to what many individuals may see as a nurse's skill set. Gender bias may be at work, as well as outdated perspectives that nurses cannot be leaders, or that nurses will be too parochial and tied to narrow interests or, conversely, too focused on only the needs of the nursing profession (Prybil et al., 2009). Interestingly, system leaders themselves may focus too narrowly on the bottom line and not appreciate the impact of safety and quality on the bottom line, or that a nursing presence is exactly what is needed to describe how quality impacts the finances, and what might be feasible options for improving quality and reducing cost.

This is not unique to nursing. Over the past 5 years, the overall percentage of seats held by women corporate directors has not noticeably changed across the world. Figure 11.1 reflects the status of women on boards in publicly traded companies or, in the case of the United States, Fortune 500 companies with at least 10% participation. Board participation for women ranges from 0% in Saudi Arabia (even Qatar has 0.3%), South Korea (1.9%), Greece (7%), and Hong Kong (9%) to 40.9% in Norway (Catalyst, 2013). Norway has a higher participation rate because it introduced a 40% quota system for corporate boards. Spain passed legislation requiring 40% board participation by women by 2015 (Reier, 2008).

Being an Effective Board Member

Once on a board or policy-setting committee, there can still be challenges. Mason (2010) identified several barriers that nurses may face in getting their good ideas, once developed, into action. These include state regulations that limit the scope of advanced practice nurses, limitations on reimbursement by payers to nonphysician providers, and adversarial policy statements from organizations such as the American Medical Association. She also identified nurse-related barriers to policy implementation, such as a lack of adequate data to support the innovation, failing to develop strategies for translating research or system improvements into practice and policy, and the inability to scale up creative innovations to broader adaptation.

Marshall (2011) has identified several additional barriers that are more personally related to the nurse's own competencies and comfort, noting that "Too many nurses opt out of policy discussions" (p. 254). This may be due to inadequate educational preparation in policy work, and/or nurses being involved so heavily in clinical practice that little time is available. Some nurses don't see the value in policy work, believing it is for others to do. The reality is that with few nurses serving on boards and curricula that are full, finding role models and opportunities to learn about serving on boards has not been an easy task that many schools have been willing to take on.

Once a nurse is on a board or major policy body, Disch (2007) advocates for nurses to hone their skills and learn the ropes, keeping in mind that the role focus is on stewardship of an organization, not to represent nursing. Strategies for success include (a) focusing on the good of the organization, (b) listening, and (c) avoiding repetition. Frame issues and questions in terms of what's good for the organization and what is consistent with its strategic plan and objectives. Although each member has particular agendas or viewpoints, do not become the "nurse board member" who brings every issue back to nursing, or the "small town board member" who relates everything to his or her home town. While nurses are not alone in this behavior, the end result is that all contributions can be tuned out. Claire Fagin, who has vast experience in board work, suggests that, in any interprofessional or business group, a nurse should first make at least two or three comments from a broad perspective before making one even remotely related to nursing (C. Fagin, personal communication, July 2013). Listen carefully to what your fellow board members are saying in discussions and seek to understand their points of view. The goal is not to talk the most but be the individual who adds a new comment or strategy to advance the cause. Finally, if you have made your point, you have made your point. Think through what you want to say before you say it, and then say it once. Those who bring up the same points, particularly advancing their own agendas, alienate their colleagues and, again, diminish their effectiveness.

PROGRAMS THAT REFLECT THE NURSING LENS

Programs providing care delivery and reflecting the nursing lens have been in existence since Florence Nightingale's time. One of the earliest in this country is the Visiting Nurse Service of New York, led by President and CEO Mary Ann Christopher, MSN, RN, FAAN. Its roots go back to 1893 when Lillian Wald, after a care experience with a young mother, worked with a colleague to receive financial and governmental support to establish a community-based care center. Wald and her colleagues provided a foundation for public health nursing by caring for poor immigrants on the Lower East Side of New York, caring for the sick, and assisting with births and deaths (Visiting Nurse Service of New York, n.d.). Realizing that individual health and community health are inseparable, she addressed issues related to women's health and their working conditions, children's health, child labor, and emergency responsiveness.

Another well-known program developed by a nurse that reflects the nursing lens is the DC Birth Center, founded by internationally known nurse midwife Ruth Lubic, EdD, RN, CNM, FAAN (Rychnovsky, 2011). Originally she was galvanized into action by the fact that Washington, DC's infant mortality rate was twice that of the nation as a whole. Lubic and her team worked to reduce that rate by providing education and health care to women and their families. The birth center provides prenatal care, childbirth education, education on preventing premature delivery, nurse midwife care (at the Center or in a hospital), postpartum care, and other health services for women and children. Currently, Dr. Lubic is president and CEO of the Family Health and Birth Center and founder and president emerita of the Developing Families Center in Washington, DC.

A third example is the work of Patty Gerrity, PhD, RN, FAAN, and colleagues at the 11th Street Family Health Services Center in Philadelphia, PA (11th Street Family Health Services, 2010). This program, affiliated with Drexel University, dates back to 1996, when the College of Nursing at MCP/Hahnemann University entered into an agreement with the Philadelphia Housing Authority to address health issues of residents in Philadelphia's 11th Street Corridor. The 11th Street Corridor in Philadelphia encompasses several public housing tracts and has historically been underserved with regard to affordable, accessible, and quality health care services. The first services from the 11th Street Health Center focused on health promotion and disease prevention. At present, diabetes education, self-efficacy programs, nutrition education, fitness classes, cooking classes, and behavioral health group support are the core program elements of the Healthy Living Center. The center also provides a venue for the education of nurses and other health professionals in culturally competent, community-based care.

These and many other examples are included in the Raise the Voice campaign, spearheaded by the American Academy of Nursing (AAN). According to the AAN website, "Health care in America today is inaccessible to many, expensive for most and fragmented for all. Enabling the system to deliver the best possible care at an acceptable cost requires not just reformation but transformation—moving American health care away from its current hospital-based, acuity-oriented, physician-dependent paradigm toward a patient-centered, convenient, helpful and affordable system. America needs a system that keeps people as healthy as possible, treats the patient promptly, comprehensively and effectively" (AAN, n.d.). Out of this belief came the *Raise the Voice* campaign to educate the public and policy makers about innovative programs that nurses are implementing to provide holistic, personalized, effective, pragmatic, and accessible care delivery options—often to individuals, families, and communities in greatest need. The campaign profiles Edge Runners, or those nurses who are practical innovators, using new thinking to create innovative models of health care delivery. The campaign not only provides evidence-based examples of creative care delivery models that are making a difference in communities across the country, but also highlights the instrumental role nurses can play and must play in developing new policies for care delivery. The *American Journal of Nursing* has begun to highlight the work of these Edge Runners; for example, Donna Torrisi, MSN, CRNP, FAAN, executive director of the Family Practice and Counseling Network in Philadelphia. The four nurse-run health centers in this network manage 19,000 patients and 85,000 visits per year (Collins, 2013). These Edge Runners along with recipients of the Magnet Prize, a program that recognizes extraordinary innovation and transformation, provide valuable lessons on how a nursing lens impacts quality and safety, and improves the lives of those entrusted to our care.

SUPPORT AND OPPORTUNITIES FOR A NURSING LENS IN POLICY

The value of and the need for the nursing lens in health policy work have received much national attention. Numerous national organizations have called for and supported an increasing nurse presence in policy development. As support for nurses is realized and health care reform is implemented, there are also new opportunities for nurses to apply the nursing lens, especially with the burgeoning area of interprofessional work.

Support

In 2007, the AHA issued a report from a Blue Ribbon Panel on Health Care Governance, urging that boards "include physicians, nurses and other clinicians on the board. Their clinical competence and viewpoints are valuable to board members and will help the board better understand the needs and concerns of several of the organization's stakeholders" (Blue Ribbon Panel, 2007, p. 13). In 2010, the Center for Healthcare Governance noted: "Because nurses have the most contact with patients, families and physicians, nurses have in-depth knowledge of healthcare delivery that could prove valuable to a board of trustees on relevant issues" (Totten, 2010).

As noted earlier, the RWJF has long advocated for nurses serving on boards and at other policy tables. With RWJF's Pipeline to Placement initiative aimed at highlighting and disseminating the important contributions that nurses make in policy issues, organizations were encouraged to include more nurses as board members (RWJF, 2007).

Furthermore, the RWJF commissioned a Gallup poll of over 1,500 policy leaders in order to assess their view of nursing's role in policy. Of the respondents, a large majority indicated that nurses have a great deal of influence on components of a quality health care system such as medical error reduction, patient safety, and patient care quality (Khoury, Blizzard, Wright Moore, & Hassmiller, 2011). In the survey, however, the leaders identified that nurses were not being perceived as key health care decision makers, which was a major barrier to nurses' influence. Reed V. Tuckson, MD, FACP, former executive vice president and chief of Medical Affairs at UnitedHealth Group in Minnetonka, Minnesota, stated, "There is a movement afoot, and that movement is saying that if we do not get nurses fully engaged at every level of this delivery system, from policy formulation to operations, that we all ultimately suffer, and we are tired of suffering" (Barclay, 2010).

Nurses bring an added dimension to research as well. This is essential not only for policy research but also for examining potential policy implications of research; this is true both when research is designed and again when research is completed. Beth Collins Sharp, when she was senior advisor for nursing at the Agency for Healthcare Research and Quality (AHRQ), noted (2012, p. 1): "We bring an on-the-ground perspective—a reality check—to studies. Ideally, nurses are involved from the beginning as questions are developed through to the end when the research gets put into practice." Carolyn Clancy, who was AHRQ director, added (2012, p. 2): "I often say that nurses are on the frontlines of care. While this is true, nurses despite their vast influence and importance have too often been in the background of health care research and policy. This is changing. … It's about time. … We're ready."

In spite of these clear mandates for the need for a nursing lens, in reality, the belief appears to be stronger for the mandate than the actuality. In *The Future of Nursing* report (IOM, 2011, p. 223), for example, the comment was made that perhaps the public views nurses as "functional doers" rather than "thoughtful strategists." In the RWJF Gallup poll of opinion leaders, not all of the findings were optimistic. In spite of the clear belief that nurses had a strong role to play and that nursing was one of the most trusted sources of health information, the respondents also perceived that nurses will have the least amount of influence on health care reform over the next 10 years (Khoury et al., 2011).

Nurses are often not at policy tables. A 2007 study found that only 0.8% of voting members of hospital and health system boards were chief nurse officers, whereas chief medical officers totaled 5.1% (Governance Institute, 2007). In a survey of community health systems, it was found that 2.3% had nurses and

22.6% had physicians on their boards (Prybil et al., 2009). A 2011 AHA survey of more than 1,000 hospital boards (Hassmiller & Combes, 2012) found that just 6% of board members were nurses; 20% were physicians. Part of this inequity may be due to misconceptions. A major one is that the physician can speak for all providers on health care issues. However, nurses and physicians have different responsibilities to and relationships with patients and families, and spend very different periods of time with them. Mary Chesney, PhD, CRNP, RN, president of the National Association of Pediatric Nurse Practitioners, describes her theory of this major barrier as being the "slice of the apple" phenomenon: "The public and legislators tend to see the physician as the big apple of health care, able to do all things and, thus, if a board or policy group has a physician in the group, this person is authorized to speak for all other health professional groups. The physician is the whole apple and every other profession is just a slice of the apple. What we need to do is to help legislators and the public see that the physician can be the apple, but the nurse is an orange. Different perspectives, some unique and some overlapping skill sets, different areas of expertise yet both are important and are needed for a full complement of services" (Chesney, M., personal communication, 2010).

On the other hand, there are hopeful signs that this may be changing. Support comes from the AHA Center on Healthcare Governance, "Because nurses have the most contact with patients, families and physicians, nurses have in-depth knowledge of healthcare delivery that could prove valuable to a board of trustees on relevant issues" (Blue Ribbon Panel, 2007). Nick Turkal, CEO of Aurora Health Care, asked, "Why would any board not have a nurse on the board?... I think it's common sense, when you look at where healthcare is delivered" (Evans, 2009). Gail Warden, president emeritus of the Henry Ford Health System, added: "I've always felt strongly that people don't understand the fact that the nurse and nursing ... is the part of the organization that is responsible for the care of the patient around the clock" (Evans, 2009). John Combes, president and CEO for Healthcare Governance, says he sees "a growing number of nurses on governing boards and credits the shift to hospital boards' increasing responsibilities." "It's not just about business and finance," he says. "Boards need directors or trustees who understand healthcare delivery and can help improve its quality and responsiveness" (Evans, 2009). The importance of the nursing lens is recognized in *The Future of Nursing* report issued by the RWJF and the IOM: "By virtue of its numbers and adaptive capacity, the nursing profession has the potential to effect wide-reaching changes in the healthcare system. Nurses' regular, close proximity to patients and scientific understanding of care processes across the continuum of care give them a unique ability to act as partners with other health professionals and to lead in the improvement and redesign of the healthcare system and its many practice environments" (IOM, 2011, p. 23).

> **EXHIBIT 11.6**   *THE FUTURE OF NURSING KEY MESSAGE 3*
>
> *Nurses should be full partners, with physicians and other health professionals, in redesigning health care in the United States.*
>
> Strong leadership is critical if the vision of a transformed health care system is to be realized. Yet not all nurses begin their career with thoughts of becoming a leader. The nursing profession must produce leaders throughout the health care system, from the bedside to the boardroom, who can serve as full partners with other health professionals and be accountable for their own contributions to delivering high-quality care while working collaboratively with leaders from other health professions (IOM, 2011, p. 36).

Opportunities

Opportunities for nurses in using the nursing lens are created by the calls for greater involvement of nurses in establishing health policy and shaping our health care system, interprofessional collaboration, and the creation of transformative programs. *The Future of Nursing* report not only recognized the value of the nursing lens, but also issued a key message that extols the centrality of nurses as partners in the process of reshaping health care in the United States (see Exhibit 11.6). This message, while seemingly simple, is complex when one considers the dynamic historical interplay of nurses and physicians. In this report, nursing leadership is called to be involved at every level, from bedside to boardroom. This call is not an issue of *parity*, such as bringing in nurses' voices as an act of generosity, or equity, but rather one of *perspective*. Nurses' viewpoints are essential if workable solutions for health care problems are to be developed, implemented, and successful.

Nurses' viewpoints are used to influence policy by lobbying, persuading legislators, and working in coalitions to get legislation passed. But that's only part of the policy-making process. What remains is actually turning policy into practice. As health care reform is implemented and health care organizations change their internal policies and procedures to comply with new laws, new care coordination environments called health care homes (HCH), patient-centered medical homes (PCMH), and accountable care organizations (ACO) are being created. Health care providers are joining and working together interprofessionally in these organizations to maximize their patients' health through more seamless, integrated provision of care, thereby reducing the unnecessary and more expensive use of hospitals and emergency departments. They all employ nurses, who can bring their unique perspectives and talents to institutionalizing the patient-centered and value-oriented transformation of health care that the new laws intend.

One arena that illustrates how the application of a nursing lens to policy is an ongoing evolutionary process is the use of nurse experts in court cases throughout the country. A topic such as this would likely have never been raised by someone solely prepared in law or medicine, or perhaps any other field. But a nurse would see the potential inconsistency here that has grave implications for nursing. See Exhibit 11.7 for a policy analysis related to nurse testimony.

The reality of interprofessional work, however, is still being written. As a result of *The Future of Nursing* report (IOM, 2011) and the RWJF/IOM collaborative launch of the Initiative on the Future of Nursing, the RWJF organized a meeting of 12 nurse and physician leaders to begin a document that outlined what collaboration between these two groups should entail (RWJF, 2013). The project ended prematurely as some physician groups withdrew their participation when the report prematurely became public. As a follow-up (in 2012), the Center for Applied Research (CFAR) staff questioned nurse and physician participants to understand what might be learned from the undertaking and to move forward with future steps toward interprofessional collaboration. The four main results were that

1. "The dialogue produced not only a document but also a new understanding between nurses and doctors, and spurred debate among members of their organizations
2. Interprofessional collaboration is already occurring on the ground—the problem is at the organizational level
3. The consensus and lessons from the dialogue can help improve such collaboration
4. The patient must be at the center of interprofessional collaboration, but challenges remain in applying that focus" (RWJF, 2013)

There are organizations, however, where interprofessional changes have helped to bring order, emphasize priorities, and provide protection for physicians, nurses, staff, and patients. Examples of two policies that arose out of nursing concerns and resulted in major organizational change were those led by Barnsteiner and colleagues at Children's Hospital of Philadelphia (2001), and Disch and Taranto at Fairview-University Medical Center (2002). In the former example, Barnsteiner, along with the nursing director of cardiovascular nursing and the chief cardiovascular surgeon, spearheaded a process for instituting a disruptive conduct policy for medical staff, a controversial policy change.

In the second example, Disch and Taranto led an organization-wide effort to institute a policy for handling emergent situations, such as in the operating room when someone present believes something is wrong and is hesitant to speak up. This work is the forerunner to the time-out practice endorsed in 2010 by the Association of periOperative Registered Nurses (AORN) when it launched the Time-Out Commitment campaign (Operating Room, 2010).

Both of these examples demonstrate key strategies that can be used in either the big "P" or little "p" of policy development when working interprofessionally. The application of the nursing lens requires persistence as well as drawing upon the diverse skill sets that are possessed by many nurses (see Policy on the Scene 11.5).

| EXHIBIT 11.7 | POLICY ANALYSIS OF NURSE TESTIMONY |

Mat Keller, BSN, JD, RN, a nurse and lawyer, wanted to examine the intersection between nursing and the law, such as how is nursing advantaged or disadvantaged by the interpretation of certain laws, and how can existing laws strengthen nursing's position as an autonomous profession? The issue here centered on negligence or malpractice actions against nurses wherein expert witness physicians are used to establish the applicable nursing standards of care. Do physicians, in fact, meet the standards for qualification as expert witnesses regarding applicable nursing standards, or is this in part a result of the societal handmaiden nurse stereotype infusing the legal community? And if physicians do indeed meet the expert witness standards as a matter of law, should they, as a matter of policy?

Federal legislation sets a fairly low standard for qualification of expert witnesses as it applies in malpractice actions—for the most part, the experts' specialized knowledge is required only to assist the jury in understanding the evidence or in determining a fact in issue. The matters to which an expert witness may testify should (logically) be limited to those areas in which the witness is qualified as an expert. Despite a pervasive belief to the contrary, nurses are not in fact trained in medicine. Rather, they are trained in the nursing process. Conversely, physicians are trained in the medical, not nursing, model, and so would seem to be unqualified as experts on the basis of their training in nursing practice. Likewise, the basis for the physician experience in nursing practice does not rise to a level that could be described as "expert." Certainly, members of the two occupations work with each other and interact on a daily basis, but only insofar as coordinating medical with nursing care. Indeed, nurses develop a workable knowledge of medical practice through their experience, but they are by no means medical experts.

Nursing's status as an autonomous profession has required that nursing establish its own standards of care as a matter of policy, just as lawyers have established their legal standards of care, accountants theirs, and dentists theirs. Nursing has done this, but it must also establish its standards of care in the courtroom as well, and be recognized as the true expert witness when testimony on expert nursing practice is needed. However, the low standard for expert witness qualification, the strong and pervasive misconceptions regarding medical versus nursing practice, and the wide discretion granted to trial judges in qualifying experts adds up to the outcome that physicians can and will continue to be qualified as experts in establishing applicable nursing standards of care. A physician's advanced medical education, traditionally respected position in society, historically paternalistic role in health care, and perhaps even gender combine to make his or her testimony exponentially more persuasive than that of a given nurse, despite the nurse's substantially higher expertise in nursing care. Despite any relevance the physician's opinion may have on an issue at hand, expert physician testimony regarding nursing standards of care should be barred both for policy reasons and in accordance with federal legislation.

Here, the nursing lens can be used to illuminate the misapplication of existing law. Federal legislation exists that supports the idea that physicians should not provide testimony regarding nursing standards of care. However, this continues to occur and compromises the profession's ability to exercise its rightful autonomy. This is an important distinction to understand (i.e., whether an issue has a legal basis, a political basis, or elements of both). A key point is that influencing policy requires understanding as to where attention should be paid (e.g., the law, the political process, public awareness, or some combination of the three).

POLICY ON THE SCENE 11.5: Applying the Nursing Lens to Integrate Services

A midwest county hospital decided to integrate its human services, a local hospital and its clinic system, a separate safety net community clinic, and a managed care organization in a demonstration project modeled after the Patient Protection and Affordable Care Act (2010) accountable care organization. All four organizations had a history of working closely with the county and shared a mission of serving people on publicly funded programs, yet inadequate communication channels and accountability mechanisms had resulted in little change, with traditional provider practices and processes continuing.

Eileen Weber, DNP, JD, PHN, RN, was invited to direct the process. Already familiar with the hospital system, she engaged in months of discussions with nurses, social workers, physicians, and managers, determining that an integrated, interactive training program and compilation of key documents into a single training manual were needed. Over the course of the next several months, Eileen (a) instituted a planning team of a diverse array of members; (b) drafted a training agenda with logical sequencing and enough content detail to stimulate productive discussion; (c) created an educational session to cover essential content (one successful component being a discussion with patients receiving services about what worked and what didn't despite strong skepticism by a non-nurse project director); (d) hosted two education sessions; (e) compiled the documents for the training manual and assigned those that were essential but nonexistent; and (f) launched monthly update sessions for care coordination teams to continue the project's momentum. Perhaps most importantly, the interprofessional and interorganizational relationships that were developed offer a foundation upon which successful, ongoing transformative care coordination can be based.

In this situation, Eileen skillfully used her nursing lens. She used her specialized knowledge, well-developed assessment skills, and clinical judgment to incorporate functional resources patients need to maximize the impact their treatments can have. She understood the concepts of care planning and coordination, and their essential place in working with Medicaid recipients. She was able to clarify and simplify the materials so that patients and care providers could better understand each other's roles. She demonstrated an appreciation for the need for structure to accomplish the group's goals and worked with them to co-create the educational sessions and the training manuals.

Her organizational skills, developed over years of multitasking as an emergency department nurse, served her well in juggling several competing priorities. Finally, she used her strong interpersonal skills to build an atmosphere of collaboration and collegiality with a diverse array of stakeholders, bringing everyone to the table, including patients.

As a nurse working to change a policy that involves several professions in a service area (e.g., women's health, emergency department), across a system or in a local community you can:

1. Bring together a diverse group of stakeholders to address the issue
2. Appoint leaders who can reflect different perspectives; for example, strong nurse and physician leadership
3. Keep the focus on what is best for the patient—and support for those providing care
4. Provide data to underscore the importance of the problem and evidence to support the legitimacy of the proposed solution
5. Identify champions within the group who can speak to various constituencies
6. Garner senior leadership support and be explicit about the meaning of that "support"
7. When needing the support of an individual who is crucial to the acceptance of a policy, send the person who has the closest relationships and greatest influence to garner support
8. Approach each discussion with a new person from the beginning, that is, state the problem, indicate why it is a concern, determine what can be done, review the proposed change, and agree on the best approach
9. Never assume that others are at the same point of embracing policy change

Shaping policy interprofessionally makes sense for patients, all professions, and organizations. A number of initiatives that reflect the nursing lens have taken hold across health care and have strong interprofessional underpinnings and are not limited to the development of these programs: Magnet Recognition Program®, National Database of Nursing Quality Indicators® (NDNQI), Safe Patient Handling Mobility (SPHM), National Priorities Partnership, National Quality Forum, and Sexual Assault Nurse Examiner (SANE). The work of each of these programs is patient centered, includes broad interprofessional collaboration, and reflects a clear application of a nursing lens. In the Option for Policy Challenge, see how a nursing lens helped address the issues presented at the beginning of this chapter.

OPTION FOR POLICY CHALLENGE:
The Nursing Lens Applied
Joanne Disch

I drew on several aspects of my nursing background to help handle this situation. The experiences that I had had in various nursing roles prepared me for identifying the aspects of the bill that I supported, and to explain these simply and compellingly to the audience members. I was able to talk in layman's terms and sincerely say that "this was a D- bill but D- is a passing grade—and here is why I support it." I could point to aspects that

I knew most members had not heard of, but could relate to, such as funding preventive health care, supporting the role of advanced practice nurses, and increasing access to the public for needed health care. In addition, it would provide financial support for medications and protect seniors from catastrophic medication expenses. My nursing background enabled me to read the body language of the participants, listen fully to their concerns, restate them at times, and offer simple responses to their questions. I was even able to provoke laughter at a few moments. Also, by acknowledging that the bill wasn't perfect—in fact, it had scored a D- in my estimation—I could demonstrate the importance of compromise and work toward better solutions while getting started with what was now possible. After the educational sessions, those of us presenting the content met informally with audience members to make sure that they had understood our message and that their feelings, even if in opposition, were respected and heard.

Nurses are particularly skilled in connecting with people from all backgrounds, translating complex topics into coherent messages, listening to what is being asked as well as what is not being said, helping people deal with monumental change and disappointment, and identifying sources of optimism and hope. This reflects a skill set that is congruent with an approach that is holistic, people oriented, realistic, big picture, and yet attuned to the small details of the human experience. This is the nursing lens.

IMPLICATIONS FOR THE FUTURE

Nurses can influence the development, implementation, and evaluation of policies at the local, organizational, and national levels in many ways. Every nurse has the opportunity to influence policy, whether it is from a formal or an informal position. More than that, as nurses they have a unique skill set that well suits them to achieve significant change in every setting. For those nurses who see the world through nursing's unique prism and are willing to act, this is their time and the future is theirs to write.

To further these efforts, nurses must see policy engagement as something that begins from the time they are in school and continues into employment, not something that is begun when they have time, when established in their work, or when they have seniority. For far too long nurses have encouraged the next generation of nurses to get established before furthering their education and experience, or becoming involved in policy. As nurses look for opportunities for practice change, full consideration must be given to policy implications of their work and consider policy as a way to bring order, emphasize priorities, and safeguard patients, nurses, and the institutions where they work. Interprofessional education and collaboration can provide the training ground for nurses to assume more significant roles in health care policy development. Nurses must set goals and develop strategies to increase the number of elected officials serving who articulate the nursing lens much as the goal has been set to increase the number of nurses on boards. In 1992 Donna Diers wrote that nurses must discard the "I am only a nurse" mentality when talking about why they chose their nursing role. It is time to argue that nurses must now discrard the "policy is to be done by someone else" mentality. All nurses must be actively involved in shaping policy.

KEY CONCEPTS

1. Nurses need to assume their rightful place in policy leadership and in partnership with others in shaping our health care system.
2. The absence of a nursing lens in policy development results in suboptimal policy outcomes.
3. A nursing lens can be brought to bear on high-profile health issues through unity and solid data.
4. Nurses are underrepresented in formal political structures both in the United States and globally.
5. The nursing lens differentiates nurses from others engaged in the political process through insights about health, illness, resiliency, and the human condition.
6. The nursing lens brings a whole-person/whole-system perspective that informs the promotion of health as well as the creation of effective systems and pragmatic solutions.
7. Political opportunities exist within formal political structures, as well as through membership on boards, committees, and task forces in associations, at work, and in communities.
8. Board service, particularly in health care organizations and organizations that have a connection to the health care industry, is a key strategy for expanding nursing's influence.
9. Strategies for being a successful board member include focusing on the good of the organization, listening, and avoiding repetition.
10. Edge Runners and Magnet Prize recipients provide exemplars of how nurses have influenced policy to make a difference in policy and the outcomes of care.
11. Support for including more nurses on health care boards comes from prominent national organizations.
12. To enhance the influence of the nursing lens, nurses need to be involved in policy throughout their careers.

SUMMARY

There are several ways in which nurses can contribute through using their nursing background and expertise—their nursing lens—when serving in key decision-making roles. Nurses are able to take complex topics and craft messages that enable stakeholders, employees, or members to understand them and see how they apply to their particular situations. Nurses even know to ask, "What are the implications for constituents or frontline workers when changes are being considered, such as reductions in benefits, elimination of services, or closing of facilities?" Nurses are holistic in their thinking so that, when policies are developed, they know to ask "What are the implications for the family, or the patient in the home, or the community?" Nurses are inclusive in their language so that policies that promote "physician" as provider offer more options when the phrase "health care provider" is used, or that "at the patient's side" is preferable to "bedside." Nurses know that implementation of exciting new technology doesn't come without significant investment in orientation and ongoing training, as with electronic health records (EHRs) or medication dispensing systems. Nurses know that what works at 2 p.m. on a weekday doesn't always work at 10 p.m. on a Saturday night: Policies have to reflect the realities of practice and patient care in all settings, at all times, with all combinations of providers. Finally, nurses know where threats to patient safety and quality exist, such as in failure to invest in adequate resources, staff support, and training.

Nurses are the largest group of health care providers in the world, and also the group with the closest connection to the recipients of service. The current health care crisis can and should be addressed in part through solutions supplied by the largest health care profession—nursing. Policy development and implementation require the active and ongoing engagement of nurses using their nursing background and expertise.

This chapter provided a definition and framework for engaging in policy work at all levels. It introduced the concept of the nursing lens and described how the nursing lens enriches policy and politics, citing several examples of nurses whose work was shaped by a view of the world through this nursing lens—and the differences that can make in improving health and health care through policy work.

LEARNING ACTIVITIES

1. Compare and contrast the legislative agendas of two prominent nursing associations. Which appeals more to your priorities and why?
2. Interview three chairs of committees/task forces where you work and ask the chairs to describe how they became chairs.
3. Identify four potential state appointments that a nurse holds in your state beyond the state board of nursing.

4. Participate in a committee meeting at work or in your community. Assess the leader's behaviors and pay special attention to those that advance the work. What is he or she doing or saying that makes a difference?

5. Review the following websites and develop your own list of tips for becoming more active in policy: http://campaignforaction.org/webinar/nurse-leaders-boardroom-skills-you-need-be-successful-board and http://community sector.nl.ca/voluntary-sector-resources/board-development/ten-tips-becoming-more-effective-board-member

6. Identify an organization whose mission you support. Explore the processes that it uses to select board or committee members.

7. Click into the Library of Leaders at www.nursing.umn.edu/densford. View the video tapes of Claire Fagin and Vernice Ferguson. Compare and contrast their approaches to leadership and policy. With whom do you resonate most? Why?

E-RESOURCES

- 2020 Women on Boards. http://www.2020wob.com
- Best on Boards. http://www.bestonboard.org/website/about.html
- Catalyst: Changing Workplaces. Changing Lives. http://www.catalyst.org
- International Council of Nurses (ICN). (2004). *Guidelines on the nurse entre/intrapreneur providing nursing service.* Geneva, Switzerland: ICN. http://www.crnns.ca/documents/Self%20Emp%20Practice/Guidelines%20 for%20Nurse%20Entrepreneurs%20%28ICN%29.pdf
- Nurse Leaders in the Boardroom—The Skills You Need to Be Successful on a Board. http://campaignforaction.org/webinar/nurse-leaders-board room-skills-you-need-be-successful-board
- Nurses on Hospital Boards—Why Is It So Important? http://www.rwjf .org/en/blogs/human-capital-blog/2013/09/nurses_on_hospitalb.html
- Power to Influence Patient Care: Who Holds the Keys? http://www .nursingworld.org/MainMenuCategories/ANAMarketplace/ ANAPeriodicals/OJIN/JournalTopics/Topic32

REFERENCES

11th Street Family Health Services: History. (2010). Retrieved from http://www.drexel. edu/11thstreet/history.asp

American Academy of Nursing (AAN). (n.d.). *Transforming America's health care system through nursing solutions.* Retrieved from http://www.aannet.org/raisethevoice

Anderson, J. (2006). *Public policymaking: An introduction* (6th ed.). Boston, MA: Houghton Mifflin.

Barclay, L. (2010, February 2). Nurses should play greater role in health policy planning, management. *Medscape Medical News.* Retrieved from http://www.medscape.com/ viewarticle/716344

Barnsteiner, J. H., Madigan, C, & Spray, T. L. (2001). Instituting a disruptive conduct policy for medical staff. *AACN Clinical Issues, 12*(3), 378–382.

Blue Ribbon Panel on Health Care Governance. (2007). *Building an exceptional board: Effective practices for health care governance: Report of the Blue Ribbon Panel on Health Care Governance.* Retrieved from http://www.americangovernance.com/resources/reports/brp/2007

Catalyst. (2013, May 31). *Board seats held by women, by country. Quick take.* Retrieved from http://www.catalyst.org/knowledge/women-boards

Clancy, C. (2012, December). From the director. *AHRQ Research Activities, 388,* 2. Retrieved from http://www.ahrq.gov/news/newsletters/research-activities/12dec/1212RA.pdf

Collins, A. M. (2013). Caring for the whole person. *American Journal of Nursing, 113*(5), 53–54.

Color of Safety Initiative, born locally, spreads nationally and to the military. (2009, October 6). *Northeast Pennsylvania Business Journal.* Retrieved from http://biz570.com/education-healthcare/healthcare/color-of-safety-initiative-born-locally-spreads-nationally-and-to-the-military-1.313280

Diers, D. (1992). One-liners. *Image: Journal of Nursing Scholarship, 24*(1), 75–77.

Disch, J. (2007). Extending your influence: Serving on the AARP Board. In D. J. Mason, J. K. Leavitt, & M. W. Chaffee (Eds.), *Policy and politics in nursing and health care* (5th ed., pp. 778–781). St. Louis, MO: Elsevier.

Disch, J. (2012). The nursing lens. *Nursing Outlook, 60,* 170–171.

Disch, J. (2014). Invite an adversary to lunch. *American Journal of Nursing, 114*(5), 8.

Disch, J., & Taranto, K. (2002). Creating change in the workplace. In D. Mason & J. Leavitt (Eds.), *Policy and politics in nursing and health care* (4th ed., pp. 333–361). St. Louis, MO: Saunders.

Evans, M. (2009). A different nursing shortage. *Modern Healthcare, 39*(15), 28–30.

Fagin, C. M. (2000). *Essays on nursing leadership.* New York, NY: Springer Publishing.

Governance Institute. (2007). *Boards x 4: Governance structures and practices.* San Diego, CA: Governance Institute.

Hassmiller, S., & Combes, J. (2012). Nurse leaders in the boardroom: A fitting choice. *Journal of Healthcare Management, 57*(1), 8–11.

Institute of Medicine (IOM). (2011). *The future of nursing: Leading change, advancing health.* Washington, DC: National Academies Press.

International Council of Nurses. (2010). *Nurse politicians network: Overview.* Retrieved from http://www.icn.ch/networks/overview

Khoury, C. M., Blizzard, R., Wright Moore, L., & Hassmiller, S. (2011). Nursing leadership from bedside to boardroom: A Gallup national survey of opinion leaders. *Journal of Nursing Administration, 41*(7–8), 299–305.

Lyttle, B. (2011). Politics: A natural next step for nurses. *American Journal of Nursing, 111*(5), 19–20.

Manojlovich, M. (2007, January 31). Power and empowerment in nursing: Looking backward to inform the future. *OJIN: Online Journal of Issues in Nursing, 12*(1) .Retrieved from http://www.nursingworld.org/MainMenuCategories/ANAMarketplace/ANAPeriodicals/OJIN/TableofContents/Volume122007/No1Jan07/LookingBackwardtoInformtheFuture.asp

Marshall, E. S. (2011). *Transformational leadership in nursing.* New York, NY: Springer Publishing.

Mason, D. J. (2010). *Nursing's visibility in the national health care reform agenda.* Paper presented at the meeting of the American Association of Colleges of Nursing Doctoral Education Conference, Captiva Island, FL.

National Association of Clinical Nurse Specialists (NACNS). (n.d.). *Guide to getting appointed to your state boards of nursing*. Retrieved from http://www.nacns.org/docs/toolkit/3B-GuideToBON.pdf

Operating Room Nurses Ask for Time Out. (2010, June 10). *Medical News Today*. Retrieved from http://www.medicalnewstoday.com/releases/191469.php

Pennsylvania Patient Safety Authority. (2005, December 14). Use of color-coded patient wristbands creates unnecessary risk. PA PSRS *Patient Safety Advisory, 2*(Suppl 2), 1–4.

Politics. (n.d.). *Wikipedia*. Retrieved from http://en.wikipedia.org/wiki/Politics

Powell, C. (2010, June 28). Ohio nurse could help solve problems with feeding tube connectors. *Akron Beacon Journal*. Retrieved from http://medcitynews.com/2010/06/ohio-nurse-could-help-solve-problems-with-feeding-tube-connectors

Prybil, L., Levey, S., Peterson, R., Heinrich, D., Brezinski, P., Zamba, G., … Roach, W. (2009). *Governance in high-performing community health systems: A report on trustee and CEO views*. Chicago, IL: Grant Thornton LLP.

Reier, S. (2008, March 21). Women take their place on corporate boards. *New York Times*.

Robert Wood Johnson Foundation (RWJF). (2007). *Putting nursing skills and experience to work in the boardroom*. Retrieved from http://www.rwjf.org/en/about-rwjf/newsroom/newsroom-content/2007/11/putting-nursing-skills-and-experience-to-work-in-the-boardroom.html

Robert Wood Johnson Foundation (RWJF). (2013). *How to foster interprofessional collaboration between physicians and nurses? Incorporating lessons learned in pursuing consensus*. Retrieved from http://www.rwjf.org/content/dam/farm/reports/program_results_reports/2013/rwjf403637

Rychnovsky, J. (2011). *Ruth Lubic: A timeliness and tireless visionary for childbearing families*. Retrieved from http://onlinelibrary.wiley.com/doi/10.1111/j.1552-6909.2011.01272.x/full

Shalala, D. E. (2012). Foreword. In D. J. Mason, J. K. Leavitt, & M. W. Chaffee (Eds.), *Policy and politics in nursing and health care* (6th ed., p. xxvii). St. Louis, MO: Elsevier.

Sharp, B. C. (2012, December). The changing role of the nurse. *AHRQ Research Activities, 388*, 1, 3–4. Retrieved from http://www.ahrq.gov/news/newsletters/research-activities/12dec/1212RA.pdf

Simmons, D., & Graves, K. (2008). Tubing misconnections-A systems failure with human factors: Lessons for nursing practice. *Urologic Nursing, 28*(6), 460–464.

Sullivan, E. (2012). *Becoming influential* (2nd ed.). Saddle River, NJ: Prentice-Hall.

Totten, M. K. (2010). *Nurses on healthcare boards: A smart and logical move to make*. Center for Healthcare Governance. Retrieved from http://www.bestonboard.org/website/pdf/MJ10_GovInsights_reprint.pdf

Visiting Nurse Service of New York. (n.d.). *Lillian Wald*. Retrieved from http://www.vnsny.org/community/our-history/lillian-wald

IV

Judging Worth and Advancing the Cause

TWELVE

Serving the Public Through Policy and Leadership

Virginia Trotter Betts
Susan Tullai-McGuinness
Loretta Alexia Williams

Two roads diverged in a wood, and I—I took the one less traveled by. And that has made all the difference.—Robert Frost

OBJECTIVES

1. Identify the common characteristics of nurse policy leaders in order to enhance one's own policy journey.
2. Explore the multiple paths to becoming a nursing leader and policy advocate.
3. Analyze strategies designed to encourage nurses' involvement in policy.
4. Create a plan for one's personal growth in leadership and advocacy.

While Florence Nightingale is often cited for her caring service to others, and her skilled clinical work as the "lady of the lamp," her more long-standing impact comes from her ability to leverage data and her effective and intensive advocacy to achieve implementation of a reform agenda that would change health care delivery forever. And Nightingale was only one of many reformers who have pioneered advocacy and leadership in nursing.

In the United States, there are also notable nurse leaders and advocates for health care reforms and improvements. Dorothea Dix advocated for reforms in the care of the mentally ill. Clara Barton founded the American Red Cross. Lillian Wald founded the Henry Street Settlement at the turn of the 20th century, which eventually grew into the Visiting Nursing Service of New York and, by the way, suggested a national health insurance plan (National Women's History Museum, n.d.). Virginia Henderson authored a classic text that defined nursing for the profession. Hildegard Peplau, a president of the American Nurses Association (ANA), formulated the interpersonal theory of nursing, providing a foundation for psychiatric nursing. M. Elizabeth Carnegie led the way in breaking down racial barriers for nurses, while Luther Christman, a long-time advocate for integration in nursing, broke down barriers for men in nursing. This formidable legacy continues with leaders whose innovative health care practices and advocacy have improved the lives of many and improved health policy, both public and private.

In this chapter, we explore the many varied paths to taking on the mantle of leadership and advocacy. We share the stories of exceptional nurse leaders, who have made outstanding achievements in health and health policy, both public and private, and in local, state, national, and global arenas. We introduce you not only to those nurses in elected or appointed government posts, but also to nurse leaders who have made extraordinary contributions to health policy through either their formal employment, their professional organizations, or their volunteer work in their communities. These leaders reflect concern for their fellow human beings and a desire to help others through advancing the nursing profession. Being a nurse leader and advocate takes many forms and provides the opportunity to have a direct role in influencing health care policy. For the author, (VTB), my deeply held beliefs that (a) the profession of nursing is *the* solution for so many health problems experienced in the United States and (b) there is no health without the consideration of mental health has fueled my passion to take on an ever-increasing role in public policy. See the Policy Challenge for details of how my passions prompted me to action.

POLICY CHALLENGE: Getting Started on the Journey to Champion Nursing and Mental Health Through Policy Activism
Virginia Trotter Betts, MSN, JD, RN, FAAN, Nashville, TN

An incredible nursing professor in my BSN education program piqued my interest in psychiatric mental health nursing as a specialty focus. Coming from a long line of public health nurses, I was also interested in public health nursing and I could have specialized in either and been content. But I chose psychiatric nursing and a graduate education stipend in return for a service commitment to work in public mental health. This was meant to be!

Psychiatric/mental health nursing was both interesting and challenging, and I loved all its aspects. I gained human behavior expertise in human and group behavior as well as communication, motivational, and collaboration skills so necessary not only to interpersonal and organizational success but also to policy work. (It is not surprising to me that quite a few of the ANA's past presidents, in addition to me, have had a psychiatric nursing background: Hildegard Peplau, Lucille Joel, Beverly Malone, and Becky Patton to name a few.)

After my MSN graduation, I worked in a state psychiatric hospital and at a community mental health center and developed programs in both facilities to provide substance abuse services which were so needed and which no one else was inclined to take on. Later, I chose law school for my doctoral education and I focused on health law and public policy, centering my project work on those areas. I wanted to be a *nurse lawyer*! Throughout my nursing career I was an active member of the Tennessee Nurses Association (TNA). This was not surprising as my roots for TNA were strong as I had been a Tennessee Association of Student Nurses officer, and my mother and my aunt had been active TNA members when I was growing up. In TNA, I served on committees, worked on position papers, and strategized on the health issues facing our state and how my profession, nursing, could be positioned to address them. These activities laid the groundwork for my election as TNA president, which led to significant opportunities to represent Tennessee nurses within the ANA.

Each phase of my career has been built upon on a strong foundation: all my previous education, work and professional experience, including a major opportunity that came when I was selected as a Robert Wood Johnson (RWJ) Health Policy Fellow (www.healthpolicyfellows.org). This extraordinary program involved a total immersion in health policy, interacting daily at the Institute of Medicine (IOM) in Washington, DC, and learning the historical foundations, theory, and practical applications of health policy while meeting with key political leaders and policy opinion makers in the nation and within the Beltway.

Dialoguing with and observing these key leaders were critical to my understanding the issues influencing policy decision making. Even the best policy solutions will not be adopted without keenly understanding the politics of the situation and working it to one's best advantage. An important portion of the RWJ Fellowship program is the placement for experiential work/application in a specific policy office or agency. While I considered numerous offers from executive branch agencies, congressional committees, and individual Senate or House members, I wanted to maintain a closer connection to my home (after all, I had a 7-year-old at home with her dad). Al Gore was then an up-and-coming senator from Tennessee, who offered me a place on his Senate staff working on health issues. In his Senate office, I learned to appreciate how very important involved, vocal people are to advancing policy initiatives. In retrospect, it didn't hurt nursing, or our professional agenda, when Senator Gore became Vice President Gore in the same year that I became ANA president. These phases of my career resulted in my building a foundation of expertise and political know how that enabled me thereafter to have the necessary vision, networks, confidence, and leadership qualities and credentials to be at the table to advance and promote the nursing profession, mental health, and health through policy activism—my professional passions.

See Option for Policy Challenge.

Research has demonstrated that nurses hesitate to become involved in policy because they believe that they have inadequate knowledge and skills in the policy arena (Boswell, Cannon, & Miller, 2005; Cramer, 2002; Taft & Nanna, 2008; Vandenhouten, Malakar, Kubsch et al., 2011; Winter, 1991). When nurses do participate in political activities, very often it is in activities such as voting and contacting elected officials rather than public speaking, participation in organizations, and active involvement in addressing a cause (Vandenhouten et al., 2011). By learning from the stories of our nurse exemplars and providing guidance for strategies for assuming a more active policy role, we hope that you are called to action to serve the public and profession by becoming passionately engaged in the policy process.

Interviews for this chapter were conducted with distinguished nurse "exemplars," who thoughtfully and reflectively responded to questions about their varied journeys in nursing leadership and health policy. See Exhibit 12.1 for a listing of these nurses and their areas of interest and expertise. The voices of these nurses, their ideas, values, and advice, are shared in this chapter to help you think about your role and opportunity in policy, as well as to inspire the creativity and passion that you have for nursing so that you can harness that energy to begin, enhance, and fulfill your commitment to advocacy.

EXHIBIT 12.1 NURSE EXEMPLARS AND POLICY EXPERTISE

NURSE EXEMPLAR	POSITION	AREA OF POLICY EXPERTISE
José Alejandro, PhD, RN-BC, MBA, CCM, FACHE	Past President, National Association of Hispanic Nurses (NAHN); Corporate Director of Case Management, Cornerstone Healthcare Group	Health care disparities; case management
Pamela Bennett, BSN, RN, CCE	Executive Director, Healthcare Alliance, Purdue Pharma, LP	Pain management; develops and manages relationships with national patient advocacy and professional associations

(continued)

EXHIBIT 12.1   NURSE EXEMPLARS AND POLICY EXPERTISE *(CONTINUED)*

NURSE EXEMPLAR	POSITION	AREA OF POLICY EXPERTISE
Michael Bleich, PhD, RN, FAAN	Maxine Clark and Bob Fox Dean, Goldfarb School of Nursing at Barnes-Jewish College	Health policy; future trends in nursing
Lois Capps, MA, RN	Congresswoman, United States House of Representatives, 24th District, California	Health policy; school health; quality and safety; workforce planning issues
Jennie Chin Hanson, MSN, RN, FAAN	CEO, American Geriatrics Society; Past President, AARP	Geriatrics; primary, acute, and long-term care community-based services
Marilyn P. Chow, PhD, RN, FAAN	Vice President, National Patient Care Services, Kaiser Permanente; First Director, Executive Nurse Fellows Program, Robert Wood Johnson Foundation	Regulation of nursing practice and workforce policy. Promotion of nurses' roles in primary care, advanced practice, and hospital-based care
Pamela F. Cipriano, PhD, RN, FAAN	President, American Nurses Association; Past Editor, *American Nurse Today*	Safety of HIT and meaningful use of HIT. Nursing standards
Cole Edmonson, DNP, RN, FACHE, NEA-BC	Chief Nursing Officer/Vice President, Texas Health Presbyterian Hospital	Leadership, succession planning, moral courage, and nurse bullying creator of http://www.stopbullyingnurses.com
Michael L. Evans, PhD, RN, NEA-BC, FACHE, FAAN	President, American Nurses Credentialing Center (ANCC); Dean, UMC Endowed Chair for Excellence in Nursing, Texas Tech University Health Sciences Center School of Nursing	Health care management, credentialing, professional association leadership

(continued)

EXHIBIT 12.1 NURSE EXEMPLARS AND POLICY EXPERTISE (*CONTINUED*)

NURSE EXEMPLAR	POSITION	AREA OF POLICY EXPERTISE
Claire M. Fagin, PhD, RN, FAAN	Senior Advisor, Jonas Center; Dean Emerita, School of Nursing, University of Pennsylvania, first woman to serve in president role of any Ivy League university; Past President, National League for Nursing	Nursing education and leadership; geriatric nursing
Kristine Gebbie, DrPH, RN, FAAN	Professor, Flinders University; First White House AIDS Policy Coordinator	Public health, disaster response and recovery, nursing policy
Susan B. Hassmiller, PhD, RN, FAAN	Senior Advisor for Nursing, Robert Wood Johnson Foundation (RWJF)	Future of Nursing Campaign for Action; public health, international primary care, disaster preparedness
Frances E. Likis, DrPh, NP, CNM, FACNM	Senior Investigator, Vanderbilt University, Evidence-Based Practice Center; Editor-in-Chief, Journal of Midwifery & Women's Health	Nurse midwifery, women's health, APRN scope of practice and reimbursment
Carol Ann Lockhart, PhD, RN, FAAN	President, C. Lockhart Associates; Professor of Nursing, University of Tennessee Health Science Center	Health systems relations and policy consultation; Medicare and Medicaid payment
Judy Murphy, RN, FACMI, FHIMSS, FAAN	Deputy National Coordinator for Programs and Policy, Office of the National Coordinator for Health IT, Department of Health and Human Services	Health informatics, health IT, electronic health records, system implementation methodologies, technology to support evidence-based practice
Barbara L. Nichols, DHL(h), MS, RN, FAAN	President and CEO, Barbara Nichols Consulting; Past President, ANA, Former CEO, Commission on Graduates of Foreign Nursing Schools (CGFNS)	Nursing regulation, workforce, professional practice standards, international migration of nurses, credentialing, ethnic minority inclusion

(continued)

EXHIBIT 12.1   NURSE EXEMPLARS AND POLICY EXPERTISE (*CONTINUED*)

NURSE EXEMPLAR	POSITION	AREA OF POLICY EXPERTISE
Ann O'Sullivan, MSN, RN, CNE, NE-BC	Assistant Dean of Support Services, Blessing-Rieman College of Nursing	Health policy, standards of nursing practice
Ellen-Marie Whelan, PhD, NP, FAAN	Senior Advisor, Innovation Center, Centers for Medicare & Medicaid Services	Innovative payment and service delivery models for primary care, accountable care, perinatal care, and population health
May Wykle, PhD, RN, FAAN FGSA	Dean Emerita and Marvin E. and Ruth Durr Denakas Professor of Nursing at Frances Payne Bolton School of Nursing, Case Western Reserve University; Past President, Sigma Theta Tau International	Leadership, nursing shortage, geriatrics, family caregiving, minority caregivers, and caregivers of patients with dementia

While these nurse exemplars are not the only policy and advocacy leaders in nursing, they all are exceptional role models. They carry the mantel of characteristics in common to many nurse professionals who have blazed a trail or left their special mark on nursing and health policy. Each has a unique set of life experiences that shaped how he or she forged his or her own particular paths. In this chapter, you will hear their voices explore their ideas, note their abiding values, and take in their honed advice and "lessons learned." All of these exemplars would say to you, "Come along—you can do this! Get involved—change the world—nursing, health care. Our patients need you. You are each needed." No one in this group became a nurse in order to be a health policy influential— yet they did. You can learn from these policy leaders and build your knowledge and skills so that you can join them. You too can lead nursing and health care forward through your own policy-oriented advocacy.

These nurse leaders blended their passion with their clinical professional knowledge and skills in advocating for health and their profession. Many went into nursing simply with the desire to help others. Nurses are able to help others on a daily basis while directly caring for patients or in any one of the numerous professional roles in nursing, serving the public as clinicians, administrators, educators, researchers, and in any number of other capacities. Many of these exemplars expanded their advocacy roles into policy because they saw and wanted to address pressing social justice issues. Assuming a more active role in policy allows for the multiplication of individual efforts that will have a broader impact on health and the profession. More than ever before, nurses are needed to serve in roles that have a direct impact on health policy.

Next, we describe critical junctures in the path of the nurse leader and health nursing activist. Each step of the way provides examples, the lessons learned of how to become a policy activist and manage the challenges of this role.

COMMON BEGINNINGS

The nurse exemplars in this chapter started their nursing careers in very similar ways to most nurses. It is easy to think, mistakenly, that something is inherently different about nursing leaders that makes them great and effective advocates. Rather, clear patterns emerge when listening to their stories that help us all identify and plan ways to become active in policy.

Many of these nurse exemplars heard the call to nursing at a very young age. Personal experiences and role models influenced them. Some were exposed to nursing or health care because of personal or family member illness; others grew up with close relatives who loved their nursing careers; others became nurses because of their volunteer work in a health care setting. During one exemplar's high school years, he observed visiting nurses in his home caring for his dying father. He witnessed "their acts of kindness and love, mixed with technology and science. Their strength, determination, and authenticity became my inspiration …." This, very often, is the spark that ignited these exemplary leaders toward nursing as a career and to action.

Other nurses made their decision to enter nursing in young adulthood but were also influenced by personal experiences and role models. They were drawn to a career where they could make a difference. While in college, one exemplar decided to change his career path from English to nursing after working as an orderly. He vividly remembers asking a nurse what she liked about her work. She replied that she was happy being a nurse because "I know that I have made a profound difference in people's lives." That comment impacted his life and his career choice.

In the 1950s, May Wykle realized that her dream of being a physician was not realistic for an African American woman. She sought a job as a nurse's aide. The health care facility in her hometown did not hire African Americans as nurse's aides; thus, she was offered a housekeeping job instead. However, she was fortunate that her family had a good relationship with a physician who intervened and helped her obtain a nurse's aide position. After she skillfully assisted in caring for a very sick patient, a nurse commented on the excellent care she had provided by stating, "You could be responsible for saving this patient's life." This experience and professional encouragement fueled countless months spent seeking nursing school admission. What an interesting start filled with the challenging roadblocks of outright discrimination for an individual whose significant contributions include serving as a dean of a leading nursing school, and as president of Sigma Theta Tau International.

Then, there are nurses who, like one of the chapter authors, despite positive family nurse role models and volunteer nurse aide experiences, decided that nursing was *not* for her. VTB became the "accidental" nursing student, but along the way she fell in love with nursing. Through rotations in public health, mental health, and maternal/child care in underserved communities, she learned that *only nursing* gets the big picture—that health care is about the patient, the family, and the community, *not* the provider. She stayed the course determined to give nursing more voice and more power to make the changes essential for the patients it serves.

What is your story? Did you always want to be a nurse for as long as you could remember or did you choose nursing as a second career when you were an older adult? Regardless of your path in nursing, all who are willing can make a difference!

COMMON AND RECURRING THEMES

The beginnings of a path to nursing may have many commonalities. However, what is striking is that once in nursing, the journey to leadership policy activism also has commonalities. Seeking advanced education and professional association involvement stood out as common characteristics of these exemplars. But, it was not just these specific acts; it was the views of these exemplars about the role of education and professional involvement as a path to influencing policy that set them apart.

Education as a Door Opener

A striking commonality among the exemplars was the critical role that education played in the career development of almost everyone. Seeking advanced degrees, formal and informal course work, certifications, continuing education, and important fellowships—all were fundamental to their career development and access to opportunities. The exemplars stated unequivocally that knowing more gave them both recognition for their expertise and knowledge and, thus, allowed them to do more. It was through education that they began to realize that the possibilities of making systemic change would require policy actions for any changes of substance. They realized "that being involved in policy making could help to make a greater impact." For example, one nurse had helped to care for dying patients as a nurse clinician. Later in her career, she served on a committee that developed and implemented advanced directives throughout a hospital. This is a great example of taking clinical expertise to the table to make policy change to enhance quality of life for those whom nurses serve.

Intellectual rigor and conceptualizing nursing as a discipline and a field of thought and substance during their education facilitated a broad view and bold horizon well beyond the boundaries of a job or an organization. Advanced nursing education equated with a path for long-term productivity that, for these exemplars, has yielded not only recognition, but tremendous satisfaction in their choice of a profession. They spoke to their beliefs that a well-educated, well-read, and well-credentialed nurse has limitless opportunities because education facilitated being open to stepping through doors of opportunity and challenge. While these exemplars pursued nursing educational specialties across the spectrum of nursing and health care, the specialties of public health, mental health, and health care administration were strongly evident in this particular group of nurse leaders. The need to get strong educational credentials is echoed in the current literature by Curran and Fitzpatrick (2013, p. 133) who advise going to the best school that you can, getting the best degrees that you can, and becoming a lifelong learner.

Professional Growth Through Associations

The exemplars looked beyond their immediate work setting for professional relationships, growth, and development. Almost everyone emphasized over and over the profound and critical role involvement with professional associations played in their professional careers. Professional association membership and involvement led them to grasp the importance of policy issues and helped them connect with other professionals interested in advocacy and policy. The associations most frequently mentioned for involvement were the ANA, state nurses associations, American Academy of Nursing, American Public Health Association (APHA), Academy of Health Care Executives, and the National Student Nurses Association (NSNA).

Professional nursing associations were described as raising the profession to new heights, protecting and/or expanding the boundaries of scope of practice, and educating other nurses and the public about the discipline of nursing and its value. The exemplars were clear that the value of the ANA and its affiliated entities was in helping set standards, creating certification criteria, and serving as think tanks for general and specialty groups to drive innovation in nursing and health care.

José Alejandro encourages all nurses "to be an active member of professional associations that are best aligned with their interests. It is critical for nurses to belong to the ANA and their specialty association." José credits his awareness of the value of professional associations to early mentors who encouraged and supported his involvement in his state's student nurses association. José's passion for improved care for Hispanic populations led him to actions and advocacy that resulted in the presidency of the National Association of Hispanic Nurses (NAHN).

Barbara Nichols was the first Black nurse elected president of the Wisconsin Nurses Association and then the ANA. As president, she represented ANA as the U.S. member at the International Council of Nurses (ICN) and became passionately interested in global health concerns. She served as a board member of the ICN and then spent a good part of her career as the chief executive officer (CEO) of the Commission on Graduates of Foreign Nursing Schools (CGFNS).

The exemplars' stories made it clear they believed nurses have the best opportunity to bring the collective power of the profession to shape health and health care in our nation through the ANA and the state nurses associations. While professional nurses are essential to health care on a one-to-one clinical basis, it is through professional organizations that nurses can feel, build, and express their power/experiences in society. One nurse exemplar stated, "Being involved in your professional association cannot be a maybe thing. It is a must if nurses want to influence policies impacting nurses."

Professional leadership and advocacy does not necessarily end with retirement. This is illustrated by Claire Fagin's wise and reasoned presence as a nurse leader in so many organizations "when they needed her more than she needed them." While others would be fully "retired," Claire is guiding the Jonas Foundation to invest significantly in nursing education and mental health nursing.

The exemplars indicated that a key advantage of association activism is the opportunity to meet and network with nurses holding a variety of positions across the country. Involvement in professional nurses organizations was described as the sources of "colleagues, information, and opportunities." As a volunteer leader, involvement in professional nurses associations helps "to improve communication, develop leadership, and enhance the ability to work in teams." Another exemplar stated that our professional associations are essential to nursing's ability to survive and thrive. "Each of us has a responsibility to contribute to those organizations in some way. At a minimum, we need to be members of the organizations that need our financial support for their work."

Early Beginnings

Most of our exemplars began their participation in professional associations when they began their careers, thus creating the opportunity to network and build relationships over time. Most held membership (and some held significant leadership positions) in other health-related professional associations, while a few were leaders of other nonprofit associations. One exemplar, Jennie Chin Hansen, was a recent president of AARP at the time the Patient Protection and Affordable Care Act (PPACA) was being developed and debated nationally. Networking across disciplines and with multiple organizations was valued. As she stated, "It expands your vision of the world; you learn new skills; and doors of opportunity open."

For many, these values had been instilled through their experiences with student nurses associations. Many of our exemplars participated during their student days as leaders in their state student nurses associations, and several held elected positions at the national level in the NSNA. Student associations served an important role in building interest in both policy and professional issues as well as a training ground for leadership development and important advocacy skills. Thus, after graduation, these exemplars held a sense that they could make a much greater difference in health care through membership in a collective and external group rather than as a single nurse working alone or in a "workplace-only" group. Their experiences with the NSNA led them to join and then aim for leadership positions in their local, state, and national nurses associations. Many of these nurse exemplars also held elected offices in several specialty organizations and/or their state nurses associations as well as the ANA.

Serving first as vice president and then president for the NSNA fueled Pam Cipriano's interest and passion for political and public policy activities. Later, Pam was elected as a reformer/transformational treasurer of the ANA. She served as the first editor-in-chief of *American Nurse Today*, the official ANA monthly publication. Pam said "yes" when asked to lead the publication. Her ability to pull together this monthly publication that gives voice and advocacy to the nursing profession demonstrated her dedication that nurses must "embrace lifelong learning." In June 2014, Pam was elected as the 35th ANA president, in which capacity she will further advance the ANA's mission and vision. She advanced the ANA vision and mission as the editor of its official monthly publication, *American Nurse Today*. Pam believes professional associations are our "backbone for promoting our advocacy for nursing and the public's health. They are our link to fulfill our commitment to society and that we have a responsibility to give back through our professional association so we strengthen nursing and ensure nurses are in the national debate to improve health care."

The policy implication for nurse educators is that students need to be introduced to and become involved in the student nurses association and professional nurses associations at the undergraduate, graduate, and doctoral levels. And, for those nurses who did not have experiences with the nursing student organization at the undergraduate level, it is never too late to seek out professional organization experiences as part of one's career development. Leadership experiences in small organizations, local chapters, or a health care organization's practice committees can provide the opportunity to develop valuable competencies that can be transferred to other settings.

MENTORSHIP

When a door opens, be sure to take other nurses along. This is manifest by the process of mentorship. All of our nurse exemplars felt strongly about the power of mentorship—having a mentor and being a mentor. The strength of nursing's numbers can only be realized when there is strength of place and position. Mentoring is a vehicle for leadership development that brings more nurses to policy tables. Without nursing at the health policy table, there will be no banquet.

Being a mentor and a role model for so many is illustrated by Marilyn Chow's path. She is well known for her leadership in nursing regulation, workforce policy, and representing nursing at the Joint Commission. Her vision and leadership were instrumental in establishing the Robert Wood Johnson Foundation (RWJF) Executive Nurse Fellows programs with a focus on providing exceptional nurses with the tools and enhanced abilities for self-knowledge, strategic vision, risk taking and creativity, interpersonal interactions and communication effectiveness, and managing change as the "pillars of leadership" (RWJF, 2011).

Many exemplars reported having formal mentors who expressed belief in their mentees' capabilities, held high expectations, and were supportive and caring. They served as career advisors and encouraged involvement in professional associations.

Mentors who bring diverse gender, racial, political, professional, and leadership perspectives to your work and career are invaluable. A mentor can help you understand the organizational culture and interpret the "rules" of an organization. See Chapter 7, "Building Capital: Intellectual, Social, Political, and Financial," for additional details on mentoring. My (STM) lifelong political mentor is my husband. Through his influence, example, and support, I have met a number of influential politicians and business leaders. These individuals were extremely important and supportive of my candidacy for the state house in Ohio in 2012 (see Exhibit 12.2 for quotes on the role of mentors in leadership development).

Though the exemplars' relationships with their mentors varied, all expressed the very acute sense of responsibility they hold in providing mentorship to others (it could be you, because each and every one of them said that

---

EXHIBIT 12.2 ROLE OF MENTORS IN LEADERSHIP DEVELOPMENT

"Mentors have the ability to share insights with you that you may not even be close to bringing to your own consciousness."

"Mentors will help set a vision, build character, offer critique and criticism as a gift of growth."

"My first mentor believed in me so powerfully that I had no choice but to succeed!"

"Mentors have been extremely important in career-defining decisions and my involvement in professional associations."

"Mentors' greatest gifts were to help me find my own answers and reinforce what I already know, but can come to doubt."

"Mentors provide diverse and sometimes harsh but realistic perspectives."

"Mentors have helped me to make connections."

"As a Black nurse in a leadership role, no one stepped forward to mentor me. Thus, I chose to observe role models from afar and supplemented through a tremendous amount of reading on leadership."

they would be open to outreach from you!). They appreciated the mentorship they received, which influenced their willingness to help others. As one nurse said, "I want to help those coming after me."

In selecting a mentor, it is important to reflect upon one's needs. Mentors provide benefits at different times in our careers. Mentors may not necessarily come to you. Select a mentor who is a match for your current needs. Continuing with the mentor will depend on how the relationship evolves over time. Important to mentorship is selecting someone whose accomplishments and tactics you admire.

THE ROAD TO POLICY ACTIVISM

Many of these exemplars started their nursing careers providing direct patient care in a clinical setting. As they continued to learn and were encouraged and mentored, their passion for participation in leading, making needed changes, and then involving themselves in practice, professional, and policy decision making grew. Many took on new roles within their own workplace and then outside the workplace and into their community. Most opportunities presented themselves because of their involvement with professional associations and other volunteer activities in communities. Their initial testing of the "I can make a change" moments gave them the opportunity to network with and be recognized by a variety of leaders, health professionals, and nurses across their community, state, and country. They took risks and accepted the challenge to create better health care on their unit, in their facility or organization, or through associations, regulatory bodies, or legislation. However, they wanted you to know that they were not alone and that is one of the reasons they shared their stories. Very frequently, the exemplars stated they had what they considered to be the invaluable guidance, support, and encouragement along the way from their mentors, family, friends, and significant others. Very often the road to public policy advocacy consisted of involvement in public health issues, taking advantage of opportunities beyond their work expectations and commitment to a great professional role for nurses. Commitment to advancing nursing and improved policy continued when these nurse exemplars assumed executive leadership roles in service, system, and academic settings.

Taking Action Through Public Health

A public health perspective was another commonality shared by these nurse exemplars. Public health in this context related to health of populations, health programs/services from a not-for-profit lens that often focused on gaps and inequities, and person-centered approaches to care. It provided many of our exemplars with policy expertise at the community level, which then was translated to endeavors at the societal level. In some ways, this is taking the nursing model on the road for an implementable systems perspective. Susan Hassmiller's interest in policy work was piqued when continuing her nursing education, "I learned about population health and the possibilities of making decisions through policy. I realized that being involved in policy making could help to make a greater impact." Susan became even more aware of its importance and impact when she became personally involved with the American Red Cross after the organization helped locate her parents after an earthquake. Her service on the board of a local chapter led to her becoming involved in the Red Cross's governance and volunteering locally, regionally, and nationally, an involvement that she continues today.

When working as a public health nurse, Jennie Chin Hansen learned "that decisions were made beyond my realm that affected many people." As a young public health nurse, she learned how to work with humility (not always having to be *the* expert) and how, rather, to enable a community to make decisions. Jennie Chin Hansen followed her path of interest that involved systems and teams. She was always interested in meeting community needs through cross-disciplinary work on behalf of her target population (the elderly), which eventually led her to leadership roles at AARP.

Carol Lockhart found that "you can't be in public health without realizing that policies set at all levels of government and within the private sector influence the health of people." While working as the Arizona state health department's coordinator for county public health, Carol learned the needs of all the counties and then used that knowledge and her intergovernmental relationships to shape the first capitated Medicaid program in the United States. Carol's work is an example of utilizing her knowledge of what communities need and then taking on a leadership role to develop systems that fund and purchase those very services and programs. Carol has been an active member of the Arizona Nurses Association, the ANA, and the APHA. Using her expertise in the economics of health care, she represented the ANA in testifying before Congress. Later she became ANA's nominee to the Physician Payment Review Commission, which has proven to be so important for payments for advanced practice nurses. Carol, using her public health nursing foundation, her advanced degree in social and economic policy, and her continuing involvement in professional organizations, positioned herself as a part of the policy-making process to shape nursing and public health policy at the local, state, national, and international levels.

Kristine Gebbie spent a long career serving as the public health director for the state of Oregon, and then Washington, a remarkable accomplishment in and of itself. Her advocacy for and criticism of AIDS policies during the Reagan era led to her being recognized by the Clinton administration to serve as the first White House AIDS policy coordinator, otherwise known as the AIDS czar. Her work focuses on emergency preparedness and developing the public health workforce. In that difficult role, she applied sound public health principles to health issues that had enormous political and cultural conflicts. Not willing to let the status quo or naysayers get in the way of good policy, she has lived by her motto: "Who said we can't do that, how do I get on that committee?" Clearly, nurses bring a larger holistic view to the policy table. Coupling that view with an attitude of figuring out how to achieve goals despite many obstacles, large and small, can yield powerful results.

Nurse Executives' Commitment to the Nursing Role

Although our nurse exemplars no longer function in the role of direct care nurse, their commitment to nursing and its indispensable value in patient care and society remains steadfast. Consider Cole Edmonson, chief nursing officer/vice president at Texas Health Presbyterian Hospital Dallas, who continues to contribute to the primary nursing role through his creation of a website aimed at decreasing nurse bullying, a pervasive issue jeopardizing unit morale and patient safety. He created a supportive environment where respect and integrity of practice are highly valued. He supports, inspires, and mentors both novice and experienced staff nurses. He is a "true nursing advocate" who believes, espouses, and actively works to create leaders at the bedside and empower them to lead.

Dr. Michael Evans's career in nursing encompasses a number of executive roles in nursing service and academia. He has demonstrated his continued commitment to nursing, serving as president of the Texas Nurses Association and as secretary and treasurer of the ANA. More recently, he is advancing nursing and policy by serving as the president of the American Nurses Credentialing Center (ANCC), which provides credentialing in nursing specialty certifications and implements the Magnet Recognition Program® in the nation's hospitals.

Academic Leaders' Commitment to the Nursing Role

Although our exemplars began their careers in the clinical setting, many found their passion in academia. Claire Fagin's commitment to nursing is demonstrated in her having led the development of landmark nursing education and research programs, including a PhD program. Her outstanding leadership for nursing education led not only to her influential term as president of the National League for Nursing, but also to her appointment as the first nurse and first female president of an Ivy League university. Additionally, as noted earlier, she is a senior advisor to the Jonas Scholar program, which provides funding to support educational development of new nurse faculty. Her extensive knowledge and experience provide guidance and insight into the Jonas Center's planning and programs designed to enhance the nursing profession.

One of the greatest rewards Ann O'Sullivan experienced in her career has been the opportunity to teach, coach, and support nursing students for more than 30 years. As an educator, she inspires and empowers her students to further nursing and quality health care. With her guidance, hundreds of students have been educated in a variety of leadership and health policy courses, making her contribution one that is ongoing and lasting. "They often contact me later and seek more information about how to stay involved and informed." Among Ann's contributions is developing a guide for educators to teach in the use of the ANA's *Nursing: Scope and Standards for Practice* (2010).

Another exemplar illustrating achievement of academic opportunities for nursing and advancing the nursing role is Michael Bleich. A nationally recognized speaker with an extensive background in all levels of nursing education, he was the only dean of a nursing program to serve on the IOM committee that issued *The Future of Nursing: Leading Change, Advancing Health* report (IOM, 2011). According to Michael, "The magnitude of policy change in areas such as scope of practice, academic competency and degree advancement, workforce supply and demand initiatives, and the like inspires my career each and every day."

Leveraging Opportunities

Progressive steps, such as ever-increasing positions of significance coupled with additional education and credentials, put nurses in the right place at the right time for leadership roles. It is always the best situation to be lucky and good in order to leverage opportunities.

It is important to recognize an opportunity when it becomes available. Jenny Chin Hansen illustrates this point: "I think I have been fortunate to, in one case, have a retiring faculty member turn to me to hand off a legacy to focus on aging that has led to my career track. I must admit, though, it was a focus of necessity since I was the only faculty member at the time to have any interest in aging and she said, 'You're it!' Not a glamorous strategy and transformative insight, but I did have a deep caring of older persons from my community health practice years." Jennie's "yes" led to the On-Lok program for seniors in the San Francisco Bay area and the Program of All-Inclusive Care for the Elderly (PACE) that provides comprehensive long-term services and support for Medicaid and Medicare enrollees. Quite a legacy indeed.

Pamela Bennett's "jump to public policy came when I attended a hearing in the Colorado legislature on the treatment of chronic pain." For Pam, who was working as a staff nurse, the testimonies of the deans of medical, nursing, and dental schools were simply not consistent with what she saw daily at the bedside. As a result of her courage in simply asking a question in such a public and unfamiliar forum, one of the senators holding the hearing followed up with her and asked her to testify at the next scheduled hearing. "I said that I couldn't because I was (just) a practicing nurse." The senator replied, "If you don't speak out for your patients, who will? And if we want legislators to make good decisions, how can that happen without knowing what is going on in the trenches?" For Pam, that first step in speaking up has led her to making a difference in quality pain management policy and a career in improving pain care practices for so many more.

Judy Murphy has a passionate belief in the power of health information technology (HIT) to ensure that patients are full partners in their care coupled with a desire to change unworkable health care cultures. When the use of computers first began on nursing units, Judy was in the right place at the right time and was curious and not afraid. Through her role in staff development, she provided education and innovation regarding clinical computer applications. Judy had the vision to recognize the potential positive value of information technology for nursing. She was insightful about the perspective that nursing brings about technological innovation and seized the opportunity to represent nursing in the information technology department in her organization. To expand her knowledge and networks, she became involved in two premier information technology organizations—the American Medical Informatics Association (AMIA) and the Health Information and Management Systems Society (HIMSS)—and assumed volunteer leadership roles in each of them. When a federal advisory committee was formed on HIT, she expanded her knowledge of federal information technology work by serving on the standards committee. Her "on-the-job training" along with professional volunteer posts led her to a senior executive position in the federal government as Deputy National Coordinator for Programs and Policy at the Office of the National Coordinator for HIT, U.S. Department of Health and Human Services.

Francie Likis started writing because "one of my former faculty members was a journal editor who asked me to submit a manuscript. That led to me joining the editorial board and working my way up to become editor-in-chief." Writing editorials is one means of influencing policy. Like many of our exemplars, Francie's policy expertise extends into several arenas. She has gained national recognition for her work on the prevention of unintended pregnancy. She serves as a senior investigator for the Agency on Healthcare Research and Quality–funded Evidence-Based Practice Center (EPC) at Vanderbilt where she leads comparative effectiveness reviews that inform clinical care. Additionally, she has leadership roles in advancing advanced practice registered nurses (APRN) practice in Tennessee. Francie promotes the idea that a part of being a policy activist is never missing a chance to let family, friends, or acquaintances know that nursing is a grand field that is limitless in opportunities for enhancing the social good through so many venues and paths.

Taking advantage of opportunities to advance policy usually involves a number of different factors that include networking, obtaining advanced education, and association involvement. These in turn led to being at the right place at the right time when opportunity knocks. When opportunity knocks, it is important to take advantage of it, even if you feel you are not *quite* ready for it.

TURNING COMMITMENT INTO ACTION

As we have seen, our exemplars have taken career paths that enabled them to put their commitment to nursing into action that advances health and health policy. Serving the public through policy and leadership involves assessment, being strategic, creating balance and garnering support, building your team and financial support, and knowing the written and unwritten rules. If we want a policy to be put in place, we can't expect others to do it for us. This means one might take a road that involves assuming a leadership role within an organization that seeks to pass legislation and ensure that certain regulations are formulated, or actually becoming a policy maker through running for formal office or seeking political appointments to key positions.

Assessing Readiness

Assessing your readiness to serve is an important step and serves two purposes: (a) providing a realistic appraisal of what you will bring to a particular position or office and (b) identifying areas for self-development. A realistic appraisal can be used to determine the match between your education, expertise, and interest in being a policy maker. Ensuring a match between the qualifications for an office and one's own qualifications is a prerequisite. These matches need not be perfect; strengths can be maximized and potential weaknesses can be addressed. Many times people are hindered by thoughts that they cannot do the job. Women are less likely than men to believe that they are qualified to run for office (Lawless & Fox, 2012). Women comprise 93.3% of nurses (U.S. Department of Health and Human Services, 2010) and the question is whether this gender bias impacts the likelihood of nurses running for office. However, nurses' experiences with patients, families, and other health care professionals in diverse and sometimes unpredictable situations make them ideal candidates for assuming an active role in policy. Exhibit 12.3 includes elements of a self-assessment for assuming a leadership role in policy.

While not all of the components of this particular readiness assessment would apply to a particular position, one needs to look at the requirements of the position and identify those elements that would be most applicable. For example, running for a position in an association will require networking and a willingness to meet with people one doesn't know and answer questions. Consider asking a close friend who can be realistic about your assets and help you strategize to strengthen your position.

Completing the assessment, while it may be tedious, provides you with realistic insight and a roadmap for preparation for your chosen course of action. Regardless of the results of your assessment, it will be important to hone your speaking and writing skills (see Chapter 10, "Working With the Media: Shaping the Health Policy Process"). Identifying areas for improvement is part of the action plan necessary to achieve the desired goals.

Being Strategic

Being strategic requires a careful analysis of your assessment as well as planning for the achievement of your goals. The analysis of your assessment can provide direction to your plan. For example, while you may wish to run for a

EXHIBIT 12.3   SELF-ASSESSMENT OF READINESS FOR A LEADERSHIP ROLE

KEY ELEMENT	QUESTIONS TO ASK YOURSELF
Interest in and knowledge of the role	What do you see as the most interesting and challenging component of the desired position? What do you know about the actual responsibilities of the role and the commitment necessary to fulfill its responsibilities?
Drive to win or obtain the position	How willing are you to talk about yourself, meet and greet people, or talk to people you have never met? Are you willing to take the necessary actions to help you to win? Do you regularly notify the public relations department of your organization about your accomplishments, publications, certifications, and so on?
Credibility	Do you have the necessary background (education, credentials, and expertise) and respect (political, ethical, and practice) in the community of interest to be credible when speaking to the issues at hand? What are your exceptional skill sets?
Electability/appointment prospects	Have you been involved in committees, community organizations, or religious organizations? Have you notified the public relations department of your organization about your accomplishments, publications, or certifications? Do you have name recognition among relevant organizational stakeholders or the community of interest? Do you have the background to be credible when speaking to the issues at hand?
Public speaking	Do you have experience in presenting and answering questions from the media? Are you willing to use opportunities to practice or get assistance with speech writing and public speaking?
Support network	Have you had crucial conversations with your family, friends, and supporters about the time commitment and change in routine that will be required? Do you have the flexibility that might be needed to assume a specific office or policy role? Can you count on your family and friends for their support?
Issues	What are the issues that you are most passionate about? How does being in the role or position you are interested in advance your goals in addressing these issues?
Risk taking and personal exposure	Are you competitive when playing games? Do you take risks? Are you willing to go public with your stance on an issue and demonstrate your vulnerability? Are you willing to lose some privacy through personal exposure?

(continued)

EXHIBIT 12.3	SELF-ASSESSMENT OF READINESS FOR A LEADERSHIP ROLE (*CONTINUED*)
Receptiveness	Are you a good listener? Are you open to different ideas? Can you be comfortable with confrontation and criticism? How do you handle positive, negative, and inappropriate comments?
Strengths and weaknesses	What are your strengths and weaknesses? How can you leverage your strengths and address your weaknesses?
Timing	Is this the right time to run in terms of your personal life? Is the timing right in terms of your visibility in the organization or political arena? Is the timing right with the issues currently at the forefront of the constituency?
Stamina and energy	Do you have the necessary energy and stamina to do the follow-through that is needed to seek the desired position?

certain office within an organization, some consideration should be given to which positions within the organization have traditionally produced candidates for the top leadership positions in the organization. Or, alternatively, determine which positions provide the most visibility and allow you to showcase your skills as a leader. On the other hand, every so often a leader comes along who sets all the traditional rules on their head by breaking stereotypes. It would be wise to determine the personal qualities of the leaders and characteristics of the organizations at the time that created the confluence of events that allowed an individual to move forward rapidly in assuming a leadership role.

Not having certain qualities according to the unwritten rules of the organization does not necessarily mean that one should not move forward with a plan, but rather, one might need to adopt different strategies in order to succeed. While it is prudent to employ strategies to achieve a particular position, one needs to recognize that a single position is not an end in and of itself, but rather it is a journey of a lifelong commitment to becoming a leader and expanding one's influence to advance policy. A successful strategy for enhancing one's expertise is becoming a policy fellow (see Chapter 15, "Taking Actions, Expanding Horizons"). As can be seen in the career trajectories of our exemplars, they did not stop their involvement with one position or one accomplishment, but used that experience to leverage opportunities to take action at a different level or different environment. Congresswoman Lois Capps knew that when she was preparing to run for Congress that her experience as a nurse would make her a great advocate for the "health community in Congress because just as nurses are the best advocates on behalf of our patients in the hospital, we are naturally inclined to be the best advocates on behalf of our patients in the Capitol."

Creating Balance

The nurse exemplars are passionate and dedicated to the nursing profession. One exemplar commented, "My professional life is very much personal. Nursing is my passion and my life's work, and that's why sometimes the line between the two can blur." Exemplars were consistent in their responses about the need to balance responsibilities. As one nurse said, "Life is nothing if not a balancing act, often out of balance but recoverable with dedication, work and support." Some talked about making sacrifices. "At least be able to name what the risks and sacrifices are in the most conscious way possible and keep balance."

Other nurses spoke of challenges rather than sacrifices. "I haven't really made sacrifices as all of these experiences have been choices I have made, and they have helped to allow me to be who I am professionally and personally." And yet another talked of prioritizing. "It's hard to learn to say no … I haven't mastered that so I am usually willing to do more to help influence policy and professional politics." And another spoke of a strategy she uses to keep her life in balance. "I do think it is very important to take time where you truly step away from work. I have to have some time every year when I am completely unplugged from work with no e-mail access."

Supportive employers played a role in the career of some of the exemplars, while supportive families played a consistent role in the interviewees' lives. One exemplar was a single parent. "My first husband died when our son was a year old. Fortunately, I was blessed with great support in child care so that I was able to do some travel with some confidence that my son was in good hands. Having spoken with him now as [a] parent himself, he luckily felt he was fine as I did the work I did."

The comments of our exemplars reflect the diversity of meaning and perspectives given to the notion of balance. Regardless of one's approach to work, the added responsibility of an executive or volunteer leadership position requires thought about how one's life might change and how to manage additional responsibilities. Some organizations might provide specifics about the time commitment involved for meetings, travel, and other responsibilities. However, this information may be oversimplified and may not fully capture the nuances inherent in the role. Thus, it is useful to speak to trusted mentors about the actual time commitments as well as the nature of the work.

The concept of balance has the connotation that one can only put so much into work without it beginning to have a deleterious effect on other aspects of one's life. For some people, this may not be an issue at all, that work is what they enjoy and what gives them satisfaction. For women, this tends to be a double-edged sword. Witness the criticisms of women holding public office regarding the negative impact on their family. Such criticisms have a decidedly gender bias. On the other hand, some of the conversations on work–life balance have been driven by the needs and values of different generations in the workforce. Regardless, it is still prudent to examine what might be different if one assumes a particular position and how to successfully incorporate the added responsibilities into one's life.

Some people are so successful in creating balance that their professional and personal lives are fully integrated, where one aspect enhances the other. For us, VTB and STM, the benefits of being able to give back to the profession we love is an immeasurable reward. However, each of us has had to give consideration to the very practical aspects of the changes in our lives incurred by taking on a leadership role in nursing. Some tips and an example of a resource for each area in achieving balance are illustrated in Exhibit 12.4.

EXHIBIT 12.4   TIPS FOR ACHIEVING BALANCE

ARENA	RATIONALE	RESOURCE
Maintaining health and physical fitness	A healthy lifestyle in terms of diet and exercise will enhance fitness and provide energy	American Nurses Association Healthy Nurse http://www.nursingworld.org/MainMenuCategories/WorkplaceSafety/Healthy-Nurse
Rearranging errands and responsibilities	Eliminating or reorganizing activities adds valuable time to your week	Easier errand running http://www.readersdigest.ca/home-garden/money/easier-errand-running
Getting adequate sleep	Energy and enthusiasm are essential for effective functioning in the role	How much sleep do you need? http://www.helpguide.org/life/sleeping.htm
Dealing effectively with energy sappers	Setting limits with emotionally draining people helps preserve emotional integrity	Are coworkers draining your energy? http://www.drjudithorloff.com/Press-Room/co-workers-draining-energy.htm
Saying no	Saying no respectfully can reduce stress	Boundaries are important. Do you set them? http://www.leadersatalllevels.com/boundaries-are-important-do-you-set-them
Managing your time	Lack of organization or overbooking can lead to stress	10 time-management tips that work http://www.entrepreneur.com
Using tools for organization	Using tools can help increase productivity	Top 15 time-management apps and tools http://www.lifehack.org/articles/technology/top-15-time-management-apps-and-tools.html

Coaching

Coaching is a strategy that can be used by the novice and the leader in advancing a professional career. Donner and Wheeler (2009) define coaching as an "interactive, interpersonal process that supports continuing personal, professional and career development through the acquisition of appropriate skills, actions and abilities that are crucial to professional practice." Coaching is usually more short term and focused, whereas a mentoring relationship is likely to be long term. Coaching can be used to develop a specific competency or skill set in order to achieve a specific goal. It can be used for nurses at different time points in their careers such as (a) helping new graduates navigate the complexities of transition to their first nursing position (Dela Cruz, Farr, Klakovich, & Esslinger, 2013; Welding, 2011), (b) engaging senior nurses in advancing their professional careers (Wendler, Fyans, & Kirkbride, 2013), (c) building interprofessional teams (Donner & Wheeler, 2009; Shunk, Dulay, Chou, Janson, & O'Brien, 2014), and (d) succession planning (Titzer & Shirey, 2013). Coaching can also be used when one transitions to a new leadership role, such as a member of a practice committee in a health care organization, or a board member. It is an integral component of the RWJF Executive Nurse Fellows program in preparing nurses to lead and shape health policy. Advanced practice nurses have used coaching to support lifestyle and behavior health changes to promote health (Robins, Kiken, Holt, & McCain, 2013) and develop specific nursing competencies (Gordon, Melillo, Nannini, & Lakators, 2103). Coaching has been used to enhance organizational effectiveness in the perioperative arena (Nigam, Huising, & Golden, 2014) and is considered an essential component of the clinical nurse leader role (Sherman & Pross, 2010).

Coaching involves the creation of a safe place for coaching conversations, the examination of readiness for change, the identification of goals, selecting action steps, evaluating progress, and sustaining change (Hess et al., 2013). Nurses can use the self-assessment in Exhibit 12.3 to select areas for a coaching intervention.

Sponsorships

More recently, attention on leadership success has turned to sponsorship. Sponsors bring another dimension to one's leadership growth. Serving the public through leadership and policy will require going beyond traditional mentorship and seeking sponsors to help achieve your goals. A sponsor is someone who actively promotes you and touts your accomplishments to others in order to advance your goals. While we may traditionally think of sponsorship as the process that is used for access to selective professional groups (e.g., American Academy of Nursing, the American Academy in Nursing Education, the American Academy of Nurse Practitioners, or the IOM) or nominations for awards, these make up only one type of the roles that can be assumed by a sponsor.

In Dan Schawbel's interview (2013) with Sylvia Hewlett about her book, *Forget a Mentor, Find a Sponsor*, she describes the role of a sponsor within the corporate world:

> If mentors help define the dream, sponsors are the dream-enablers. Sponsors deliver: They make you visible to leaders within the company—and to top people outside as well. They connect you to career opportunities and provide air cover when you encounter trouble. When it comes to opening doors, they don't stop with one promotion: They'll see you to the threshold of power.

According to Hewlett (2013), the relationship with a sponsor is reciprocal—while you may need a sponsor to help you get connected in the right places, the sponsor also expects that you can deliver for him or her. The reciprocal nature of the relationship between the sponsor and protégé roles is illustrated in Figure 12.1.

While some corporations have developed sponsorship programs, these types of programs need to be expanded to the health care sector (Travis, Doty, & Helitzer, 2013). Regardless, you can seek out a sponsor, have a frank conversation about your goals, and develop plans. Sponsors can help you navigate difficult waters and advocate for your success.

Qualities in a sponsor that would be desirable for someone embarking on a policy journey include (a) being familiar with your accomplishments, (b) benefiting from something you do for them or their organization, and (c) having the capacity to advance your career (Hewlett, 2013).

In order to advance one's competencies in policy leadership, one may garner the assistance of a number of different people in the journey. While our exemplars highlighted the role of mentors in their professional journeys, coaches and sponsors are important for different reasons and can be used to enhance your career process.

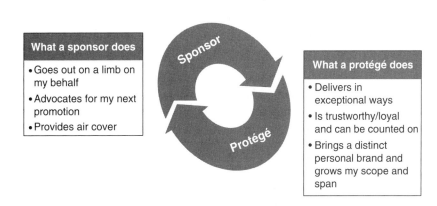

FIGURE 12.1 The two-way street.
Reprinted by permission of *Harvard Business Review* from Hewlett (2013, p. 41).

Resources

Assuming an active role in policy leadership will at some point require an assessment of resources necessary to move one's plan forward. Financial resources may be critical to success. Nurses, because of their particular career trajectories, may not be familiar with the need to obtain financial or other resources such as media expertise or the need to engage in fundraising. Obtaining financial resources will require basic skill in financial management. While some of these functions can be outsourced to members of a team, the ultimate responsibility for such resources rests with you. For example, if you are running for a political office or seek an appointment, it is important that you understand and know the rules that apply. These can include nomination or filing deadlines, or campaign finance rules. Many times, the public learns about the unraveling of a campaign with a candidate claiming ignorance of the details. Aside from an organization's website, numerous websites are available to assist with the general or specific details. Needless to say, ignorance of the details does not absolve one of the responsibilities for the outcome or the consequences of one's actions.

Assuming a leadership role may also involve fundraising, being a donor, and leveraging assets, as well as being a responsible steward. Fundraising is not only necessary for political office, but may also be needed when campaigning for elected office in an association (see this chapter's E-Resources for additional information). If seeking an appointment to a community or nonprofit board, one is expected to attend not only board meetings, but also various community or association events. New nurse board members may be surprised when asked to make a donation to an association's charitable arm or political action committee. These donations are important when hoping to influence key policy makers (Twedell & Webb, 2007). Nursing has been fortunate to have non-nurse champions who have supported and advanced nursing goals. However, these donors will want to know that the board of an association or charitable organization has 100% participation in giving to the mission of the organization and commitment to the association's causes. Leveraging assets may include such tasks as determining which individuals or groups may be the best choice to tackle a particular task at a given point in time. Finally, it may be necessary to seek additional education and training to make responsible decisions for resources whether it is one's own campaign or an organization's finances. See Policy on the Scene 12.1 for STM's description of her campaign experiences in acquiring needed competencies and resources.

Think about how you can make an impact in seeking elected or appointed positions. Nursing must have "friends" in the legislature. If you have the desire to run for office, start or continue to build your base of potential financial and volunteer supporters. Think strategically about the timing of your efforts. Join your local political party and attend meetings. Find a political mentor who will help you strategize as to how to reach your goal. You need someone who knows

POLICY ON THE SCENE 12.1: Taking on a New Role, Political Candidacy
Susan Tullai-McGuinness, PhD, MPA, RN

Wanting to make a difference inspired me to run for public office. Over the years, my education, work and life experiences, and our professional associations opened my eyes to the role a legislator can play in creating healthy communities. I wanted to have "a seat in the Ohio House of Representatives" and participate in creating legislation that would ensure affordable, quality education and health care for everyone; protect our environment; support job creation; and protect our safety.

Timing played a significant part in my decision to run for the Ohio House in 2012. The Democratic party was seeking a candidate to run against the incumbent who supported very conservative issues. However, no one was willing to take on this incumbent known for running negative campaigns. I felt it was time for me to come forward and express my interest in running. I thought I was well positioned to win because of my community and professional nursing activities. My husband and I served on different community boards, attended local fundraisers, and networked well together. In fact, my husband has long served as my political mentor. He supported my decision to run and to this day reminds me that I am a "nurse," a member of the most trusted profession. In addition, the Ohio Nurses Association (ONA) supported my decision to run. I have been an ONA member for more than 25 years and have served on a number of elected and appointed positions at the local, state, and national levels.

I learned how to run a campaign by attending a program sponsored by the state party and listening to a number of previous candidates, current office holders, party leaders, union officials, and my husband who insisted that I need a consultant, which I hired. I think that running a campaign is much like running a business. You need a plan, capital, messaging, loyal customers (supporters), and hard work. My successes were my capacity for raising money and connecting with voters at their doors. It was the ONA that provided most important early financial support. I also requested and received contributions from individual nurses whom I have met over the years through membership in the ONA, ANA, other professional nursing organizations, and the Ohio Democratic Nurse Caucus. Nursing prepared me to communicate effectively with individuals. I was able to quickly build a rapport with voters when I was canvassing.

There were campaign challenges. I had a few nurses, family members, and friends who helped me canvass, but I found that it was difficult to recruit local volunteers to canvass. In addition, I did not feel comfortable speaking in sound bites on every issue, such as K–12 education funding and evaluation. It took time for me to be at ease with the press. And I did not always listen to my advisors. I came short on votes but raised more money, knocked on more doors, and received more votes that many thought I would.

Many have said to me "you need to try again." I am keeping my options open. Good luck in your political efforts. Contact me if you would like to "have a seat at the legislative table and want a coach."

the local politics. Then reach out to the state party and ask about the campaign training programs they offer. Most importantly, "pay your dues." Help others on their campaigns, canvass, attend fundraisers, and help your candidates win nursing's vote and financial support. Winning a race takes timing, hard work, and patience. Tips for getting elected to an office or appointed to a board or committee are given in Exhibit 12.5.

Every position, whether it be elected or appointed, whether it is the first effort or a re-election, has a different set of circumstances that requires a different action plan. Each time that you take on an advocacy role, you bring your expertise to the table and you take something away as you advance professionally. Each time that you take on a new role in policy, it gets easier, and you develop new skill sets which, in turn, enable you to take on new challenges. Having the opportunity to experience professional growth and doing something that you enjoy while advancing the profession has great rewards. Ellen-Marie Whelan began her advanced practice career in an adolescent primary care center in West Philadelphia. She assumed progressively more responsible clinical, then system, then policy roles, and now assists in the design and implementation of delivery system and payment reform at the Centers for Medicare and Medicaid Services (CMS).

EXHIBIT 12.5 **TIPS FOR GETTING ELECTED TO AN OFFICE OR APPOINTED TO A BOARD OR COMMITTEE**

1. Identify what qualifications and experiences make you the best person for the office
2. Validate required qualifications
3. Be strategic; for example, consider timing for seeking position
4. File all the necessary forms early
5. Contact your friends for support
6. Form a campaign committee
7. Develop a fund-raising plan with key donors and supporters
8. Prepare media messages; for example, elevator and campaign speeches and/or written support letters
9. Make personal contacts, including key leaders and representatives of voter blocks
10. Listen to your friends and supporters
11. Learn about the written and unwritten rules of the organization

For VTB, the challenge and opportunity was being in on the ground level in the achievement of mental health parity, a lifelong vision for eliminating one type of disparity in health care (see the Option for Policy Challenge for details about her advocacy journey).

OPTION FOR POLICY CHALLENGE: Coming Full Circle: Policy Is an Ongoing Process
Virginia Trotter Betts

All my education and my earlier work in nursing and professional organizations—law and policy—laid the foundation for subsequent policy leadership roles inside nursing, health care organizations, and government including chairing the task force that developed Nursing's Agenda for Health Care Reform (1991). This agenda was used as organized nursing's health care reform blueprint during the 1992 presidential election campaign so that I, as the newly elected ANA president, could clearly articulate what nurses thought would be the best reform principles for the nation. After the election, when First Lady Hillary Clinton spearheaded the Clinton–Gore health care reform initiative (Health Security Act [HSA] of 1993), I was able to work closely with her and her reform team to advance the role/scope/autonomy of the professional nurse in a health system with improved access and quality and controlled costs. As ANA president, I certainly reaped the benefit of the completion of ANA's move from Kansas City to Washington, DC, which provided more opportunities for ANA and nurses to be visible and at the table to advance key health policy issues/options being debated throughout the nation during President Clinton's first term.

I am rarely shy nor afraid to take strategic risks and take on totally new roles or challenges. After my ANA presidency (1992–1996), I co-chaired the health desk for the Clinton–Gore re-election campaign. And then, when Donna Shalala, Secretary of Health and Human Services (HHS), invited me to join the HHS executive team as a senior advisor on nursing and policy, I again said yes.

Building on earlier health care activism relationships, I collaborated with David Satcher, MD, PhD, whom I had worked with prior to his appointment as assistant secretary of health and the 16th surgeon general. Now in Washington, I chaired Dr. Satcher's planning process for his term as surgeon general. One priority became the development of the first ever surgeon general's report on mental health (U.S. Public Health Service, 1999), which was later used to provide the public health foundation of mental health parity legislation that was passed in 2008.

After leaving HHS, I returned to Tennessee and became involved in the 2002 election process, bringing nursing and health care issues to

(continued)

the attention of candidates of both parties on behalf of TNA and the TNA Governmental Affairs Committee. Personally, I worked to win support of health care professionals for Phil Bredesen, D-TN. When newly elected Governor Bredesen appointed me as commissioner of the Department of Mental Health and Developmental Disabilities, I became the first nurse to serve in a cabinet post in Tennessee. Being a past ANA president was *just* the right preparation for my commissioner post (leading an effort with complex issues and with insufficient resources for a very worthy cause).

I am so fortunate to have had a career that has allowed me to focus professionally on my life's passions: professional nursing, mental health and health policy, and politics. I have experienced positive outcomes that reflect a full circle of health care problems with policy solutions. Some examples include development of Nursing's Agenda for Health Reform and then using it to guide my work with the Clinton HSA task force; advocacy as ANA president for legislation for direct Medicare reimbursement for APRNs; and then being a senior HHS staff member participating in shaping its regulatory implementation. After working for decades in a variety of clinical settings, organizations, and government positions urging parity coverage of mental illness and substance abuse services, I served as the president of the National Association of State Mental Health Program Directors (NASMHPD) when the landmark Mental Health Parity and Addiction Equity Act of 2008 was passed and, working through NASMHPD, seeing that parity on steroids became available within PPACA.

In *so* many ways, for *so* many years, I have found a way to be an advocate and a leader, to productively participate in professional nursing, mental health nursing, and health policy. I hope that I will leave all three better off than when I found them.

IMPLICATIONS FOR THE FUTURE

When asked their views about the future of nursing, the exemplars' responses were positive, but pointed out the challenges ahead along with caveats for the nurse leaders of tomorrow—YOU. They seemed to agree that, with an increased number of people entering the health care system as the PPACA is implemented, more primary health care providers, including and especially advanced practice nurses, will be needed, and these APRNs will need to know more. Transformation of the U.S. health care system is creating, and will continue to create, more opportunities for professional nurses. Positions are opening in care coordination, chronic disease management, and quality improvement—all of which require skills in team building, population health, evidence-based practice, collaboration, leadership, and advocacy. These exemplars strongly expressed the critical importance of nurses being able to use their education to practice at their full scope of authority. For this full practice authority to be realized, legal and regulatory barriers must be overcome, and nurses must be consistently and powerfully at federal, state, and local policy tables; in addition, they must be able and willing to speak with one voice.

Nurses will assume a greater role in leading and advancing change in the health care system recommended by *The Future of Nursing* report (IOM, 2011). As recommended by Fyffe (2009), in her analysis of nurses' roles in policy in the United States and the United Kingdom, greater coordination of efforts in order to maximize influence will be needed. Nurses will continue to gain prominence and influence in the transformation of health care. Nurses will help to address our nation's most pressing health care challenges—access, quality, and cost. As payors and providers actively deconstruct the care hierarchies and transform them into care circles around patients, families, and communities, the barriers to professionals serving at the top of clinical education and training practices across health care will be eliminated.

KEY CONCEPTS

1. Nurse leaders have made extraordinary contributions to health policy in a variety of roles in the public and private sector.
2. The stories of nurse exemplars provide valuable guidance and inspiration to nurses who may be hesitant to embark upon the path of policy leadership.
3. It is possible to blend one's passion for nursing with serving the public through policy advocacy.
4. Advanced education and professional association involvement are some of the commonalities among nurse policy leaders that led to long-term policy advocacy.
5. Having mentors and serving as mentors are important aspects of policy leadership development.
6. Public health is a common pathway to policy leadership because of its focus on population health, health care disparities, and identifying systemic solutions to population problems.
7. Nurse executives and academic nurse leaders are in prime positions to use their roles to advance policy at a societal level.
8. It is important to recognize and leverage opportunities to advance nursing and health policy.
9. Assessment of readiness for policy activism provides a realistic appraisal of one's strengths and areas needing improvement.

10. Creating balance involves integrating one's professional and personal lives as well as examining strategies to make leadership roles and policy work possible.

11. Seeking a coach is a strategy that can be used to acquire or enhance specific competencies necessary for the policy role.

12. Sponsors are important in achieving one's policy career goals by touting accomplishments and providing connections to career opportunities.

13. A realistic appraisal of needed resources and their acquisition are important for leveraging assets to achieve goals.

14. Involvement in policy making leads to additional opportunities to continue to make an impact on policy.

15. Leadership and advocacy are important in creating the preferred future for nursing and creating a health care system responsive to the needs of the public.

SUMMARY

Serving the public through leadership and policy is a role/goal/requirement for every nurse regardless of the particular position he or she occupies at a given moment in time. Our exemplars are not only role models—they willingly share their wisdom. According to Michael Evans, "Success in leadership is a mixture of academic progression, progressive work experience, and learning to lead oneself, then others with humility, grace, respect, integrity, and honesty. ... Servant leadership builds the leaders for the world of today and tomorrow. There is no organization, no hospital, and no business without the people who create, maintain, and innovate it. Today, you have to be a culture builder, a builder of people and to do that you need to first invest in yourself ... your soul must match the role. You must know who you are before you try to know others .... Be well rounded, be big, be broad, and accept no limits to your thinking on your abilities. First go about breaking all the rules. Be daring, and be someone's superhero .... More of us are leaders than we know, so find your inner leader and bring it out, the world needs more courageous leaders."

Let's let Congresswoman Lois Capps provide a last word, "Get involved! My advice to any nurse who wants to get involved in policy advancement is to get out there and be heard. When I began my career as a nurse, nurses were never asked or expected to be involved in federal policy making but now we have to be. You do not need to run for Congress to have an impact on policy—there are many ways to be involved in advocacy with local and national organizations. But no matter how you get involved, nurses are the backbone of our health care system and your input is as essential as elected officials legislate on related issues."

LEARNING ACTIVITIES

1. Identify a nurse policy leader and interview that person about how he or she became involved in policy and what that person believes is his or her most important policy accomplishment.
2. Complete the self-assessment in Exhibit 12.3 in relation to an identified position.
3. Identify a potential coach, mentor, and sponsor. Describe a specific goal for establishing each relationship.
4. Identify three individuals that you could coach, mentor, and sponsor. Identify a specific strategy that would enhance each individual's involvement in policy.
5. Develop an elevator speech about why you would be the best candidate for an appointment to a committee, office within an association, political appointment, or elective office within an association or your community (e.g., school board, local community group, and church group).
6. Complete a 100- to 200-word description of your qualifications for an elected office for an association position.
7. Develop a strategic plan to seek an elected or appointed position with specific steps and a strategy for each step.

E-RESOURCES

- Academy of Medical-Surgical Nurses/Mentoring. http://www.amsn.org/professional-development/mentoring
- Center for American Women and Politics: Ready to Run. http://www.cawp.rutgers.edu/education_training/ReadytoRun
- Center for Talent Innovation. http://www.talentinnovation.org
- Community Catalyst. http://www.communitycatalyst.org
- Crotty, C. Campaign Guide. http://www.completecampaigns.com/article.asp?articleid=13
- Emerging RN Leaders Blog. http://www.emergingrnleader.com
- Green Dog Campaigns. http://www.greendogcampaigns.com/areyouready.html
- Ignite: Political Power in Every Young Woman. http://ignitenational.org/programs/college
- Institute on Women: Mentorship vs. Sponsorship. http://instituteonwomen.org/mentors-vs-sponsors
- Ron Faucheaux: Running for Office. http://www.monkeysee.com/play/6658-what-personal-and-family-considerations-should-I-think-about-before-running-for-political-office
- Stop Bullying Nurses. http://www.stopbullyingnurses.com
- Young, R. D. Volunteerism, benefits, incidence, organizational models and participation in the public sector. University of South Carolina Institute for Public Service and Policy Research. http://www.ipspr.sc.edu/publication/Volunteerism%20FINAL.pdf

REFERENCES

American Nurses Association. (2010). *Nursing: Scope and standards of practice* (2nd ed.). Silver Spring, MD: Author.

Boswell, C., Cannon, S., & Miller, J. (2005). Nurses' political involvement: Responsibility versus privilege. *Journal of Professional Nursing, 21*(1), 5–8.

Community Catalyst. (2013). *Advancing health reform by inclusion: Engaging communities of color in creating policy change.* Boston, MA: Author. http://www.communitycatalyst.org/doc-store/publications/Advancing-Health-Reform-by-Inclusion_Jan2013update.pdf

Cramer, M. E. (2002). Factors influencing organized political participation in nursing. *Policy, Politics and Nursing Practice, 3*(2), 97–107.

Curran, C., & Fitzpatrick, T. (2013). *Claiming the corner office: Executive leadership lessons for nurses.* Indianapolis, IN: Sigma Theta Tau International.

Dela Cruz, F. A., Farr, S., Klakovich, M. D., & Esslinger, P. (2013). Facilitating the career transition of second-career students into professional nursing. *Nursing Education Perspectives, 34*(1), 12–17.

Donner, G., & Wheeler, M. M. (2009). *Coaching in nursing: An introduction.* Indianapolis, IN: Sigma Theta Tau International.

Fyffe, T. (2009). Nurses shaping and influencing health and social care policy. *Journal of Nursing Management, 17*(6), 698–706.

Gordon, S. J., Melillo, K. D., Nannini, A., & Lakators, B. E. (2013). Bedside coaching to improve nurses' recognition of delirium. *Journal of Neuroscience Nursing, 45*(5), 288–293.

Hess, D. R., Dossey, B. M., Southard, M. E., Luck, S., Schaub, B. G., & Bark, L. (2013). *The art and science of nursing coaching: The providers' guide to coaching scope and competencies.* Silver Spring, MD: American Nurses Association.

Hewlett, S. A. (2013). *Forget a mentor, find a sponsor: The new way to fast-track your career.* Boston, MA: Harvard Business School Publishing.

Institute of Medicine (IOM). (2011). *The future of nursing: Leading change, advancing health.* Washington, DC: The National Academies Press.

Lawless, J. L., & Fox, R. L. (2012). *Men rule: The continued under-representation of women in U.S. politics.* Washington, DC: Women & Politics Institute.

National Women's History Museum. (n.d.). *Lillian D. Wald (1867–1940).* Retrieved from http://www.nwhm.org/education-resources/biography/biographies/lillian-wald

Nigam, A., Huising, R., & Golden, B. (2014). Improving hospital efficiency: A process model of organizational change commitments. *Medical Care Research and Review 71*(1), 21–42.

Robert Wood Johnson Foundation (RWJF). (2011). *Robert Wood Johnson Executive Nurse Fellows: A RWJF national program.* Retrieved from http://www.rwjf.org/content/dam/farm/reports/program_results_reports/2011/rwjf69782

Robins, J. L., Kiken, L., Holt, M., & McCain, N. L. (2013, November 21). Mindfulness: An effective coaching tool for improving physical and mental health. *Journal of the American Association of Nurse Practitioners.* Epub ahead of print.

Schawbel, D. (2013, September 10). *Sylvia Ann Hewlett: Find a sponsor instead of a mentor.* Retrieved from http://www.forbes.com/sites/danschawbel/2013/09/10/sylvia-ann-hewlett-find-a-sponsor-instead-of-a-mentor

Sherman, R., & Pross, E. (2010). Growing nurse leaders to build and sustain healthy work environments at the unit level. *OJIN: Online Journal of Issues in Nursing, 15.* Retrieved from http://nursingworld.org/MainMenuCategories/ANAMarketplace/ANAPeriodicals/OJIN/TableofContents/Vol152010/No1Jan2010/Growing-Nurse-Leaders.html

Shunk, R., Dulay, M., Chou, C. L., Janson, S., & O'Brien, B. C. (2014). Huddle-coaching: A dynamic intervention for trainees and students to support team-based case. *Academic Medicine. 89*(2), 244–250.

Taft, S. H., & Nanna, K. M. (2008). What are sources of health policy that influence nursing practice? *Policy, Politics and Nursing Practice, 9*(4), 274–287.

Titzer, J. L., & Shirey, M. R. (2013). Nurse manager succession planning: A concept analysis. *Nursing Forum, 48*(3), 155–164.

Travis, E. L., Doty, L., & Helitzer, D. L. (2013). Sponsorship: A path to the academic medicine C-suite for women faculty. *Academic Medicine, 88*(10), 1414–1417.

Twedell, D. M., & Webb, J. M. (2007). The value of the political action committee: Dollars and influence for nurse leaders. *Nursing Administration Quarterly, 31*(4), 279–283.

U.S. Department of Health and Human Services. (1999). Mental health: A report of the surgeon general. Rockville, MD: U.S. Department of Health and Human Services, Substance Abuse and Mental Health Services Administration, Center for Mental Health Services, National Institutes of Health. Retrieved from http://profiles.nlm.nih.gov/ps/access/NNBBHS.pdf

U.S. Department of Health and Human Services, Health Resources and Services Administration. (2010). *The registered nurse population: Initial findings from the 2008 National Sample Survey of Registered Nurses.* Retrieved from http://bhpr.hrsa.gov/healthworkforce/rnsurveys/rnsurveyinitial2008.pdf

Vandenhouten, C. L., Malakar, C. L., Kubsch, S., Block, D. E., & Gallagher-Lepak, S. (2011). Political participation of registered nurses. *Policy, Politics & Nursing Practice, 12*(3), 159–167.

Welding, N. M. (2011). Creating a nursing residency: Decrease turnover and increase clinical competence. *Medsurg Nursing, 20*(1), 37–40.

Wendler, M. C., Fyans, P. M., & Kirkbride, G. (2013). No more "fumbling alone": Effect of a nurse-led academic advising service in a Magnet® hospital. *Journal of Continuing Education of Nursing, 44*(5), 218–224.

Winter, K. (1991). Educating nurses in the political process. *Journal of Continuing Education in Nursing, 22*(4), 143–146.

THIRTEEN

Evaluating Policy Structures, Processes, and Outcomes

Sean P. Clarke

Continuous improvement requires systematic evaluation. Continuous improvement requires unfiltered evaluation.—Anonymous

OBJECTIVES

1. Identify the place of research and evaluation in the policy cycle.
2. Explain the process of evaluating policy using a structure, process, and outcome framework.
3. Describe the use of outcomes research as an influence on policy.
4. Compare and contrast program evaluation and outcome evaluation.
5. Analyze proposed policies for intended and unintended consequences.

The use of evidence to examine outcomes for ongoing policy evaluation and monitoring—the focus of this chapter—expands upon the centrality of the use of evidence highlighted in previous chapters. Using a structure, process, and outcome framework, the anticipated and unanticipated outcomes of implemented policies are examined with discussion of how to leverage evaluation data as the basis for discontinuing, amending, or expanding policy. Policy making is an ever-turning process that can lead to more initiatives like advocating for greater investments for a particular strategy or wider uptake of a specific initiative. Minimally, evaluation is fundamental to policy making that is accountable, no matter whether one is involved at the little "p" or big "P" of policy.

Evaluators ask common questions and take similar steps when gathering and interpreting data to determine the effectiveness of policy. These questions and steps apply across a variety of policies whether national, state, local, or organizational. The heart of this work is the process of collecting and reviewing evidence to determine whether a policy or program meets its intended goals. It involves taking stock of the inputs and outputs of an activity. For nurses, the idea of evaluation often involves assessment of a patient's status after an intervention, clinical trials of drugs and equipment, performance appraisals, or institutional accreditation from bodies like the Joint Commission. *Evaluation* is a general term that can refer to examining the outcomes—the end results or consequences—of a project, a program, or a package of services for one or more stakeholder groups. These stakeholders usually include both the recipients of a program and its providers. Evaluation may include looking at interventions or programs as a whole or examining the impacts of a policy on various individuals or society at a higher level.

An important example of evaluation that is significant to nurse and patient safety is policy work related to needle safety and injury prevention. The following Policy Challenge illustrates some successes realized to date and highlights the ongoing evolution of policy work.

POLICY CHALLENGE: Needle Safety Outcomes

Successful workplace advocacy by professional nursing associations is exemplified by the story of the policy work connected with the reduction of needlestick injuries. Since the 1980s, with the rise of the HIV/AIDS epidemic, the risk to nurses—numerically speaking, the most affected group of health care workers of blood-borne pathogen transmission from contact with used sharps—gained much prominence. Nurses who injured themselves on the job feared contracting incurable, debilitating, and possibly fatal diseases. Public health workers and occupational health epidemiologists documented the extent of the problem in the 1990s, and it turned out to be strikingly common. They quickly identified major risk factors: recapping of sharps after use and improper disposal techniques and containers. Discouraging recapping and ensuring widespread access to needle disposal containers were important outcomes of recognizing this trend. Over time, medical equipment manufacturers began making specially designed needles and other sharps that had features reducing the time health workers are exposed to the sharp ends of needles or instruments. Evaluation studies found that workers learned to use new equipment as it was developed, thus contributing to a decrease in injury rates in settings where special devices were employed. Also vital were policies developed at organizational, state, and country levels. These include sharps disposal regulations; appraisal and selection of equipment to protect patients and providers; education; tracking, evaluating, and keeping records of needlestick injuries; vaccinations; postexposure protocols; and regulation and enforcement of policies. In spite of this work, the most recent estimates are that over one third of a million exposures occur every year (Centers for Disease Control and Prevention [CDC], 2008). HIV/AIDS and several types of hepatitis are just some of the 20 estimated known pathogens that can occur from a needlestick injury.

See Option for Policy Challenge.

THE LANGUAGE OF POLICY EVALUATION

Evidence is important in the policy-making process and all types of evidence are used, as indicated in previous chapters. Before beginning a more in-depth discussion of the questions to ask and steps to follow in evaluating and modifying policy, a brief review of evaluation in relation to research is in order (see Chapter 5, "Harnessing Evidence in the Policy Process").

Research, simply put, is the discovery of new knowledge, including descriptions and explorations of the nature of phenomena and the relationship of variables to each other. Researchers have a toolkit of techniques, including carefully collecting and analyzing data, to uncover patterns that offer answers to larger questions in a scientific field depending on the approach. In the clinical and social sciences, the two major families of research methods are the qualitative and quantitative traditions. Nurses engaged in evaluation use many of the same techniques as conventional researchers, including interviews, observations, and surveys, depending on the nature of the policy and the best method for obtaining outcome data. Evaluation, such as research, can be designed prospectively or retrospectively. It is common for policy at the little "p" level to be examined retrospectively.

Evaluation

In evaluation, the purpose is to understand systems of services or policies that are put together to address various issues or problems. Often in direct care nursing, policies relate to health, safety, quality patient care, and/or provider effectiveness. Evaluation is necessary to make judgments about a policy's effectiveness and to render a decision as to whether it is sufficient, needs modification, or should be discarded.

Evaluation is pragmatic and some features that "academic researchers" might consider important in a research design are not always seen as critical in evaluation. The primary audiences for evaluation findings are people in charge of planning, implementing, and making decisions about services. They are most concerned with the practicalities of getting sound data at the most reasonable cost and in the timeliest manner as they need to know, often quickly, how well a policy or program is achieving its intended outcomes. In practice, there is a great deal of overlap between research and evaluation. Many researchers engage in evaluation projects as part of their portfolio activities; sometimes, carefully designed evaluation projects using approaches discussed in this chapter are considered to have broader applicability and scientific value and are disseminated in the same venues that more conventional and less practically oriented research appears.

Policy Analysis

Policy analysis research is done to assess how well a policy has achieved its intended outcomes and to determine if there have been unintended outcomes, as noted in Chapter 5. Policy research is often seen as the role of social scientists and sometimes more specifically of political scientists. However, policy is not just conducted at the country and state levels. Nurses in practice must be able to carry out analyses (Hewison, 2007). Policies at these levels impact day-to-day care, and it is policies at the little "p" level that intersect practice where most nurses work. Policy creates the work environment in which nurses practice and advance care for the betterment of patients.

Policy analysis often comes up in everyday nursing practice when a question or a problem with a policy is identified or when new practices are started that require an accompanying policy. Many health care employers, for example, have policies on computer, Internet, cell phone, and social media use during work hours. They are designed to protect patients and workers, prevent unethical or illegal work activity, and avoid productivity issues. Indeed, the misuses of electronic devices and social media have been reported to regulatory boards, associations, other groups of health professionals, and the media. There are many ways these modalities can also be used to help nurses provide better care. So how are these policies analyzed and who is involved in the analysis? From an organizational standpoint, these types of policies are best examined, as are many in health care, from a multidisciplinary approach. Often, this process involves contacting colleagues at other organizations, or searching the literature and the web for current practices as well as information about their effectiveness. Nurses can be informed by these practices and they can seek guidance from professional groups. For example, the National Council of State Boards of Nursing (NCSBN, 2011) has issued social media guidelines and the American Nurses Association (ANA) (2011) has developed principles for social networking media use. Each of these documents has been endorsed by the other organization. This aspect of the work environment does not easily lend itself to investigation. However, the results of such policies may become manifest in nurse satisfaction outcomes.

Policy analysis research examines specific criteria to evaluate a policy and includes developing policy alternatives, assessing the possible outcomes of each alternative, and selecting an alternative from the projected choices. The policy analysis process includes specific steps quite familiar to nurses: define the problem, establish evaluation criteria, identify policy choices among alternative solutions, formulate the chosen policy, implement the policy solution, and evaluate the policy. The practice of policy evaluation in many settings is often not as formal as research and its sequencing is less rigorous. It is often iterative with backward and forward movement in varying phases. An often-cited practical process for policy analysis is the work of Bardach (2012), who developed the eightfold path that includes the following steps: (a) define the problem, (b) assemble evidence, (c) construct alternatives, (d) select criteria, (e) project outcomes, (f) confront tradeoffs, (g) decide, and (h) tell your story. Obviously, these steps are similar to the nursing and research processes.

Quality Improvement and Benchmarking

Two important terms for further discussion are quality improvement and benchmarking. Batalden and Davidoff (2007) define *quality improvement* as concerted efforts over time by all of the stakeholders in health care to improve the health status of the population, care system functioning, and professional development or learning. We usually think of quality improvement in terms of the efforts of managers or even specifically designated work units within health care organizations responsible for measuring and improving care system functioning, but Batalden and Davidoff's definition encompasses broader activities and could even be thought of as encompassing the policy realm. Quality improvement draws on ideas from research methodology and evaluation but is yet another pursuit—and is in some ways a practical endeavor that is often understood across disciplines and therefore sometimes easier to get done when quality data are available.

Benchmarking is comparing an object, an organization, or even a society against some sort of standard on a measure or measures. In health care contexts, benchmarks are used to situate a health care system (or a subset of the system, like a clinic or nursing unit). The standard can be national or international norms for staffing or patient outcomes or a "best in class" performance level. Organizations can even benchmark against their own performance over time. Benchmarks are obviously a major part of quality improvement, highlighting what managers need to act upon. They also provide a stimulus for higher level policy makers to confront and address reasons why their organizations may not be performing well, and spur leaders to match or better the performance of peer organizations or even health care systems internationally. A good international-level example is work comparing Organization for Economic Cooperation and Development (OECD) data on numerous topics across countries. For example, Squires (2013) compares numerous countries on topics like health care expenditures, mortality, and quality. Numerous sources of benchmarking are also used in health care and within nursing today. Some common examples that nurses in hospital and home care work with on a regular basis include the National Database of Nursing Quality Indicators® (NDNQI®) and the Outcome and Assessment Information Set (OASIS).

Indicators are specific measurements that are benchmarked. Nurses in all settings and across all roles are using and are often judged on some indicators, for example, exam scores, number of publications, and clinical practice benchmarks. Indicators related to quality and safety in clinical care areas are very familiar to nurses working in hospitals, clinics, and home health care today. Patient falls, for example, are often benchmarked. NDNQI, in particular, specifically measures nursing quality and provides nurses with unit- and hospital-level measurement for benchmarking across state, regional, and national data.

EVALUATING STRUCTURE, PROCESS, AND OUTCOME

A variety of models for describing program or policy evaluation have emerged over the years. A structure, process, and outcome approach originated by Avedis Donabedian, a health services research scholar who wrote highly influential papers and books on health service quality, has been very popular in health care circles for decades. Donabedian's framework pushes clinicians, managers, and researchers to think about the services provided by professionals or the interactions with them that affect patients and communities and figure out raw materials use in terms of people, time, facilities, and equipment needed to deliver services (Donabedian, 1980, 1988). His structure, process, and outcome evaluation model is classic and remains current and applicable today.

Donabedian's framework breaks down the components of a service or program into the observable and measureable: structures, processes, and outcomes. Exhibit 13.1 illustrates how these may be applied in terms of high-level policy (big "P") as well as local service delivery (little "p").

While by no means the only evaluation framework available, Donabedian's structure–process–outcomes framework, makes intuitive sense to health care managers, practitioners, direct care providers, and program designers, and by extension is useful for thinking about health policy. The framework can be used to study outcomes in health care settings and to examine the environment, as well as the personnel and work processes in those environments. One example is when a public health nursing team doing community outreach visits (structure) does various types of teaching and connects at-risk families with resources (process) intending to facilitate coping and teaches healthy behaviors and parenting skills to at-risk families (proximal outcome) with the intention of promoting child development and long-term family functioning (higher level, long-range outcomes). Another example is when a community health nursing team works with legislators to introduce regulation (structure) to reduce the population's risk for illness (process) due to secondhand smoke exposure with the intent of downstream illness prevention (outcome).

Structure

When people speak of structure, they usually mean what one might call "basic ingredients" of health care (i.e., people and things) as well as the

EXHIBIT 13.1 EXAMPLES OF STRUCTURE, PROCESS, AND OUTCOME IN POLICY

COMPONENT	DEFINITION	LITTLE "p" EXAMPLE	BIG "P" EXAMPLE
Structure	Attributes of settings in which health care is delivered: material resources and human resources, organizational structure	Hospital unit staffing, policies, procedures	Financial, space, and structural resources to establish statewide emergency response systems
Process	What is actually done in the process of care delivery	Method of falls screening implementation; falls prevention methods	Method of recording and transmitting falls and pressure ulcer data to National Database of Nursing Quality Indicators (NDNQI)
Outcome	Effects of care on health status of patients and communities	Nosocomial pressure ulcer prevalence per 1,000 patient-days for a specific unit	Community mortality and morbidity measures

conditions or contexts of care provision. Structure encompasses human resources—the individuals who work to provide care and those who support this work, as well as the way health care workers are selected, trained, organized, and managed. Structures can also be physical resources; for example, equipment, supplies, and the physical space where care is provided. Finally, structure can also include management of settings beyond human resources needed at the point of care. Thus, structure can also encompass the organizational structure and decision-making mechanisms, the selection and support of managers, and management practices. Examples of structures cutting across both big "P" and little "p" in terms of policy are the implementation of *The Future of Nursing* report recommendations (Institute of Medicine [IOM], 2011) that the proportion of nurses with baccalaureate degrees be increased to 80% by 2020, and that residency programs be implemented for new nurses, new advanced practice nurses, and nurses transitioning to new practice areas.

Process

Processes are the elements of the care or services actually provided to a patient or client population—the services intended to improve health. The activities of health care workers, the order in which they are carried out, and their quality or content are normally included here. At the simplest level, it might include whether sterile technique for dressing change was done correctly. There have been some departures and popular reframing of structure, process, and outcomes over the years from Donabedian's original writings. Some also would include management practices under the banner of "processes" but at least in the original formulation, management approaches would normally fall under "structures." Using the 80% baccalaureate preparation of nursing staff example mentioned earlier, a process evaluation of this proposal might include an evaluation of the ways that the bachelor of science in nursing (BSN) degree can be obtained for registered nurse (RN) staff and the barriers and facilitators of that process. In a hospital setting, the evaluation of the processes in play when rapid response teams are called and implemented is another example of process evaluation.

Outcome

Outcomes are downstream end points of care. Donabedian's work considers these primarily from a clinical point of view. These include "objective" health outcomes such as the incidence of illness, illness severity, complications, and mortality. However, there are many "subjective" patients' and families' perspectives on health situations that are also important to consider. The notion of quality of life is an important subjective measure. It allows for individually interpreted ratings of health states and their impacts as well as their perceptions of the quality of the care they have received and their satisfaction with their experiences.

Access and quality are elements of health care system outcomes that work the same way in that perspectives vary with one's position in the system, with consumers caring on a case-by-case basis about their personal experiences of care and managers and policy makers tending to look at experiences of many measured at a distance in an aggregated manner. Access can refer to "theoretical access" or the availability of personnel and facilities in the community with or without examining whether there are enough "spaces" to meet demand. It can refer to "practical" access—affordable services available within reasonable travel distances (Roberts, Hsiao, Berman & Reich, 2008). Similarly, quality of services can refer to the extent to which care reflects "best practices" and it can also refer to "positive outcomes" and the absence of negative, presumably preventable ones.

Quality can be considered in terms of the degree to which the package of services is in line with what are thought of as best practices (frequently the clinical point of view), but it may also be thought of in terms of the positive or desirable end points that are achieved (recovery of function, return home, and enhanced long-term survival) or negative end points (such as complications) that are avoided in the delivery of a service.

Thus, there are also a number of important outcomes related to health system performance. Clearly these take on different forms when considered through the perspectives of various stakeholders in a health care system. Outcomes can be framed from the point of view of the resources consumed to bring a patient to a certain health state. Financial outcomes, seen from the perspective of a health care consumer (patients and families), will usually relate to costs of their insurance coverage (through taxes, insurance premiums, or both), as well as any out-of-pocket costs that are not covered by insurance, such as additional copayments or bills above and beyond what their insurance plan covers, and expenditures like travel expenses and lost income. Through the eyes of a health care provider, outcomes will relate to the expenses sustained in delivering services relative to the reimbursements they receive and whether or not there are deficits that must be compensated for by other revenue-generating activities—for instance, other health care services. For a government or insurance payer, financial outcomes are a balance between the outlays relative to the end points that they are responsible for producing for their clients or citizens. These outcomes may be the total costs of treating a patient with a specific condition or care that is acceptable to covered individuals.

Interconnectedness

The connections between *structures, processes,* and *outcomes* are very important. Altering processes of care that have limited or highly indirect connections to desired outcomes is highly unlikely to produce improvements. Likewise, hoping to improve processes of care without ensuring that a critical mass of structures is in place to allow sound practices to be consistently carried out is equally misguided. Some experts believe the first step in planning and evaluating a service or an initiative is to construct a diagram (one such type of diagram is called a *logic model*) that lays out what the various moving parts of an intervention or policy are, what the preconditions for the outputs are in terms of actions of the participants, and then move backward to identifying what basic resources need to be put in place to make these actions possible. See Figure 13.1 for a comparison of Donabedian's framework and a simple logic model for a hypothetical program involving teaching self-care to individuals living with diabetes.

Some also call such a series of relationships a *program theory*. A program theory or logic model not only is a convenient tool for explaining the proposed project to those interested in understanding the reasoning behind it, but also provides a road map for evaluating interventions down the line.

Health is a complicated phenomenon having many facets that can be studied at many different levels from an individual level through the community and society levels; it has various components and facets that are influenced by a multitude of factors like genetics, one's developmental and life history, the social and physical environment, and of course health care received. In health policy, the aim is often to use government powers to influence population health, usually, but not always, by just influencing what happens in health service delivery.

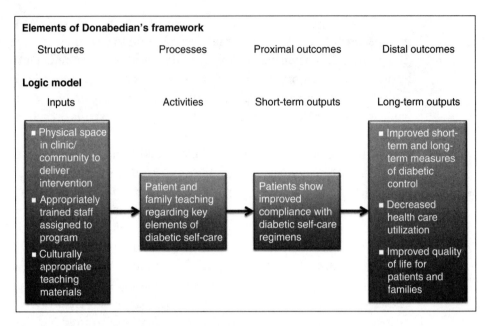

FIGURE 13.1 A comparison of Donabedian's framework and a logic model.

The Patient Protection and Affordable Care Act (PPACA) is a legislative intervention intended to influence financing (structure), increase patient access to health care (process), and improve health (outcome) in the U.S. system. This complex act, from its inception, has stimulated a great deal of evaluation and study by researchers and policy analysts. Opinions regarding the legislation are very strong and do vary, but many in organized nursing have advocated for these reforms, especially the elements of the law that involve access to care, quality and cost of care, and more effective utilization of the nurse workforce. Outcomes like overall system costs, health insurance coverage of individuals across age groups, quality of care, health outcomes, and emerging roles are closely interconnected through the structure, process, and outcome components of the act. The jury will be out for many years regarding the impacts of this legislation, but changes in public opinion about the legislation, consumer experiences, and insurance carrier and health care provider responses to the legislation are already being tracked.

Another example of the interconnectedness of these factors comes from research on nurse staffing and patient falls. In some studies, higher nurse-staffing ratios have been linked to decreased patient falls. Of particular importance to this discussion is work done by Kalisch, Tschannen, and Lee (2012), who used the "missed nursing care model" to anchor their study on falls by positing that care not done would lead to more patient falls. Staffing was the structural variable, missed nursing care was the process variable, and falls was the outcome measure. The Kalisch team found that lower levels of nurse staffing and missed care were linked to in-patient falls. Policy on the Scene 13.1 illustrates how structure, process, and outcome data are being used at the local and national levels.

POLICY ON THE SCENE 13.1: Impact on Quality Measures
Isis Montalvo, MBA, MS, RN, Nursing Consulting Partners, LLC
Franklin, WI, Former Director of ANA's National Center for
Nursing Quality

The interconnectedness among structure, process, outcome, and the importance of using meaningful data with evaluation provide a roadmap to achieving improved outcomes. More than ever before the national focus is on improving quality and patient outcomes. One of the nursing's solutions was the creation of an NDNQI that records measures sensitive to nursing interventions. This database allows comparisons of nursing quality measures nationally, regionally, and locally, even to the unit level. Donabedian's structure–process–outcome framework has been instrumental in guiding improvements in outcomes such as decreasing falls and pressure ulcer rates.

With Centers for Medicare and Medicaid Services (CMS) changes in reimbursement, the call to action to improve outcomes will only increase. And while the increased demand for quality outcome data spans decades, legislation, regulation, and their media coverage have created higher expectations of quality for consumers, providers, and payers. Trending and evaluation of NDNQI data are making a difference. Nurses can use the data locally and researchers can use the data nationally not only to track and report but also to examine what specific interventions are effective for reducing pressure ulcers and improving other outcomes.

Improvements could not have been attained without making policy and practice modifications at the bedside. The significance and importance of using indicators and evaluating them at the unit level cannot be underestimated. The following graph of actual data from a community hospital illustrates a comparison of trend data at the unit level with national-level data. This particular medical–surgical unit maintained a fall rate below the NDNQI comparable bed size benchmark mean for all quarters shown. However, not all units at this particular facility did as well. Using these data as a baseline, the staff implemented more targeted falls prevention interventions that continue to be trended.

At the national level, numerous published studies have shown how NDNQI data can be used (Bouldin et al., 2013; Lake, Shang, Klaus, & Dunton, 2010; Staggs & Dunton, 2013). At the local level, there are numerous examples of how nurses use quality data (Duncan, Montalvo, & Dunton, 2011; Dunton & Montalvo, 2007, 2009). However, ongoing research is needed to determine the effect on outcomes post-policy implementation. A CMS public–private partnership working to improve quality, the

(continued)

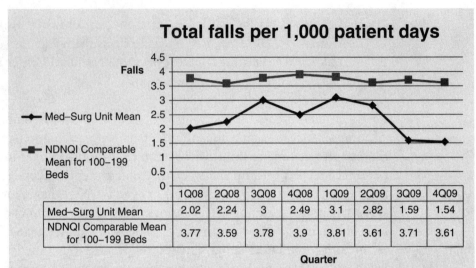

Total falls per 1,000 patient days

	1Q08	2Q08	3Q08	4Q08	1Q09	2Q09	3Q09	4Q09
Med–Surg Unit Mean	2.02	2.24	3	2.49	3.1	2.82	1.59	1.54
NDNQI Comparable Mean for 100–199 Beds	3.77	3.59	3.78	3.9	3.81	3.61	3.71	3.61

Quarter

Partnership for Patients, is very promising with close to 4,000 hospitals participating. Its ambitious goals are to reduce hospital-acquired conditions by 40% and hospital readmissions by 20% (Partnership for Patients, n.d.). Falls is an example of only one nurse-sensitive indicator collected by NDNQI. Using NDNQI in its entirety provides a comprehensive interconnected evaluative approach that gives the provider information needed to gain knowledge and make additional changes to achieve target goals.

In cases where service delivery is not the direct focus of attention, government-level health policy may be aimed at increasing one of the other determinants of health (i.e., income, social and physical environments, or health-related behaviors). Most public health and social policy interventions fall into this category (see also Chapter 14, "Eliminating Health Inequities Through Policy, Nationally and Globally"). In either case, staff time, basic resources, or raw materials (structures) are transformed into services or contacts with a clientele that is expected to impact changes in their circumstances and then ultimately influence health-related outcomes. Policies of local agencies usually target narrower aspects of office, unit, or service functioning, but relate to the way structures are used to accomplish the day-to-day work of an organization; the outcomes often relate to smooth organizational function or movement toward an organizational goal. In this local example, the health status of the population is a tacit, or implied, downstream goal.

MEASURING CHANGE

Evaluation is generally summative, formative, or a combination of both. Summative evaluation is appraisal occurring after policy implementation or at the end of a program. Formative evaluation occurs as a policy or program is implemented, so feedback is more immediate and in some cases changes can be made in response to the evaluation. No matter the format of evaluation, realizing a change in outcomes most often takes time.

Understanding Change Over Time

The heart of research design is identifying differences in features of a situation—over time or across conditions, notably, what variables do and do not vary, and which variables change alongside differences in the main variable of interest. For instance, we could imagine a clinical research study asking whether health status, using any number of evaluative measures, changes when a specific drug or treatment protocol is given to patients. Perhaps health status moves in different ways after receiving treatment depending on the gender or age of the patient. We might be interested in a research study in examining how hospital length of stay or inpatient mortality varied across patients, across hospitals, across regions, or over time. The Agency for Healthcare Research and Quality's (AHRQ) Healthcare Cost and Utilization Project (HCUP) (www.ahrq.gov/research/data/hcup/index.html) data set is ideally suited to answer such questions. This U.S. database is a nationwide longitudinal collection; state-by-state hospital care data can be searched on a range of indicators. In addition, national patient registries can provide population-specific data for use in tracking outcomes over time (Taha, Ballou, & Lama, 2014).

Demonstrating change, which is the goal of evaluation, is merely highlighting differences in a phenomenon of interest over a time period that included a change in actions or contexts. The evaluation of a policy involves assessing changes in structures or processes (or both) that are related to policy implementation along with possible changes in outcomes among people targeted by a program or policy.

Think now of a specific policy initiative involving the implementation of home visits by community nurses after the arrival of new babies in socially and economically vulnerable families such as the well-established nurse–family partnership (Olds et al., 2010). The aim might be to improve short- and long-term child development. In this case, development of the children in targeted families would be measured before and after their participation in the program. When outcomes change after implementation of a policy or program that has also affected the structures or processes in a system and competing explanations for outcomes improvements can be ruled out (e.g., mere passage of time, other changes in the environment that were independent from the interventions), we can make statements with relative confidence that the initiative was responsible for the change. Change data are needed to determine whether a policy or program is effective. In the home visit example, if the families receiving the intervention had considerable contact with nurses and the content of those interactions was closely aligned with providing information about optimal parenting techniques, anticipatory guidance, and timely referrals, this would strengthen confidence that any improvements seen were due to the policy. Also, showing that the improved outcomes were seen only when nurses and not lay community workers conducted the intervention would suggest that it was relationship building with a trusted educated professional and not merely supportive presence of a friendly individual that was connected with improved outcomes for families and children (Bornstein, 2012).

Using Quantitative and Qualitative Approaches to Evaluation

In many cases, we are trying to untangle what would happen without the intervention or initiative—without actually being able to conduct a formal experiment. For situations when trials and other forms of experimentation are not possible for one reason or another, researchers in the social and health sciences have assembled many approaches that attempt to answer the question of what would have happened without a specific initiative in place. This has sometimes included finding groups or situations that provide a possible "control" or "comparison" group outside the research or evaluation initiative to gauge the outcomes of those targeted by a policy or initiative against. It could involve examining outcomes for a comparable group of vulnerable families in areas of the same region who did not participate in the home visit program, for instance.

Posttest evaluation designs that involve measurements only after enactment of a policy or program are extremely common. The numbers of competing explanations there might be for any patterns seen complicates drawing conclusions from the data obtained from such designs. The ideal approach would involve a pretest followed by a posttest after the policy is implemented. Lack of planning and resources, both human and financial, contributes to the common use of posttest-only designs for evaluating policy.

It is important and perhaps not surprising to realize that in many evaluations the main outcome of interest fails to change or show differences, probably for several reasons. First, most outcomes are the product of complex and often interrelated factors. Second, interventions or initiatives can only hope to address a small handful of the factors, and we may not understand the mechanisms involved as well as we think. Third, data measurement may not be as specific as we would like for the measurement we are after. This situation is sometimes found in large, preexisting data sets or when data can only be accessed after a policy has been implemented. An example of proxy data is using education level for health literacy or self-rated health status for disease state. Fourth, sometimes data are collected and theoretically available for use in evaluation but access to them is greatly restricted, ostensibly to protect the privacy of patients or providers, with the end result that those who are interested have no access and are unable to analyze the data. Many compromises have been made, including using proxy data in order to evaluate programs, but with compromises come debates about data quality that can render evaluations open to critique.

Thus, quantitative approaches to evaluation are not always the best choice. The preceding paragraphs describe approaches to evaluation that are based on measurement and the quantitative paradigm. A large and growing contingent of researchers and evaluators, as well as policy makers, recognize that measurement is not the only approach for understanding the implementation and impacts of a program. They apply methods from qualitative research, including content analysis of various types of documents, as well as conduct interviews, focus groups, and field observation, to gain insights into the experiences of participants and stakeholders. Donabedian's framework and the elements of structures, processes, and outcomes are equally relevant here—addressing quality of the structures, evaluating changes in processes (or behavior changes of providers or citizens), and understanding the outcomes perceived and lived by all involved are possible through quantitative or qualitative approaches. Some see quantitative evaluations that use well-structured quasi-experimental designs as providing more robust evidence for policy analysis, but most are agreed that multiple forms of data are needed for guiding policy.

Both quantitative and qualitative data are expensive to collect. This is a basic reality of all research. It is uncommon that all the types of data needed to evaluate a program or a policy initiative are or can even be collected. Money, energy, and time must nearly always be invested to gather necessary data. The main constraints evaluators face relate to the costs of data collection, and one of the main problems encountered by evaluators of all programs, is the lack of measures or assessments of key variables (structures, processes, or outcomes) before a policy is implemented.

FINDING EXISTING DATA SOURCES

All data collection approaches in health care or other types of evaluation fall into a small handful of categories: Evaluators can collect data themselves for the explicit purpose of assessing program function; individuals involved in some element of care delivery or its outcomes can be asked questions about their perceptions or experiences; routine tracking data like demographics can be gathered in the course of care delivery; or data can be obtained as part of managing or tracking finances or for making decisions about different sectors than health care. These methods result in two interconnected sets of issues around collecting outcomes data: Logistical and methodological issues must be overcome. Logistical issues involve energy and the human and financial resources that must be invested and barriers that must be overcome. Methodological issues include ensuring that the data collected are of consistent quality and are reliable and measure what they are intended to track. For data to be collected, stakeholder interests in gathering information must outweigh the costs and potential risks involved. These issues have been alluded to in the previous section, but they hold particular meaning for nursing since, in many cases, the impacts of policies involving nursing and nursing care are difficult to track.

For over two decades, the National Sample Survey of Registered Nurses, a federally sponsored, carefully planned representative survey of licensed RNs across the United States, was conducted every 4 years. It had a strikingly high response rate and was considered the authoritative source for understanding trends in the entry and exit from the profession as well as educational and career paths of nurses and thus was a key factor in planning state and national workforce policy (Spetz, 2010). The survey was "defunded" by the Health Resources and Services Administration after the 2008 data collection cycle and there are no immediate plans to restart it (Spetz, 2013). The career paths of nurses in the workforce are now very difficult to track and it will be much more difficult to justify and evaluate investments in the nurse workforce. Similarly, until recently, systematic data about the trajectories of patients through the health care system and many aspects of patients' lives and perceptions about their health were rarely gathered or were collected so inconsistently as to be of questionable value.

In health care, nursing is often seen as invisible as variables that represent the factors that nursing directly influences have not been routinely collected. As a partial answer to that issue, nurse-sensitive indicators have been developed that are distinct from medical indicators and reflect the outcomes that nursing care can prevent or change. These measures are found in NDNQI, established by the ANA in 1998. It is the largest global quality nursing database available to assist nurses and hospitals to improve quality care and evaluate outcomes, and helps make nursing's impact much more visible. Over 2,000 hospitals participate domestically and internationally. Donabedian's structure–process–outcome quality framework is used in the database. See Exhibit 13.2 for a listing of the measures in the NDNQI database and the relationship to the Donabedian framework.

INCORPORATING ACCOUNTABILITY AND OVERSIGHT

Health care systems are stunningly complex webs of providers, organizations, and programs. The resources invested are huge—and the stakes are high for all involved. However, consumers/citizens often feel they have limited choices about how and where they seek care and have limited inputs into the decisions around the design and payment of services. In addition to incorporating the voices of service users at the local level, such as patient and family councils and inviting community members to serve on boards, a number of approaches have emerged to address such concerns.

EXHIBIT 13.2	NATIONAL DATABASE OF NURSING'S QUALITY INDICATOR (NDNQI) MEASURES BY TYPE	

MEASURE	INDICATOR COMPONENTS	TYPE OF MEASURE(S)
1. Nursing hours per patient day*,^	a. Registered nurses (RN) b. Licensed practical/vocational nurses (LPN/LVN) c. Unlicensed assistive personnel (UAP)	Structure
2. Nursing staff skill mix: Percent of total nursing hours supplied*, ^	a. RNs b. LPN/LVNs c. UAP d. Percentage of total nursing hours supplied by agency staff	Structure
3. Nurse turnover rate	a. Advanced practice registered nurse (APRN) b. RN c. LPN/LVN d. UAP	Structure
4. Hospital readmission rate		
5. RN education/ certification	a. Highest level unit-based, direct care RN degree b. Direct-care, unit-based RNs with nursing specialty certifications	Structure
6. Pain assessment, intervention, reassessment (AIR) cycle	a. Pain assessment b. Pain intervention c. Pain reassessment	Process
7. Patient falls*, ^	a. Fall assisted by employee b. Unassisted fall	Process and outcome
8. Patient falls with injury*, ^	a. Injury level	Process and outcome
9. Pressure ulcer prevalence*, ^	a. Community acquired b. Hospital acquired c. Unit acquired	Process and outcome
10. RN satisfaction and work environment survey options*,^,†	a. Job Satisfaction Scales b. Practice Environment Scale (PES) ^	Process and outcome

(continued)

EXHIBIT 13.2	NATIONAL DATABASE OF NURSING'S QUALITY INDICATOR (NDNQI) MEASURES BY TYPE (*CONTINUED*)	
11. Peripheral intrave-nous infiltration	a. Peripheral infiltration b. Peripheral extravasation	Outcome
12. Physical assault/ injury	a. Type of assault by patient (i.e., physical, sexual, or both) b. Injury level (staff members, students, other patients, or visitors)	Outcome
13. Restraint prevalence^	a. Physical restraints (e.g., limb, waist, roll belt, vest, or side rails)	Outcome
14. Catheter-associated urinary tract infection (CAUTI) ^	a. CAUTI as defined by the Centers for Disease Control and Prevention (CDC)	Outcome
15. Central line-catheter-associated blood-stream infection (CLABSI)*, ^	a. CLABSI as defined by the CDC	Outcome
16. Ventilator-associated pneumonia (VAP) ^	a. VAP as defined by the CDC	Outcome
17. Ventilator-associated events (VAE)	a. VAE as defined by the CDC	Outcome

*Original American Nurses Association (ANA) nursing-sensitive measure.
^National Quality Forum (NQF) endorsed nursing-sensitive measure.
†The RN survey is annual, whereas the other measures are quarterly.
Adapted from the ANA (2012), Montalvo (2007), and Press-Ganey (2014).

The accountability movement aims to put information about the resources expended and outcomes obtained in the hands of consumers of the services and hold local managers and system policy makers responsible for the results generated. This movement is not unique to health care by any means; it has well-known forms in elementary and secondary education and is coming of age in many other areas of public and social services, including policing and the justice system.

Accountability for outcomes of policy makers and executives/managers is part of a broader move toward "transparency"—a willingness to submit program outcomes to outside examination. Public reporting of health care structures, processes, and outcomes is increasingly common. Review or reporting of staffing levels in health care facilities; accreditation processes that focus on the verifiable presence of various types of equipment, supplies, and operating procedures; training and management practices; review of patient records and even inspection of care practices; and public reporting of outcomes are all examples of measurement of structures, processes, and outcomes and their publication or diffusion to various audiences either in the form of individual measures or in summarized form. Data, for example, are routinely made public that compare the price of comparative surgeries across a state, a region, a country, or even the world.

Data are available from a large number of hospitals on the most deadly hospital-acquired complications. The CMS routinely publishes results that compare data on each of the following settings: nursing homes, Medicare-certified hospitals, and home care (see data.medicare.gov/about).

There is a move toward providing managers and clinicians with additional incentives for meeting targeted standards or attaining certain outcomes by tying performance to some portion of remuneration or agency funding. This movement, known as "pay for performance," exists in various forms in health care. In October 2012, reimbursement based on performance under the Medicare Hospital Value-Based Purchasing (VBP) program began for acute care hospitals throughout the United States (Ryan & Blustein, 2012). VBP can be traced to the Medicare Prescription Drug, Improvement, and Modernization Act (MMA) of 2003 and the Deficit Reduction Act (DRA) of 2005 that started with voluntary public reporting of measures. With the passage of the PPACA in 2010, an inpatient hospital VBP was mandated providing rewards for how well hospitals meet selected quality measures. One example of VBP is that all patients who potentially are experiencing a heart attack must receive care within 90 minutes. Initially, incentives will be based on clinical process and patient experience measures; subsequently, they will be based on outcomes such as 30-day mortality (Ryan, 2013).

At least two major issues relate to high-stakes measurement that is reported publicly, used to drive payment or worker compensation, or used for both purposes. The first relates to differences in the clienteles served by various health care agencies that may make it challenging to interpret variability in outcomes. Should health care providers serving patients or clients with more complex or challenging conditions be compared alongside those serving clients with less complicated conditions on their outcomes or financial performance? Performing statistical adjustments to outcomes that take patient or institutional characteristics into account and that soften the impact of treatment "failures" on the indicators is called *risk adjustment*. For instance, it is arguably important to consider the age and disability status of patients or their clinical stability and backgrounds before drawing conclusions about the possible significance of nosocomial pressure ulcer or infection data as an indicator of the quality of nursing care. The debates are not simple ones—arguably more challenging cases deserve tailored care, and clients and their communities often experience negative events as failures, whether or not some cases are inherently "harder" than others. Preliminary data after the first year of VBP show that hospitals caring for more disadvantaged patients had a worse financial impact (Ryan, 2013). These results indicate that processes for determining payments need further refinement.

The second issue relates to understanding meaningful differences across health care providers or in the same health care providers over time. Much can be made of very small differences that may be trivial, the result of minor fluctuations or the result of relatively small numbers of cases going into the calculation of event rates. Related to both of these issues is the tension between the professional organizations, consumers, and health care agencies about the public availability of data. As health care reform pushes for data transparency it is believed that consumers, if they can easily access and understand the outcome data, will choose providers with good track records on quality and who offer lower prices. In a study done of almost 1,500 employees, it was found that cost was a major factor in choosing providers (Hibbard, Greene, Sofaer, Firminger, & Hirsch, 2012). Many in the Hibbad study avoided providers who were less expensive as there seemed to be a perception that high cost equated with high quality. However, when the employees were presented with cost data and easy-to-understand information about provider and service quality, more consumers indicated they would choose quality over basing decisions on cost.

Accountability and transparency are arguably forces that work in favor of increased investments in nursing. In many organizations, nursing services are considered overhead. Relying on financial accounting approaches with a misunderstanding of what are truly equivalent care structures and processes and without considering care outcomes can lead to decisions that cut staffing and other nursing resources but ultimately increase service costs. Widening the indicators tracked and reported/used to drive reimbursement to include more process and outcomes measures influenced by nursing care could support investments or reinvestments in structures of care. What is needed is a paradigm shift such that the financial bottom line is not the only outcome that should determine action.

In the case of nursing, we need to analyze in what ways nursing offers value to the public in terms of keeping citizens healthier, including helping individuals to enjoy greater quality of life and health within the context of illness. This involves identifying how outcomes for the public can be made tangible through measurement, exploring how nurses produce these outputs and what types of structures and processes are needed to achieve these outcomes, and considering whether and how measurement of structure and process should be undertaken. It also involves helping the public demand outcome data. Next, the logistics of data collection need to be resolved. Finally, ways of putting data in the hands of appropriate stakeholders need to be decided upon in terms of how data are tabulated or graphed and what media are used to transmit the messages. It should be kept in mind that although structures, processes, and outcomes and their relationships to each other are all important, many stakeholders beyond clinicians and managers are almost exclusively interested in "hard" patient and financial outcomes. Structure and process data seem to be much more important to the architects of policy and the managers of services than to many other stakeholder groups. This is perhaps why transitional care interventions by advanced practice nurses that facilitate coordination of services between community and institutional settings were fully embraced only when their impacts on outcomes like hospitalizations and overall service use were demonstrated (see Chapter 7, "Building Capital: Intellectual, Social, Political, and Financial"). Another example highlighting the work of nurses beyond cost can be found in care coordination, the value of which has been well demonstrated (Camicia et al., 2013). The ANA (2013) has published a framework identifying the structural components and measurement context for nurses' contributions to care coordination. The latter includes system, institutional, and individual/population contributors, impacting the ability of nurses to deliver high-quality care.

Historically, because the types of data that are most easily extracted from secondary data have involved negative outcomes assumed to be preventable with more nursing staff and investments in nursing care structures, such as falls and pressure ulcers, such measures have been emphasized in data collection schemes to date. However, many researchers and leaders are working to develop and refine measures that cover more areas and domains of nursing practice and assess what nurses do to facilitate positive outcomes, rather than only examining a narrow range of negative outcomes. Down the line, we can only hope for more nursing-relevant measures that can inform resource allocation decisions by suggesting where investments in health care settings should be increased to improve outcomes.

Despite the promise of the accountability movement to provide leverage for the nursing profession by helping it assert its value and argue for investments in nursing services, special emphasis on indicators, especially outcome measures alone, can be a double-edged sword and can result in unintended consequences, as will be discussed briefly here and in more depth later in this chapter. Boiling down the outputs of systems for delivering care to single measures, or a collection of indicators, even if only for the sake of clarity, starts to draw lines between important and less important aspects of system performance. This division can distract individuals from aspects of care activities that are "unpaid." These activities, if seen as expected by management but not affecting reimbursement, can create ambiguity for staff. Furthermore, emphasizing grades or scores can force health care workers in direct care as well as managers to reallocate efforts without improving patient outcomes. For instance, increasing the burden on health care providers to maintain certain types of records can increase costs and divert attention from necessary work. Chasing favorable outcomes can persuade individuals and organizations to pursue any number of strategies that involve steering outcomes to avert fraud. For the public, even if they don't realize it, steering attention and other resources away from aspects of care influencing their well-being or experience of care and playing up activities toward practices that will not be of benefit to them is a real possibility.

Accountability programs have much popular appeal even if their implementation is complicated and raises many concerns. Speaking out against accountability is risky because professionals and agencies can construe it as an avoidance tactic—a ploy to protect themselves and dodge responsibility for results. It may be risky even if it's intended to warn consumers and policy makers about the unintended consequences of using poor measures. Within health care, rating schemes developed by organizations such as the Leapfrog Group, which distill a great deal of data regarding patient safety down to a single, easily interpreted letter grade, generate similar anxiety in leaders and clinicians—and some of their criticisms seem warranted (Castillo, 2012). Arguably, nursing as a profession needs to take on a greater role in developing outcomes science. Developing meaningful measures, cost-effective means for tracking data, and an understanding of the web of factors influencing the components of evaluation are necessary to ensure the public's safety.

QUANTIFYING THE IMPACT OF POLICIES FOR NURSING

Quantifying the impact of policy actions for the profession is first and foremost identifying how patients' well-being is influenced by nurses' actions. But it also means understanding how outcomes are influenced by nursing-related processes and/or how nursing actions are promoted or impeded by structures and then understanding to what extent the actions or policies in question affect the ability of nurses to act. It has been argued for some time that what is "good for nurses" in terms of influencing their satisfaction at work and other aspects of their work lives influencing their mental or physical health is also in patients' best interests. The Magnet Recognition Program, which identifies institutions applying best practices in nursing workplaces and patient care, has shown the promise of this idea in the research literature. A growing body of literature shows more favorable outcomes for hospitals that have achieved Magnet status when compared with non-Magnet hospitals (Kelly, McHugh, & Aiken, 2011). Drenkard (2010) makes a compelling business case for the Magnet program. This work is important at this time of profound change in the health care system with so many nurses experiencing displacements in their careers, and concerns about the costs of health care as blanket statements about return on investments in single professions like nursing are challenged more often.

Costs

As costs of health care have risen, consumer expectations have risen, and payers, government agencies, legislators, and advocacy groups are debating the ability of health care expenditures to continue at current levels. Economic evaluation, or the assessment of options in health care in terms of their costs and consequences from a financial viewpoint, has therefore become increasingly important. There are a number of different types of evaluation. The two most common approaches are (a) cost-effectiveness analysis, where ratios of the total costs to the same measurable health outcomes obtained—lives saved, infections prevented, unit drops in blood pressure, or quality-adjusted life years—are calculated and compared for different treatment/care options, and (b) cost–benefit analysis, which assigns monetary values to the different health states resulting from various health care approaches and analyzes them in relation to the costs of these treatments (Glick, Polsky, & Shulman, 2010; Stone et al., 2002).

Economic evaluation is complicated by a number of features. Economic analysis is always about the comparison of different approaches to care or investments in services to each other. Selecting which conditions to put side by side can be both methodologically and politically challenging. Another issue is finding consistent and accurate means of tracking all relevant costs and outcomes and not restricting attention to those costs and outcomes for which data are most readily available. For instance, even though it is fairly simple to learn what hospitals are billing for their services, charges or billings by health care providers have only a weak connection to what careful analysis might show to be the real costs of providing the services, which are notoriously much higher than what providers actually collect. Given uncertainties surrounding health outcomes as well as differences across individuals in what outcomes or health states are desirable, it is often also difficult to assign values to different health states. Deciding on the frame of reference for analysis in terms of whose costs and benefits and over what time frames given both the plurality of stakeholders and the long-time horizons for many benefits of health care is a further challenge.

The steps in an economic evaluation are relatively simple—but the resources required for accomplishing them and the technical considerations involved can be considerable. First, an attempt is made to measure all relevant benefits or to assign values to health states, and then all relevant costs are measured. Next, how costs vary, across treatment options or situations where a program exists and one does not, is determined. Then, the ratio between outcomes and costs is calculated, and finally an attempt is made to see how much this ratio is affected by assumptions that needed to be made about how services are delivered, the most important elements of the costs and benefits to consider, and what could be ignored. The last step is quite important; good economic evaluations always provide a sense of how the conclusions might be affected by making different assumptions.

Economic analyses are technical and costly in time and expertise and incorrectly conducted analyses can reach unhelpful and even damaging results. Economic analyses with insufficient attention to time horizons and the positions of the stakeholders (or that are read without attention to these subtleties) can reach counterintuitive conclusions. For instance, in accounting for the added costs of hospitalization for individuals who experience adverse outcomes, it can appear more cost-effective to make choices that lead to death (and death early in patients' hospital stays) than create conditions that allow for situations that require prolonged hospital stays to treat.

Conclusions about costs and benefits are also often meaningfully different for different stakeholders. Cost savings or value added for a provider of health care or insurer may not be value added by a patient's reckoning. One analysis concluded that the net benefits of improved nurse staffing on patient outcomes may really accrue to patients and society rather than to individual hospitals

(Dall, Chen, Seifert, Maddox, & Hogan, 2009). This suggests that policy strategies for improving nurse staffing may need to consider where motivations can be leveraged—that is, at the societal level.

The literature linking nurse staffing with patient safety outcomes in acute care hospitals has been at the heart of more than 15 years of advocacy work on the part of many, including nurses' professional associations in a number of countries, trying to fend off dramatic cuts in funding for nurse staffing and increases in nurse–patient workloads. These efforts have led to more explicit examination of the unintended consequence of changes in nurse staffing whether due to nurse shortages or hospital cost cutting of staff. One such unintended consequence that is receiving increasing scrutiny is nurse rationing of care. Policy on the Scene 13.2 presents data from several recent nursing studies that examine the links between decreased nurse staffing hours and the rationing of patient care.

Analyzing Intended and Unintended Consequences

A central concept in public policy is the notion of unintended consequences. Policies may fail to achieve the outcomes targeted by their originators in many ways. Policy initiatives may be based on incomplete or misinformed ideas about the factors that influence the outcomes being targeted, or various political forces may lead to policies being adopted that are not the ones most likely to produce desired responses. Downstream, implementation of measures may also be incomplete or inconsistent—that is, structures not being put in place or failing to influence processes in the manner expected. Furthermore, attempting to engineer complex social systems with multiple actors can produce any number of reactions as stakeholders attempt to maximize or maintain their benefits and minimize their costs or inconveniences. The PPACA, which was designed to increase coverage of working-age adults by requiring employers of 50 or more employees to offer health insurance coverage to all employees working 30 or more hours per week, is an example of these polarities. There are some pundits who claim that this measure will end up creating a disincentive to employers to create new jobs and to give more weekly hours to employees scheduled at the 30-hour per week threshold. This of course is bad news in a time of economic challenges when workers need hours and jobs and society is in need of job creation (McVeigh, 2013). It is not yet clear whether this is in danger of happening on a large scale (FactChecking, 2013). What is, however, clear, as a general principle, is that stakeholders can and do shift their energies or resources into alternative behaviors that can undermine the original intent of a policy or program. As a result, consequences of implementing a policy may fall well short of the expected or intended ones and the possibility of new desirable and undesirable effects that were never foreseen must be kept in mind.

POLICY ON THE SCENE 13.2: Nurse Rationing—A Developing Concept for Staffing Plans and Ratios

Nurses in direct care are often heard saying, "There is not enough time." They report not having time to get patient care done and that they go home at the end of their work day worrying about what did not get done. While much attention has been given in the past 15 years to staffing, the notion of bedside rationing as a result of staffing and time resources is relatively new. "Bedside rationing in nursing care refers to withholding or failure to carry out certain aspects of care because of limited resources such as time, staffing or skill mix" (Papastavrou, Andreou, & Efstathiou, 2013, para 1). Studies on staffing and skill mix have most often focused on safety issues and quantifiable negative outcomes like medication and treatment errors and adverse clinical incidents, including patient falls, pressure ulcers, unplanned patient readmissions, restraint use, and nurse injury. As early as 2001, evidence emerged that nurses were not getting all of their work done. Canadian, U.S., and German nurses reported that basic tasks like skin care were not being performed for lack of time. While there were differences among the countries, at least 34% of the surveyed nurses reported that two tasks—comforting patients and care-plan updating—were being left undone when necessary. (Aiken et al., 2001). More recently, a systematic review of 17 quantitative studies on rationing of care and nurse–patient outcomes revealed areas where some patterns were seen: features of the care that were rationed, reasons for the rationing, and nurse and patient outcomes resulting from rationing (Papastavrou et al., 2013).

Staffing ratios and staffing policies are continuing to unfold as research evidence continues to inform policy. Since California adopted the first state-level legislation related to staffing, a number of states have developed laws or regulations on staffing. The variation in approaches reflects the complexity of policy makers' interpretation of these outcomes in the context of their political climate. The ANA maintains a website on the current status of staffing legislation and regulation in the United States (nursingworld.org/MainMenuCategories/Policy-Advocacy/State/Legislative-Agenda-Reports/State-StaffingPlansRatios).

Unintended consequences are not always bad, however. There are times when outcomes that were not targeted by a program or policy can be positive. One example of a positive unintended consequence is found in examining health information exchanges (HIEs). HIEs, electronic-based exchanges that allow organizations, systems, and providers to share health information, are a direct result of the legislation, The American Recovery and Reinvestment Act of 2009. In spite of concerns about privacy invasion, at least one positive unintended consequence is new possibilities for syndromic surveillance. Clinicians, officials, and researchers using syndromic surveillance are able to identify patterns of conditions and diseases that might point to a developing public health problem sooner, providing the opportunity for earlier response and intervention (McGowan, Kuperman, Olinger, & Russell, 2012). Of particular interest to policy is that nurses may be restricted from full access to HIEs. Thorn and Carter (2013), for example, compellingly argue for critical importance of access for nurses and point to the relevance of this access in the emergency department, where individual hospital policies may specifically prohibit that access.

A full evaluation of a policy tracks and tallies both costs and benefits and attempts not only to identify whether expected changes are observed in targeted outcomes but also to track what other related factors may be affected by the intervention. Commonly intended consequences of policies and programs include improved service quality, cost efficiencies, and health outcomes; increased and expanded access to services; and enhanced quality of life. Unintended consequences can be found by anticipating them both when developing policy and examining a policy once it is in place for both positive and negative outcomes. See Exhibit 13.3 for a classification system for unintended consequences based on the work of Smith (1995) and Rambur, Vallett, Cohen, and Tarule (2013). Their work was designed specifically for use in examining performance metrics but has been reworked to what we call "traps" to missing unintended consequences. These traps can provide a cautionary note when both evaluating and planning for policies. Involving

---

EXHIBIT 13.3 TRAPS TO MISSING UNINTENDED CONSEQUENCES

Tunnel vision: Evaluating effectiveness based primarily on financial benefits

Measure fixation: Focusing on a metric such as 30-day readmission without full consideration of the patient

Acontextual actions: Choosing patients who will give you the best results when implementing a policy

Misrepresentation: Managing outcomes so that only selected outcomes are presented, either positive or negative or either expected or unexpected

Gaming: Changing behavior to get the best results; for example, patients are told how to respond on satisfaction surveys

Myopia: Focusing only on short-term results

Suboptimization: Pursuing limited number of outcomes and those that are the most favorable

Ossification: Deterring innovation with overemphasis on strict positive outcomes

those directly impacted by the policies helps in anticipating potential consequences.

Deep knowledge of the targeted health problem or care delivery issue with an understanding of the community and critical unbiased eyes is needed to draw up a complete list of consequences and select variables to include in an evaluation. Evaluations that leave out important consequences may sell the successes of a policy short or overestimate its benefits. Equally critical, evaluations perceived as omitting important considerations will be particularly vulnerable to claims of bias. Nurses by virtue of their role are well positioned to observe and advise how to correct for unintended consequences (Rambur et al., 2013).

DETERMINING SUSTAINABILITY

Sustainability refers to the ability of a change in conditions following an intervention to continue after an initial investment of resources. As we noted earlier in this chapter, many program or policy evaluations fail to identify the hoped-for improvement in the main outcome of interest. Even fewer evaluations are able to demonstrate sustained improvement in outcomes over time. People fatigue of messages and fail to be motivated by inducements or penalties; overall, systems have a tendency to revert to their original states over time (Swerissen & Crisp, 2004). At the little "p" level in hospitals, the incidence of falls, restraint use, lack of hand hygiene, and alarm fatigue are examples where old habits tend to recur and complacency is common.

Whether the resources normally available in a system will be sufficient to cover the ongoing costs or expenses of a policy initiative is a recurring question. Can a regulation be enforced to a sufficient extent over time? Will behavior become widespread enough or will people in various roles have enough knowledge and intrinsic motivation over time to continue proceeding in a certain way? Could the benefits of an initiative balance the costs and eventually lead to it "paying for itself"? If regulation is used as a means of influencing patients, providers, and health care payers and systems, will resources for inspection and enforcement of these regulations be available in the long term? Will the benefits of the policy, whatever it is, be sufficiently clear to maintain a critical mass of support over time?

Obviously, careful evaluation of a policy initiative can provide important information for making a case that an intervention is sustainable. Thinking about sustainability is critical from the moment a policy is developed. If the structures needed to implement a policy are not thought through or are incompletely measured, the long-term costs and benefits of the intervention will be underestimated. Because of this problem, evidence-based practice (EBP) models include a final step of ongoing monitoring and/or evaluation. Without ongoing monitoring and evaluation, initial improvements often fade away.

STRATEGIZING NEXT STEPS

The policy process is a cycle, as others have alluded to in earlier chapters. From problem identification, through agenda setting, policy formulation, selection, and implementation, often some type of evaluation takes place even if it is on an informal basis and involves stakeholders gathering impressions and drawing conclusions about whether their aims were met and beginning the cycle anew. In terms of strategizing next steps, a number of basic options are available: to do nothing, that is, to cease interventions and to let "natural" conditions take or retake hold; to maintain the current course; to increase investments or expand the scope of a policy; to change course by withdrawing financial support or repealing regulations; to introduce new policies that proceed in a different direction; or to let others do something that takes the policy in a different direction.

People seeking to influence the policy process must decide which of the previous options they wish policy makers to address. Formal analysis of a policy indicating the extent to which a policy measure has achieved its intended ends and what its other consequences have been can be useful tools in figuring out how to move forward and as supports for arguments.

Many argue that evaluation is a fundamentally political process and that data will nearly always be seen as the tool of one side or another in a policy debate. Perhaps this is true, but using data in a principled way and avoiding intentionally overstating or misstating facts in the long run is best for credibility of advocates as well as the future of using data to inform policy in the future.

DEVELOPING POLICY SCHOLARSHIP IN NURSING

The future of health care will increasingly require health professionals to confront dilemmas about how to offer high-quality services that are accessible to the public at reasonable cost. As the pace of change in terms of social and economic forces hitting health care shows no sign of abating, nurses and others will have to understand and in some instances attempt to steer local- and higher-level policy impacts on their work.

Most health professionals and researchers still have an uncomfortable relationship with policy and politics. They consider it, at best, a distraction from "higher yield" direct service to clients and, at worst, partaking of a convoluted and often distasteful process of manipulation and strategizing. However, many are now realizing that keeping our distance from policy is no longer a viable option. Beyond becoming informed about the policy process in general, it is important to learn about specific policies at various levels and eventually to share our experiences in advocacy, implementation, and evaluation.

Relatively few academic policy evaluations specialize in health care issues, and even fewer nurse researchers are involved in this area. There are some notable examples, however, at a few major centers across the country. If we turn our attention briefly to local policy initiatives, many are never formally evaluated at all; among those where some data are collected and/or analyzed, few are ever formally reported in any consistent or retrievable manner. Given the understandable emphasis in the nursing literature on updating clinicians on clinical matters and publishing reports of research studies, it is easy to see how policy-focused articles are less often written or sought. As a result, there is mostly an informal method of passing along information about what has worked in local policies and programs and certainly around nursing involvement in policy and its results.

Contexts and history are important for anyone who would seek to generalize approaches used in other communities or around other policy issues to new settings, but data of some sort—preferably health outcomes data—tend to be quite influential. While articles appear about political involvement and state and national policy issues affecting nursing, as well as policy

OPTION FOR POLICY CHALLENGE: Charting a Wider Path for Needlestick Safety

The history of needle safety presented in the opening policy challenge and the most current figures on needlestick injury point to the importance of continuing work on this important issue. As recently reported by ANA president, Karen Daley, almost two out of three nurses reported an accidental needlestick in a 2008 ANA survey; she went on to highlight the findings of Dr. Jagger and her colleagues (2010), revealing that in some areas such as operating rooms, sharps injury rates have increased over previous years (Daley, 2011). This, coupled with the underreporting of sharps injuries, clearly indicate that legislation and enforcement are not enough. Ongoing efforts at the big "P" and little "p" levels remain crucial.

A feature of North American legislation, for example, was that institutions track sharps injuries and document that the selection process for equipment was a structured one that involved staff. However, nurses were not always put on committees making decisions about equipment choice, and policing compliance with legislation was not always easy. The question now is what types of policy might be required to produce further improvements and if the perceptions of the risk run by health care providers are sufficient to interest policy makers in continuing action on this issue. One answer may lie in turning to research. Research evidence was a

(continued)

key part of policy success in the history of legislation being adopted. How might we use evidence again?

Continuing active research, sharing research results, and practice and policy changes at all levels are vital to preventing the complacency that often sets in once policies are in place. In 2010, a conference, the Tenth Anniversary of the Needlestick Safety and Prevention Act: Mapping Progress, Charting a Future Path, was held and this very sharing took place. As a result, a consensus statement and call to action was issued and the following areas were identified for continuing improvement: (a) sharps safety in surgical settings, (b) understanding and reducing exposure risks outside hospitals, (c) frontline health care workers' involvement in selecting safety devices, (d) safety device innovation, and (e) education and training in all health care settings as well as nursing and medical schools (Staff, 2012).

While this consensus statement helps direct future options, it is up to each nurse to examine the research, or in some cases conduct and share it; in other cases, it may mean nurses need to help ensure policies are followed, or in some cases rewritten. What is the nurse's role: Is he or she working as an administrator, educator, manager, or direct care nurse, or is his or her specialty home care, informatics, or policy analysis?

advocacy efforts involving nursing, in publications such as the *American Journal of Nursing, American Nurse, American Nurse Today, OJIN: Online Journal of Issues in Nursing,* and *Politics, Policy and Nursing Practice*; and anecdotal experiences with implementing policies and programs are dotted throughout the management and clinical literatures, it is probably time to begin thinking in some new ways to report these kinds of experiences. A number of scholars and journal editors developed the Standards for Quality Improvement Reporting Excellence (squire-statement.org) to assist groups in reporting their local experiences implementing and evaluating programs in a complete and rigorous manner, keeping in mind that there is likely to be a fair degree of variation in the nature of programs and content of evaluations. Perhaps nurses, nurse scientists, and leaders need more encouragement to write up their experiences and more recognition needs to be given to those who share their experiences in local and higher level policies with broad professional audiences.

Developing the science of measurement of nursing's structures, processes, and outcomes, and developing and maintaining data sources, is a second major challenge. Ensuring that mandates and funding for collecting key types of data that highlight the impacts of policies on nurses and nursing care will be a major challenge for nurses and the profession in the next years. It will require careful planning. If unsuccessful, a long history of nursing being largely invisible in policy circles will continue, evaluation of nursing-related policy and policies that impact nurses will be hampered, and advocacy for nursing-related health policy will be rendered more difficult.

IMPLICATIONS FOR THE FUTURE

Outcomes and evaluation research are important tools in policy development and advocacy. Increasing debates about the role of government and of regulation in ensuring health care quality will mean that in the future, arguments for new health policies (or that justify existing programs) will increasingly need support with data. Educating the public about outcomes and their role as empowered consumers will be increasingly important. Of course, many have become increasingly cynical about the shaping of political messages and the selective reporting or overt misrepresentation of facts, including research and evaluation data, in the fight for public opinion. In the past decades, there have been massive investments in research projects and the conclusions that could be drawn from these have often been somewhat softer or nuanced than many would like. The next years will probably see many stakeholders being more realistic in their expectations of program evaluations to guiding policy and more understanding that the synthesis or summarizing of evidence may need to proceed in a different direction than expecting a small handful of studies to provide "the" answers to complex and often very polarizing health policy debates and challenges.

KEY CONCEPTS

1. Evaluation of outcomes is an integral component of accountable policy making at all levels.
2. Evaluation takes many forms from the examination of specific interventions to the impact of a policy on society.
3. Evaluation uses many of the same techniques of conventional researchers, for example, quantitative and qualitative methods; prospective and retrospective approaches.
4. The purpose of evaluation is to understand systems and services or policies that address various issues or problems.
5. Policy analysis research assesses how well a policy has achieved its intended outcomes.
6. Benchmarking is a comparison against a stand of performance or level of quality.
7. Indicators are specific measurements that are benchmarked.
8. Nurse-sensitive indicators are outcomes that are believed to be particularly influenced by nursing.
9. Structure, process, and outcome is a frequently used framework for evaluation that takes into consideration people, facilities, equipment, and the delivery of services.

10. Evaluation may be summative (after a policy is implemented) or formative (while a policy is implemented).
11. Demonstrating differences in outcomes is difficult because of the complexity of factors and their relationships, lack of complete understanding of involved factors, imprecise measurement, and data access restrictions.
12. Outcome measurement may have both positive and negative unintended consequences that impact direction for policy.
13. Pay-for-performance schemes and public reporting are examples of high-stakes outcome measurement initiatives.
14. Economic evaluation focuses on the comparison of different approaches to investments in care or services and how the results vary based upon different assumptions.
15. The sustainability of outcomes needs to be included in the initial development of policy.
16. Development of the science of measuring structures, processes, and outcomes, and developing and maintaining data sources, is critical to enhancing visibility in policy circles.

SUMMARY

Sound data have enormous potential to influence the creation of worthwhile policies as well as to assist stakeholders in evaluating the impacts of policies on key outcomes. Frameworks that describe how structures and processes for providing services influence outcomes are critical for designing outcomes, and time spent determining whether the connections between various elements of a policy or program are logical tends to be well spent. Obtaining data that will assist in policy or program planning is often costly and complicated, but possibilities almost always exist to leverage at least one of the major strategies. Documenting and presenting the contribution of nursing services to the public's well-being is a challenging but worthwhile pursuit; economic analyses of policies and programs are becoming more common; and certainly an awareness of concepts like sustainability and unintended consequences is key to using evaluation data for policies. Future challenges for nursing relate to developing a tradition of nursing scholarship around how we know policies have been successful, and ensuring that data sources are available in the future to guide our efforts.

LEARNING ACTIVITIES

1. Identify a little "p" or big "P" health policy related to an issue of interest to you. List the intended and unintended consequences.
2. Obtain a policy evaluation report and compare and contrast the elements of the policy evaluation with the elements described in this chapter. Describe

the stated conclusion about the effectiveness of the policy in the report and the next relevant steps. Identify why you support or do not support the conclusions of the report based on the data presented in the report.

3. Select a little "p" policy at work or in your educational program and discuss how outcomes for the policy are being formally measured. Discuss how the measures are reported and what changes for maintaining or modifying the measures and their reporting you would make and why.

4. Reexamine Exhibit 13.2 and select a policy you would like to change. Make a list of four to five questions that you would ask to determine if the unintended consequences have not been fully explored because of the potential traps identified in the table.

5. Discuss the interconnectedness of structure, process, and outcome using a current health policy to illustrate the concepts.

6. Identify two research or EBP questions related to an issue in your practice setting that would yield important outcomes in providing direction for policy.

E-RESOURCES

- Agency on Healthcare Research and Quality Healthcare Cost and Utilization Project (HCUP). http://www.ahrq.gov/research/data/hcup/index.html
- Agency on Healthcare Research and Quality: Patient Safety and Quality: An Evidence-Based Handbook for Nurses. http://www.ahrq.gov/professionals/clinicians-providers/resources/nursing/resources/nurseshdbk/index.html
- American Public Health Association: Policy Evaluation. http://www.apha.org/programs/cba/CBA/resources/Policy+Evaluation.htm
- Centers for Disease Control and Prevention: Office of the Associate Director for Program (OADPG). http://www.cdc.gov/eval/materials/Developing-An-Effective-Evaluation-Report_TAG508.pdf
- Centers for Medicare and Medicaid Services. https://data.medicare.gov/
- Centers for Medicare and Medicaid Services: Hospital Value-Based Purchasing Program. http://www.cms.gov/Outreach-and-Education/Medicare-Learning-Network-MLN/MLNProducts/downloads/Hospital_VBPurchasing_Fact_Sheet_ICN907664.pdf
- Health Indicators Warehouse. http://www.healthindicators.gov
- Needlestick Safety and Prevention Act of 2000, Pub. L. 106-430. https://www.govtrack.us/congress/bills/106/hr5178
- NDNQI™ Quality Improvement Solutions From the ANA. http://www.nursingquality.org
- Outcome and Assessment Information Set (OASIS). http://www.cms.gov/Medicare/Quality-Initiatives-Patient-Assessment-Instruments/OASIS/index.html
- Patient Safety—Quality Improvement Website of the Department of Community and Family Medicine at Duke University. http://patientsafetyed.duhs.duke.edu/module_a/module_overview.html

- Robert Woods Johnson, Evaluation 101: Why We Do Evaluation. http://www.youtube.com/watch?v=E14fU2jYk7o
- SQUIRE Standards for Quality Improvement Reporting Excellence. http://squire-statement.org

REFERENCES

Aiken, L. H., Clarke, S. P., Sloane, D. M., Sochalski, J. A., Busse, R., Clarke, H., … Shamian, J. (2001). Nurses' reports on hospital care in five countries. *Health Affairs, 20*(3), 43–53.

American Nurses Association. (2011). *ANA's principles for social networking and the nurse: guidance for registered nurses.* Silver Spring, MD: Author.

American Nurses Association. (2012). *NDNQI Indicator Manual.* Silver Spring, MD: Author.

American Nurses Association. (2013). *Framework for measuring nurses' contributions to care coordination.* Retrieved from http://www.nursingworld.org/Framework-for-Measuring-Nurses-Contributions-to-Care-Coordination

American Recovery and Reinvestment Act of 2009, Pub. L .111-5. 123 Stat. 115.

Bardach, E. (2012). *A practical guide for policy analysis: The eightfold path to more effective problem solving* (4th ed.). Thousand Oaks, CA: CQ Press.

Batalden, P. B., & Davidoff, K. (2007). What is "quality improvement" and how can it transform health care? *Quality & Safety in Health Care, 16*(1), 2–3.

Bornstein, D. (2012, May 16). *The power of nursing.* Retrieved from http://opinionator.blogs.nytimes.com/2012/05/16/the-power-of-nursing/?_r=0

Bouldin, E. L., Andresen, E. M., Dunton, N. E., Simon, M., Waters, T. M., Liu, M., … Shorr, R. I. (2013). Falls among adult patients hospitalized in the United States: prevalence and trends. *Journal of Patient Safety, 9*(1), 13–17.

Camicia, M., Chamberlain, B., Finnie, R. R., Nalle, M., Lindeke, L. L., Lorenz, L., … McMemamin, P. (2013). The value of nursing care coordination: A white paper of the American Nurses Association. *Nursing Outlook, 61*(6), 490–501.

Castillo, M. (2012, November 28). *Study on safest hospitals shows some surprising results.* Retrieved from http://www.cbsnews.com/8301-204_162-57556061/

Centers for Disease Control and Prevention (CDC). (2008). *Workbook for designing, implementing and evaluating a sharps injury prevention program.* Retrieved from http://www.cdc.gov/sharpssafety/pdf/sharpsworkbook_2008.pdf

Daley, K. (2011). Complacency erodes sharps safety gains. *Hospital Employee Health, 30*(8), 91–92.

Dall, T. M., Chen, Y. J., Seifert, R. F., Maddox, P. J., & Hogan, P. F. (2009). The economic value of professional nursing. *Medical Care, 47*(1), 97–104.

Deficit Reduction Act of 2005. Pub. L. 109-171. 120 Stat 4 (2006).

Donabedian, A. (1980). Methods for deriving criteria for assessing the quality of medical care. *Medical Care Review, 37*(7), 653–698.

Donabedian, A. (1988). The quality of care. How can it be assessed? *JAMA, 260*(12), 1743–1748.

Drenkard, K. (2010). The business case for Magnet. *Journal of Nursing Administration, 40*(6), 263–271.

Duncan, J., Montalvo, I., & Dunton, N. (2011). *NDNQI case studies in quality improvement.* Silver Spring, MD: American Nurses Association.

Dunton, N., & Montalvo, I. (2007). *Transforming nursing data into quality care: Profiles of quality improvement in U.S. health care facilities.* Silver Spring, MD: Nursesbooks.org.

Dunton, N., & Montalvo, I. (2009). *Sustained improvement in nursing quality. Hospital performance on NDNQI indicators, 2007–2008.* Silver Spring, MD: American Nurses Association.

"FactChecking 'Pernicious' Obamacare Claims." (2013, September 25). In *Articles/Featured Posts.* Retrieved from http://www.factcheck.org/2013/09/factchecking-pernicious-obamacare-claims

Glick, H. A., Polsky, D. P., & Shulman, K. A. (2010). Trial-based economic evaluations: An overview of design and analysis. In M. Drummond & A. McGuire (Eds.), *Economic evaluation in health care: Merging theory with practice* (pp. 113–140). New York, NY: Oxford University Press.

Hewison, A. (2007). Policy analysis: A framework for nurse managers. *Journal of Nursing Management, 15*(7), 693–699.

Hibbard, J. H., Greene, J., Sofaer, S., Firminger, K., & Hirsch, J. (2012). An experiment shows that a well-designed report on costs and quality can help consumers choose high-value health care. *Health Affairs, 31*(3), 560–568.

Institute of Medicine (IOM). (2011). *The future of nursing: Leading change, advancing health.* Washington, DC: The National Academies Press.

Jagger, J., Berguer, R., Phillips, E. K., Parker, G., & Gomaa, A. E. (2010). Increase in sharps injuries in surgical settings, versus nonsurgical settings after passage of national needle-stick legislation. *Journal of the American College of Surgeons, 210*(4), 496–502.

Kalisch, B. J., Tschannen, D., & Lee, K. H. (2012). Missed nursing care, staffing, and patient falls. *Journal of Nursing Care Quality, 27*(1), 6–12.

Kelly, L. A., McHugh, M. D., & Aiken, L. H. (2011). Nurse outcomes in Magnet* and Non-Magnet hospitals. *Journal of Nursing Administration, 41*(10), 428–433.

Lake, E. T., Shang, J., Klaus, S., Dunton, N. E. (2010). Patient falls: Association with hospital Magnet status and nursing & unit staffing. *Research in Nursing and Health, 33*(5),413–425.

McGowan, J. J., Kuperman, G. J., Olinger, L., & Russell, C. (2012). *Strengthening health information exchange: Final report HIE Unintended Consequences Work Group.* Retrieved from http://www.healthit.gov/sites/default/files/hie_uc_workgroup_final_report.pdf

McVeigh, K. (2013, September 30). *US employers slashing worker hours to avoid Obamacare insurance mandate.* Retrieved from http://www.theguardian.com/world/2013/sep/30/us-employers-slash-hours-avoid-obamacare

Medicare Prescription Drug, Improvement, and Modernization Act of 2003. Pub. L. 108-173.

Montalvo, I. (2007). The National Database of Nursing Quality Indicators* (NDNQI*). *OJIN: The Online Journal of Issues in Nursing, 12*(3), Manuscript 2. Retrieved from http://www.nursingworld.org/MainMenuCategories/ANAMarketplace/ANAPeriodicals/OJIN/TableofContents/Volume122007/No3Sept07/NursingQualityIndicators.ht

National Council of State Boards of Nursing (NCSBN). (2011). *White paper: A nurse's guide to the use of social media.* Advance online publication. doi:10.1037/a0028240. Retrieved from https://www.ncsbn.org/Social_media_guidelines.pdf

Olds, D. L., Kitzman, H. J., Cole, R. E., Hanks, C. A., Arcoleo, K. J., Anson, E. A., … Stevenson, A. J. (2010). Enduring effects of prenatal and infancy home visiting by nurses on maternal life course and government spending. *JAMA Pediatrics, 165*(5), 419–424.

Papastavrou, E., Andreou, P., & Efstathiou, G. (2013, January). Rationing of nursing care and nurse-patient outcomes: A systematic review of quantitative studies. *International Journal of Health Planning and Management.* Advance online publication. doi:10.1002/hpm.2160

Partnership for Patients. (n.d.). About the partnership. Retrieved from http://partnershipforpatients.cms.gov

Patient Protection and Affordable Care Act of 2010. Pub. L. 111-148, 124 Stat 119-1025.

Press-Ganey Associates, Inc. (2014). *NDNQI*™. *Our research gives you the advantage*. Retrieved from http://www.nursingquality.org/About-NDNQI/Research-Advantage

Rambur, B., Vallett, C., Cohen, J. A., & Tarule, J. M. (2013). Metric-driven harm: An exploration of unintended consequences of performance measurement. *Applied Nursing Research, 26*(4), 269–272.

Roberts, M. J., Hsiao, W., Berman, P., & Reich, M. R. (2008). *Getting health reform right: A guide to improving performance and equity*. New York, NY: Oxford University Press.

Ryan, A., & Blustein, J. (2012). Making the best of hospital pay for performance. *New England Journal of Medicine, 366*(17), 1557–1559.

Ryan, A. M. (2013). Will valued-based purchasing increase disparities in care? *New England Journal of Medicine, 369*(26), 2472–2474.

Smith, P. (1995). On the unintended consequences of publishing performance data in the public sector. *International Journal of Public Administration, 18*(23), 277–310.

Spetz, J. (2010). The importance of good data: How The National Sample Survey of Registered Nurses has been used to improve knowledge and policy. *Annual Review of Nursing Research, 28*, 1–18.

Spetz, J. (2013). The research and policy importance of nursing sample surveys and minimum data sets. *Policy, Politics & Nursing Practice, 14*(1), 33–40.

Squires, D. A. (2013). *Multinational comparisons of health systems data, 2012*. New York, NY: The Commonwealth Fund. Retrieved from http://www.commonwealthfund.org/Publications/Chartbooks/2013/Mar/Multinational-Comparisons-of-Health-Data-2012.aspx

Staff of the International Healthcare Worker Safety Center and Steering Committee for 10th Anniversary of the Needlestick Safety and Prevention Act: Mapping Progress, Charting a Future Path. (2012). *Moving the sharps safety agenda forward in the United States: Consensus statement and call to action*. Charlottesville, VA: University of Virginia.

Staggs, V. S., & Dunton, N. (2013). Associations between rates of unassisted inpatients falls and levels of nurse staffing. *International Journal for Quality in Health, 26*(1), 87–92. doi:10.1093/intqhc/mzt080

Stone, P. W., Bakken, S., Curran, C. R., & Walker, P. H. (2002). Evaluation of studies of health economics. *Evidence-Based Nursing, 5*(4), 100–104.

Swerissen, H., & Crisp, B. R. (2004). The sustainability of health promotion interventions for different levels of social organization. *Health Promotion International, 19*(1), 123–130.

Taha, A., Ballou, M. M., & Lama, A. E. (2014). Utilization of national patient registries by clinical nurse specialist: Opportunities and implications. *Clinical Nurse Specialist, 28*(10) 56–62.

Thorn, S. A., & Carter, M. A. (2013). The potential of health information exchange to assist emergency nurses. *Journal of Emergency Nursing, 39*(5), e91–e96.

FOURTEEN

Eliminating Health Inequities Through Policy, Nationally and Globally

Shanita D. Williams
Janice M. Phillips
Josepha E. Burnley

Health inequities arise because of a toxic combination of poor social policies, unfair economic arrangements and bad politics. These, in turn, affect the circumstances in which people are born, grow, live, work and age.—Sir Michael Marmot (2008)

OBJECTIVES

1. Explain the link between social and economic conditions and population health inequity in the United States and globally.
2. Describe U.S. inequities and present the global context in which health inequities exist.
3. Analyze the health impact of the social determinants of health (SDOH).
4. Evaluate the social, structural, economic, and health policy determinants of health inequities.
5. Recommend potential policy solutions for health inequities in the United States and globally.

Health is a human right, and social inequities are indeed a matter of economics and social justice. Yet, persistent social and economic inequities in health and health care exist both in the United States and on a global scale. Throughout the world, health inequities are inextricably linked to the unequal distribution of social and economic resources. Socially and economically disadvantaged groups are less likely to be in good health, less likely to have access to quality health care services, and more likely to die prematurely when compared with the socially and economically advantaged. In the United States, those who live in poverty, the uninsured, the disabled, and people of color bear the brunt of the health inequities burden.

Registered nurses at 2.8 million strong (nurses reporting their occupation as a registered nurse) comprise the largest segment of the U.S. professional health workforce (U.S. Department of Health and Human Services [USDHHS], 2013). Nurses are at the heart of the interface between health systems and patients, families, and communities, and are strategically positioned to serve as key actors to advocate for the health and well-being of the nation. Therefore, championing the elimination of health and health care inequities through political advocacy and a commitment to policy development is an essential element of professional nursing practice.

When people learn about health care inequities, they may assume that issues related to inequities do not exist in their own communities. However, one need not travel very far to observe the adverse impact of inequities on health and policies that perpetuate the status quo. Addressing national and global health inequities requires "upstream" long-range approaches at the big "P" level to address their underlying causes. However, there are numerous opportunities where nurses advocating for better health outcomes can address inequities in their local communities at the little "p" level to make a more immediate impact on the health of people in need.

This chapter presents a broad overview of the link between social and economic policy and health inequities and highlights the health impact of social determinants on populations in the United States and across the globe. In the United States, the nature of health inequities has traditionally focused on racial, ethnic, and socioeconomic status (SES)/class inequities with regard to health care access and health outcomes. This chapter aims to extend the health inequities discussion beyond the U.S. borders to include a global context that allows us to describe the social, structural, economic, and health policy determinants underlying health inequities both within the United States and among nations. We conclude with a discussion of potential policy approaches that may contribute to the elimination of health inequities in the United States. See the Policy Challenge, which illustrates the all too familiar story of the intersection of poverty and health in America.

In this familiar story of life in rural, poverty-stricken Appalachia, the systemic and pervasive intergenerational health inequities highlight the root causes or true underlying nature of health inequities—lack of critical material and social resources that are necessary to ensure health and well-being across generations. However, Gina and her daughter's story does not have to end in such a predictable way. The right policies and appropriate interventions can interrupt the cycle of poverty, low educational achievement, teenage pregnancy, and LBW infant outcomes that continue to feed upon itself across generations. The key question for nurses then becomes … what implications does Gina's story have for U.S. and global policies on health and health care inequities?

POLICY CHALLENGE: The Case of Gina: Living at the
Intersection of Social and Economic Determinants of Health
(Poverty, Low Education) and Health Inequities (Teenage
Pregnancy and Low-Birth-Weight Health Outcomes)

Gina, a 14-year-old girl (the daughter and granddaughter of teenage mothers), gives birth to a low-birth-weight (LBW) infant in a rural Appalachian region of the United States. The newborn infant girl (whose mother and grandmother are uninsured) is transferred to a regional acute care facility and receives extensive, technologically advanced, neonatal intervention and treatment that exceeds $150,000. The health system, a safety net provider, writes this cost off as an uncollectable debt under their state-supported public funding program.

At 6 months of age, Gina's daughter is diagnosed with cognitive deficits, and at 12 months she is determined to be developmentally delayed. Four years later, Gina is now a 19-year-old third-generation teenage mother, and an unemployed high school dropout. Gina fails to enroll her 5-year-old in preschool. Later, the 5-year-old child is enrolled in school as a first grader with no previous exposure to a structured educational environment. Consequently, the child lacks critical social and developmental skills necessary to do well in the first grade. The child is quickly marginalized in the resource-poor county's underperforming public school. Gina's low SES, low level of education, lack of social and material resources, and lack of family and community support put her at risk. It may not be surprising that Gina's daughter is now failing the first grade.

If history is to repeat itself, it is very likely that Gina's first grader will also grow to become a 14-year-old poor, pregnant, high school dropout, with no health insurance or access to care, and no clear prospects for employment. Hence, the cycle of poverty and disadvantage is poised to repeat itself into the fourth generation.

See Option for Policy Challenge.

WHAT ARE HEALTH INEQUITIES?

The World Health Organization (WHO) broadly defines *health inequities* as systematic and unfair differences in the health status of different population groups. Health inequities have significant social and economic costs to both individuals and societies (WHO, 2008). However, Healthy People 2020 (U.S. Department of Health and Human Services [USDHHS], 2014) defines the concept of health disparities as "a particular type of health difference that is closely linked with economic, social, or environmental disadvantage"—the assumption that the health differences are unjust or unfair more closely aligns with the WHO "health inequity" language. *Health inequalities* refer to population health summary measures that are associated with group- or individual-level attributes such as income, education, or race/ethnicity (Asada, 2010).

> Health inequities adversely affect groups of people who have systematically experienced greater social or economic obstacles to health based on their racial or ethnic group, religion, socioeconomic status, gender, age, or mental health; cognitive, sensory, or physical disability; sexual orientation or gender identity; geographic location; or other characteristics historically linked to discrimination or exclusion. (U.S. Department of Health and Human Services [USDHHS], 2013, 2014)

National and Global Health Inequities

There are no biological or genetic reasons to explain why socially disadvantaged groups, whether residing in wealthy or poor countries, experience significantly poorer health outcomes compared with the socially advantaged (Friel & Marmot, 2011). Nevertheless, those who have increased access to material and social resources—the educated, employed, socially connected—in almost every society on the globe experience better health and longer life. Furthermore, this health advantage is patterned along a social and economic gradient whereby as one's status on the social and economic hierarchy increases, health progressively improves. Gender and environment are two areas important for nurses advocating for the elimination of national and global health inequities.

Clearly, there are inequities in health for women and girls globally. The WHO has made it a priority to improve the health of girls and women as a gateway for improved overall health of families and communities, productivity of its citizens, and the disease burden for the individual and the country as a whole. As with many inequities, numerous interrelated factors play a role in a spiral of decline that limits realizing one's full potential that frequently leads to premature death and disability. According to the Global Commission on Women's Health of the WHO (1996), "A blackboard and piece of chalk can be as influential as antibiotics and contraceptives in protecting health." A U.S. Global Health Initiative (n.d.) priority (among others) for improving the health of women focuses on empowering women as care providers, caregivers, and decision makers in health systems from the local to national levels. While gender is a nonmodifiable factor, education has been identified as a powerful tool in improving the health of girls and women. See Policy on the Scene 14.1 later in this chapter, for the impact of strategies to address gender inequity.

The environment is receiving much more attention globally. What is often not included in the discussion is health inequities associated with environmental exposures. For example, in some instances there is a fivefold increase in exposure for the disadvantaged in comparison with the advantaged (WHO, 2012). These include exposures associated with secondhand smoke, housing, injuries, noise, sanitation, and water supply. These problems are not limited to developing countries but can be found in our communities (see Chapter 1, "Leading the Way in Policy").

Race, Ethnicity, and U.S. Health Inequities

Social, economic, and class inequities that are pervasive and systemic across nations are frequently articulated in the United States as racial and ethnic disparities. Race and ethnicity in the United States historically have served as a proxy (or substitute) for SES and class primarily because racial and ethnic minority groups in the United States are consistently overrepresented among the poor and disenfranchised. The United States has traditionally collected data on ethnic and racial groupings, which has facilitated tracking disparities by these categories rather than by social class (Panel on the Department of Health and Human Services [DHHS] Collection of Race and Ethnic Data, 2004). Yet, race and ethnicity are complex social phenomena in the United States that have been consistently shown to have real health impacts that are not fully explained by biological, genetic, or environmental determinants.

Take, for example, the case of Hispanic/Latino ethnicity and health outcomes in the United States. Researchers have shown that generally Whites in the United States experience improved health outcomes when compared with racial and ethnic minorities. Jones and colleagues (2008) further explored this fairly consistent finding in a study that examined discordance between self-identified race and ethnicity (What race/ethnicity do you consider yourself?), socially assigned race and ethnicity (What race/ethnicity do others classify you?), and self-rated health outcomes (Do you rate your health as poor, fair, good, or excellent?). They found that Hispanics/Latinos who were socially assigned as "White" although they classified themselves as Hispanics/Latinos experienced large and statistically significant advantages in health status relative to self-identified Hispanics/Latinos who were also socially classified as Hispanics/Latinos (Jones et al., 2008). Furthermore, the socially assigned "White" Hispanics/Latinos experienced health outcomes that were statistically the same as U.S. Whites. The author's major conclusion was that socially assigned categories of ethnicity had a significant and measurable impact on an individual's self-rating of health status.

The significant point about the findings of Jones and colleagues (2008) is that self-rated health has been consistently shown throughout the literature to be a good proxy indicator of physical health outcomes, including morbidity and mortality (DeSalvo, Bloser, Reynolds, He, & Muntner, 2006; Idler & Benyamini, 1997). This example of self-identified versus socially assigned ethnicity is also important in that it reveals one mechanism by which socially assigned race and ethnicity in the United States can impact the physical health outcomes of members of a social group.

In the United States, it is the complex meaning of race and ethnicity and the manner in which it is used to assign value and life opportunities in society that poses the greatest challenge to eliminating health inequities—particularly those health inequities that are driven by race, ethnicity, and socioeconomic/class differences among populations. However, the global context allows us to understand more fully that in the United States, health inequities are not simply about race and ethnicity. A global assessment of socioeconomic/class patterns of health inequities confirms the role of broader societal-level factors, such as human development, gender inequality, gross national product, income inequality, and health care system infrastructures, as the fundamental determinants of health inequities among populations and among nations (Azuine & Singh, 2012).

SOCIAL DETERMINANTS OF HEALTH INEQUITIES

The moral test of government is how that government treats those who are in the dawn of life—the children; those who are in the twilight of life—the elderly; those who are in the shadows of life—the sick, the [poor], and the [disabled]—Hubert H. Humphrey, 1977

There is general consensus among social and public health researchers that widespread health inequities experienced by social groups in the United States and throughout the world cannot be solely explained by individual-level determinants such as health-related behaviors. As a consequence, there have been increased efforts to better understand factors that lie outside of an individual's control such as social-, economic-, and policy-related factors that contribute to persistent and inequitable health outcomes.

SDOH can be understood as the conditions in which people are born, grow, live, work, and age—including the health system—and are shaped by the distribution of money, power, and resources at global, national, and local levels, which are themselves influenced by policy choices (WHO, 2012). Research on SDOH and its contribution to population health disparities emphasizes the complex role that social structures and economic systems play in the health of populations. The WHO confirmed in its landmark 2008 Commission on the Social Determinants of Health report (CSDH, 2008) that the SDOH are indeed mostly responsible for health inequities—the unfair and avoidable factors in health status—within and among countries. By examining the individual factors that collectively form the composite measure of SES—income and employment, education, and access to care and health insurance—we can illustrate the potential health impacts of social determinants on populations in the United States.

Income and Employment

Income and employment opportunities are critical to achieve and maintain optimal health and access health care services (Adler & Newman, 2002; Fiscella & Franks, 2000). Income and employment are directly related to morbidity and mortality outcomes in almost every health outcome. Health-related diabetes, cardiovascular disease (CVD), cancer, and infectious disease outcomes each follow a consistent income and employment gradient—as income and employment increase, mortality and morbidity decrease. Subramanian and Kawachi state, "income poverty is a risk factor for premature mortality and increased morbidity" (2004, p. 78). Take, for example, the well-established association between income and CVD and its associated risk factors such as hypertension, cholesterol, smoking, diabetes, and physical inactivity. Collins, Liu, and Davis (2012) examined the impact of education, employment, income, and stress on CVD clinical risk factors in rural and urban men over the age of 18 years. Collins and colleagues reported that lower education, unemployment, lower income, and general stress were each significantly correlated with the presence of two or more CVD risk factors. In an earlier study of CVD risk and late career involuntary unemployment, researchers found that displaced workers who lost their jobs late in their careers were more than twice as likely to have a myocardial infarction and stroke as compared to employed persons (Gallo et al., 2006). The investigators recommended that health care providers consider involuntary unemployment a significant risk factor for CVD.

One of the challenges in income and employment for U.S. citizens is the lack of intergenerational income mobility or movement into the middle class as illustrated by the Policy Challenge, *The Case of Gina*. Disadvantaged groups are not able to rise out of poverty and mitigate its attendant health risks. A recent study examined the degree to which children can rise out of poverty. Factors having a positive impact on increasing income mobility included (a) greater geographical dispersion of the middle class, (b) better-than-average schools, (c) higher proportion of two-parent households, and (d) engagement with community and religious organizations (Chetty, Hendren, Kline, & Saez, 2013).

Education

Educational attainment is closely aligned with income and employment and reliably influences future earning potential and employment opportunities. Level of education is also closely linked to population health outcomes in the United States and globally. Different groups are disadvantaged because of their lack of access to education. For example, nearly twice as many adults with disabilities do not complete high school as the general population and similarly twice as many people with disabilities live below the poverty level (Centers for Disease Control and Prevention [CDC], 2011).

Another group that experiences multiple inequities is women. There is a common expression, "when you educate a girl, you educate a family." Extensive national and international data show that women who are educated and can obtain meaningful work are more likely to delay childbirth, to increase spacing between births, and are less likely to deliver LBW infants. Hence, educated women are more likely to experience healthy maternal and childbirth outcomes (Li & Keith, 2011; Matijasevich et al., 2012; Singh & Kogan, 2007). The CDC, aware of the link between education and teenage pregnancy, launched a social media campaign targeting teenage youths to promote high school graduation as an effective intervention to reduce rates of teenage pregnancies and improve opportunities for increased income and employment opportunities.

Infant mortality rate (IMR) is considered to be an important outcome of a nation's health (CDC, 2012; Singh & van Dyck, 2010). It is an indicator that is commonly and consistently measured throughout the world, providing local and global comparative health care outcome data. In the United States, IMRs are highest among racial and ethnic minorities, the poor, and women living in the South (see Figure 14.1). As with maternal outcomes, infant mortality is also closely linked to education.

And as shown in Figure 14.2, there is a clear inverse association between educational attainment and IMR—as a woman's educational attainment increases, IMRs decrease. The IMRs among mothers with less than a high school diploma are more than twice those of mothers with a bachelor's or higher degree (NCHS, 2013a; Singh & Kogan, 2007). Researchers have shown that education status and race and ethnicity interact and result in cumulative disadvantage such that racial and ethnic minority women with low educational attainment experience the highest IMR among all women in the United States (Li & Keith, 2011; Singh & Kogan, 2007).

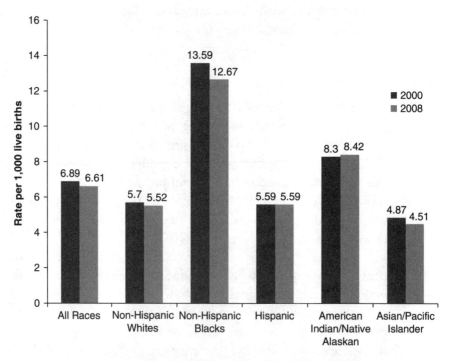

FIGURE 14.1 U.S. infant mortality rate by race and ethnicity, 2000 and 2008.
Source: National Center for Health Statistics (2013b).

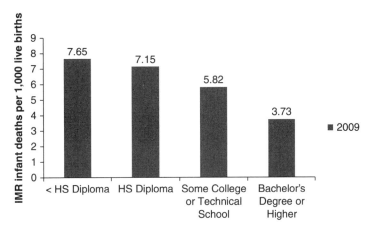

FIGURE 14.2 U.S. infant mortality rate by mother's educational attainment, 2009.
Source: National Center for Health Statistics (2013a).

Access to Care and Health Insurance

Health insurance in general, and private, employer-based insurance specifically, is the gateway to accessing health and health care services in the United States. Higher status occupations and jobs are correlated with employer-based insurance, which is associated with increased access to health providers. And yet private, employer-based insurance, while considered the preferred method of payment by health care systems and its providers, can frequently lack key coverage provisions that require additional co-pays and deductible and other out-of-pocket costs. Furthermore, private insurance plans that are not employer based have even greater out-of-pocket-related expenses. In the United States, 62% of women with private insurance that was not employer based lacked maternity coverage (Assistant Secretary for Planning and Evaluation [ASPE], 2011). Consequently, women in the United States with private health insurance average $3,400 in out-of-pocket pregnancy-related expenses (Rosenthal, 2013).

Often, persons in lower status occupations often lack employer-based health insurance and frequently do not have the resources available to pay for private insurance. As a consequence, low-status occupations such as service-oriented, trade, and labor sectors populate the ranks of the uninsured in the United States. The type of health insurance is a key indicator of SES and class status in the United States. Type of health insurance status is also strongly correlated with race, ethnicity, and SES (see Figure 14.3 for comparisons in relation to the federal poverty level (FPL)). Public insurance or Medicaid is the primary source of health insurance for racial and ethnic minorities and the poor—primarily because they are unemployed or hold part-time or full-time positions within the lower sector occupations that frequently do not offer health insurance to their employees (Mead et al., 2008). Several studies have shown that persons with public insurance or Medicaid experience decreased access to care

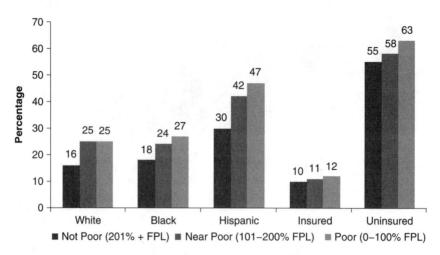

FIGURE 14.3 No regular source of health care among adults aged 18–64 by race/ethnicity and insurance coverage by poverty status, 2006–2007.
Source: National Center for Health Statistics (2009).

and poor health outcomes that are comparable to uninsured population in the United States. In essence, having public health insurance or Medicaid offers no health advantages over having no insurance coverage (LaPar et al., 2010).

Health care workers are not immune from these effects. Approximately 11% of the U.S. health care workforce lacks health insurance, with ambulatory care workers being 3.1 times more likely and residential workers 4.3 times more likely to be uninsured; service workers are 50% more likely to lack insurance than workers involved in diagnosing and treating illness (Chou, Johnson, Ward, & Blewett, 2009). Similar results were found in an earlier study with 23.8% of health aides, 14.5% of licensed practical nurses, 5% of registered nurses uninsured; and for employment setting: 20% of nursing home workers, 8.2% of medical office workers, and 8.7% of hospital workers (Case, Himmelstein, & Woolhandler, 2002). Very often, per-diem nurses and adjunct nurse faculty have several part-time positions and thus do not have health insurance. In terms of impact on health outcomes, younger health service workers have 19 times the rate of severe obesity as younger health diagnosing workers, indicating these trends are similar to those for the U.S. health workforce in general (Lee et al., 2012).

Cancer survival is another example of health insurance status and health inequities. Niu, Roche, Pawlish, and Henry (2013) found that for breast, colorectal, lung, non-Hodgkin lymphoma (NHL), bladder, and prostate cancers, uninsured and Medicaid-insured patients had significantly higher risks of death than privately insured patients. Similarly, Robbins and colleagues (2010) reported in a study of patients with rectal cancer that those with Medicaid insurance or no insurance were more than twice as likely to die in 5 years as patients with private insurance. The researchers found that the disparity in risk of death from cancer by insurance status was approximately 15.5 times larger than the disparity in risk of death from noncancer causes (Robbins et al., 2010).

Furthermore, insurance status is associated with not only inequities in cancer survival but also differences in cancer stage at diagnosis and treatment options. Shavers and Brown (2002) found that although African American cancer patients had access to employer-based and other private health insurance, the type of care experienced was of a lower quality. African Americans received less efficacious forms of treatment and were less likely to be referred to a specialist despite having adequate insurance coverage. Cancer appears to be an ideal example of the impact of health insurance status on health outcomes because it highlights the role of insurance as a gateway to health care services and perhaps exposes the cumulative effects of disadvantage over the life course—whereby cancer's prolonged time from cancer initiation to detection can be a marker of cumulative disadvantage.

Illness, therefore, can be a path to poverty. In the United States, 62% of personal bankruptcies filed in 2007 were related to medical problems (Himmelstein, Thorne, Warren, & Woolhandler, 2009). The same study found that 78% of the bankruptcy filers had health insurance when they first became ill, in contrast to 8% in 1981; 60.3% did not have Medicare or Medicaid, but instead had private insurance.

In addition to racial and ethnic minorities and the poor, other vulnerable populations such as the nation's disabled populations and low-income seniors also depend upon Medicaid as both a primary and secondary source of health insurance. Persons with disabilities and low-income seniors are continually threatened by the potential of inequities in health care access and lower quality care services. Hence, quality, coordinated, and accessible care are critical issues with all uninsured vulnerable populations as well as those dependent on Medicaid. The projected Medicaid expansion within the Patient Protection and Affordable Care Act (PPACA) is expected to have a significant impact on improving the health and well-being of our most vulnerable and underserved populations. Expanding access to care through Medicaid and ensuring that Medicaid users receive equitable health care is necessary to ensure greater equity in health coverage and health care services. Nurses are in a key position to advocate for equitable, quality care for all persons regardless of insurance status. For a detailed discussion of Medicaid-related issues and current priorities for the expansion of Medicaid via the PPACA as presented by the Kaiser Family Foundation, please visit kff.org/medicaid.

HEALTH POLICY: GLOBAL AND THE UNITED STATES

Health policy is a subcategory within social policy, and social policy is located within the larger framework of public policy. Public policies inform social policies, which in turn shape health policy, whether at the local, state, national, or global levels; they frequently reflect unspoken values, and are in turn shaped by the economic and political climates of countries. Policy efforts can be directed to act at the level of the individual within countries or can influence action on the SDOH, which operates outside the level of the individual and across nations. Yet policy making is insignificant unless policies are implemented within society.

What will it take to interrupt the cycle of social and economic disadvantage that is so closely linked with health inequities throughout the world and the United States? There is growing national and international consensus that addressing health inequities will require cross-sector policy solutions that span the continuum of health and health care and indeed the life course (WHO, Robert Wood Johnson Foundation [RWJF], MacArthur Foundation). Put simply, eliminating health inequities requires equitable access to material and social resources necessary for health. Therefore, effective U.S. and global policies to eliminate health inequities must contain, to some extent, elements of effective education, employment, and housing policies, among others.

Global Policies to Reduce and Eliminate Health Inequities

Globally, several countries have mobilized and formed regional alliances to develop frameworks that address the SDOH and health inequity with the context of a nation's political, social, and economic systems. In a call for public health advocates for public policy to address social inequities throughout the world, Annas (2013, p. 967) writes, "the health and human rights movement should be able to make a difference by focusing public health advocacy on promoting a universally accepted framework of government obligations. Evidence-based public health advocates should loudly and insistently make the case for governments to put population-based prevention programs, such as vaccination, clean water, decent sanitation, basic medical care, and a universally available safety net, as budgetary priority items—ones that should be protected and even expanded in times of economic recession and depression, when vulnerable populations are most at risk."

Many resource-poor and developing nations around the globe are working in concert with governmental and private sector entities to develop public health infrastructures to deliver necessary population health care services to meet the needs of the public (Council on Foreign Relations, 2013). Private foundations are taking a leading role as well. For example, the Clinton Foundation (n.d.) began an initiative in 2002 to address the HIV/AIDS crisis in developing nations. This has been expanded to include work on malaria, access to new vaccines, and efforts to lower infant mortality. The Bill and Melinda Gates Foundation (n.d.) is working to address hunger and poverty through investment in science and technology. In the United States, the public health infrastructure is also in need of increased funding and coordination of multiple sectors and resources to meet the public health needs of the U.S. population.

History of U.S. Federal Policy Efforts to Reduce and Eliminate Health Inequities

In the early 20th century, African American leaders and abolitionists first sounded the alarm that the United States was a nation divided—separate and unequal with wide gaps in health and life expectancy between Whites and Blacks. William Edward Burghardt (W.E.B.) Du Bois (1899) and Booker T. Washington (1914; as cited in Quinn & Thomas, 2001) lamented the lack of access to quality health care experienced by Blacks during the early emancipation period. However, the early documentation of health inequities was recorded as far back as 1840 when female Black slaves experienced disproportionately high rates of maternal and infant mortality (Dell & Whitman, 2011). During the period of slavery in the United States, it was argued that the disparate maternal and child health outcomes were biological (Dell & Whitman, 2011). W.E.B. Du Bois countered the biological hypothesis and instead argued that the maternal and child inequities were a result of a combination of social exclusion, racism, and widespread poverty (Dell & Whitman, 2011). Over a century later, researchers and scientists began again, in earnest, to extensively document the persistent unequal care and disparity in life expectancy between Whites and Blacks in the United States.

The data were compelling—widespread racial, ethnic, and socioeconomic inequities in health care access and health outcomes remain.

In 1985, with the publication of the Report of the Secretary's Task Force on Black and Minority Health (DHHS, 1986), a federal focus on racial and ethnic health inequities emerged. This landmark report sounded the alarm regarding the magnitude of disparities among Black and minority populations and led to the creation of the Office of Minority Health, a critical step for developing policies and programs dedicated to improving the health of racial and ethnic minority populations (DHHS, 1986).

Several policy-driven initiatives, reports, and legislative activities have emerged at the federal level since the Secretary's 1985 report on Black and Minority Health. In 2003, the Institute of Medicine's (IOM) report, *Unequal Treatment: Confronting Racial and Ethnic Disparities in Health Care*, further documented the seemingly entrenched and systemic inequities in health care and health outcomes. The IOM report focused specific attention on health care system factors that contributed to the racial and ethnic inequities (Institute of Medicine, 2003). The Agency for Healthcare Research and Quality (AHRQ), in a recent annual *National Healthcare Disparities Report* (2013), revealed that between 2002 and 2008, 50% of the health care access disparity measures showed no improvement and 40% of the measures

EXHIBIT 14.1	KEY REPORTS SHAPING HEALTH INEQUITY POLICY DISCUSSIONS AND DEVELOPMENT	

YEAR	KEY REPORT
1986	Secretary's Task Force on Black and Minority Health http://archive.org/details/reportofsecretar00usdepar
2000	Healthy People 2010 http://www.healthypeople.gov/2010
2002	Unequal Treatment: Confronting Racial and Ethnic Disparities in Health Care http://www.iom.edu/Reports/2002/Unequal-Treatment-Confronting-Racial-and-Ethnic-Disparities-in-Health-Care.aspx
2006	Examining the Health Disparities Research Plan of the National Institutes of Health: Unfinished Business http://iom.edu/Reports/2006/Examining-the-Health-Disparities-Research-Plan-of-the-National-Institutes-of-Health-Unfinished-Business.aspx
2010	Healthy People 2020 http://www.healthypeople.gov/2020/about/new2020.aspx
2013	CDC Health Disparities and Inequalities Report-United States, 2013 http://www.cdc.gov/mmwr/preview/ind2013_su.html#HealthDisparities2013
2013	AHRQ National Healthcare Quality and Disparities Report http://www.ahrq.gov/research/findings/nhqrdr/nhqr13/index.html

showed a widening quality gap whereby health inequities appeared to worsen (AHRQ, 2013). See Exhibit 14.1 for a listing of key reports shaping health inequity policy discussions. Therefore, despite increased interest and investments in efforts to reduce population inequities, progress toward eliminating social and economic health inequities has been slow (Fiscella, 2008; Voelker, 2008).

To date, key federal legislation has focused on numerous efforts to decrease inequities. See Exhibit 14.2 for milestones that have shaped discussions and initiatives focused on eliminating health inequities. Some diversity efforts have included increasing minority and underrepresented persons in health care and research, as well as increasing minority recruitment and retention into federally funded research studies. Minority health legislation has focused, expanding health care coverage and affordability, which results in improving health outcomes among racial and ethnic minority and vulnerable populations. Efforts have been made to improve coordination of the documentation and evaluation of minority health initiatives at the state and

EXHIBIT 14.2	SNAPSHOT OF U.S. HISTORIC POLICY MILESTONES RELATED TO HEALTH INEQUITIES, 1986–2010	
1986	Office of Minority Health (OMH)	Created a federal office to improve the health of racial and ethnic minority populations through the development of health policies/programs that help eliminate health disparities.
1993	National Institutes of Health (NIH) Revitalization Act, 1993	Included women and minorities in clinical research unless well justified, reported, and approved by the NIH. Amended in 2001 (PL 103-43).
1994	Disadvantaged Minority Health Improvement Act of 1990	Developed the capacity of health care professionals to address the cultural and linguistic barriers to health care delivery and increase access to health care for limited English-proficient people. This office was reauthorized by the PPACA in 2010 (PL 101-527).
2000	Minority Health and Health Disparities and Education Act	Created the National Center on Minority Health and Health Disparities (NCMHD) at the National Institutes of Health. This law also provided the definition for health disparities, which is used by many today (PL 106-525).
2000	Minority Health and Health Disparities Research and Education Act	Established the National Center on Minority Health and Health Disparities (NCMHD) to expand the infrastructure of Institutions committed to health disparities research and to encourage the recruitment/retention scientists in the fields of biomedical, clinical, behavioral, and health services research (PL 106-525).
2003	Healthcare Equality and Accountability Act of 2003	Aims to reduce the proven disparities in health care and access to medical service between minority communities and other Americans. Members of Congress announce legislation to improve health care for Asian Americans and Pacific Islanders. Reintroduced.
2010	Indian Health Improvement Act of 1976	Received permanent reauthorization. The Indian Health Improvement Act (IHCIA) serves as the statutory foundation of the government's responsibility to provide health care to Native Americans. This provision aims to improve the health promotion and prevention services and access to modernized care facilities, where American Indians and Alaska natives receive care. (PL 94-437)

(continued)

EXHIBIT 14.2	SNAPSHOT OF U.S. HISTORIC POLICY MILESTONES RELATED TO HEALTH INEQUITIES, 1986–2010 (*CONTINUED*)	
2010	The Patient Protection and Affordable Care Act (PPACA)	Aids in eliminating health disparities by including provisions such as expanding health care coverage, improving access to care. Reauthorized the HHS Office of Minority Health and established Offices of Minority Health within six agencies of HHS. Reauthorized the Indian Health Care Improvement Act (PL 111-148).

federal levels, as well as the development of standards for data collection on race and ethnicity.

More recently, the United States has begun to align its health equity efforts and agenda with a larger global strategy to address social and economic inequities in health through targeted actions on the SDOH. The U.S. federal government, in concert with a number of stakeholders, is increasingly integrating the social determinants into policies designed to reduce and eliminate health inequities.

Healthy People 2020

The United States' expanded focus on the social determinants is reflected in Healthy People 2020's (USDHHS, 2014) aim to achieve health equity, eliminate disparities, and improve the health of all groups. The Healthy People 2020 aim is an expansion of the Healthy People 2010 disparities objective, which aimed to "eliminate, not just reduce, health disparities" (USDHHS, 2014).

The Healthy People 2020's health equity goal includes a "health in all policies" approach. Former U.S. Surgeon General and member of the influential WHO Commission on the Social Determinants of Health, Dr. David Satcher, advocated for the inclusion of social determinants in all efforts to reduce health inequities. The "health in all policies" approach requires stakeholders to establish collaborative partnerships with a variety of sectors beyond health care and include private, industry, education, transportation, economic, and the justice system sectors (Satcher, 2010). In fact, several agencies within state and federal governments have established a framework and identified resources to move forward with a "health in all policies" approach to eliminate health inequities.

For example, the use of health impact assessments (HIAs) holds promise for reviewing and evaluating social policies designed to improve the health and well-being of populations. The HIA process has been used in European countries and is now outlined in Healthy People 2020 as well (USDHHS, 2014).

The Patient Protection and Affordable Care Act

> ... health care systems are social and cultural institutions, that are built out of the existing social structure, and carry its inequities within them. (Mackintosh, 2001, p. 175)

Health care systems, therefore, play a key role in generating and perpetuating social group health inequities. The U.S. health care system is a complex amalgamation of private, for-profit, and public entities (e.g., military and veterans) with various health service and delivery goals that may include delivering quality health care services to meet the health needs of the population, increasing access to care for disadvantaged and underserved populations, and decreasing health and health care inequities. Furthermore, the health system has to interface and balance the interests of patients and consumers, businesses and purchasers, labor, health plans, clinicians and providers, communities and states, and suppliers. Too frequently, however, the U.S. health system enables exclusionary and inequitable practices that limit access based on health and health care by insurance status. Limiting care based on payment methods or inability to pay routinely results in inequitable health care experiences.

The PPACA (2010) is one of the most comprehensive pieces of legislation enacted in the past 40 years with direct implications for eliminating health inequities. The passage of the PPACA presented new opportunities for implementing cross-cutting interventions and strategies that are driven by economic and educational policy framed in the context of the SDOH. The PPACA intentionally created a paradigm shift from a focus on disease management to health promotion. This shift not only addressed health care reform, but also created more opportunities to eliminate health inequities. Included among other provisions are specific efforts to address minority health within the federal government. Offices of Minority Health were created within six federal agencies: the AHRQ, the CDC, the Centers for Medicare and Medicaid Services, the Food and Drug Administration, Health Resources and Services Administration (HRSA), and the Substance Abuse and Mental Health Services Administration.

The National Prevention Strategy (NPS) was created by the PPACA. Under the leadership of the U.S. Surgeon General and Chair of the National Prevention, Health Promotion, and Public Health Council, the National Prevention Council will oversee the implementation of the various priorities outlined in the NPS. These activities are designed to reduce the leading causes of preventable death and major illness through tobacco-free living, prevention of drug abuse and excessive alcohol use, healthy eating, active living, injury and violence-free living, reproductive and sexual health, and mental and emotional well-being. In addition to these priorities, four strategic directions were identified (see Exhibit 14.3), and five steps to address health disparities were developed (see Exhibit 14.4). The NPS was developed by the National Prevention Council, which consists of 17 federal agencies, including housing, transportation, and labor. Thus, involvement of many sectors of the federal government is necessary in improving health and health outcomes for individuals, families, and society.

EXHIBIT 14.3	NATIONAL PREVENTION COUNCIL STRATEGIC DIRECTIONS FOR A PREVENTION-ORIENTED SOCIETY
Building Healthy and Safe Community Environments	Health begins in communities, which include homes, schools, public spaces, and work sites
Expanding Quality Preventive Services in Both Clinical and Community Settings	When people receive preventive care services, such as immunizations and cancer screenings, they experience better health and lower health care costs
Empowering People to Make Healthy Choices	Access to actionable and easy-to-understand information and resources empowers individuals and communities to make healthier choices
Eliminating Health Disparities	Eliminating disparities in achieving and maintaining health can lead to improved quality of life for individuals, families, and communities

Source: National Prevention Council (2011).

EXHIBIT 14.4	FIVE STEPS TO ADDRESS HEALTH DISPARITIES

1. **INCREASE AWARENESS** About Health Disparities
   - Blog or tweet about health disparities in your community or share information via Facebook.
   - Contact the media with stories about health disparities in your community.
   - Write a letter to the editor or an opinion article for your local newspaper.
   - Speak at health fairs, PTA and school board meetings, civic meetings, faith-based events, and other community gatherings.
   - Take the NPA Pledge to end health disparities.
   - Issue a statement from your organization in support of the NPA.

2. **BECOME A LEADER** for Addressing Health Disparities
   - Educate others about disparities and share stories about model programs with local organizations or community leaders, as well as the NPA.
   - Start a petition to get local citizens to support policy recommendations and submit the petition to the appropriate elected officials.
   - Organize a meeting of local organizations representing diverse sectors and work together to ensure health disparities are on the local and state health agenda.
   - Form coalitions with local organizations representing diverse sectors and leaders from different racial, ethnic, and other groups affected by health disparities to address common barriers and join the NPA.
   - Serve as a mentor to a young person in your family, neighborhood, or community. Educate him or her on the issues, encourage him or her to make healthy lifestyle choices, and guide him or her to resources.

(continued)

EXHIBIT 14.4 FIVE STEPS TO ADDRESS HEALTH DISPARITIES (*CONTINUED*)

3. **SUPPORT HEALTHY AND SAFE BEHAVIORS** in Your Community

- Be a role model and serve nutritious foods at work or social functions.
- Involve your employees in a group physical activity or challenge. Participate in National Health Observances—such as AIDS Awareness Days—by sponsoring local health events or encouraging loved ones and colleagues to take action to address their health.
- Host seminars in your local library, school, workplace, or other venue to discuss health disparities in your community. Topics could include reducing asthma triggers in the home, managing obesity and chronic illnesses, or indicating how to enroll in public health insurance programs.
- Join the First Lady's Let's Move! initiative to raise a healthier generation of kids, the President's Challenge, and other similar initiatives.
- Join the Consumer Product Safety Commission's Pool Safely Campaign to help prevent drowning, which occurs at higher rates among racial and ethnic minorities.

4. **IMPROVE ACCESS** to Health Care

- Partner with a local health care provider or employer to offer free health screenings in your workplace or place of worship.
- Ask local health care providers to translate health and health care information or connect them to an individual or organization who can provide translation services.
- Establish a Community Health Worker or *Promotoras de Salud* program in your community.

5. **CREATE HEALTHY NEIGHBORHOODS**

- Advocate for more sidewalks, bike lanes, and recreation facilities in your neighborhood.
- Encourage local schools, workplaces, and assisted living facilities to provide healthier lunch and snack options.
- Ask your neighborhood supermarket to provide fresh fruit and vegetables to the local food bank, ask local restaurants to provide healthy menu options, or organize a farmers' market that accepts food stamps.
- Work with your local government and organizations in your community to collect and track data about health disparities and monitor changes over time.

Note: These potential strategies build on the four goals of the NPS Stakeholder Strategy for Achieving Health Equity.
Source: National Partnership for Action to End Health Disparities (n.d.).

While there are a number of federal initiatives to reduce health inequities, opportunities to reduce health inequities also exist on the local level. The first step is becoming aware of resources within the community through governmental agencies, community, and religious organizations. Next is to take steps to ensure one's own cultural competence within one's practice arena, modeling desirable behaviors for others, and advocating for the resources so that all health care providers are culturally competent. Nurses can share with legislators, the media, and decision makers their firsthand knowledge of how low income, lower educational attainment, and limited access to care negatively impact health outcomes. Nurses can advocate for the provision of resources to underserved populations in their own communities. While we have focused much of our discussion on infant mortality and maternal outcomes, we need to recognize that the problem of health inequities cuts across all health care settings and populations. Initiatives to reduce health inequities can only be strengthened with nurse involvement and nurse advocacy.

The PPACA illustrates how the big "P" intersects with the little "p" at the community level. A key provision in the 2010 PPACA legislation is an $8.6 billion over 20-year investment in the HRSA to support the Nurse-Family Partnership (NFP) and similar programs. The NFP program links a public health nurse with a vulnerable, low-income, first-time mother to enable a healthy pregnancy, improve pregnancy outcomes, reduce rates of high-risk and subsequent pregnancies, reduce childhood injuries and abuse, and reduce developmental and cognitive delays. Public health nurses are the key providers in the evidence-based, community health program. The NFP program has already been shown to be cost-effective and touts family and societal benefits by improving the long-term health of children and families (NFP, n.d.).

At the community level, public health nurses conduct home visits as part of the NFP program. The nurses provide holistic care and empower first-time mothers and young families by providing basic childrearing information and resources. The Policy on the Scene 14.1 story about Lisa is one example of the many cases of the NFP strengthening families and improving health outcomes. This story illustrates how big "P" policies are implemented at the little "p" or local level.

POLICY ON THE SCENE 14.1: Nurse–Family Partnership: Intersection of Big "P" and Little "p"

Lisa is a 17-year-old high school junior who found out she was pregnant 1 month after the death of her mother. Her only source of support was her boyfriend, the father of her unborn child, who himself was a high-school dropout. The nurse from the NFP program supported this young couple by functioning as a role model, mentor, friend, health care provider, educator, confidant, and cheerleader. With the help of the visiting public health nurse, Lisa was able to graduate from high school and begin taking classes at a local junior college. The nurse also engaged the young father to actively participate in the childrearing of the newborn in addition to his role of providing financial support to his young family. An assessment of Lisa's baby 6 months after birth revealed a thriving infant that was meeting and exceeding all of his developmental milestones. Lisa's story is not the typical outcome for many young teenage mothers and reflects the successful engagement of nurses in the NFP program. Additional success stories and information can be found on the NFP website: http://www.nursefamilypartnership.org/first-time-moms/stories-from-moms.

OPTION FOR POLICY CHALLENGE: The Case of Gina: Potential Policy Solutions to Break the Cycle of Social and Economic Disadvantage in the United States

The story of Gina is significant in that it highlights independent and overlapping cumulative social determinants of low SES—low educational attainment, lack of income and employment opportunities, no health insurance, and no social support along with the impact of these SDOH across generations. Life course researchers and epidemiologists suggest that the seeds of health inequities are planted generations before an infant is born. There is growing longitudinal evidence to support the hypothesis that the SES and the health of the maternal grandmother is a significant predictor of a newborn's health risk (Baker, 2012). Other studies have reported that a mother's SES is the primary determinant of whether a child lives in poverty (Duncan & Magnuson, 2011). A mother's SES also shapes the life opportunities of her children and perhaps grandchildren (Duncan & Magnuson, 2011) in subsequent generations.

Evidence-based strategies that have been shown to be effective in addressing poverty-associated inequities in children's cognitive and developmental outcomes include providing high-quality educational experiences directly to preschoolers (Baker, 2012) and a combination of home visits to vulnerable mothers and children and educational interventions (Baker, 2012). For example, the CDC's *Legacy for Children* program is a federally supported, community-based strategy to improve child health and developmental outcomes among families raising children in poverty (CDC, 2013; Kaminski et al., 2013). Similarly, programs such as the Chicago Parent Program (2012) have documented the value and effectiveness of parent and teacher training programs in building positive parent–child relationships and reducing behavioral problems in high-risk, low-income children in urban communities (Breitenstein et al., 2012; Gross et al., 2003).

IMPLICATIONS FOR THE FUTURE

We have presented considerable evidence of the nature and impact of health inequities in our society. The following are trends that can have a powerful impact on health inequities: (a) increased demands for improved quality of health care; (b) greater recognition of the role of community in reducing health inequities; (c) implementation of health care reform, specifically PPACA; (d) great emphasis on health promotion and prevention of illness; (e) increased use of technology; and (f) greater recognition of environmental impacts on health. These trends will impact how nurses can and should work in the future.

We have seen an increase in demands and accountability for improving quality in the delivery of health care. With the advance of technology and the use of electronic health records, it is increasingly possible to use data-mining techniques to drill down to very specific outcomes and interaction effects. Consequently, it will be increasingly apparent that health outcomes will not improve without bringing along all sectors of society into an improved high-quality health care delivery system. In other words, without addressing unequal treatment, racism, prejudice, and stigma, care cannot rise to a high level of quality. Programs to address cultural competency may be helpful in increasing awareness and addressing unconscious biases. However, health care organizations and systems will need to focus on intentionally using these resources to decrease health inequities within their own communities.

The use of technology will increase not only by health care organizations and individual health care providers, but also by individual consumers. We have nurse researchers who are creatively exploring the use of soap opera videos and text messages to create tailored health messages (Jones et al., 2008; Kim & Glanz, 2013) as health care providers are implementing integrated electronic health records. We can only expect an acceleration of changes and innovations in this arena. As with the implementation of any technology, some segments of society and some segments of the health care delivery system will lag behind because of a lack of resources. On the other hand, technology has been used to collect epidemiological data in underdeveloped countries and there is no reason to believe that the potential of technology could not be thoughtfully and creatively applied to reducing health inequities.

Our society is increasingly interconnected. While overall population health indices have improved, we have failed to make progress in certain counties in increasing life expectancy (U.S. Burden of Disease Collaborators et al., 2013). With an ever-growing body of research indicating that where one lives matters in terms of health and how communities influence health and health behavior, greater focus will be on ensuring that our communities are healthy places to live and work. Success in improving health and reducing inequities will require engagement and commitment at a local level. Our communities will become increasingly important in addressing the underlying causes of health inequities such as access to education, a safe place for children to play, and work environments that are free of health hazards.

Recognizing that health inequities harm everyone will result in an increase in collaborative partnerships of all types: government–private, local–state, education–health, business–government, to name a few. Employers will increasingly recognize that a healthy workforce will result in a more productive workforce and that a focus on reduction of employee health benefits is counterproductive without partnering with their employees to improve their health and the health of their families (Partnership for Prevention, 2009). These partnerships will bring together key stakeholders who recognize that each sector of the community has resources and expertise that can be used together to improve health. The NFP highlighted in this chapter illustrates the potential success of these approaches.

The PPACA has specific provisions designed to provide health insurance and eliminate health inequities by creating a legislative framework that protects the right to health, representing a turning point in U.S. health care (Majette, 2012). These provisions include the expansion of community health centers, oral and behavioral health care services, school-based health centers, nurse-managed health clinics, and community health teams to support medical homes. As these provisions are implemented, we will see changes in the number of people who have insurance. As of this writing, there is variation in the beginning stages of implementation of health insurance exchanges at the state level impeding access to health insurance. Furthermore, having health insurance does not necessarily equal access to health care. And having health insurance does not address unequal treatment when there is access. As can be expected, we will have new and somewhat unknown challenges as the PPACA is implemented. Unfortunately, debate surrounding the implementation of the PPACA may result in further polarization and marginalization of those who have been traditionally disadvantaged in our society.

Increasingly, our efforts at improving the health of society will focus on the promotion of health and the prevention of disease. The PPACA and other initiatives will accelerate this process. Many health inequities have to do with the underlying conditions that have resulted in greater risk for maternal and infant mortality, physical inactivity, obesity, air pollution, violence, and tobacco and alcohol consumption (Wang et al., 2013). The emphasis on evidence-based strategies for addressing these health problems and their underlying antecedents will only grow exponentially.

The incidence of natural disasters will have an impact on communities and in particular the most vulnerable in our communities, not only on physical health, but also on mental health. These events, as we have seen in recent years, will add additional burden to any safety net provided by our communities and its health care infrastructure. Thus, any efforts to address health inequities must be coupled with efforts to address the effects of environmental impacts on health including climate change. Access to basic human needs, clean air, safe drinking water, sufficient food, and safe shelter are impacted by climate change and these are most pronounced for those living in the margins of our society.

It is important for nurses to be aware of these trends and capitalize on the potential for promoting positive health outcomes for all people. Nurses, as widely respected and trusted members of health care teams, their workplace, and their communities, are in key positions to take a leadership role in working to reduce health inequities and their root causes. As nurses, they are in an ideal position to change the health outcomes for future generations. It is more than just a consideration, it is nurses' responsibility. Implementing *The Future of Nursing* (IOM, 2011) recommendations with its call to action for nurses to further their education and to step up to the plate in assuming leadership roles can serve as a vehicle to accelerate the necessary work to reduce health inequities.

KEY CONCEPTS

1. Health is a human right.
2. Health and social inequities are a matter of economics and social justice.
3. Nurses need to be knowledgeable about health care and social policies that create inequities to be effective advocates for the populations and communities they serve.
4. SDOH are the conditions in which people are born, grow, live, work, and age—including the health system—and are shaped by the distribution of money, power, and resources at global, national, and local levels, which are themselves influenced by policy choices.
5. Social and economic determinants drive population health inequities.
6. SDOH have important implications for the U.S. and global health policy.
7. Health inequities are unfair differences in the health status of different populations that are closely linked with historical social and economic disadvantage.
8. There are no biological or genetic reasons to explain why socially disadvantaged groups experience significantly poorer health outcomes compared with the socially advantaged.
9. The type of health insurance is a key indicator of SES and class status in the United States. Type of health insurance status is also strongly correlated with race, ethnicity, and SES.
10. SES has a direct influence on the type of health insurance one is able to obtain, and health insurance has a direct impact on health outcomes.
11. Effective health policy strategies should include education, housing, labor, commerce, urban development, and environmental initiatives.

12. Public health programs like the nurse home-visiting programs for low-income and resource-poor pregnant women have been shown to improve maternal, infant, and family outcomes.

13. Partnerships that extend beyond the boundaries of nursing and health care to include education, housing, and economic sectors must be engaged to effectively address population health inequities.

SUMMARY

Political advocacy and policy engagement on behalf of people, families, and communities are essential role functions for professional nurses. In the United States, social and economic health inequities are indeed real and present threats to the nation's health. Given the urgency of health inequities, it is important that today's nurses are prepared to actively engage in all aspects of the policy-making process where discussions and decisions take place regarding the SDOH and health care. However, the health inequity problem cannot be solved solely by nursing—and despite being the largest workforce in the United States, nurses will not be able to eliminate health inequities by working in isolation. Rather, nurses will have to work to create partnerships with other nurses and with other professions that not only span the health care landscape but also extend beyond the borders of health care. Diverse cross-sector partnerships will enable nursing to acquire the necessary knowledge, skills, language, and expertise to address the social and economic determinants of health inequities.

Once those partnerships are formed, we then must continue to work to better understand the complexity of the deep-rooted drivers of inequities in health among social groups. To be effective and influential in seeking solutions to the persistent inequities in health, it is imperative that nursing secures diverse cross-sector partnerships. To address the complexity of SDOH, partnerships with government, academia, business, industry, public and private partners, community, and faith-based organizations, to name a few, are needed. In recent years, the call for a partnership approach to advance health by the nursing community has gained momentum (IOM, 2011; Shalala & Vladeck, 2011). The value of diverse perspectives in addressing health and nursing-related issues is reflected in the committee membership for the landmark report, *The Future of Nursing: Leading Change, Advancing Health* (IOM, 2011). The report committee was comprised of a cadre of professionals from areas such as business, academia, health care delivery, and health policy. Each member of this diverse coalition collectively provided unique perspectives and experiences when shaping the robust action-oriented report on the future of nursing. Shalala and Vladeck echoed a similar call to action when they emphasized the need for nursing to develop allies from a wide variety of fields in order to effectively garner the political support and capital to implement the recommendations outlined in *The Future of Nursing* report.

Next, we must maintain our commitment to develop effective policies and interventions to address and redress societal health inequities. Developing effective policy and following up with policy implementation actions through policy-directed initiatives and strategies is the way to move forward to achieve the goal of health equity for all.

LEARNING ACTIVITIES

1. Discuss two areas of social and economic health inequities in the patient population you serve and the role nursing can play in closing the gap in one of the inequities.
2. Identify the annual income and the life expectancy for men and women for the county/parish where you live. Then, identify the counties/parishes in your state that have the highest and lowest annual income and the life expectancy for men and women for the county/parish where you live. Compare these life expectancies in your state with two affluent countries such as Japan and Switzerland and then compare these results with two less affluent countries such as Algeria and Bangladesh.
3. Prepare a list of partnerships in your area that have developed programs for health inequities. Discuss nursing's roles and visibility or lack of roles and visibility in these partnerships.
4. Investigate a common health problem for a hospital, clinic, or community agency based on admissions per year or visits per year and discuss how health inequities may contribute to the prevalence of the problem. Examples might include obesity, preterm pregnancy, or a specific chronic health condition like asthma. Identify one strategy that can be used for this problem.
5. Find one article that highlights a nurse-led initiative to help the underserved with health inequities and identify the lessons learned for your specialty area.
6. Identify an upstream strategy to address health inequities related to one of the WHO Millennium Development Goals.
7. Describe the type of project that you could develop if you served as an intern with the WHO that related to the reduction of health inequities.

E-RESOURCES

- Centers for Disease Control and Prevention (CDC). *April Is Minority Health Month.* http://www.cdc.gov/minorityhealth/observances/MHMonth/Evolution.html
- Ethnic Minority Fellowship Program. http://www.emfp.org
- Frist, W. H. (2005). Overcoming disparities in US health care. *Health Affairs, 24*(2), 445–451. http://content.healthaffairs.org/content/24/2/445.full
- GovTrack.us. Tracking the Activities of the United States Congress. http://www.govtrack.us
- Healthy People 2020. http://www.healthypeople.gov/2020/default.aspx

- HHS Action Plan to Reduce Racial and Ethnic Health Disparities, 2011. http://minorityhealth.hhs.gov/npa/templates/content.aspx?lvl=1&lvlid=33&ID=285
- The Joint Commission. (2010). *Advancing effective communication, cultural competence, and patient-and family-centered care: A roadmap for hospitals.* http://www.jointcommission.org
- Kaiser Family Foundation. http://www.kff.org
- Kaiser Family Foundation. (2010). *Health care reform and communities of color.* http://kff.org/disparities-policy/issue-brief/health-reform-and-communities-of-color-implications
- Kaiser Family Foundation (KFF). (2013). *Medicaid: A primer—Key information on the nation's health coverage program for low-income people.* http://kff.org/medicaid/issue-brief/medicaid-a-primer
- Medicaid. http://www.medicaid.gov
- The Minority Health and Health Equity Archive. http://health-equity.pitt.edu/541
- National Association of County and City Health Officials Roots of Health Inequity. http://www.naccho.org/topics/justice/roots.cfm
- National Conference of State Legislatures. http://www.ncsl.org/issues-research/health/health-disparities-laws.aspx
- National Partnership for Action. National Stakeholder Strategy for Achieving Health Equity. http://minorityhealth.hhs.gov/npa/templates/content.aspx?lvl=1&lvlid=33&ID=286
- Office of Minority Health. *The National CLAS Standar*ds. http://minorityhealth.hhs.gov/templates/browse.aspx?lvl=2&lvlID=15
- Peragallo, N. (2009). The future of nursing in eliminating health disparities. http://www.iom.edu/~/media/Files/Activity%20Files/Workforce/Nursing/2009-NOV-2/Peragallo.pdf
- Substance Abuse and Mental Health Services Administration. http://www.samhsa.gov
- Tomer, J. (n.d.). Health disparities: The beginning of the end. *The Minority Nurse*. http://www.minoritynurse.com/article/health-disparities-beginning-end
- World Health Organization. Global Health Observatory (GHO). Health Equity Monitor. http://www.who.int/gho/health_equity/en/index.html
- World Health Organization. Millennium Development Goals. http://www.who.int/topics/millennium_development_goals/en
- World Health Organization. Ten Facts on Health Inequities and Their Causes .http://www.who.int/features/factfiles/health_inequities/en

ACKNOWLEDGMENTS

The views expressed are the authors' and not necessarily those of the Health Resources and Services Administration or the U.S. Department of Health and Human Services.

REFERENCES

Adler, N. E., & Newman, K. (2002). Socioeconomic disparities in health: Pathways and policies. *Health Affairs, 21*(2), 60–76.

Agency for Healthcare Research and Quality (AHRQ). (2013). *2012 National healthcare disparities report*. Rockville, MD: AHRQ Publication No. 13-0003. Retrieved from http://www.ahrq.gov/research/findings/nhqrdr/index.html

Annas, G. J. (2013). Health and human rights in the continuing global economic crisis. *American Journal of Public Health, 103*(6), 967.

Asada, Y. (2010). A summary measure of health inequality for a pay-for-population health performance system. *Preventing of Chronic Diseases, 7*(4), A72.

Assistant Secretary for Planning and Evaluation (ASPE). (2011, December 16). Essential health benefits: Individual market coverage. *ASPE Issue Brief*. Retrieved from http://aspe.hhs.gov/health/reports/2011/IndividualMarket/ib.shtml

Azuine R. E., & Singh, G. K. (2012). Addressing global health, development, and social inequalities through research and policy analyses. *International Journal of MCH and AIDS, 1*(1), 1–5.

Baker, C. (2012, October 22). Fighting poverty with education; hope for breaking the cycle of multi-generational poverty. *Deseret News*. Salt Lake City: Utah. Retrieved from http://www.deseretnews.com/article/765613268/Fighting-poverty-with-education-hope-for-breaking-the-cycle-of-multi-generational-poverty.html?pg=all

Bill and Melinda Gates Foundation. (n.d.). *What we do*. Retrieved from http://www.gatesfoundation.org/what-we-do

Breitenstein, S. M., Gross, D., Fogg, L., Ridge, A., Garvey, C., Julion, W., & Tucker, S. (2012). The Chicago Parent Program: Comparing 1-year outcomes for African American and Latino parents of young children. *Research in Nursing and Health, 35*(5), 475–489.

Case, B. G., Himmelstein, D. U., & Woolhandler, S. (2002). No care for the caregivers: Declining health insurance coverage for health care personnel and their children, 1988–1998. *American Journal of Public Health, 92*(3), 404–408.

Centers for Disease Control and Prevention (CDC). (2011, January 14). CDC health disparities and inequalities report (CHDIR) United States, 2011. *Morbidity and Mortality Weekly, 60*, s1-s116. Retrieved from http://www.cdc.gov/mmwr/preview/ind2011-su.html

Centers for Disease Control and Prevention (CDC). (2012). *Infant mortality*. Retrieved from http://www.cdc.gov/reproductivehealth/MaternalInfantHealth/InfantMortality.htm

Centers for Disease Control and Prevention (CDC). (2013). *Legacy for children*. Retrieved from http://www.cdc.gov/ncbddd/childdevelopment/legacy.html

Chetty, R., Hendren, N., Kline, P., & Saez, E. (2013). *The economic impacts of tax expenditures: Evidence from spatial variation across the US*. Retrieved from http://obs.rc.fas.harvard.edu/chetty/tax_expenditure_soi_whitepaper.pdf

Chou, C. F., Johnson, P. J., Ward, A., & Blewett, L. A. (2009). Health care coverage and the health care industry. *American Journal of Public Health, 99*(12), 2282–2288.

Clinton Foundation. (n.d.). *Clinton health access initiative*. Retrieved from http://www.clintonfoundation.org/main/our-work/by-initiative/clinton-health-access-initiative/about.html

Collins, R. K., Liu, J., & Davis, S. K. (2012). Social determinants of cardiovascular disease risk factor presence among rural and urban Black and White men. *Journal of Men's Health, 9*(2), 120–126.

Commission on the Social Determinants of Health (CSDH). (2008). *Closing the gap in a generation: Health equity through social determinants of health. Final Report of the Commission on Social Determinants of Health.* Geneva: World Health Organization. Retrieved from http://www.who.int/social_determinants/thecommission/finalreport/en/index.html

Council on Foreign Relations. (2013). *The Global Health Regime.* Retrieved from http://www.cfr.org/world/global-health-regime/p22763

Dell, J. L., & Whitman, S. (2011). A history of the movement to address health disparities. In S. Whitman, A. M. Shah, & M. R. Benjamins (Eds.), *Urban health: Combating disparities with local data* (pp. 8–30). New York, NY: Oxford University Press.

Department of Health and Human Services (DHHS). (1986). *Report of the secretary's task force report on black and minority health volume I: Executive summary.* Washington, DC: Government Printing Office. Retrieved from http://minorityhealth.hhs.gov/assets/pdf/checked/1/ANDERSON.pdf

DeSalvo, K. B., Bloser, N., Reynolds, K., He, J., & Muntner P. (2006). Mortality prediction with a single general self-rated health question. A meta-analysis. *Journal of General Internal Medicine, 21*(3), 267–275.

Dubois, W. E. B. (1899). *The Philadelphia Negro: A social study.* Philadelphia, PA: University of Pennsylvania Press.

Duncan, G. J., & Magnuson, K. (2011). The long reach of early childhood poverty. *Pathways of the Sanford Center on Poverty and Inequality, Winter,* 22–27.

Fiscella, K. (2008). Achieving the Healthy People 2010 goal of elimination of health disparities: What will it take? In L. Helmchen, R. Kaester, & A. Lo Sasso. (Eds.), *Beyond public health insurance: Public policy to improve health in advances in health economics and health services research* (p. 19). Bringley: Emerald.

Fiscella, K., & Franks, P. (2000). Individual income, income inequality, health, and mortality: What are the relationships? *Health Services Research, 35,* 307–318.

Friel, S., & Marmot M. G. (2011). Action on the social determinants of health and health inequities goes global. *Annual Review Public Health, 32,* 225–236.

Gallo, W. T., Teng, H. M., Falba, T. A., Kasl, S. V., Krumholz, H. M., & Bradley, E. H. (2006). The impact of late career job loss on myocardial infarction and stroke: A 10-year follow up using the health and retirement survey. *Occupational Environmental Medicine, 10,* 683–687.

Gross, D., Fogg, L., Webster-Stratton, C., Garvey, C., Julion, W., & Grady, J. (2003). Parent training of toddlers in day care in low income urban communities. *Journal of Consulting and Clinical Psychology, 71*(2), 261–278.

Healthy People 2010. *Leading indicators at a glance.* Retrieved from http://www.cdc.gov/nchs/healthy_people/hp2010/hp2010_indicators.htm

Himmelstein, D. U., Thorne, D., Warren, E., & Woolhandler, S. (2009). Medical bankruptcy in the United States, 2007: Results of a national study. *American Journal of Medicine, 122*(8), 741–746.

Idler, E. L., & Benyamini, Y. (1997). Self-rated health and mortality: A review of twenty-seven community studies. *Journal of Health and Social Behavior, 38*(1), 21–37.

Institute of Medicine. (2003). *Unequal treatment: Confronting racial and ethnic disparities in health.* Washington, DC: National Academies Press.

Institute of Medicine (IOM). (2011). *The future of nursing: Leading change, advancing health.* Washington, DC: National Academies Press.

Jones, C. P., Truman, B. I., Elam-Evans, L. D., Jones, C. A., Jones, C. Y., Jules, R., … Perry, G. S. (2008). Using socially assigned race to probe white advantages in health status. *Ethnicity and Disease, 18*(4), 496–504.

Kaminski, J. W., Perou, R., Visser, S. N., Scott, K. G., Beckwith, L., Howard, J., ... Danielson, M. L. (2013). Behavioral and socioemotional outcomes through age 5 years of the legacy for children public health approach to improving developmental outcomes among children born into poverty. *American Journal of Public Health, 103*(6), 1058–1066.

Kim, B. H., & Glanz, K. (2013). Text messaging to motivate walking in older African Americans: A randomized controlled trial. *American Journal of Preventive Medicine, 44*(1), 71–75.

LaPar, D. J., Damien, J., Bhamidipati, C. M., Mery, C. M., Stukenborg, G. J., Jones, D. R., ... Ailawadi, G. (2010). Primary payer status affects mortality for major surgical operations. *Annals of Surgery, 252*(3), 544–551.

Lee, D. J., Fleming, L. E., LeBlanc, W., Arheart, K. L., Ferraro, K. F., Pitt-Catsouphes, M., ... Kachan, D. (2012). Health status and risk indicator trends of the aging U.S. healthcare workforce. *Journal of Occupational and Environmental Medicine, 54*(4), 497–503.

Li, Q., & Keith, L. G. (2011). The differential association between education and infant mortality by nativity status of Chinese American mothers: A life-course perspective. *American Journal of Public Health, 101*(5), 899–908.

Mackintosh, M. (2001). Do health care systems contribute to inequalities? In D. Leon & G. Walt (Eds.), *Poverty, inequality and health* (pp. 175–193). London: Oxford University Press.

Majette, G. R. (2012). Global health law norms and the PPACA framework to eliminate health disparities. *Howard Law Journal, 55*(3), 887–936.

Matijasevich, A., Victora, C. G., Lawlor, D. A., Golding, J., Menezes, A. M., Araújo, C. L., ... Smith, G. D. (2012). Association of socioeconomic position with maternal pregnancy and infant health outcomes in birth cohort studies from Brazil and the UK. *Journal of Epidemiology and Community Health, 66*(2), 127–135.

Mead, H., Cartwright-Smith, L., Jones, K., Ramos, C., Woods, K., & Siegel, B. (2008). Racial and ethnic disparities in U.S. health care: A chartbook. *The Commonwealth Fund.* Retrieved from http://www.commonwealthfund.org/usr_doc/Mead_racialethnicdisparities_chartbook_1111.pdf

National Center for Health Statistics. (2009). *No regular source of care among adults 18–64 by race/ethnicity and insurance coverage by poverty status, 2006–2007.* Retrieved from http://www.cdc.gov/nchs/health_policy/adults_no_source_health_care.htm

National Center for Health Statistics. (2013a). *US infant mortality rate by mother's educational attainment, 2009.* Retrieved from http://www.cdc.gov/nchs/data/nvsr/nvsr61/nvsr61_08.pdf

National Center for Health Statistics. (2013b). *US infant mortality rate by race/ethnicity 2000–2008.* Retrieved from http://www.cdc.gov/nchs/data/nvsr/nvsr61/nvsr61_08.pdf

National Partnership for Action to End Health Disparities. (n.d.). *Toolkit for community action.* U.S. Department of Health and Human Services, Office of Minority Health. Retrieved from http://minorityhealth.hhs.gov/npa/files/Plans/Toolkit/NPA_Toolkit.pdf

National Prevention Council. (2011). *National Prevention Strategy.* Washington, DC: U.S. Department of Health and Human Services, Office of the Surgeon General. Retrieved from http://www.surgeongeneral.gov/initiatives/prevention/strategy/report.html

Niu, X., Roche, L. M., Pawlish, K. S., & Henry, K. A. (2013). Cancer survival disparities by health insurance status. *Cancer Medicine, 2*(3), 403–411.

Nurse-Family Partnership (NFP). (n.d.). Pregnancy assistance for first-time moms. Retrieved from http://www.nursefamilypartnership.org/first-time-moms

Panel on DHHS Collection of Race and Ethnic Data, Ver Ploeg, M., Perrin, E. (Eds.), & National Research Council. (2004). *Eliminating health disparities: Measurement and data needs.* Washington, DC: National Academies Press.

Partnership for Prevention. (2009). *Healthy workforce 2010 and beyond.* Retrieved from http://www.prevent.org/Publications-and-Resources.aspx

Patient Protection and Affordable Care Act of 2010, Pub. Law No. 111-148.

Quinn, S. C., & Thomas, S. B. (2001). The National Negro Health Week 1915–1951: A descriptive account. *Minority Health Today, 2*(3), 44–49. Retrieved from http://health-equity.pitt.edu/541/

Robbins, A. S., Chen, A. Y., Stewart, A. K., Staley, C. A., Virgo, K. S., & Ward, E. M. (2010). Insurance status and survival disparities among nonelderly rectal cancer patients in the National Cancer Data Base. *Cancer, 116*(17), 4178–4186.

Rosenthal, E. (2013, June 30). American way of birth: Costliest in the world. *New York Times.* Retrieved from http://www.nytimes.com/2013/07/01/health/american-way-of-birth-costliest-in-the-world.html?pagewanted=all&_r=0

Satcher, D (2010). Include a social determinants of health approach to reduce health inequalities. *Public Health Reports, 125*(Suppl 4), 6–7.

Shalala, D., & Vladeck, B. (2011). Leading change: How nurses can attract political support for the IOM Report on the future of nursing. *Nurse Leader, 9*(6), 38–39, 45.

Shavers, V. L., & Brown, M. (2002). Racial and ethnic disparities in the receipt of cancer treatment. *Journal of the National Cancer Institute, 94*(5), 334–357.

Singh, G. K., & Kogan, M. D. (2007). Persistent socioeconomic disparities in infant, neonatal, and postneonatal mortality rates in the United States, 1969–2001. *Pediatrics, 119*(4), e929–e939.

Singh, G. K., & van Dyck, P. C. (2010). *Infant mortality in the United States, 1935–2007. Over seven decades of progress and disparities.* Rockville, MD: U.S. Department of Health and Human Services, Health Resources and Services Administration, Maternal and Child Health Bureau.

Subramanian, S. V., & Kawachi I. (2004). Income inequality and health: What have we learned so far? *Epidemiological Reviews, 26*(1), 78–91.

U.S. Burden of Disease Collaborators, Murray, C. J. L., Abraham, J., Ali, M. K., Alvarado, M., Atkinson, B. S., … Lopez, A. D. (2013). The state of US health, 1990–2010. Burden of diseases, injuries, and risk factors. *JAMA, 310*(6), 591–608.

U.S. Department of Health and Human Services (USDHHS). (2014). *Healthy People 2020. Disparities.* Retrieved from http://www.healthypeople.gov/2020/about/disparitiesAbout.aspx

U.S. Department of Health and Human Services, Health Resources and Services Administration, National Center of Health Workforce Analysis. (2013). *The US health workforce chartbook. Part I: Clinicians.* Retrieved from http://bhpr.hrsa.gov/healthworkforce/supplydemand/usworkforce/chartbook/chartbookpart1.pdf

U.S. Global Health Initiative. (n.d.). *Global Health Initiative supplemental guidance on women, girls, and gender equality principle.* Retrieved from http://www.ghi.gov/principles/docs/wgge_principle_paper.pdf

Voelker, R. (2008). Decades of work to reduce disparities in health care produce limited success. *JAMA, 299*(12), 1411–1413.

Wang, H., Schumacher, A. E., Levitz, C. E., Mokdad, A. H., & Murray, C. J. L. (2013). Left behind: Widening disparities for males and females in US county life expectancy, 1985–2010. *Population Health Metrics, 11*, 8.

World Health Organization. (2012). *Environmental health inequalities in Europe.* Assessment report. Geneva: WHO. Retrieved from http://www.euro.who.int/en/what-we-publish/abstracts/environmental-health-inequalities-in-europe.-assessment-report

World Health Organization. (1996, April 26). *Global Commission on Women's Health to promote health security.* [Press release]. Retrieved from http://scienceblog.com/community/older/archives/L/1996/A/un960828.html

World Health Organization, Commission on Social Determinants of Health. (2008). *Closing the gap in a generation: Health equity through action on the social determinants of health.* Retrieved from http://www.who.int/social_determinants/thecommission/finalreport/en

FIFTEEN

Taking Actions, Expanding Horizons

Rebecca M. Patton
Margarete L. Zalon
Ruth Ludwick

People often say, with pride, "I'm not interested in politics." They might as well say, "I'm not interested in my standard of living, my health, my job, my rights, my future or any future."...
If we mean to keep any control over our world and lives, we must be interested in politics.—Martha Gelhorn, journalist (1984)

OBJECTIVES

1. Identify the critical role of all nurses in advancing policy for quality, safety, and access to health care, in addition to advancing the profession.
2. Identify leadership strategies to facilitate nursing's policy influence.
3. Compare and contrast the development of policy roles for nurses in different settings and different points in one's career in relation to one's personal goals.
4. Explore how to leverage your role in nursing and health care organizations for political activism.

Advancing nursing and health requires that nurses take action and expand their horizons beyond the daily activities of practice by becoming involved in policy. When each nurse takes one step and joins with other nurses, we can have more than 3 million nurses taking steps together to strengthen nursing, improve health, and fulfill our contract with society to advocate for the "... care of individuals, families, groups, communities, and populations" (American Nurses Association [ANA], 2010, p. 5). The policy involvement of all nurses provides the best strategy for creating the preferred future of how nursing evolves and health is advanced. Numerous strides have been made in policy when nurses are involved, but in reality, to keep pace with the numerous changes in health care, it is vital that all nurses across all settings are involved.

Nurses with managerial authority, nurse educators, and nurse researchers have a tremendous opportunity and responsibility to influence future generation of nurses. They must not only be involved individually, but they also have a broader obligation as leaders to help put in place the structural and process components that encourage and support nurses in a variety of direct care roles to become involved in policy making. Thought leaders in nursing in the United States and beyond have called for nurses' more active involvement in policy (Benton, 2012; Institute of Medicine [IOM], 2011; Kunavikitul, 2014). Widespread involvement will require a paradigm shift whereby nurses' active involvement in policy becomes the established norm; in the ideal situation, large numbers of nurses are active in policy, tackling the issues and solving problems at work, in the community, nationally, and globally. Becoming a policy advocate, to echo the words of Dwight Eisenhower, our 34th president, ought to be the part-time profession of every nurse who would protect and advance the health of his or her patients. And hopefully, for increased numbers of nurses, policy work will be a full-time commitment. The purpose of this chapter is to more closely examine the creation of a paradigm shift to nurses' greater involvement in policy, creating the structures and processes to facilitate such involvement. We hope to engender a commitment from you, our readers, about the active roles that should be taken in policy now and in the future as your career evolves. The following Policy Challenge illustrates how the military emphasizes, fosters, and expects leadership behaviors in order to advance health care.

POLICY CHALLENGE: Getting Started in Influencing Policy
Bonnie Mowinski Jennings, PhD, RN, FAAN, Colonel
U.S. Army (Retired) Professor, Nell Hodgson Woodruff School of Nursing
Emory University, Atlanta, GA

Even as a nursing student, I knew when I graduated I wanted to do something different to start my career. I ultimately decided to join the Army Nurse Corps (ANC). A real incentive, given that I was paying for my own education, was they would commission me as a second lieutenant—right then—meaning I would make second lieutenant pay in the last semester of my senior year. It was a pittance by today's standards, yet it was an opportunity that snagged me, along with the chance to serve my country and see the world!

When I joined the ANC, policies were being examined that would require the bachelor of science in nursing (BSN) as the required education for entering practice for officers. There was pushback and negotiation, yet ultimately, in 1976, the BSN was mandated as the educational standard for entering the ANC. As such, my military career was largely spent in a setting where BSN-prepared nurses were in the majority, creating a practice setting that held staff to a high professional standard. Collaboration and teamwork were not just words, but a cultural norm and ethic. I recall rounding and participating in what now would be referred to as interprofessional meetings. Perhaps that cultural stance is fueled by the continuing recognition of how advanced education yields stronger, more dynamic patient-centered care teams. Today, for instance, the BSN continues as the entry standard with 35% of ANCs holding master's degrees.

Little did I know that along with funding to pursue my doctorate, the ANC would afford me a wealth of opportunities, all derived from the philosophy that a career in the ANC is built upon a series of progressive assignments designed to develop individuals as leaders and assume positions of increased responsibility. In my case, along with becoming an excellent clinician, I also had opportunities to develop skill as an educator, researcher, administrator, health policy analyst, and health care executive. My career was filled with formal education in leadership as well as daily opportunities to practice leadership and hone my leadership skills. There is an explicit career development plan that is followed to help each military nurse acquire the knowledge, skills, and attributes of a leader. Military nursing is inherently about leadership; it stems from a system in which there is a basic expectation for you to step up to the plate—and lead—whether that is at the bedside or in the boardroom. In my case, that leadership also took me into the halls of the Pentagon.

Early in my career, as a staff nurse, I had an opportunity to lead a rather massive policy change for the military system, although I didn't realize the significance of the situation at the time. When I entered the ANC, married female officers could not get family member identification (ID) cards for their husbands, yet married male officers could get family member ID cards for their wives. The military ID is your passport into the military grocery store, department store, and health care. I thought this was quite unfair and I raised my voice to register concern. Most people were truly not aware of these gender-based discrepancies. In any case, I filed an official complaint with the help of an army lawyer. I was quite surprised when my plea was not supported. I was even more surprised some years later when I learned my complaint was pooled with others in a class action suit that changed policy: It was a turning point in the military system—married female officers could get ID cards for their husbands. Taking action did not yield immediate change, yet ultimately change happened. This experience taught me how essential it is to make your voice heard—a key feature of leadership and policy.

(continued)

> I also had opportunities to develop new care delivery processes, putting in place the second Ambulatory Surgery Center (ASC) in the army. I used a systems approach for designing and implementing the ASC. This ties into collaboration and teamwork and reflects leadership as well. All stakeholders were engaged in conversations about how best to make the ASC work—from anesthesia providers, to surgeons, pharmacists, food service, housekeeping, and nurses from the operating room and postanesthesia care unit to leaders in the larger military community who could help me communicate with the beneficiaries who would be using the service. Today, the ASC is a common way of delivering care. At that time, it was a very novel approach to care delivery that was just taking hold.
> *See Option for Policy Challenge.*

As illustrated in the Policy Challenge, increasing the engagement of nurses in policy is really about strengthening the leadership competencies of nurses within the context of health policy advocacy.

NURSES' CRITICAL ROLE IN ADVANCING POLICY

There are far too many examples at the little "p" and big "P" levels where nurses have not had the interest or clout to prevent the implementation of policies with negative or unintended consequences. Some policies have long-standing implications for how nursing is practiced and have influenced the direction of the profession. Nurses have a critical role in advancing policy that directly impacts the profession and also for achieving the Institute for Health Care Improvement's (IHI, n.d.) triple aim of quality and safety, improved health, and reduced cost.

Advancing Policy for the Profession

Every day nurses face issues related to how to practice. Some are more obvious than others. Regardless, nurses need to recognize the need to be proactive; ignoring or not addressing issues can have significant policy implications. Title protection and practice barriers are two areas related to practice that bear active monitoring and ongoing advocacy. Sunset laws described in Chapter 3, "Navigating the Political System," are another example. A final example described in the following section is the nurses' work environment.

Title Protection

It is easy to take the title "nurse" for granted. Most nurses are not aware that the title "nurse" is still not protected in 11 states, meaning that anyone can call himself or herself a nurse (ANA, 2013) (see Figure 15.1). This is a common occurrence in health care provider offices where medical assistants might be called nurses or refer to themselves as a "doctor's nurse." Some will perform

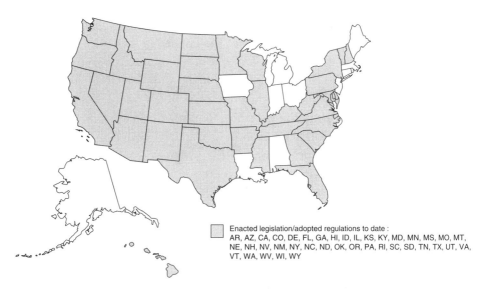

Enacted legislation/adopted regulations to date :
AR, AZ, CA, CO, DE, FL, GA, HI, ID, IL, KS, KY, MD, MN, MS, MO, MT,
NE, NH, NV, NM, NY, NC, ND, OK, OR, PA, RI, SC, SD, TN, TX, UT, VA,
VT, WA, WV, WI, WY

FIGURE 15.1 States with title "nurse" protection.
Reprinted with permission from the ANA (2013).

activities outside their scope of practice. An example of a little "p" activity for nurses is to raise questions as the recipients of care in these settings. When people who are not nurses call themselves nurses, it minimally creates confusion in the eyes of the public. It may in some cases be unethical, deceitful, and harmful. Having title protection is an important step, but it does not provide immunity from challenges to nursing practice that may take the form of other professionals using the definition of nursing or a portion of it as they seek recognition for their disciplines, or limitations to nurses carrying out long-standing responsibilities such as pressure ulcer assessment. Each of us has a duty to identify ourselves as a registered nurse or as an advanced practice nurse in all of our interactions with the public and other health care providers. Likewise, advanced practice registered nurses (APRNs) may not be familiar with the details of language regarding their titling and practice. The term *mid-level provider* does not reflect the roles and responsibilities of APRNs and continues a focus on hierarchy instead of interprofessional collaboration. Do we call anyone high-level or low-level providers? Using this term and allowing the continued use of this term create confusion for the public, insurers, and other key stakeholders.

Practice Barriers

Full practice authority for APRNs is not a reality across the United States. As with the practice of nursing, each state or territory has its own laws, rules, and regulations governing advanced practice, in addition to federal laws, rules, and regulations that also impact advanced practice. Careful attention needs to be paid in each jurisdiction so that APRNs can practice in accordance with their education and expertise. The challenge is that each different scenario has a different set of stakeholders, a different history and perspective that needs to be addressed, keeping in mind the unique circumstances in that jurisdiction, as we are reminded by Tip O'Neill Jr.'s quote that all politics is local. For example, recently the Veterans Health Administration (VHA) has proposed a system-wide policy revision in its nursing handbook that designates all APRNs as independent practitioners. The proposed revision will allow APRNs (nurse practitioners [NPs], certified registered nurse anesthetists, clinical nurse specialists, and certified nurse midwives [CNMs]) to work independently regardless of the location of the VA facility, using the federal supremacy of the constitution as the basis for its decision.

While the initiatives of the military and the VHA pave the way for nurses and APRNs, the complexity of how each advanced practice situation plays out at the state level might be different. Not all advanced practice nurses are solely regulated by the nurse board within each state. Some states have joint regulations, some have joint regulations for the administration of medications, and, in some instances, one type of advanced practice nurse is regulated by the board of nursing and another is regulated by the board of medicine. Uniformly changing regulatory oversight of the nurse board is not without its challenges. For example, in Pennsylvania, CNMs are regulated by the medical board and may delegate since delegation regulations are in place under the medical practice act. However, no delegation regulations are in place for nurses in Pennsylvania; thus, moving regulatory authority to the nurse board would restrict the ability of CNMs to delegate, specifically their delegation to lay midwives. Thus, it is important to keep a watchful eye on proposed regulations, and also be at the table when initial drafts of proposed regulations are requested. Legislative and regulatory changes could, at the same time, enhance one area of practice, but inadvertently create a stumbling block that impedes practice or access to care elsewhere.

Work Environment

Title recognition and barriers to practice are just two issues faced by the profession. Beyond legislative and regulatory details governing these issues, policies are also important to nurses delivering high quality and safe care. In order for nurses to deliver high quality and safe care, policies need to be in place allowing for the realization of that potential. Published research has indicated that the work environment of nurses is related to the quality of care (Aiken et al., 2012; Djukic, Kovner, Brewer, Fatehi, & Cline, 2013). If policies are not in place within organizations to achieve a positive work environment, then remedies to address the work environment issue have been sought through policy implementation in the larger arena at the state or national level. Staffing legislation is an example where a number of different proposals have been put forth reflecting the beliefs and values of different constituencies within nursing. Regardless of the desirability and/or evidence supporting the proposed methodology, staffing legislation is a policy solution that would improve the quality of nurses' work environment and has demonstrated impact on patient care. No matter what arena, be it improving quality through nurse staffing within an organization or improving quality through staffing standards accomplished with legislation or regulation, it requires nurses to be engaged in the policy process.

While many nurses and APRNs work within larger health care systems, many nurses also work in small-scale, and many times underresourced, settings. Establishing structures that foster policy advocacy in these environments may be more challenging. Therefore, strengthening the foundation for advocacy in educational settings becomes more critical because we are counting on nurses as individuals to engage in policy activism with limited resources and perhaps against the prevailing tide within a health care facility. For example, ASCs and endoscopy centers typically have less regulatory oversight. Yet, each of these settings employs nurses who are witness to the implementation of its policies and procedures. One of the worst infection control lapses occurred at the Nevada endoscopy clinics owned by a single gastroenterologist. This lapse created a public health crisis of enormous proportions, where up to 63,000 patients might have been exposed to hepatitis C. One nurse who was employed at the clinic for only 3 days reported her concerns to a regulatory body (Leary & Diers, 2013). In this environment rife with breakdowns in practice standards, nurses were intimidated with regard to their advocacy responsibility to address these concerns.

With care expansion in primary settings, attention is now being drawn to factors critical to establishing a positive work environment in these settings. Not surprisingly, these include NP–physician relations, independent practice and autonomy, professional visibility, organizational support, and NP–administrative relations (Poghosyan, Nannini, Stone, & Smaldone, 2013). Creating a work environment that ensures nurses have the opportunity to take an active role in controlling their practice and positively influences the critical factors in that work environment will entail policy knowledge and work.

The challenge as a profession is helping nurses to understand the policy implications of day-to-day practice and how organizational, legislative, and regulatory initiatives can in turn impact policy in everyday practice. The issues discussed earlier will need continued activism and equally important is watching for new issues that are on the horizon as the nature of health care and the myriad of providers evolve.

Advancing Policy for Quality, Safety, and Access to Health Care

Improving quality, safety, and access to health care requires much more of nurses than "just" being excellent direct care nurses; it requires being the thought leaders and drivers of change and policy in health care organizations in order to keep pace with an ever-changing complex health care environment. Chapter 13,

"Evaluating Policy Structures, Processes, and Outcomes," discussed in depth how nurse-sensitive quality indicators are directly linked to the work of nurses and discussed the importance of economic evaluation. Showing not only improved quality but also economic value helps make the case much stronger when nurses seek policy changes and want to enforce policy. Hospital-acquired infections (HAIs) are one nurse-sensitive indicator that can be used to illustrate this interplay between cost, quality, and the need for policy, as the annual costs linked to HAIs are projected as high as $45 billion, and thus have a major impact on the rising costs of health care (Scott, 2009). When studying nosocomial infections and cost-effectiveness, researchers found that many intensive care units did not have good staff adherence to infection prevention policies. Percent adherence rates for policies related to central line-associated bloodstream infections (CLABSI), ventilator-associated pneumonia (VAP), and catheter-associated urinary tract infections (CAUTI) varied widely within each infection category, across infection categories, and in types of intensive care units. The lowest adherence to policy was for CAUTI, which ranged from "6% to 27%" (Stone et al., 2014, p. 96). This statistic is not only low, but it also illustrates wide variation in adherence within infection-specific guidelines.

Safety is another area where nurses' policy input is critical. Nurses are at the sharp edge of safety, frequently the first to make note of safety issues and often first to take action in preventing harm to a patient. Safety is intimately intertwined with quality and the work environment as noted earlier.

However, to achieve a safety culture, nurses are needed not only to advocate on behalf of their individual patients, but also to feel safe in speaking up within their organizations and beyond. Being silent in an organization has been recognized as a serious threat to patient safety (Henriksen & Dayton, 2006). Being a leader requires being an advocate. Nurses can be the leaders and drivers of change in advancing policy related to safety initiatives. While there is much value in implementing safety programs, nurses need to be at policy tables setting the agenda for efforts to improve safety. An example of a safety practice being adopted in some hospitals where nurse advocacy is needed is the adoption of red rules, that is, rules that cannot be broken. If these rules are broken, the outcome may be serious patient harm. The practice of red rules was adopted from highly reliable industries (e.g., airlines), but they should not be confused with organizational policies like infection control. A common red rule across a hospital might be patient verification technique or time-out before an invasive procedure. An important role for nursing in the development of red rules is the guidance they can provide in making sure that the rules are not used to improve adherence to policies already in place or to replace policies that are not working; another is working to ensure the approach to evaluating a red rule is applied uniformly across departments.

Nurses have a long history of being at the forefront of promoting access to care with leaders like Lillian Wald and Myra Breckenridge. Nurses in public health and nurses providing care in community-based clinics engage in strategies to promote access on a daily basis. Issues related to access to care are played out in nurse-managed centers, and the walk-in clinics for health care being established across the country in drugstores and supermarkets. These market forces bring in additional stakeholders who have an interest in removing practice barriers for NPs. Nurses must be politically astute to capitalize on these opportunities in the interest of promoting access to care (see Chapter 14, "Eliminating Health Inequities Through Policy, Nationally and Globally").

The ANA has supported the development of nurse-delivered primary care in retail-based health clinics and has voiced the opinion that these clinics provide a creative access point for patients. The ANA (2009) supports the American Academy of Nurse Practitioners' (2007) position statement, *Standards for Nurse Practitioner Practice in Retail Clinics* (www.aanp.org/images/documents/publications/StdsforNPRetail-BasedClinics.pdf). No differences in quality or return visits to primary care providers have been demonstrated in care provided in retail clinics compared with other settings (Mehotra et al., 2009; Rohrer, Angstman, Garrison, Pecina, & Maxson, 2013). Despite this, efforts are being taken by organized groups to sway public opinion not to use these clinics (Committee on Practice, 2014). These actions require the vigilance of nurses' groups as well as nurses' advocacy efforts to counter these barriers to practice that impinge upon access to care.

While we typically think of the removal of barriers to practice in the context of advanced practice nurses, in order to achieve access to care, nurses at all levels are needed to practice at the full scope of their education and abilities. More will be expected of nurses, including the ability to demonstrate health policy competencies set forth by the American Association of Colleges of Nursing (AACN) in their Essentials Series for nursing education at the baccalaureate, master's, and practice doctorate levels (AACN, 2006, 2008, 2011; www.aacn.nche.edu/education-resources/essential-series). The goal or the final end point or outcome of access to care is better health. While there are great strides being made in access to care, there are parts of the country where access to care is being increasingly limited, where the death rates and other indicators of population health are worse than the rest of the country and even worse than in previous years. Many of these same regions are those with significant practice barriers for APRNs. See Figure 15.2 for a map of restrictive collaboration requirements by state for certified nurse practitioners (CNPs).

Shaping social policy is not only critical for access to care, but an ethical responsibility of all nurses, not just a dedicated few. The challenge is to increase the commitment of all nurses; not only those working in tandem for broader issues, but also those working on issues germane to a practice specialty area in order to advance health.

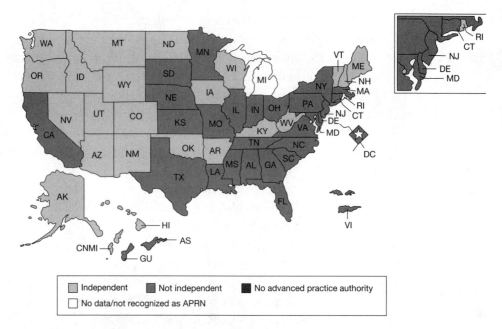

FIGURE 15.2 Independent practice for nurse practitioners by state.
Reprinted with permission from the National Council of State Boards of Nursing (2014).

LEADERSHIP STRATEGIES TO ADVANCE NURSING'S POLICY INFLUENCE

Leadership strategies to advance nurses' policy influence include understanding the policy competencies of new nurse graduates and new hires of an organization; increasing participation in health policy through professional development; and fostering membership and active involvement in associations, organizations, or specialty interest groups in nursing, across disciplines and with the public. In the previous chapters, we have largely focused on how an individual nurse can become involved in policy and strategies that can be taken at each step of the policy-making process. Nurses' collective impact is much greater when we maximize the potential in nursing's power of numbers. Thus, one step at the time taken by an individual nurse can become 3 million steps taken together. Getting to 3 million steps together requires nurse leaders, at every level and in every setting, creating the expectation that nurses will be policy activists.

Policy Competencies of New Graduates and New Hires

A first step in expanding the number of nurses involved in policy is for nurse leaders to understand the beginning competencies of nurses with regard to health policy. Being familiar with the AACN's Essentials Series that defines specific competencies with regard to health policy for graduates of baccalaureate, master's, and doctoral programs is a starting point for launching nurses' policy roles with consideration to nurses' educational foundations in policy. The Essentials documents for each education level describe the foundational knowledge of the practitioner of nursing with regard to policy, with expectations for the policy role of nurses expanding at each successive educational level. Exhibit 15.1 illustrates selected key action-oriented competencies from a longer comprehensive list of strategies related to knowledge and attitudes about policy making.

The health policy competencies as identified by the AACN provide specific actions that are grounded in the *Code of Ethics for Nurses* (ANA, 2001). *Ethically*, nurses are expected to participate in improving health care environments, collaborating with others in meeting health care needs, and shaping social policy. All of these expectations require nurses to take an active role in policy. Being familiar with these competencies will enable leaders to incorporate these expectations into the orientation process for new nurse hires and for yearly and/or merit performance reviews like professional advancement programs, sometimes called clinical ladders. Incorporating expectations in work environments will help bridge the often-noted gap between education and practice.

Understanding the health policy competencies of nurses is a first step in marshaling the strength of numbers. The profession can ill afford the hard-earned health policy competencies to be left at the door as nurses graduate from educational programs and move into their new roles. These competencies can be marshaled by taking a lesson from our colleagues in the military, where the

EXHIBIT 15.1	**COMPARISON OF SELECTED ACTION-ORIENTED POLICY COMPETENCIES AT EACH EDUCATIONAL LEVEL**
Baccalaureate	• Participate as a nurse in political processes and grass-roots legislative efforts to influence policy • Advocate for consumers and for the nursing profession
Master's	• Participate in policy development and implementation at each level • Interpret research for policy makers • Advocate for policies that improve the health of the public and the profession of nursing
Doctoral	• Analyze health policy proposals • Influence policy makers • Educate policy makers and others • Advocate for nursing within policy and health care communities • Lead in development and implementation of health policy at all levels • Provide leadership for health policy for health financing, regulation, and delivery • Advocate for social justice, equity, and ethical policies in health

Sources: American Association of Colleges of Nursing (2006); American Association of Colleges of Nursing (2008); American Association of Colleges of Nursing (2011).

expectation is not only that nurses develop and refine their skills for a specific clinical role, but also that nurses assume leadership roles to take policy action.

The growth of nurse residency programs provides a ready-made mechanism for incorporating the expectation of leadership and policy engagement. While the IOM report, *Future of Nursing: Leading Change, Advancing Health* (2011), recommends the establishment of residencies for new nurses, new advanced practice nurses, and nurses switching to a new specialization, developers of these programs can also include content and experiential learning activities supporting the policy role of nurses at the little "p" level within an organization and beyond. This can be accomplished by transitioning some of the structured activities of nurse residency programs to add a focus on policy involvement. Likewise, expectations for professional growth, which have been increasingly incorporated into job descriptions, can include involvement in professional activities. This involvement creates more informed nurses, who bring their knowledge to the practice arena to strengthen nursing within their own health care organizations. Thus, when nurses advance their education through formal program enrollment, or advance in organizational leadership, involvement in policy will not be a brand new competency needing development; instead, policy advocacy can be built upon a strong foundation.

Health Policy Professional Development

Numerous programs exist to enhance the professional development of nurses in health policy. Some programs are of a general nature and are open to nurses with a requirement to develop a specific area of expertise. Others, such as the Robert Wood Johnson Nurse Executive Fellowship and the American Academy of Nursing/American Nurses Foundation/American Nurses Association Institute of Medicine Scholar-in-Residence, are specifically available to nurses. In Chapter 7, "Building Capital: Intellectual, Social, Political, and Financial," Lauren Inouye describes her experience in the Nurse in Washington Internship (NIWI).

However, there are many more opportunities for gaining policy expertise. Each of these has a defined focus that can be used as a stepping stone to wider policy involvement. It is important that nurses are well represented in these programs and take advantage of the available opportunities (see Chapter 12, "Serving the Public Through Policy and Leadership"). See Exhibit 15.2 for a selected listing of fellowship programs. Policy fellowships are also available in public health through the Centers for Disease Control (CDC), as well as health services research. Some states have policy fellowships available as well.

Fostering Membership and Active Involvement in Associations and Policy

Increasing the numbers of nurses involved in policy is vital to leveraging our full policy potential as nurses. Much of our policy work is accomplished through

EXHIBIT 15.2 SELECTED HEALTH POLICY FELLOWSHIP PROGRAMS

PROGRAM	WEBSITE
American Academy of Nursing/ American Nurses Foundation/ American Nurses Association Institute of Medicine Scholar-in-Residence	http://www.iom.edu/Activities/ Education/NurseScholar.aspx http://www.aannet.org/menu-iom
American Hospital Association– National Patient Safety Foundation Comprehensive Patient Safety Leadership Fellowship	http://www.hpoe.org/PSLF/PSLF_ main.shtml
Health and Aging Policy Fellows	http://www.healthandaging policy.org
Robert Wood Johnson Executive Nurse Fellows	http://www.executivenurse fellows.org
Robert Wood Johnson Foundation Health Policy Fellows	http://www.healthpolicyfellows.org

numbers achieved by membership in associations, specialty organizations, or groups. Whether a nurse is an educator who requires student nurses to attend professional meetings or encourages them to join nursing (e.g., National Student Nurses Association [NSNA]) or other student groups, an agency manager or administrator who fosters staff nurses' involvement in shared governance (as described in Chapter 9, "Activating the Advocacy Plan"), or a staff nurse who covers for a nurse who wants to attend a meeting or who invites a colleague to attend a shared governance or professional meeting, all nurses have a role in fostering engagement and involvement in policy.

Policy involvement provides nurses with the opportunity to learn about practice standards and to engage with other nurses to obtain guidance and information about addressing policy issues of serious concern. Whether taking concerns to a professional association would have made a difference in the hepatitis C case in Nevada that was described earlier is unknown, but nurses can work together in creating a paradigm shift so that practice problems are acknowledged, discussed, and addressed. Nurses who participate in professional associations build upon the policy advocacy foundation begun in educational programs and bring back their expertise to enhance the environments in which they live and work. Many times nurses become inspired about an issue, but are not familiar with the processes for advancing the policy process. While this book outlined many of the steps in policy making, the ANA, state nurses associations, specialty associations, and their affiliates have their own spheres of influence and provide critical expertise on the nuances of policy processes within that sphere.

Nursing has the numbers to be a powerful influence. It has a respected national association with state and local affiliates. Nursing also has a proliferation of associations at the national, state, and local levels addressing the special interests of nurses. Working together, these groups can be leveraged to strengthen nursing's influence across health care at the organizational, local, state, national, and international levels. Considerable effort has been made through the Nursing Community, a coalition of over 60 associations representing over 1 million nurses, and also the Campaign for Action, at the Center to Champion Nursing in America (CCNA), to expand nursing's influence. Nurses associations are also working on key appointments at the state level. However, this needs to be expanded to all segments of nursing (Fyffe, 2009) and into all the communities where nurses live and work.

An important strategy to help foster involvement is to recognize the policy work that nurses carry out. This recognition can take a number of forms, including individual recognition and, engaging groups through selected activities, as well as through promotion of a particular policy (see Chapter 10, "Working With the Media: Shaping the Health Policy Process"). The purpose is not only to provide recognition for an individual's contributions to particular policy efforts, but also to enhance visibility in a selected community. Recognition within organizations or associations creates excitement and fosters member engagement. It also provides additional opportunities to bring the policy to the attention of key stakeholders. Most importantly, recognizing the work of policy activists creates a culture where policy advocacy becomes the norm rather than the exception.

Additional opportunities for recognition can take place through the development of conferences and other activities that highlight the work of nurse policy makers. An example is provided by the ANA Policy Conference, *Nursing Care in Life, Death and Disaster*, that resulted in the development of a policy paper (ANA, 2008). State associations, specialty associations, educational institutions, health care systems, and other groups have convened summits and other high-level visibility activities to heighten the publicity around a particular issue, along with the attendant media activities.

For nurses whose work cuts across disciplines like gerontology, there are opportunities through conferences that highlight policy. One example is the Gerontological Society of America (GSA) that has a solicitation for policy work at their conference. This is a solicitation for symposia called Social Research, Policy, and Practice (SRPP). Opportunities for interprofessional collaboration in policy are available in nearly every specialization; for example, critical care, cardiovascular care, pain management, patient safety, and long-term care, to name just a few.

POLICY ROLES

Policy activities and expectations can be incorporated into existing structures within educational institutions and organizational structures. There is a role for all nurses to help foster policy activities and expectations. Here, we focus on the roles of educators and nurses with graduate education that hold managerial and advanced practice roles, as the work of both groups is necessary to avoid a continuing gap between education and practice related to policy.

Nurse Educator

In order for more nurses to become policy experts and increase their policy skill level, a required concerted effort is needed to ensure that educational strategies are substantive and meaningful. It includes adequate preparation of faculty teaching this content. Educators would not think about having someone teach a clinical content course without the requisite background. The same consideration needs to be given to faculty assigned to teach policy. Someone who has never been involved in policy or is not a member of a professional association is not qualified.

Current status suggests that the involvement of new nurses or new advanced practice nurses in policy is limited, that the focus in the first year after graduation is on the development of competencies related to the provision of direct care. There is evidence that nurses do not feel prepared for political participation (Cramer, 2002; Vandenhouten, Malakar, Kubsch, Block, & Gallagher-Lepak, 2011) and do not see the connections between the service role of nurses and political action (Rains & Barton-Kriese, 2001; Zauderer, Ballestas, Cardoza, Hood, & Neville, 2008). Evidence also indicates that a strong foundation in policy led by educators who are well grounded in policy has the potential to increase the policy competencies of nurses (Byrd et al., 2012; Primomo, 2007). These complementary findings indicate that significant investment in the value of policy education for nurses with the actual implementation of policy content in nursing curricula has the potential to reap rewards for the profession.

Strengthening policy-related activities in nursing educational programs can include a range of activities: establishing and strengthening of health policy courses, integrating policy learning activities across courses, creating expectations for professional association involvement, and expanding the emphasis on civic or service learning that focuses on upstream activities that advance health advocacy. Nurse educators have demonstrated the value of health policy courses in changing nurses' or future nurses' attitudes toward policy involvement (Hahn, 2010; Hearne, 2008; Houck & Bongiorno, 2006; Primomo, 2007; Wall, Novak, & Wilkerson, 2005). The activities described in these studies provide guidance to nurse educators who are rapidly gearing up to develop and strengthen their doctor of nursing practice (DNP) program offerings.

Education for policy can take place in dedicated coursework in both nursing and with other disciplines as well as through experiential learning accomplished with professional activities and involvement in specific policy issues germane to clinical content. Incorporating policy activities always begs the question: If we add to the curricula, what might be deleted or changed?

While adding to health policy curricula might be a long-term solution, there are opportunities to incorporate a policy focus within the existing curricula. These include service learning activities as well as strengthening the support for leadership activities through the student nurses association.

Courses with a heavy clinical content focus can include policy implications drawn from health care disparities, genetics, and access to care, as well as quality and safety initiatives. The latter will almost always include implications for policy. Other health care professional groups have the same issues in preparing their workforce for policy activism amid calls to action by their leaders. A policy course can include formal lectures and classroom exercises, integration of real-world experiences, guest lecturers with direct policy experience, and a culminating experiential learning activity (Hearne, 2008).

Infusing policy-related content into nursing curricula can be accomplished by incorporating a policy focus into clinically oriented discussions. At the undergraduate level, this can be accomplished on a regular basis in the clinical setting as students learn about the processes of care. An example of changing students' awareness of safety includes the work of Currie and colleagues (2007) in the development of a patient safety curriculum. Students were asked to anonymously report safety breaches online. While these reports generated an analysis of the types of safety breaches, they also heightened awareness of potential safety issues (Currie et al., 2007). The next step in moving observations into action might involve students systematically identifying and analyzing the policy implications of their observations of safety issues in nursing care. Likewise, students' policy awareness can be enhanced by consistent inclusion of health policy implications in classroom discussions. Incorporating policy discussions into clinical conferences also means those adjunct faculty who often provide much of the clinical teaching also need to be well versed in policy. Policy content and expectations may need to be developed for preceptors.

Infusing policy-related content can also be accomplished at the master's level in clinical practicums. Interest and involvement in policy by nurse faculty serve as important modeling of policy activist behaviors. An exemplar of effective role modeling for professional development in relation to policy is the American Association of Nurse Anesthetists (AANA). The AANA maintains a membership penetration well over 90%, enabling it to have a large presence in Washington with one of the largest health care Political Action Committee funds. Much of this is accomplished with a strong educational foundation in health policy in nurse anesthetist educational programs. Given AANA's membership penetration, it is likely that this phenomenon is replicated in their state affiliates across the nation. And, as has been demonstrated, important policy advances for the profession occur at the state level. At the level of the doctorate, many opportunities for policy work present themselves. In DNP programs, the final scholarly project or capstone might focus on a policy issue or minimally include policy implications of the project (see Chapter 5, "Harnessing Evidence in the Policy Process").

The growth of programs offering nursing doctorates with an emphasis on the health policy and leadership roles of nurses provides unique opportunities for strengthening policy advocacy. Policy courses and capstone courses in policy provide the opportunities for immersion experiences in policy, allowing students to explore issues in depth and engage in multiple steps of the policy-making process. The growth of these programs also creates the need to develop the policy competencies of faculty across the curriculum.

Service learning activities, which have been widely incorporated into nursing curricula, can increase students' sensitivity and awareness of social justice issues. Very often, these activities focus on providing individual service to members of disadvantaged communities. Systematically expanding this focus to include upstream activities designed to have a larger, more proactive approach can help students learn about the important role of policy making in advancing health. A community and/or health promotion focus can be used as a service learning structure for development of health policy competencies at the undergraduate level (Broussard, 2011; O'Brien-Larivée, 2011). Similarly, the NSNA's *Leadership University* provides a structured mechanism for providing course credit for leadership-related learning activities that include, among others, shared governance, legislation, and community health and disaster projects (NSNA, n.d.). Creating an expectation of policy advocacy and involvement needs to occur across a curriculum in order to internalize the value of advocacy in health policy. When health policy is only a strategy that is mentioned or addressed in a final capstone course, students will have difficulty understanding the connections to their daily practice and see participation in health policy advocacy as an unnecessary impediment to the development of the competencies required to transition to a new practice role.

Nurses With Advanced Organizational Roles

Equally important to the full realization of nurse policy engagement is the role of nurses in organizations where care is delivered; for example, hospitals and the community. Nurse managers and nurses with advanced degrees like APRNs have not only critical roles individually for active policy engagement but also in mentoring, coaching, role modeling, and creating structures and processes that facilitate direct nurse care involvement in policy. As the group of nurses most often responsible for developing, monitoring, evaluating, and changing policy, nurses with advanced organizational roles are in a unique position to help nurses understand policy within the work setting, but also outside of the organization in associations and community work. Their advanced role and often advanced education provide opportunities for engagement that direct care nurses frequently or readily do not see. Policy on the Scene 15.1 is an exemplar with which many who have written policy will identify. It demonstrates how even writing and updating hospital policy can lead to unforeseen policy issues.

POLICY ON SCENE 15.1: Whose Job Is It Anyway?
Linda Griggs MSN, RN-BC, ACNS-BC, Medical-Surgical Educator
NICHE Coordinator Aultman Hospital, Canton, Ohio

I began the workday reading a note left by my boss, "Linda. Thank you for your help with the accreditation visit. Great job with updating policies—I know that is a thankless job at times. Appreciate what you do!"

Oh, hospital policies! Reviewing and revising them can be a thankless, time-consuming job. My latest challenge was a pap smear policy. When this policy first appeared on my task list, I thought "Great, this is a one page to the point policy. No big deal. I'll type it in the new format, send it to the Policy & Procedure Committee for approval and off my task list it will go." Little did I know the maze it would begin for me.

I read over the policy and asked myself, "Do we offer pap smears to every female patient 18 years and older as the policy states?" I accessed the electronic documentation system and looked at the admission history form. Nothing was there. I asked a few staff nurses, who told me it disappeared from the form months ago and most patients refused it anyway due to insurance coverage issues. Next, I looked up the Ohio Revised Code reference to see if the policy was current. The reference number didn't match. I kept searching and couldn't find what I needed so I contacted a nurse in risk management (asking myself, who knew reference numbers change from year to year?). The nurse offered to look up the current Ohio Revised Code reference number and also suggested I call the vice president over Women's and Children's Services, who previously worked on earlier versions of this policy. I did so and discovered the policy had been reassigned to me because they don't perform pap smears in her area. She also pointed out the policy didn't follow current practice guidelines. Next, I searched and found guidelines from the American College of Obstetricians and Gynecologists (ACOG) and the Report of the U.S. Preventative Services Task Force, Guide to Clinical Preventative Services that recommend starting cervical screening at the age of 21 years, not 18.

I now sit at my desk with this overdue policy mirroring Ohio law, which does not follow current practice guidelines, in which we are non-compliant and ponder "Is it my responsibility to contact a local government representative to get the law updated? Really?? Whose job is it anyway?"

This Policy on the Scene demonstrates not only the complexity of "doing policy" in organizations, but it also raises ethical issues—what happens when you uncover an issue that was bigger than you ever expected? The nurse writing the policy is not a women's health expert, so what might she do?

Some policy roles of organizational nurse leaders have been alluded to in previous sections of this chapter, like incorporating policy expectations into orientation, residency programs, performance reviews, and other similar activities. But a strong commitment is called for from organization nurse leaders to help direct-care nurses connect their work in shared governance to policy. The shared governance model provides structure for nurses to have input into their practice and work environment and the input related to policy that is one of the vital elements to success. Through shared governance, nurses are empowered to use their clinical intellectual capital and to use and gain social capital, which are necessary skills to move policy advocacy from the little "p" to the big "P."

The challenge in the day-to-day care of patients for nurses who are paid an hourly rate and often are facing staffing issues is how to foster direct-care nurse involvement as he or she may feel unprepared to address policy issues. Others may not want to be part of politics as they believe that they chose a profession where service and hard work in care delivery are the only requirements of the profession. However, health care is not a world unto itself that is devoid of policy and politics. No matter what we do, policy and the concomitant politics that go with the formulation, development, implementation, and evaluation of policy have a pervasive influence over practice. Policies drive our practices. Our interactions with patients involve policy, or our understandings of policies.

As laws are implemented through regulations and as regulations are interpreted in practice settings, policy and politics drive the strategies designed for the implementation of care. Likewise, if we are not at the table to influence policies that impact our practice and the profession's ability to promote quality, safety, and access to health care for all, others are ready to step up to the plate, perhaps in a way that might not be productive for nursing or health care. Our policy work is to not only provide policy solutions to address particular health care or professional needs, but also to keep the public's health at the forefront of policy makers' decision-making processes.

It is, therefore, necessary to make sure nurses know the shared governance structure of the nursing organization and that they not only can tell you where the documents are that describe it, but can identify all the parts and the interconnections. More importantly, it is necessary that they see the value of the structure for each of them, know the location (e.g., department or unit), and know the organization's nurse leaders' value-shared governance. Then, nurses need to know how to get involved and have the support needed (e.g., time back, coverage, and paid time) to attend and to carry out the work of the council or committee of shared governance to which they belong. These activities require organizational leaders to demonstrate their belief in the value of shared governance and that they are willing to expend resources and energy to implement and provide ongoing support for shared governance. This support starts with the chief nurse officer and extends across to all leaders. These resources include professional development for direct care nurses so they better understand shared governance and the necessary space, time, and financial resources. With the increasing emphasis on interprofessional practice and shared governance for patient care across disciplines, it is important that the voice and perspective of nursing are not lost (see Chapter 12).

A clear example of when the organization has failed in shared governance is when whistle-blowing occurs. This issue can be seen in the hepatitis C story shared under the section "Work Environment." This story is a clear example of why internal policies to address nurse concerns are vital to protect patients and nurses. Shared governance makes it hard for nurses to work in silos and working in silos makes it easier for bad behavior to go undetected and reports of bad behavior to be unreported. As Fletcher, Sorrell, and Silva (1998) succinctly state, "Our underlying premise is that when whistleblowing occurs there is an institutional failure" (para 11).

Organizational nurse leaders can also help build a culture that values policy advocacy by using several strategies: role modeling, coaching, and mentoring. First, as a leader, take inventory of your policy activities and memberships for self-evaluation and also for the potential they may have for being shared. If, for example, you are an APRN, consider inviting a nursing student who works at your agency or that you precept in your advanced practice area to attend a local membership meeting. For new members of shared governance committees, remember to have an established orientation process (see Chapter 11, "Applying a Nursing Lens to Shape Policy").

Lastly, providing recognition for nurses involved in policy, while noted earlier, bears repeating, specifically as it relates to the organization. Through organizational and unit newsletters, the accomplishments in policy, appointments to boards, memberships, and offices held should be noted. Imagine working in periOperative nursing and not knowing a colleague was on a national subcommittee of the American Association of periOperative Registered Nurses (AORN). Names of nurses sitting on shared governance councils or committees should be highlighted in the area they work and posted on easily accessible resources like an organization's Intranet and/or Internet site.

All nurses have roles in policy and nurses with advanced education have not only individual roles but roles in assisting direct care nurses in policy advancement. Public health nurses, nurse informaticists, nurse case managers, and every nursing position one can identify require policy advocacy. In chapters throughout this book, we have detailed some of these roles; for example, in Chapter 5, researchers' roles were highlighted, and in Chapter 9 administrators' roles were discussed. The important contributions of nurses to the development of policy occur at the local, state, and national levels. In an increasingly global society, it is noted that nurses around the world face similar challenges in advancing health policy, within the context of their unique environments. Leadership development provides a foundation for the development of competencies in policy. And, it is not only the development of leaders that is important, but also a paradigm shift and the creation of a culture that creates expectations and rewards nurses for their active engagement in policy (see the Option for Policy Challenge). The challenge for the future is for all nurses individually to recognize and embrace their roles and to support each other individually and in groups to move our policy agenda for our profession and for health forward.

OPTION FOR POLICY CHALLENGE: Expectations of Leadership as the Path to Policy
Bonnie Mowinski Jennings

In civilian life today I find myself involved with educating health care clinicians and helping them with examining existing policies and, where appropriate, implementing new ones. Serendipitously, for example, I had the opportunity to engage with nursing and medical students and teach an interprofessional course on quality and patient safety. This change sounds simple and yet it was not because of academic silos and asynchronous schedules. Yet with leadership and determination, policies were established to make this course a reality. I also had the opportunity to lead the development of a program of study about health systems leadership. This program helps to meet the call for action from the IOM to educate more nurse leaders; this program benefits from my career in the ANC where leadership was an expectation regardless of one's position in the organization.

Today, I also continue to pursue my interest in health systems research. A recent discovery from an ethnography study conducted during my postdoctoral fellowship at the University of North Carolina at Chapel Hill has gained the attention of individuals in the policy arena. Findings about patient turnover[1] illustrate that not only is midnight census an inadequate metric for describing workload, but features of admissions and discharges make them nonequivalent events. For instance, whereas nurses have some control over discharges, admissions are unpredictable; they require the nurse's immediate attention. Moreover, the pattern of admissions influences workload, with admissions that are clustered creating more work intensity than staggered admissions. In addition, admissions that occur in the proximity of a shift change also create more intensity. The opportunity

(*continued*)

to use these findings to potentially lead to changes in policies that relate to workload, staffing, and patient safety fuels my excitement!

What I learned throughout my military career, and what I apply on a daily basis now, is that, while education is foundational to leadership development, the real lessons in becoming a leader occur by practicing leadership. Leadership is about relationships and communication. Leadership is about listening and also about speaking in ways to be heard—and understood. Leadership is about advocating effectively—in a calm, confident, knowledgeable way that inspires others to follow. Leadership is about stepping out of the way to let followers develop as leaders, lending a hand in their development, and taking pride when the follower's abilities exceed those of the leader from whom the follower has learned.

[1]Jennings, Sandelowski, and Higgins (2013).

IMPLICATIONS FOR THE FUTURE

The next great frontiers in health care influenced by nursing practice will depend on the extent to which nurses are actively involved in policy. A number of issues will have a critical impact on nursing. Nurses in all settings will need to be vigorously monitoring, refining, and developing health care policy at the little "p" and big "P" levels so that we are seen as not only the most trusted health professional but also most trusted for health policy and advocacy. Pioneering efforts will be needed to develop new competencies and skills for future health policy work given the increasing complexity of the world. Leading the way in policy is an immersion experience in life that it is not easy; it is often messy and evolving, and it requires opening the doors of opportunity without waiting for an invitation. Redesigning sustainable health reform care cannot be successful without its largest provider group, nursing, being fully engaged. See Figures 15.3 and 15.4, which reflect how the role of nurses in health care reform has changed since the 1960s. Does the future hold the promise of a nurse as a leader of the executive office?

Building solutions for closing the gap between expected new graduate competencies and expected and rewarded performance competencies will increasingly focus on leadership development as well as interprofessional collaboration that includes policy roles.

Specific policy initiatives will focus on safety, the workplace environment, and the needs of our communities with regard to basic supplies of

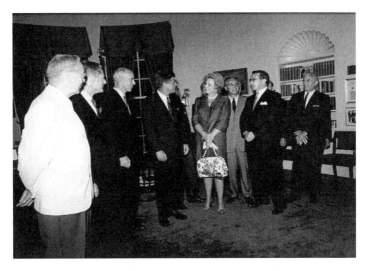

FIGURE 15.3 Early health care reform discussion in the Oval Office with President Kennedy and one nurse, ANA president, Margaret Dolan.

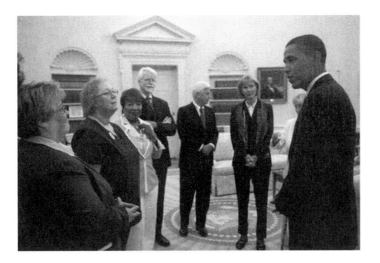

FIGURE 15.4 Fifty years later, President Obama in the Oval Office discussing health care reform with members of Congress including nurse representatives, Lois Capps, RN, Eddie Bernice Johnson, RN, and Carolyn McCarthy, RN, along with ANA president, Rebecca M. Patton and other ANA members.

food, water, air, and housing. As we have seen with natural disasters and health inequities, our own communities where we live and work provide opportunities for nurses to be actively involved in policy activities related to quality, safety, and access to health care for all, as well as health care cost containment. Additional safety initiatives will focus on finding the balance among being at the sharp end of safety, where nurses are often the last professional to have an interaction with a patient before a threatening event, and developing the network of skills while also moving science and policy forward to protect the public. The economic value of nursing will increasingly be reflected in discussions and decisions made at policy tables. Therefore, nurses will be called upon to participate and contribute to the economic evaluation of their care.

KEY CONCEPTS

1. All nurses in all settings need to be actively engaged in policy in order to capitalize on the potential of over 3 million nurses taking steps together to advance health.
2. Strengthening policy competencies is about fostering the expectation that all nurses are leaders.
3. Language matters in advancing practice, removing practice barriers, and protecting the public.
4. Removal of practice barriers is a complex ongoing process that involves multiple layers of legislation and regulation at the local, state, and national levels.
5. All nurses need to be involved in policy issues at their place of work to enhance quality of care and make improvements in practice and the work environment.
6. Daily practice provides numerous opportunities to shape and advance practice in promoting quality, safety, and access to health care for all.
7. Nurses need to be at policy tables formulating policy rather than only serving as the implementers of policy.
8. Nurse organizational leaders play a key role in advancing the policy competencies of nurses through role modeling, education, and providing opportunities to participate in policy formulation, implementation, and evaluation.
9. Shared governance provides numerous opportunities for nurses to develop policy competencies.
10. Policies created at the local, state, and national levels may not necessarily be synchronous with the advance of the profession and practice policies at the organizational level.
11. The development of policy competencies needs to be embedded in routine activities such as evaluation, as well as orientation, nurse residencies, and other specialized programs.
12. Leadership development requires a paradigm shift away from a primary focus on the attainment of clinical competencies to a focus that also includes a concomitant development of policy skills.
13. Exemplars of leadership development can be used as models for the development of policy competencies.

14. Nurses need to be involved in professional associations to realize the potential of strength in numbers because it is these groups that are concerned with and are actively engaged in addressing nursing practice issues at the state and national levels.

15. Organizational nurse leaders have an important role in building a culture in nursing that values and fosters policy advocacy.

SUMMARY

The roles of nurses individually and collectively are basic to health care transformation and the necessary policy that is needed for the triple aim of quality, safety, and access. It is indefensible for a nurse to be told or to believe that his or her only duty for care is direct service. Ethically, we are bound to be at the policy table. If not invited, we must knock loud and hard on the door and when necessary just walk in. The strategies to achieve more nurse involvement will rest with the best educated who not only have the competencies but often hold a position of leadership that can most easily effect change. New structures and processes in education and work settings are needed that will facilitate the professional development of policy for all nurses commiserate with their roles. The gap between education and practice needs to be bridged for nurses to fully take action and expand policy horizons.

LEARNING ACTIVITIES

1. Using the resources for building intellectual capital as a model (see Chapter 7), identify at least five resources that are available related to an issue that is of particular interest to you.

2. Sign up for at least one mailing list service related to policy for the duration of this class and critique its usefulness to your practice.

3. Compare the state BSN essentials with those of graduate nurses and explore how, as a nurse with advanced education, you can support BSN nurses in activities in policy at the big "P" and little "p" levels.

4. Develop a plan for two policy activities at any level that you can achieve within 6 months and then within 1 year. Identify the amount of effort it will take and your strategies for accomplishing the activities and the rationale for selecting the activities.

5. Make a list of all the policy activities that you have participated in during the past 5 years and critically analyze your participation for growth personally and your contribution to the association, cause, or organization that you helped.

6. Describe potential responses to nurses who indicate they are not involved in associations because they don't believe in policy activity.

E-RESOURCES

- American Association of Colleges of Nursing Essentials Documents. http://www.aacn.nche.edu/education-resources/essential-series
- American Association of Nurse Practitioners' Position Statements and Papers. https://www.aanp.org/publications/position-statements-papers
- American Nurses Association Position Statements. http://www.nursing world.org/positionstatements
- Barton Associates Scope of Practice Laws: Interactive Nurse Practitioner (NP) Scope of Practice Law Guide. http://www.bartonassociates .com/nurse-practitioners/nurse-practitioner-scope-of-practice-laws
- Future of Nursing Campaign for Action at the Center to Champion Nursing in America. http://campaignforaction.org
- The Huffington Post, Life Expectancy Shortest in Southern "Poverty Belt" (INFOGRAPHIC), Death and the Poverty Belt. http://www .huffingtonpost.com/2013/07/19/life-expectancy-_n_3624495.html
- Impact 101: Best Practices for Communicating With Policy Makers. https://www.academyhealth.org/Training/ResourceDetail.cfm?Item Number=2314
- The Nursing Community. http://www.thenursingcommunity.org

REFERENCES

Aiken, L. H., Sermeus, W., Van den Heede, K., Sloane, D. M., Busse, R., McKee, M., … Kutney-Lee, A. (2012). Patient safety, satisfaction and quality of hospital care: Cross-sectional survey of nurses and patients in 12 countries in Europe and the United States. *BMJ, 344*, e1717.

American Academy of Nurse Practitioners. (2007). *Standards for nurse practitioner practice in retail clinics.* [Position Statement]. Retrieved from https://www.aanp.org/images/documents/publications/StdsforNPRetail-BasedClinics.pdf

American Association of Colleges of Nursing. (2006). *The essentials of doctoral education for advanced nursing practice.* Washington, DC: Author.

American Association of Colleges of Nursing. (2008). *The essentials of baccalaureate education for professional nursing practice.* Washington, DC: Author.

American Association of Colleges of Nursing. (2011). *The essentials of master's education in nursing.* Washington, DC: Author.

American Nurses Association. (2001). *Code of Ethics for Nurses with interpretive statements.* Silver Spring, MD: Nursebooks.org.

American Nurses Association. (2008). *Adapting standards of care under extreme conditions: Guidance for professional during disasters, pandemics, and other extreme emergencies.* Silver Spring, MD: Author.

American Nurses Association. (2009, December 11). *Additional access to care: Supporting nurse practitioners in retail-based health clinics.* Retrieved from http://nursingworld.org/MainMenuCategories/Policy-Advocacy/Positions-and-Resolutions/ANAPositionStatements/Position-Statements-Alphabetically/Additional-Access-To-Care-Supporting-Nurse-Practitioners-In-Retail-Based-Health-Clinics.html

American Nurses Association. (2010). *Nursing's social policy statement The essence of the profession* (3rd ed.). Silver Spring, MD: Nursesbooks.org.

American Nurses Association. (2013, December 12). *Title "Nurse" Protection*. Retrieved from http://www.nursingworld.org/MainMenuCategories/Policy-Advocacy/State/Legislative-Agenda-Reports/State-TitleNurse

Benton, D. (2012). Advocating globally to shape policy and strengthen nursing's influence. *OJIN: The Online Journal of Issues in Nursing, 17*(1), Manuscript 5. Retrieved from http://www.nursingworld.org/MainMenuCategories/ANAMarketplace/ANAPeriodicals/OJIN/TableofContents/Vol-17-2012/No1-Jan-2012/Advocating-Globally-to-Shape-Policy.html

Broussard, B. B. (2011). The Bucket List: A service-learning approach to community engagement to enhance community health nursing clinical learning. *Journal of Nursing Education, 50*(1), 40–43.

Byrd, M. E., Costello, J., Gremel, K., Schwager, J., Blanchette, L., & Malloy T. E. (2012). Political astuteness of baccalaureate nursing students following an active learning experience in health policy. *Public Health Nursing, 29*(5), 433–443.

Committee on Practice and Ambulatory Medicine. (2014). AAP principles concerning retail-based clinics. *Pediatrics, 133*(3), e794–e797.

Cramer, M. E. (2002). Factors influencing organized political participation in nursing. *Policy, Politics, & Nursing Practice, 3*(2), 97–107.

Currie, L. A., Desjardins, K. S., Stone, P. W., Lai, T. Y., Schwartz, E., Schally, R., & Bakken, S. (2007). Near-miss and hazard reporting: Promoting mindfulness in patient safety education. *Studies in Health Technology and Informatics, 129*(Pt 1), 285–290.

Djukic, M., Kovner, C. T., Brewer, C. S., Fatehi, F. K., & Cline, D. D. (2013). Work environment factors other than staffing associated with nurses' ratings of patient care quality. *Health Care Management Review, 38*(2), 105–114.

Fletcher, J., Sorrell, J., & Silva, M. (1998). Whistleblowing as a failure of organizational ethics. *Online Journal of Issues in Nursing, 3*(3), Manuscript 3. Retrieved from www.nursingworld.org/MainMenuCategories/ANAMarketplace/ANAPeriodicals/OJIN/TableofContents/Vol31998/No3Dec1998/Whistleblowing.aspx

Fyffe, T. (2009). Nursing shaping and influencing health and social policy. *Journal of Nursing Management, 17*(6), 698–706.

Hahn, J. (2010). Integrating professionalism and political awareness into the curriculum. *Nurse Educator, 35*(3), 110–113.

Hearne, S. A. (2008). Practice-based teaching for health policy action and advocacy. *Public Health Reports, 123*(Suppl 2), 65–70.

Henriksen, K., & Dayton, E. (2006). Organizational silence and hidden threats to patient safety. *Health Services Research, 41*(4 Pt 2), 1539–1554.

Houck, N. M., & Bongiorno, A. W. (2006). Innovations in the public policy education of nursing students. *Journal of the New York State Nurses Association, 37*(2), 4–9.

Institute for Health Care Improvement (IHI). (n.d.). *The IHI Triple Aim Initiative: Better care for individuals, better health for populations, and lower per capita costs*. Retrieved from http://www.ihi.org/engage/initiatives/TripleAim/Pages/default.aspx

Institute of Medicine. (2011). *The future of nursing: Leading change, advancing health*. Washington, DC: National Academies Press.

Jennings, B. M., Sandelowski, M., & Higgins, M. K. (2013). Turning over patient turnover: An ethnographic study of admissions, discharges, and transfers. *Research in Nursing & Health, 36*, 554–566.

Kunavikitul, W. (2014). Moving towards the greater involvement of nurses in policy development. *International Nursing Review, 61*(1), 1–2.

Leary, E., & Diers, D. (2013). The silence of the unblown whistle: The Nevada hepatitis C public health crisis. *Yale Journal of Biology and Medicine, 86*(1), 79–87.

Mehotra, A., Liu, H., Adams, J. L., Wang, M. C., Lave, J. R., Thygeson, N. M., ... McGlynn, E. A. (2009). Comparing costs and quality of care at retail clinics with that of other medical settings for 3 common illnesses. *Annals of Internal Medicine, 151*(5), 321–328.

National Council of State Boards of Nursing (NCSBN). (2014). *APRN maps.* Retrieved from https://www.ncsbn.org/2567.htm

National Student Nurses Association. (n.d.). NSNA Leadership University: Giving credit where credit is due. Retrieved from http://www.nsna.org/Membership/FrequentlyAskedQuestions.aspx

O'Brien-Larivée, C. (2011). A service-learning experience to teach baccalaureate nursing students about health policy. *Journal of Nursing Education, 50*(6), 332–336.

Poghosyan, L., Nannini, A., Stone, P. W., & Smaldone, A. (2013). Nurse practitioner organizational climate in primary care settings: Implications for professional practice. *Journal of Professional Nursing, 29*(6), 338–349.

Primomo, J. (2007). Changes in political astuteness after a health systems and policy course. *Nurse Educator, 32*(6), 260–264.

Rains, J. W., & Barton-Kriese, P. (2001). Developing political competence: A comparative study across disciplines. *Public Health Nursing, 18*(4), 219–224.

Rohrer, J. E., Angstman, K. B., Garrison, G. M., Pecina, J. L., & Maxson, J. A. (2013). Nurse practitioners and physician assistants are complements to family medicine physicians. *Population Health Management, 16*(4), 242–245.

Scott, R. D. II. (2009). *The direct medical costs of healthcare-associated infections in US hospitals and the benefits of prevention.* Retrieved from http://www.cdc.gov/HAI/pdfs/hai/Scott_CostPaper.pdf.

Stone, P. W., Pogorzelska-Maziarz, M., Herzig, C. T., Weiner, L. M., Furuya, E. Y., Dick, A., & Larson, E. (2014). State of infection prevention in U.S. hospitals enrolled in the national health and safety network. *American Journal of Infection Control, 42*(2), 94–99.

Vandenhouten, C. L., Malakar, C. L., Kubsch, S., Block, D. E., & Gallagher-Lepak, S. (2011). Political participation of registered nurses. *Policy, Politics, & Nursing Practice, 12*(3), 159–167.

Wall, B. M., Novak, J. C., & Wilkerson, S. A. (2005). Doctor of nursing practice program development: Reengineering health care. *Journal of Nursing Education, 44*(9), 396–403.

Zauderer, C. R., Ballestas, H. C., Cardoza, M. P., Hood, P., & Neville, S. M. (2008). United we stand: preparing nursing students for political activism. *Journal of the New York State Nurses Association, 39*(2), 4–7.

Index